Health Care Needs Assessment

the epidemiologically based needs assessment reviews

Second series

Edited by

Andrew Stevens
Professor of Public Health Medicine, The University of Birmingham

(formerly Senior Lecturer in Public Health Medicine,
The Wessex Institute for Health Research and Development)

and

James Raftery
Professor of Health Economics,
Health Services Management Centre
The University of Birmingham

(formerly Senior Health Economist,
The Wessex Institute for Health Research and Development)

Produced by

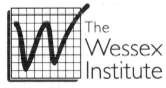

for Health Research & Development
incorporating Public Health Medicine

RADCLIFFE MEDICAL PRESS
OXFORD and NEW YORK

Radcliffe Medical Press Ltd
18 Marcham Road, Abingdon, Oxon OX14 1AA, UK

Radcliffe Medical Press, Inc.
141 Fifth Avenue, New York, NY 10010, USA

British Library Cataloguing in Publication Data

A cataloguing record for this book is available from the British Library.

ISBN 1 85775 199 X

Library of Congress Cataloging-in-Publication Data is available.

Typset by Tradespools Ltd, Frome, Somerset
Printed and bound in Great Britain by Redwood Books, Trowbridge, Wiltshire

Contents

Introduction
A Stevens, J Raftery

1 Accident and Emergency Departments
B Williams, J Nicholl, J Brazier

2   Child and Adolescent Mental Health

SA Wallace, JM Crown, M Berger, AD Cox

3 Low Back Pain

P Croft, A Papageorgious, R McNally

4   Palliative and Terminal Care

I Higginson

5 Dermatology

HC Williams

6 Breast Cancer

P Dey, E Twelves, CBJ Woodman

7   Genitourinary Medicine Services

A Renton, S Hawkes, M Hickman, E Claydon, H Ward, D Taylor-Robinson

8 Gynaecology

CDA Wolfe

Foreword

Everyone involved in the purchasing, planning and prioritization of health care needs accurate, comprehensive and well-packaged information to answer at least four crucial questions. With what population or patients are we concerned? What services are provided? What is the evidence of the effectiveness of services? What is the optimum set of services? In other words: What is the need and how can it be best met?

These questions are answered in part by epidemiological literature and in part by the products of the evidence-based health care movement. The *Health Care Needs Assessment* series neatly combines these two elements and offers a perspective across an entire disease or service area. A purchaser or practitioner reading one of these chapters is rapidly brought up-to-speed with the whole spectrum of care.

Many positive comments, including evidence supplied to the House of Commons' Health Committee, have demonstrated the value and importance of the first series. The additional topics in the second series extend the range of information available covering both areas where the assessment of need and effectiveness of services has long been discussed, such as aspects of gynaecology and low back pain, and ones in which there has been less interest, such as dermatology. The new series will be welcomed by purchasers of health care in the United Kingdom but it should also be of value to all those concerned with assessing and meeting health care needs, from central government to individual practitioners.

Graham Winyard
Medical Director, NHS Executive
September 1996

Preface

This book forms the second series of health care needs assessment reviews. The first series, published in 1994, comprises reviews of 20 diseases, interventions or services selected for their importance to purchasers of health care. Importance is defined in terms of burden of disease (mortality, morbidity and cost), the likely scope for changing patterns of purchasing and the wish to see a wide range of topics to test the method used for needs assessment. The first series also includes an introductory chapter, explaining the background to needs assessment and a conclusive chapter, bringing together the main findings of the disease reviews.

The eight reports set out in this book have been chosen, using the same importance criteria to increase the coverage of all health service activity. There has been a small change in emphasis, away from disease groups (strictly *Breast Cancer* only), to services and in some cases entire specialties (*Dermatology* and *Gynaecology*). The change has been partly to maintain coverage of substantial areas in each report (where otherwise a relatively small disease group would now require an individual chapter) and also to reflect the wishes of the users for the topic areas to be consistent with the scope of purchasing plans if at all possible.

As before the authors have been selected on the basis of academic expertise and each chapter is the work of individual authors. The chapters do not necessarily reflect the views of the National Health Service Executive that sponsored the project, nor indeed the current professional consensus. Each chapter should be in no way regarded as setting norms; rather it should be used as a valuable source of evidence and arguments on which purchasing authorities may base their decisions.

There have been other changes since the first series which have influenced the range of chapters and the content of individual chapters. First districts have merged and a population base of 250 000 is no longer the norm. Denominators are now expressed as per 100 000, or per million population. Second the term purchasers no longer strictly means just district health authorities. Some small steps have therefore been taken in the direction of making the material relevant to primary care purchasing. This is particularly so in the *Low Back Pain* chapter, in which the focus is on the presenting symptom as in general practice rather than on a confirmed diagnosis following secondary care. Third the science of systematic reviews and meta-analyses has developed remarkably since the production of the first series. While this important development has been of great use to purchasers, the role of the needs assessment in covering entire disease and service areas remains unique. Both objectives of providing baseline information for purchasers to assist with the knowledge-base of all the processes around purchasing and designing a method for needs assessment have largely been vindicated by comments received on the first series and the demand for a second series.

The editors wish to acknowledge the contribution of those who helped with the origination of the project: Graham Winyard, Mike Dunning, Deirdre Cunningham and Azim Lakhani; and also members of the current Steering Group: Mark Charny, Anne Kauder and Graham Bickler; as well as those at Wessex who have enabled the project to run smoothly: Ros Liddiard, Pat Barrett and Melanie Corris.

Contributing authors

Berger, Dr M
Consultant Clinical Psychologist
Department of Clinical Psychology
Lanesborough Wing
St George's Hospital
Blackshaw Road
LONDON SW17 0QT

Brazier, J
Director of Health Economics
Sheffield Centre for Health & Related Research
University of Sheffield
30 Regent Street
SHEFFIELD S1 4DA

Claydon, Dr E
Clinical Director, Genitourinary Medicine
St Mary's NHS Trust
Praed Street
LONDON W2 1NY

Cox, Professor AD
UMDS
Department of Adolescent Psychiatry and Psychology
Bloomfield Centre
Guy's Hospital
London Bridge
LONDON SE1 9RT

Croft, Professor P
Professor of Epidemiology
Industrial & Community Health Research Centre
School of Postgraduate Medicine
University of Keele
Hartshill Road
STOKE-ON-TRENT ST4 7NY

Crown, Dr JM
Director
South East Institute of Public Health
Broomhill House
David Salomon's Estate
Broomhill Road
TUNBRIDGE WELLS TN3 0XT

Dey, Dr P
Lecturer in Public Health Medicine
Centre for Cancer Epidemiology
University of Manchester
Christie Hospital NHS Trust
Kinnaird Road
Withington
MANCHESTER M20 4QL

Hawkes, Dr S
Honorary Clinical Research Fellow
Department of Epidemiology & Public Health
Imperial College School of Medicine at St Mary's
Norfolk Place
LONDON W2 1PG

Hickman, M
Epidemiologist and Research Fellow
Department of Epidemiology & Public Health
Imperial College School of Medicine at St Mary's
Norfolk Place
LONDON W2 1PG

Higginson, Professor I
Department of Palliative Care and Policy
The Rayne Institute
King's College School of Medicine and Dentistry
Bessemer Road
LONDON SE5 9PJ

McNally, R
Information Officer
Arthritis & Rheumatism Council Epidemiology Research Unit
Stopford Building
The Medical School
University of Manchester
Oxford Road
MANCHESTER M13 9PT

Nicholl, Professor J
Director
Sheffield Centre for Health and Related Research
University of Sheffield
30 Regent Street
SHEFFIELD S1 4DA

Papageorgious, A
Study Co-ordinator
Arthritis & Rheumatism Council Epidemiology Research Unit
Stopford Building
The Medical School
University of Manchester
Oxford Road
MANCHESTER M13 9PT

Renton, Dr A
Senior Lecturer in Public Health Medicine
Department of Epidemiology & Public Health
Imperial College School of Medicine at St Mary's
Norfolk Place
LONDON W2 1PG

Taylor-Robinson, Professor D
Department of Genitourinary Medicine & Communicable Disease
Imperial College School of Medicine at St Mary's
Norfolk Place
LONDON W2 1PG

Twelves, E
NW Regional Breast Screening Quality Assurance Co-ordinator
West Pennine Health Authority
Westhulme Avenue
Oldham
OL1 2PL

Wallace, Dr SA
Senior Registrar in Public Health Medicine
South East Institute of Public Health
Broomhill House
David Salomon's Estate
Broomhill Road
TUNBRIDGE WELLS TN3 0XT

Ward, Dr H
Senior Lecturer in Public Health Medicine
Department of Epidemiology & Public Health
Imperial College School of Medicine at St Mary's
Norfolk Place
LONDON W2 1PG

Williams, Professor B
Department of Public Health Medicine & Epidemiology
University Hospital
Queen's Medical Centre
NOTTINGHAM NG7 2UH

Williams, Dr HC
Senior Lecturer in Dermatology
Dermato-Epidemiology Research Unit
University Hospital
Queen's Medical Centre
NOTTINGHAM NG7 2UH

Wolfe, Dr CDA
Senior Lecturer in Public Health Medicine
Department of Public Health Medicine
Division of Public Health Sciences
United Medical & Dental Schools of Guy's & St Thomas' Hospitals
Block 8 (South Wing)
Lambeth Palace Road
LONDON SE1 7EH

Woodman, Professor CBJ
Professor of Public Health Medicine & Cancer Epidemiology
Director of the Centre for Cancer Epidemiology
University of Manchester
Christie Hospital NHS Trust
Kinnaird Road
Withington
MANCHESTER M20 4QL

Introduction

A Stevens, J Raftery

Needs assessment means different things according to who uses the term, when and where. Some of these uses are reviewed in this introduction. Our understanding of needs assessment stems from the wish to provide useful information for those involved in the priority setting and purchasing of health care.

We are concerned with population health care need and define it as 'the population's ability to benefit from health care'[1,2,3] as did Culyer 20 years ago.[4] Mention of health care is important because for the purposes of commissioning health services it is crucial that there be some benefit from the interventions that follow from the assessment of need. The benefit can be immediate or in the future, physical or psychological, personal or communal. The intervention can concern health promotion, diagnosis, or palliation as well as treatment. We argue that needs are worth assessing when something useful can be done about them. The two essential determinants of a population's ability to benefit are the:

- incidence and/or prevalence of a health problem
- effectiveness of the interventions available to deal with it.

These two components form the core of the protocol used in the chapters that follow.

Current service provision although not a determinant of need is also highly relevant if needs assessment is to have any value in action. We need to know how things stand before we can change them. The reliance of our approach on these three elements is shown in Figure 1. The effectiveness corner of the triangle includes cost-effectiveness because this allows us to consider the *relative* priority of different needs.

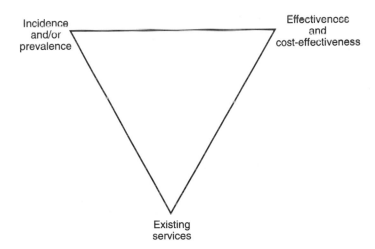

Figure 1: The elements of health care needs assessment.

We also distinguish need from demand (what people would be willing to pay for or might wish to use in a system of free health care) and from supply (what is actually provided).[1,2,3] This helps to classify health service interventions according to whether they reflect need, demand or supply (or some combination). It also highlights the need for caution in the use of information sources which often say more about supply (e.g. utilization rates) or demand (e.g. patient preference surveys) than they do about need. It also reminds health care commissioners of the importance of drawing together needs, supply and demand as shown in Figure 2. The central area of overlap is the optimum field for service provision, i.e. where need, supply and demand are congruent.

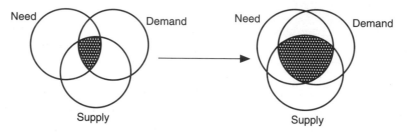

Figure 2: Drawing need, demand and supply together: the role of the purchasers of health care.

We also suggest three practical tools for health care needs assessment (see page xxxvi):

1 epidemiological
2 comparative
3 corporate.

Alternative approaches

There is a considerable range of alternative approaches to needs assessment depending on their purpose and context.

Social services assessment

In UK public policy the community care reforms which have stressed individual needs assessment for social care. Local authority social services departments must assess the needs of individuals for personal social services that mainly cover the elderly, the mentally ill and people with learning disabilities.[5]

Individual health care needs assessment

In health care too, the mentally ill have become subject to increased individual assessment through the care programme approach which is designed to cover all severely mentally ill individuals who are about to be discharged from hospital.[6] However individual health care needs assessment has existed as long as medicine and is the key feature of much of health care. The clinical focus regards need as the best that can be done for a patient in a particular setting. In primary care the establishment of routine health checks in the UK, especially for the over 75s, is an example of formalized individual needs assessment, which raised controversy in its imposition of mass individual needs assessment that includes people who are not necessarily in any need.[7,8]

Participatory priority setting

In the US needs assessment is often used as a term for participatory priority setting by organizations, which are usually public sector or voluntary rather than for profit These involve three elements: defining the needs of organizations or groups, setting priorities and democratic involvement,[9] At state level the now famous Oregon approach to priority setting has much in common with needs assessment for health care commissioning in the UK but the explicit use of the participatory democratic element in the US was striking.[10] Even in the UK health policy since 1991 has attributed growing importance to the role of the public. This has been both in the form of central exhortation[11,12] and in local practice as many district health authorities have tried to involve the public in priority setting.[13] Public involvement has also occurred unintentionally through the media: a series of controversial cases, notably Child B who was denied a second NHS funded bone marrow transplant for leukaemia on the basis of the likely ineffectiveness of the treatment, have raised national debates.[14]

Primary care approaches

Other approaches, some imposed from above and some experimental from below are emerging from attempts to establish needs assessment in primary care. The routine assessment of the over 75s is an example of a top-down initiative and is unusual in requiring individual needs assessment by general practitioners of an entire age group.[7,8] Bottom-up experimental approaches tend to be based around data gathering through different means including for example rapid participatory appraisal, the analysis of routinely available small area statistics and the collation of practice-held information.[15,16] The analysis of small area statistics has a long tradition, including the use of Jarman indicators[17] and belongs to the comparative method of health care needs assessment – principally identifying a need for further analysis. Examining practice-held information including the audit of general practice case notes has had a growing role and is potentially much more relevant to population needs assessment than audit in secondary care. Because primary care case notes have a wide population coverage (90% of a practice population in three years) and each primary health care team has a relatively small population, it is possible for a primary health care team to expose practice population needs (given a knowledge of the effectiveness of interventions) through case note analysis. The development of computerized case notes in general practice could dramatically increase the scope for this approach.

Local surveys

In health authorities the use of local surveys has increased. These can cover multiple client groups and involve the collection of objective morbidity data. Local bespoke surveys of morbidity[18] can be supplemented by the interpretation of semi-routine data from national surveys such as the General Household Survey[19] and the OPCS Disability Survey.[20,21] Directors of Public Health annual health reports often include both local surveys and elements of such data. These can collect valuable information, although there is a risk that when local surveys are both limited to a selective range of client groups, and are centred around subjective information, they will give disproportionate importance to a selective range of interests.

Specialty-specific documents

Documents setting out the service requirements of client groups of an individual specialty are sometimes also treated as needs assessments. These often recommend the augmentation of services (within that specialty). Their validity as needs assessment documents depends on the explicitness and thoroughness of their research base.

Clinical effectiveness research

Finally, perhaps the most important contribution to needs assessment has been the major expansion of clinical effectiveness research in the UK and elsewhere. In the UK the Department of Health's research programme and especially its emphasis on 'health technology assessment' is a major attempt to evaluate the effectiveness of many health care interventions and therefore inform the health care needs which underlie them.[22,23]

In determining the differences between these various approaches to needs assessment it is helpful to ask the following questions:

1 **Is the principal concern with health or social services?** The effectiveness component of need for social services is often not recognized. The reason for this may be that there is seldom a clear-cut distinction between what works and what does not. More housing or more education is seldom seen as undesirable. In health care, by contrast, some interventions work spectacularly well but a point arises at which increased intervention *is* undesirable. Excessive medication or surgery may not only be of no benefit but can be harmful. It could be argued that in social care the potential open-endedness of benefit and therefore of spending makes it more important to assess the effectiveness of interventions and make a judgement of what the need is. The spectre of rationing in a politically charged context often deters such explicitness.

2 **Is the needs assessment about population or individuals?** Many approaches to needs assessment are necessarily concerned with individuals. Local authority social services programmes and primary care health checks focus on individuals. Traditional clinical decision making and also some purchasing decisions such as extra-contractual referrals concern individuals. The media focus is almost always on the individual. Although individual needs assessment can be seen as the opposite end of the spectrum from population based needs assessment the underlying logic is the same.

   The purchaser (population needs assessor) is concerned with meeting the aggregate needs of the population. For some client groups where individuals are either few or prominent in their health care costs, such as in the case of mentally disordered offenders they may well need to be individually counted or even individually assessed to provide the population picture.[24,25] Wing *et al.* consider the purchaser's population view and the individual clinical view of mental health need to be 'largely identical'.[26] In part they say this because individual needs can be aggregated but in part they recognize the importance of service effectiveness as integral to the need equation.

3 **Is there a clear context of allocating scarce resources?** Needs assessments that fail to acknowledge resource limitations are common but are of restricted value to health care commissioners. This can be a problem with individual clinical needs assessment, which can put great pressure on health budgets and squeeze the care available to patients with weak advocates. However clinicians work within an (often) implicit resource framework. Population health care needs assessment makes that framework explicit. Some population approaches also fail to acknowledge resource issues. This can be a problem with population surveys if they are neither set in the context of effectiveness, nor make it clear that they are

exploratory. It is also a difficulty with specialty-specific documents recommending levels of service within the specialty.[27] Examples abound as many specialties are anxious to protect or enhance the resources available to them.[28] This may be justified but they risk being little more than a group extension of an unbounded clinical decision making procedure.

4   **Is the needs assessment about priority setting within the context of a variety of competing needs or is it about advocacy for a single group or individual?** This is closely related to the resource context question. Specialty-specific documents, client group surveys and even policy directives which focus on single groups often represent advocacy rather than balanced contributions to priority setting. Surveys about, for example, the needs of a particular ethnic minority are of limited help in guiding purchasers unless seen in the context of equivalent surveys of other groups. Whether a policy directive is advocacy based or priority based depends on how it comes about. A set of recommendations based on lobbying will be much more prone to distorting resource use than one based on research. Arguably the Child B case moved from a priority setting to an advocacy framework when the debate moved from the health authority to the law courts.

5   **Is the needs assessment exploratory or definitive?** Some approaches to needs assessment are exploratory in that they highlight undefined or under-enumerated problems. This is particularly true of lifestyle surveys that estimate the size of risk groups such as alcohol abusers or teenage smokers. Surveys of the needs within specific client groups can also fall within this category but they differ from population surveys in that they often involve advocacy. If effectiveness of interventions has been determined prior to a population survey then this approach is compatible with epidemiological health care needs assessment.

6   **Is the determination of the most important needs expert or participatory?** The epidemiological approach to needs assessment is essentially an expert approach (with a population perspective). It seeks to be as objective as possible although no judgement of relative needs can be truly objective. Interpretation of data is partly subjective and the rules for decision making are inevitably value-laden. However the setting of priorities using an epidemiological and cost-effectiveness framework is markedly different from a process based on democratic consensus. Attempts to merge the two as in Oregon and in the local experience of many health authorities can have merit but the outcome will nearly always depend on the relative emphasis given to the provision of objective information and the extent to which participants can interpret them. As a general rule the expert approach to priority setting is more viable the further it is from the clinical decision making. At one extreme the World Health Organization's assessment of relative need operates by very clear cost-effectiveness rules.[29] At the other extreme the individual clinical decisions are rightly very open to patient views. District health authorities have to reconcile the two.

Underlying all of these questions is the further question: 'Who carries out the needs assessment and for what purpose?' Provided the assessment's aims and context are clearly stated and clearly understood there is a place for all of these approaches to needs assessment. Many can be subsumed within the approach used in this book in that they provide information about:

- numbers in a particular group, i.e. incidence and prevalence
- the effectiveness and cost-effectiveness of interventions
- the distribution of current services and their costs.

There is more information available on these elements of epidemiology-based needs assessment. Epidemiological studies contribute to the first point in the list above; effectiveness and outcomes research, i.e. evidence-based health care, to the second and assessments of current services to the third. The bringing together of the three themes in this book has been supported elsewhere at the extremes of individual and global needs assessments. For example Brewin's approach to measuring individual needs for mental health care identifies need as present when *both* function is impaired *and* when it is due to remedial cause.[30] Bobadilla *et al.*, in prescribing a minimum package for public health and clinical interventions for poor and middle income counties across all disease groups, identify both 'the size of the burden caused by a particular disease, injury and risk factor and the cost effectiveness of interventions to deal with it'.[29] Table 1 summarizes different approaches to health care needs assessment using the criteria discussed above.

Tools

In the first series of health care needs assessment we suggested three tools for needs assessment:

1   the epidemiological
2   comparative
3   corporate approaches.[2,3]

The definition of health care needs as the 'ability to benefit' implies an epidemiological approach. That is an assessment of how effective, for how many and, for the purposes of relative needs assessment, at what cost. However comparisons between localities (the comparative approach) and informed views of local service problems (the corporate approach) are important too.

The value of the 'comparative approach' is well demonstrated in the assessment of need for renal replacement therapy.[31] Increases in dialysis and transplantation in the UK closer to levels seen in better-provided European countries has been demonstrated over time to meet real needs. The need to change replacement levels from 20 per million in the 1960s, to 80 per million was suggested by both the comparative and epidemiological approach, i.e. of identifying incident end-stage renal failure and the effectiveness of renal replacement therapy. The comparative method does not however easily lead to cost-effectiveness considerations and is less successful in assessing which modality of renal replacement therapy is to be preferred; as the different balance between haemodialysis, peritoneal dialysis and transplantation rests on a variety of factors. The cost-effectiveness of different modalities is critical to priority setting. The comparative approach can however prompt key questions and therefore sets the priorities for more detailed analysis.

Almost every chapter of the first series of health care needs assessment expressed doubts about the extent and reliability of much of the routine data available for comparative analysis. The data on activity and prescribing, for example, would need to be linked to disease codes to represent faithfully true disease episodes. Disease registers such as those provided by the cancer registries can be invaluable and developments in information technology and unique patient numbers offer great scope for improved comparative analyses.

The 'corporate approach' involves the structured collection of the knowledge and views of informants on health care services and needs. Valuable information is often available from a wide range of parties, particularly including purchasing staff, provider clinical staff and general practitioners. Gillam points out that 'the intimate detailed knowledge of health professionals amassed over the years is often overlooked' and he particularly commends the insight of general practitioners, a suggestion well taken by many health authorities.[32] The corporate approach is essential if policies are to be sensitive to local circumstances. This approach might explore: first, a particularly prominent local need – such as the identification of severely mentally ill patients discharged from long-stay mental hospitals and lost to follow-up; second, consequences of local service considerations such as the balance between secondary and primary and local authority community care – as has been noted in the case of district nursing services;[33] third, where local needs differ from expectations based on national averages or typical expectations (due to local socioeconomic or environmental factors); and fourth, local popular concerns which may attach priorities to particular services

Table 1: Different approaches to health care needs assessment

Criterium	Health/social focus	Individual population based	Resource/scarcity clear	Competing needs/advocacy	Definitive/exploratory	Expert/participatory
Population health care needs	Health	Population	Yes	Competing	Definitive	Expert
Individual health care needs	Health	Individual	Sometimes	Either	Definitive	Expert
Social services assessments	Social	Individual	Sometimes	Competing	Both	Both
Participatory planning	Social	Population	Sometimes	Competing	Definitive	Participatory
Oregon-style planning	Health	Population	Yes	Competing	Definitive	Both
Primary health care checks	Health	Individual	No	Competing	Exploratory	Expert
Primary health care case note audit	Health	Individual	No	Competing	Both	Expert
Population surveys	Health	Population	No	Competing	Exploratory	Expert
Client group surveys	Health	Population	No	Advocacy	Exploratory	Both
Specialty recommendations	Health	Population	No	Advocacy	Definitive	Expert
Effectiveness reviews	Health	Population	Yes	Competing	Definitive	Expert

or institutions (effectiveness considerations being equal). The need for cottage hospitals as opposed to large primary care units or other modes of community service provision might be an example. Clearly the potential pitfalls of informal corporate assessment of need are bias and vested interest that could cloud an objective view of the evidence. Nevertheless corporate memory should not be ignored.

The 'epidemiological approach' has been described fully.[3] It is worth reiterating that the epidemiological approach goes wider than epidemiology. It includes reviews of incidence and prevalence and also evidence about the effectiveness and relative cost-effectiveness of interventions, which, for service planners is increasingly seen as a focal concern. The epidemiological approach to needs assessment has helped pioneer what is now a sea-change towards evidence-based health care purchasing.

Evidence-based health care requires some rating of the quality of evidence. The first series required contributors to assess the strength of recommendation as shown in Table 2 adapted from the US Task Force on preventive health care.[34] This is now a mainstay of evidence-based medicine and it is retained in the present series.

Table 2: Analysis of service efficacy

Strength of recommendation	
A	There is good evidence to support the use of the procedure
B	There is fair evidence to support the use of the procedure
C	There is poor evidence to support the use of the procedure
D	There is fair evidence to reject the use of the procedure
E	There is good evidence to support the rejection of the use of the procedure
Quality of evidence	
(I)	Evidence obtained from at least one properly randomized controlled trial
(II-2)	Evidence obtained from well-designed cohort or case controlled analytic studies, preferably from more than one centre or research group
(II-3)	Evidence obtained from multiple timed series with or without the intervention, or from dramatic results in uncontrolled experiments
(III)	Opinions of respected authorities based on clinical experience, descriptive studies or reports of expert committees
(IV)[a]	Evidence inadequate owing to problems of methodology, e.g. sample size, length or comprehensiveness of follow-up, or conflict in evidence

Table adapted from US Task Force on Preventive Health Care.
[a]The final quality of evidence (IV) was introduced by Williams *et al.* for the surgical interventions considered in the first series.[35]

The changing background

Health care needs assessment was thrown into the spotlight in 1989 by the National Health Service Review.[36] The review, by separating purchasers and providers, identified population health care purchasing and therefore health care needs assessment as a distinct task. Since the beginning of the 1990s however a variety of circumstances has changed including the activities and research encompassed by health care needs assessment.

District health authority changes

The nature of the purchaser of health care at district health authority has changed in several ways. First, district mergers have resulted in larger purchasing units. Second the amalgamation of district health authorities with family health services authorities has extended the scope of purchasing and encouraged a more integrated approach to primary and secondary care services. Third the abolition of regional health authorities has necessitated careful purchasing of specialist services (these were formerly purchased regionally). Fourth the relationship between purchasers and providers of health care is showing some signs of maturing, as it has become obvious that large monopsonists (dominant purchasers) and monopolists have to work fairly closely together. Fifth there has been increased involvement of general practitioners (see below). These changes make districts potentially more sophisticated assessors of health care needs – although in practice such sophistication has been slowed by the administrative upheaval caused by the changes.

Cost containment

The second critical background circumstance affecting health care needs assessment is the increasing recognition of the need for cost containment. Although costs have always been constrained by the NHS allocation, new pressures have resulted from a variety of sources.

- Increased patient expectations – some of which have been encouraged centrally – particularly those concerning waiting times.
- New technologies with either a high unit cost, e.g. new drugs such as Beta Interferon for multiple sclerosis and DNase for cystic fibrosis, or which widen the indications for treatment, e.g. new joint replacement prostheses which have a longer life-span and can be given to younger patients.[37,38]
- New pressures at the boundaries between day health and social care in the problems of community care, and more recently with the criminal justice system – in the case of mentally disordered offenders.[39]

In theory the logic of needs assessment allows the identification of over-met need – in the sense of relatively ineffective and expensive services – as easily as undermet needs. In practice the former is more difficult to identify and much more difficult to correct. This further focuses attention on a limited number of areas and especially on a limited number of the most important cost pressures such as Beta Interferon.

General practitioner fundholding and GPs in purchasing

The third major background change has been the growing relative importance of general practice fundholding as a purchasing entity. In 1991 GP fundholding covered only around 10% of the population. One of the more striking aspects of the NHS reforms has been the expansion of fundholding which now (1996) covers more than half the population of England and Wales.[40] The scope of standard fundholding has been extended to cover the bulk of elective surgery outpatient care (except maternity and emergencies), community nursing and various direct access services. Some 70 total purchasing pilots have been established where GPs take on the entire NHS allocation for their patients. Side by side with these experiments in budget delegation is a variety of schemes whereby GPs are consulted, or otherwise involved in the commissioning of services.

Health care needs assessment in this book was designed primarily with district health authorities in mind. This reflected the dominant status of health authorities as purchasers at the time and also the size of the populations they covered. A population perspective makes more sense the larger the population, not least because the expected numbers of cases and their treatments are more predictable in larger populations. This is an issue for locality purchasing in general[41] and has even been a problem for district health authority purchasing when it comes to tertiary services and the rarer secondary services. The average GP sees only one case of thyroid cancer every 25 years and only eight heart attacks every year.[42] General practitioner fundholders cover populations ranging from 7000 to around 30 000. The total purchasing pilots which cover populations up to 80 000 only slightly ameliorate this. For GPs needs assessment as defined in this series is most likely to be applicable at the level of consortia with a large population. But taken together with GP involvement in profiling the population through case note audit and other means, needs assessment in primary care offers fruitful possibilities.

Evidence-based health care

The fourth main background change is in the drive from the research community itself. The evidence-based medicine and knowledge-based purchasing movement has been partly driven by imperatives to cost containment against a background of increasing health care costs as technology advances and by the acknowledgement that not all health care is effective[22,43] and by the differences in cost-effectiveness. The result is that needs assessment and cost-effectiveness assessment have become very closely related.

Use of the health care needs assessment series

Evidence for the usefulness of the epidemiological approach has come from the results of a survey of directors of public health in the UK[45], a Department of Health focus group on the first series, the House of Commons Health Committee's[46] review of the process by which authorities set priorities, and a national survey of contracting.[47] Two contrasting themes arising from these sources emerge.

1 There is an increasing appetite in health authorities for reliable material which assists priority setting. Health care purchasers are increasingly establishing a knowledge base across the whole range of health care, even if change is most effectively carried through by being reasonably selective.
2 Contracts themselves are not (yet) disease-based – usually built up from specialties they lack a starting point from which needs assessment can play a part. Thus although needs assessment has a role in setting the perspective for contracting, the guarantee that detailed implementation will take place is lacking. In part this reflects staffing shortages and the competing claims of other foci for purchasing (mergers, extra contractual referrals, waiting list initiatives, efficiency drives etc.). In part early attempts to develop disease-specific foci were hampered by poor quality data on patient treatment and particularly costs. This will become less of a problem not just with the growth of health technology assessment to provide the evidence base but also with initiatives such as the National Steering Group on Costing which has led to the costing of health care resource groups (HRGs) in six specialties.[48,49]

These surveys and experience with the first and second series have confirmed the usefulness of the protocol for health care needs assessment. Its six main elements remain:

1 a statement of the problem (normally a disease or intervention)
2 identifying the relevant sub-categories

3 the incidence and prevalence of the condition
4 the nature and level of service provided
5 the effectiveness (including the cost-effectiveness) of the service or treatments
6 models of care.

In addition authors have considered appropriate outcome measures, targets, the routine information available and current research priorities.

To extend the coverage and to link health care needs assessment more closely to the specialty basis of service planning this second series has moved away from single interventions and diseases to include groups of interventions (terminal and palliative care), groups of diseases/problems (sexually transmitted diseases, child and adolescent mental health) and whole specialties (gynaecology, dermatology and accident and emergency services) (Table 3). Only one chapter, on breast cancer, is defined as a disease group. Several of the chapters however use diseases as sub-categories. Back pain is defined more by the diagnostic cluster it represents than a disease group or aetiology.

Table 3: Health care needs assessment topics

	Series 1	Series 2
Cause	Alcohol misuse Drug abuse	
Diagnosis		Low back pain
Intervention	Total hip replacement Total knee replacement Cataract surgery Hernia repair Prostatectomy for benign prostatic hyperplasia Varicose vein treatments	
Group of interventions	Family planning, abortion and fertility services	Terminal and palliative care
Disease	Renal disease Diabetes mellitus Coronary heart disease Stroke (acute cerebrovascular disease) Colorectal cancer Dementia Cancer of the lung	Breast cancer
Heterogenous group of diseases/ problems	Lower respiratory disease Mental illness	Genitourinary medicine services Child and adolescent mental health
Service/specialty	Community child health services	Gynaecology Dermatology Accident and emergency departments
Client group	People with learning disabilities	

We believe that each of the authors of the eight chapters of this book has admirably matched the task of reviewing the components of health care needs assessment of their disease topic. Furthermore the original protocol has stood up well in its first few years. This has been so against a turbulent background in health care purchasing and a background of only slow progress in the development and availability of health care information. At the same time epidemiologically-based needs assessment has been reinforced by its overlap with other initiatives towards effective health care as well as by its uniquely wide coverage of entire diseases, groups of interventions and specialties.

References

1 Stevens A, Gabbay J. Needs assessment, needs assessment. *Health Trends* 1991; **23**: 20–3.

2 National Health Service Management Executive. *Assessing Health Care Needs*. London: Department of Health, 1991.

3 Stevens A, Raftery J. Introduction. In *Health Care Needs Assessment, the epidemiologically based needs assessment reviews. Vol. 1*. Oxford: Radcliffe Medical Press, 1994.

4 Culyer A. *Need and the National Health Service*. London: Martin Robertson, 1976.

5 *House of Commons NHS and Community Care Act*. London: HMSO, 1990.

6 *Department of Health Care Programme Approach Guidelines*. London: Department of Health, 1990.

7 Gillam S, McCartney P, Thorogood M. Health promotion in primary care. *Br Med J* 1996; **312**: 324–5.

8 Harris A. Health checks for people over 75. *Br Med J* 1992; **305**: 599–600.

9 Whitkin B, Altschuld J. *Planning and conducting needs assessments. A practical guide*. California: Sage, 1995.

10 Oregon Health Services Commission. *Prioritisation of health services*: Salem: Oregon Health Commission, 1991.

11 National Health Service Management Executive. *Local voices*. London: Department of Health, 1992.

12 Mawhinney B. Speech at the National Purchasing Conference. 13 April 1994, Birmingham.

13 Ham C. Priority setting in the NHS: reports from six districts. *Br Med J* 1993; **307**: 435–8.

14 Price D. Lessons for health care rationing from the case of child B. *Br Med J* 1996; **312**: 167–9.

15 Murray S, Graham L. Practice based health need assessment: use of four methods in a small neighbourhood. *Br Med J* 1995; **310**: 1443–8.

16 Shanks J, Kheraj S, Fish S. Better ways of assessing health needs in primary care. *Br Med J* 1995; **310**: 480–1.

17 Jarman B. Underprivileged areas: validation and distribution scores. *Br Med J* 1984; **289**: 1587–92.

18 Gunnell D, Ewing S. Infertility, prevalence, needs assessment and purchasing. *J Public Health Med* 1994; **16**: 29–35.

19 Office of Population Censuses and Surveys. *General Household Survey*. London: HMSO, 1992.

20 Martin J, Meltzer H, Elliott D. *The prevalence of disability among adults*. London: HMSO, 1988.

21 Higginson I, Victor C. Needs assessment for older people. *J R Soc Med* 1994; **87**: 471–3.

22 Advisory Group on Health Technology Assessment. *Assessing the effects of health technologies, principles, practice, proposals*. London: Department of Health, 1993.

23 Standing Group on Health Technology. *Report of the NHS Health Technology Assessment Programme 1995*. London: Department of Health, 1995.

24 Courtney P, O'Grady J, Cunnane J. The provision of secure psychiatric services in Leeds; paper I, a point prevalence study. *Health Trends* 1992, **24**: 48–50.

25 Stevens A, Gooder P, Drey N. *The prevalence and needs of people with mental illness and challenging behaviour and the appropriateness of their care*. (In press.)

26 Wing J, Thornicroft G, Brewin C. Measuring and meeting mental health needs. In *Measuring mental health needs* (eds G Thornicroft, C Brewin, J Wing). London: Royal College of Psychiatrists, 1992.

27 Sheldon TA, Raffle A, Watt I. Why the report of the Advisory Group on osteoporosis undermines evidence based purchasing. *Br Med J* 1996; **312**: 296–7.

28 Royal College of Physicians. Care of elderly people with mental illness, specialist services and medical training. London: RCP, RCPsych., 1989.

29 Bobadilla J, Cowley P, Musgrove P *et al*. Design, content and finance of an essential national package of health services. In *Global comparative assessments in the health care sector* (eds C Murray, A Lopez). Geneva: World Health Organization, 1994.

30 Brewin C. Measuring individual needs of care and services. In *Measuring mental health needs* (eds G Thornicroft, C Brewin, J Wing). London: Royal College of Psychiatrists, 1997.

31 Beech R, Gulliford M, Mays N *et al.* Renal disease. In *Health Care Needs Assessment, the epidemiologically based needs assessment reviews. Vol. 1.* Oxford: Radcliffe Medical Press, 1994.

32 Gillam S. Assessing the health care needs of populations – the general practitioners' contribution. *Brit J General Practice* 1992; **42**: 404–5.

33 Conway M, Armstrong D, Bickler G. A corporate needs assessment for the purchase of district nursing: a qualitative approach. *Public Hlth* 1995; **109**: 3337–45.

34 US Preventive Services Task Force. *Guide to clinical preventive services. An assessment of the effectiveness of 169 interventions.* Baltimore: Williams and Wilkins, 1989.

35 Williams M H, Frankel S J, Nanchahal K *et al.* Total hip replacements. In *Health Care Needs Assessment, the epidemiologically based needs assessment reviews. Vol. I.* Oxford: Radcliffe Medical Press, 1994.

36 Department of Health. *Working for patients.* London: HMSO, 1989.

37 Stevens A (ed.). Health technology evaluation research reviews. *Wessex Institute of Public Health Medicine. Vol. 2*, 1994 (248 pp) and *Vol. 3*, 1995 (285 pp).

38 Raftery J, Couper N, Stevens A. *Expenditure implications of new technologies in the NHS – an examination of 20 technologies.* Southampton: WIPHM, 1996.

39 Department of Health, Home Office. *Review of health and social services for mentally disordered offenders and others requiring similar services: final summary report.* London: HMSO, 1992. (The Reed Committee report).

40 Audit Commission. *What the doctor ordered. A study of GP fundholders in England Wales.* London: HMSO, 1996.

41 Ovretveit J. *Purchasing for health.* Buckingham: Oxford University Press, 1995.

42 Fry J. *General practice: the facts.* Oxford: Radcliffe Medical Press, 1993.

43 Chalmers I, Enkin M, Keirse M (eds). *Effective care in pregnancy and childbirth.* Oxford: Oxford University Press, 1989.

44 Neuburger H. *Cost-effectiveness register: user guide.* London: Department of Health, 1992.

45 Stevens A. *Epidemiologically based needs assessment series evaluation results.* 1993, unpublished.

46 House of Commons Health Committee. *Priority setting in the NHS: purchasing.* Minutes of evidence and appendices. London: HMSO, 1994.

47 *Purchasing Unit Review of Contracting – the third national review of contracting 1994–5.* Leeds: National Health Service Executive, 1994.

48 *Costing for contracting FDL(93)59.* Leeds: National Health Service Executive, 1993.

49 *Comparative cost data: the use of costed HRGs to inform the contracting process. EL(94)51.* Leeds: National Health Service Executive, 1994.

1 Accident and Emergency Departments

B Williams, J Nicholl, J Brazier

1 Summary

Introduction

Hospital accident and emergency (A and E) departments manage major illness, minor illness, major trauma and minor trauma. Currently there is a move towards:

- having fewer commissioning agencies and major provider units
- treating minor conditions in less specialized facilities or in general practice
- role-sharing between doctors and nurses
- the establishment of regional centres to deal with major trauma.

This chapter reviews and forecasts the nature and volume of demand for A and E department services, assesses the costs and effectiveness of the component parts and presents three models of organization which may be appropriate for particular geographical circumstances.

Structures

There were 237 major hospital A and E departments in England in 1993 and 198 minor or peripheral units. A major unit served a 196 000 catchment population on average and some covered 600 000–900 000. 99% had a 24-hour radiology service, 98% a pathology service, 94% an intensive therapy unit (ITU) on site and half had associated short-stay facilities. Nearly half lacked computerized tomography (CT) scanning facilities. 15% were in hospitals having cardiovascular surgery and 12% in hospitals with neurosurgery. By 1994/95 there were 216 Type 1 A and E departments defined as having medical staff on site, each open 168 hours a week.

Minor and peripheral units are mainly in community hospitals and some are developing in closed or downsized general hospitals, or in extended primary care centres and polyclinics.

There are approximately 2500 doctors in A and E medicine. Around 265 are consultants. The number of consultants has increased considerably since 1990. The British Association for Emergency Medicine in 1993 estimated an average of 1 : 225 000 population, with the range among major provider units 1 : 60 000–1 : 500 000. Designated nurse practitioners worked in 9% of major units and managed 3% of the new caseload.

Incidence of conditions giving rise to demand

With the introduction of more safety measures in the occupational environment and transportation, the incidence of serious injury from these sources is falling, but this is offset to some extent by the rise in criminal violence. The trend in incidence of minor conditions which make up the bulk of the work of an A and E department is unknown. The incidence of emergency medical and surgical conditions is increasing as the numbers and proportions of the middle-aged and elderly increase. This is demonstrable in respect of acute myocardial infarction and fracture of the neck of femur.

Activity

In 1994/95 there were nearly 12 million new attendances at A and E departments in England (246 per thousand population; regional range 188 to 295 per thousand). The numbers of new attendances are again increasing annually. Seven new attendances yield one reattendance on average. There were fewer than 35 000 first attendances annually in 54 Type 1 units, many serving scattered rural populations, but others were in the same or contiguous urban districts. Only 55 Type 1 units had 65 000 first attendances, or more.

The number and proportion of emergency admissions are increasing steadily. In some departments these patients are admitted through the A and E department, inflating new attendance numbers.

First attendance rates are highest among children, young adults and the elderly age groups, and among people in Social Class V. Inner-city A and E departments see proportionately more single people, commuters, migrants and the homeless.

A minimum data set is currently being adopted in A and E departments. No nationally representative information has hitherto been available on case-mix and case management. An overview of studies in individual units and areas suggests however that the new caseload of major A and E departments is mainly of low urgency. It includes:

1 in 1000	with major trauma
1 in 100	with life-threatening illness or injury, of which 75% is major illness, 15% trauma, 3% drug over-dose
1 in 4	whose condition does not require the facilities of a major A and E department
9 in 10	who attend without first consulting a GP
1 in 6 or 7	who is admitted as inpatient
1 in 4 or 5	is a child
1 in 700	dies in the A and E department

Demand is spread evenly over the days of the week and is higher during the summer. It is very low between midnight and 0800 (around 4%) but major trauma is more evenly spread, most cases presenting outside the well-staffed 'office hours'.

Effectiveness

The effectiveness of A and E department services can be judged in terms of health gain or how patient demand is managed.

Structures

- **Size** Some studies show that major units in small hospitals are equally effective, clinically, as those in large hospitals for a range of conditions. US studies indicate better outcomes for major trauma in larger hospitals, with less frequent procedural mistakes and fewer avoidable deaths.
- **Observation wards** These are reported to be associated with improved processes of care in the elderly and patients with head injuries.
- **Dedicated operating departments** Delays in surgical intervention can lead to poorer outcomes in cases of major trauma.
- **Triage** In emergency conditions, pre hospital triage to appropriate expertise and facilities improves outcomes. In hospital, triage into patient categories (hospital doctor, nurse practitioner, GP) improves the processes of care. Triage into degrees of urgency results in a tendency to 'over-triage' into more urgent categories, so that fewer admissions are actually seen urgently

Clinical management

- **Major trauma**
  a) Regional trauma systems based on regional trauma centres have been shown to be effective in the US trauma setting. Such a system was shown not to be more effective nor cost-effective in the one situation in the UK where it has been evaluated.
  b) Specialists needed on site. Secondary transfer of cases, especially of head injuries, is associated with poorer clinical outcome. If neurosurgery is not available on site there should be locally agreed guidelines for the rapid transfer of cases to the appropriate facilities.
  c) Trauma teams. Early mobilization of senior medical (A and E, anaesthetist, surgical specialists) and nursing staff, with rapid assessment and resuscitation improves outcome.
  d) Advanced trauma life support (ATLS). The value of having a casualty team trained in ATLS is widely accepted.
  e) CT scanning. This is effective in improving the management and outcome for head injuries. The value for other injured parts is less clear cut.
  f) Radiographic service. A 24-hour radiographic service with senior radiological assessment improves outcome.
- **Minor trauma**
  a) Nurse practitioners (NPs). There is no evidence from prospective randomized, controlled trials that NPs manage minor conditions as, or more effectively than junior doctors.
  b) Minor injury units (MIUs). There is no evidence about the effectiveness of MIUs in managing minor trauma relative to major A and E departments or the general medical services.
- **Major illness**
  a) Disease management protocols. The value of following protocols for major medical conditions such as acute asthma and severe chest pain is established and they should be adopted.
  b) Basic life support. This improves survival chances in emergencies.
- **Minor illness**
  a) On-site GP services in major departments. Patients with minor conditions are managed comparatively more appropriately using on-site GP services rather than traditional junior casualty officers.
  b) Polyclinics and extended primary care centres. The effectiveness of these arrangements for managing minor illness and injury compared with other arrangements is unknown.

Costs

There are very few reports in the literature of relative costs of different methods of catering for accidents and emergencies, nor of the component parts of the service. In particular it is rare for the cost consequences of an A and E attendance to the health service or to the individual to be considered. Moreover there is currently no information system which provides the means of estimating the workload and hence the costs associated with each type of case.

Structures

- **Size of department** The average cost of a new attendance at an A and E department in England is about £45.00. The cost varies little and inconsistently among departments according to the annual number of new attendances.
- **Amalgamation of units; full or partial closure of units** No follow-up studies have been reported of the cost consequences to the health services. Whether or not hospital cost savings are achieved is not known. However when A and E department services are centralized additional costs fall on ambulance services and patients.

Clinical management

- **Major trauma**
  a) The additional cost of the first regionalized trauma system to be evaluated, including establishing and operating a regional trauma centre, was £0.5 million per annum. The cost consequences for contiguous A and E departments were small as the numbers of cases diverted were very small.
  b) Trauma teams, ATLS. Published data on the costs of these developments are not available.
- **Major illness** Data specific to the A and E department management of major illness are not available.
- **Minor injury, minor illnesses** The comparative costs of treating these conditions together with the other caseload in major A and E departments or of managing them in separate minor units are unknown. Where GPs are employed in major A and E departments to manage minor conditions there is a saving of more than one-third per case compared with management by doctors of senior house officer grade.

Cost-effectiveness

Estimates of the size of the health effects and the costs of different configurations of A and E services are generally either unreliable or non-existent.

Models of care

Three models are proposed which purchasers and providers will consider in relation to different geographical circumstances. There can be no generally applicable model for an A and E department and its associated services.

- Preservation of existing major A and E departments with progressive development of alternative ways of dealing with some of the minor injury caseload; that is, a near status-quo position.
  This model may apply best where population densities and levels of attendance at major A and E departments are low.

- Reduction in the number of major A and E departments with simultaneous development of alternative facilities for dealing with minor injuries and illnesses.

  The major A and E departments will rarely receive less than 50 000 new attendances annually and commonly receive 70 000–100 000 from a catchment area of 300 000–600 000. Above 100 000 new attendances it would be difficult to provide the necessary volume of inpatient support facilities.
- Regionalizing trauma care services.

  In this model the treatment of major trauma would be concentrated in regional trauma centres serving 2.5 to 3.0 million people on average. This would provide a three-tier system, comprising regional trauma centres, other major A and E departments (though fewer than the present number) and stand-alone facilities for treating minor conditions.

Outcomes and targets

Outcomes

Clinical outcomes are affected by pre-hospital management as well as any subsequent inpatient and post-hospital care. The one system of clinical outcome measurement specific to an A and E department is its performance compared with other A and E departments in avoiding mortality in cases of major trauma, defined in a standard way. The Major Trauma Outcome Study system, or a development of it, can be used to monitor the effectiveness of care in the provider units and purchasers will probably wish to stipulate its use.

Desirable intermediate outcomes include having the condition of each patient assessed for urgency within five minutes of arrival and a low ratio of total to first attendances (no more than 1.2 : 1).

Targets

- **Major A and E departments**
  a) Specialty mix. Opinion varies about the mix of specialties which should be on site or close to a major A and E department. As a minimum there might be:

  general medicine; paediatrics; acute psychiatry; general surgery (including vascular surgery) with 24-hour major theatre availability; trauma and orthopaedics; obstetrics and gynaecology; anaesthetics; intensive care; radiology (including CT scanning facilities) and pathology.

  Children should not normally receive A and E department services in hospitals which do not have paediatric specialists and inpatient facilities on site.
  b) Staffing. In order to provide 24-hour cover at senior clinical level the recommendation of the British Association of Emergency Medicine for four A and E consultants, eight middle-grade doctors and 20 senior house officer grade doctors in a department seeing 100 000 new patients annually should be seriously considered.
- **Minor injury services** No population based, quantitative targets can be suggested for the provision of these facilities. Local opportunities, initiatives and preferences will determine their developments.

Information

The national minimum data set should be provided by A and E provider units as soon as possible. Regional and national overviews of provider performance should be arranged by suitable downloading of data.

Attempts should be made to identify more fully the discrete costs of major and minor A and E departments and their component services. Providers should collaborate with other agencies in collecting a standard core data set on accident cases.

Research needs

The relative cost-effectiveness of the various configurations of arrangements for dealing with major and minor conditions is an under-researched area which should be addressed as soon as possible.

2 The problem and its context

The public needs a service for dealing with accidents and emergencies, 24 hours a day throughout the year. The district general hospital A and E department is the main institutional provider of emergency treatment for major accidents and illness. However A and E departments deal with the entire gamut of injury and illness and social as well as medical problems.

The Accident and Emergency Reference Group of the London Implementation Group defined the *primary* tasks of an A and E department as to provide the following.

- Resuscitation and immediate treatment for the critically ill and injured and to refer patients as appropriate.
- A diagnostic and treatment service for the less seriously ill and injured patients who merit urgent hospital attention and to refer patients on as appropriate.
- A diagnostic and treatment service for those with conditions which allow them to be subsequently discharged.[1]

A and E departments have traditionally fulfilled these functions.

This chapter looks at a variety of institutionally-based ways of providing A and E services. It does so in the context of purchaser–provider contracts. It attempts to take into account technological changes in the ways the acutely sick and injured are managed and changes in the roles and professional development of health care providers. The relevant issues include the following.

Move towards fewer, larger commissioning agencies and providers

The National Audit Office identified 235 A and E departments in NHS hospitals in England in 1991, approximately one for every 196 000 inhabitants and more than one per health district, on average.[2] In inner London in 1993, before any mergers or closures, there was an A and E department for every 160 000 resident population and very few people lived more than two miles from the nearest A and E department. In contrast in Leicestershire one major A and E department serves a resident population of over 900 000. As health districts merge and larger commissioning agencies are formed the numbers of major A and E departments required and their distribution are being reconsidered. As some of these A and E departments close, alternative ways of coping with the residual demand for treatment of minor injuries and ailments are being introduced or considered.

Management of major trauma

There is greater public and media concern about the quality of care in A and E departments than over almost any other sector of health care. This increases when professional opinion focuses on their shortcomings, as did the Royal College of Surgeons' consensus view that at least one in every five deaths from trauma was avoidable and that inadequate clinical care in A and E departments was a major contributor.[3] This has led to the recommendation that major trauma should be dealt with in regional trauma centres, each serving 2.5–3 million population on average, where a concentration of appropriate medical skills can be made available on a 24-hour basis. Following its report, an experimental regional trauma system was set up in the North West Midlands based around a regional trauma centre in Stoke-on-Trent. Although this experimental system has been evaluated and found not to be cost-effective,[4] questions remain about the role of regional trauma systems in other areas of the country where different conditions apply.

Introducing regional trauma centres would have consequences for the location of regional clinical specialties and for the range of professional experience and training opportunities available in the remaining A and E departments.

Role sharing

In A and E departments, as in other areas of health care provision, roles are becoming blurred. In particular nursing roles are broadening to include the management of minor illness and injury. This has coincided with a reduction in the number of hours for which junior doctors are contracted to work. Nurses are fulfilling these functions, officially or unofficially, in an increasing number of A and E departments, especially in minor injury units and single-specialty hospitals.[5] Nevertheless senior house officers will continue to provide the bulk of the medical workforce in consultant-led A and E departments.[6]

General practice–hospital interface

The introduction of the 1990 GP Contract[7] followed by the NHS reforms[8] extended the scope and availability of general medical services. Investment in a diversity of practice staff and premises has meant that more of the relatively minor conditions which A and E departments dealt with hitherto can now be treated at practice level.

GPs in rural areas have always provided first-contact emergency services. Primary care emergency centres are being developed, especially in urban areas, providing a wide range of services out-of-hours to aggregated practice populations, both on a walk-in and bookable basis.[9] These are already operating in Denmark and Sweden. If introduced widely they may influence the workload of A and E departments appreciably.

Pre-hospital care

Pre-hospital emergency care is outside the scope of this chapter. However its organization and operational efficiency influences the case-mix which presents to an A and E department.

By the end of 1995 every emergency ambulance crew was due to include at least one member trained to paramedic standards. The prevalence of advanced life support skills among ambulance crews is increasing[10] as is the sophistication of their diagnostic, resuscitation and communication equipment. Response-time targets are set for ambulance services according to the densities of the populations served, although this will change in the future.[11] Rapid transit of single paramedics by small non-patient carrying vehicles is now not uncommon in many regions.

Emergency services in the field can communicate directly with A and E department staff. Protocols are being considered for deciding when and where to transfer certain types of case. The most severely injured patients can then be conveyed directly to the most appropriate facilities, such as coronary care units or hospitals with neurosurgical facilities. Helicopter-ambulances are being used in London and by some rural ambulance services to transfer seriously ill or injured patients from the incident scene to hospital (primary transfer) and between hospitals (secondary transfer).

As a result of these developments the workload of some A and E departments may be increased by seriously sick and injured patients who previously would not have survived to reach hospital.

Patient perspectives

Patients are concerned with many aspects of A and E department services such as reception, privacy and support for victims and the bereaved[12] and targets have been set in the Patient's Charter for the management of patients in these situations.[13] Information technology is evolving which can produce data to audit the prioritization of patients for attention and their clinical management.

Services for children

Children have distinct needs[14] both in pre-hospital[15] and hospital care and providing paediatric emergency care may need different facilities and training. A central concern is whether appropriate services can be provided within adult A and E departments or whether different facilities and personnel are needed.

Wider hospital context

An A and E department operates in the context of an entire hospital, the parts of which are interdependent in functions. Not all emergency medicine involves A and E departments. However any case presenting to an A and E department has the potential to involve other specialist departments. Some specialties are essential on site. Others need to be rapidly accessible. When contemplating changes in the nature or volume of A and E department activity therefore, the capacity of other departments in the hospital to accommodate these changes has to be taken into account.

The clear and concise analyses of the management and organizational problems of the A and E departments contained in the reports of the National Audit Office[2], the Audit Commission[16] and the Clinical Standards Advisory Group[17] have helped to crystallize many of the planning and strategic issues involved. The present needs assessment for A and E departments does not attempt to duplicate that work. Rather it focuses on the ways in which A and E services are organized and examines the evidence for the effectiveness of different models relative to their costs. This leads on to a series of suggestions and recommendations on the structuring of A and E services.

3 Sub-categories

A and E departments deal with a wide range of illness and injury; from the individual walk-in patient who needs only reassurance about a trivial complaint, to the simultaneous arrival of several casualties with severe, multisystem injuries from a major incident. The particular case-mix will influence the way a department is organized.

Case-mix

Complexity

A simple classification of the clinical case-mix is:

- major injury
- major illness
- minor injury
- minor illness.

There are no precisely agreed definitions of these categories. 'Major' has the connotation of being potentially life-threatening, while 'minor' does not.

Although A and E departments are among the most intensively used parts of the health service, the only systematic data about their functioning are the annual numbers of new and total attendances.[18] It is not possible to characterize routinely the caseload of many A and E departments, still less to show how the case-mixes of different departments vary. Consequently it is impossible to produce a template of the level of patient dependency to fit all A and E departments and hence the mix and volume of skills needed; hourly, daily or seasonally.

The caseload is predominantly of low urgency, that is, not life threatening nor requiring the use of technically complex diagnostic or treatment facilities. The A and E department at Hull Royal Infirmary is capable of producing routinely an analysis of clinical activity. The cases first attending the department between 1990 and 1993 were, by local standards, predominantly minor in nature (Table 1).

Table 1: Number of patients attending Hull Royal Infirmary A and E department according to severity of condition

Category of severity	1990	1991	1992	1993
major	16 852	16 962	17 389	17 735
minor	61 286	55 761	53 703	57 084
Total	78 238	72 723	71 092	74 819

Source: Gosnold J (personal communication)

In an Edinburgh study 90% of attenders scored less than five on a 0–10 scale of urgency where ten represented the greatest degree of urgency (Figure 1). Older patients had higher ratings for urgency, as did ambulance-borne patients.[19]

It has been claimed that only one case in a thousand presents with major trauma[20-23] and in a review of A and E services in London in 1993 only an estimated 1% of new attenders had severe injuries or life threatening conditions. Conversely 40% had conditions which could have been managed in primary care settings.[24]

Appropriateness

'Inappropriate' demand is sometimes defined in terms of problems which could have been dealt with in general practice, or for which consultation was not justifiable in any setting. The difficulty in defining such cases is reflected in the wide range of estimates which have been made of the prevalence of inappropriate attendance in A and E departments – from 6.7%[25] to 64–89%.[26] The proportion depends upon the method used. When patients' cases are reviewed on the basis of the processes of care they actually received, an estimated one in four is found not to have needed the facilities of a major department.[27]

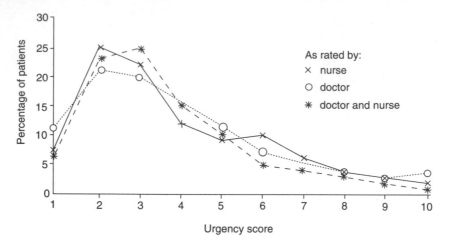

Figure 1: Urgency distribution for all patients attending the Royal Infirmary, Edinburgh A and E department. (Reproduced by kind permission of Blackwell Scientific Publications.)

Nine out of ten patients attend without first having consulted their own GPs.[28] Among the reasons for this are that they perceive their problems to be more appropriate to A and E departments and that their GPs are unavailable.[29,30] Some of these patients use the A and E department for primary care, therefore. The clientele in urban areas, particularly city centres, characteristically includes commuters with no immediate access to their usual primary care services, patients who are not registered with GPs and homeless persons. A problem which is 'inappropriate' for an A and E department clinically in terms of its minor nature may not be so when the patient's circumstances are taken into account.

In part, patients' perceptions and circumstances will always determine whether or not they use A and E departments. Short of attempting to change public perceptions there is little that can be done other than to arrange to cater for such patients, though not necessarily always in a major hospital facility as extensively equipped as a district general hospital A and E department. Ways in which this 'inappropriate' demand is catered for are described in section 5.

Special groups

The demographic patterns of attendance at A and E departments reflect largely those of their catchment area populations. Four groups need special consideration.

Children

Children need to be shielded from the disturbing situations sometimes to be seen in A and E departments and to be cared for in suitably staffed and equipped facilities.

Patients behaving aggressively or antisocially

These patients need to be managed effectively and with minimum inconvenience to others.

Bereaved

The bereaved need to express their grief and to be comforted.

Patients whose first language is not English

These patients may have additional needs related to their degree of understanding of what the service can do and the procedures to which they will be subjected.

Needs assessment for A and E departments is largely about clarifying the volume and the severity of the problems presented and about the special considerations which relate to certain patient groups and conditions.

4 Incidence and prevalence of conditions needing A and E department management

Accidents, poisonings and violence

The numbers and rates of fatalities from accidents, poisonings and violence have decreased over the past 20 years (Table 2). This may of course also reflect improvements in treatment which have occurred, irrespective of trends in incidence. However there is not yet a comprehensive information system capable of describing representative trends in incidence. Paradoxically as factors which caused severe accidents and injury in the past have been modified the demand for A and E department services has risen. The scale of heavy industry has declined sharply. Workplaces and work routines are safer; the accident rate at work has declined in all the major industries since 1971.[31] In 1986/87 a total of 499 fatal and 35 960 major injury casualties arose as a result of work and these numbers had declined by nearly 20% to 400 fatal and 29 531 major casualties in the seven years to 1994/95.[32] Road users are better protected now than at any previous time. Road traffic injuries reported to the police by the Department of Transport have decreased steadily from a peak in 1966. There were 59 034 fatal and serious road accidents in England in 1981 (126 per 100 000 population). By 1992 this number had fallen to 35 751 (74 per 100 000).[33] Violent crime has increased. Instances of violence against the person notified to the police in England and Wales rose from 100 200 in 1981 to 205 100 in 1993.[31] However the injuries which result from these offences make up only a very small part of an A and E department's caseload.

Table 2: Deaths from injury and poisoning

Year	Number (million)[a]	Rate (million)[a]
1970	22 701	466
1980	20 296	409
1990	17 943	354

[a] Data for England and Wales.

Source: *OPCS Mortality Statistics.* Serial tables. Series DH1, No. 25. 1992, London, HMSO.

Fracture of neck of femur

A predictable, age-related component of an A and E department's major injury caseload is the incidence of fracture of the neck of femur. Its occurrence virtually always results in transfer to an A and E department for assessment and then nearly always leads to hospital admission. The discontinuity in data from the discharge-based, Hospital Inpatient Enquiry (HIPE) which last reported in 1985 and the Hospital (Consultant) Episodes System (HES) summary which replaced it in 1989/90 complicates any attempt to observe trends. Formerly a discharge may have represented more than one episode of consultant-led care in one period as an inpatient. Nevertheless the numerical trend in recent years was upward; from 38 260 discharges or deaths in hospitals in England in 1980,[34] to 43 050 discharges or deaths in 1985;[35] to 54 041 episodes in 1989/90[36] and 58 970 in 1993/94[37] (Table 3). The incidence rate of fracture of the neck of femur rises with age. Numerically although the age-specific incidence is no longer rising,[38] a rise in demand until the year 2020 can be expected, when the number of persons aged 75 or over is expected to stabilize.

Table 3: Inpatient cases by main diagnosis NHS Hospitals in England

| Year | Main diagnosis, short-list[a] | | | |
	270 Acute myocardial infarction	323.2 Asthma	473 Fracture of neck of femur	53 Poisonings and toxic effects
1989/90	115 598	100 188	54 041	101 117
1990/91	119 718	93 277	55 748	101 667
1991/92	116 518	99 717	57 143	97 363
1992/93	119 049	96 659	58 959	103 445
1993/94	116 776	103 324	58 970	104 766

[a] Ordinary admissions and day cases. All persons, all ages.

Source: *Hospital Episodes Statistics.*

Wrist trauma

Data from a population-based survey in Odense, Denmark, which has a population structure similar to that of England's urban population, indicated that 690 per 100 000 inhabitants aged 15 years or over presented in a year to a hospital's emergency room. 580 per 100 000 received radiographic investigation; 270 per 100 000 had distal radial fractures; but those presenting to hospital represented only 56% (95% confidence interval 31% : 78%) of all occurrences in the population.[39]

Deliberate self-harm

In 1990 in the A and E department at Hull Royal Infirmary, 1185 patients presented who had deliberately harmed themselves in some way. Based on a planning population of 400 000, this represented an occurrence rate of 296 per 100 000 population of all ages. By 1993 the number had risen to 1788 (447 per 100 000); of whom 6% were under the age of 15 years; 53% were between the ages of 15 and 29; 25% between 30 and 44 and the remaining 16% were middle aged or elderly (Gosnold J, personal communication).

Studies in Oxford and Edinburgh in the 1980s reported declining rates of occurrence of self-poisoning, especially among the young.[40] These findings were based on hospital inpatients. However the volume of inpatient activity for poisonings and other toxic effects among the 48 million population of England is rising slightly in the 1990s (Table 3). Studies of self-harm based only on inpatients underestimate the true incidence of A and E department-managed self-poisoning. Of 200 adolescent self-harm patients treated in the A and E department at Leicester Royal Infirmary in 1989, 89 (44%) were admitted.[41] Studies in one of England's largest-volume A and E departments, at the University Hospital in Nottingham, in the 1980s showed a small decline in the episodes of deliberate self-poisoning between 1981/82 (1444 episodes) and 1987/88 (1407). The rates of presentation fell from 272 to 255 per 100 000 population of all ages. This masked a rise in the rate for the 15–34 year age group from 429 to 456 per 100 000, and corresponding falls in patients older than this.[42]

Using the figures from these surveys it may be estimated for planning purposes that about 300–450 patient episodes of deliberate self-harm per 100 000 population will need A and E department treatment annually; 250–300 per 100 000 will relate to deliberate self-poisoning, of which around 45–50% will lead to inpatient care and these will be among the 200–220 per 100 000 population treated as inpatients annually for poisonings and toxic effects.

Other major medical conditions

Since there is a lack of representative data about the incidence of the majority of diagnostic conditions the impact of any change in the incidence on the demand for A and E services cannot be predicted accurately. The London Ambulance Service's 1991 survey showed that 1% of all new attenders at London A and E departments had life threatening conditions which required urgent transportation for immediate care. This represents the most severe end of the spectrum of illness and injury. At least 75% of these were due to medical (i.e. non-surgical) conditions, another 16% to trauma and 3% to drug overdose.[43] The incidence of serious illness in the population is the main determinant of urgent need for A and E department services. This is determined largely by the proportions of the population who are middle-aged or elderly and hence at greatest risk of becoming acutely ill.

Acute myocardial infarction

Age-specific mortality rates for acute myocardial infarction are generally falling. The number of admissions for acute myocardial infarction has changed little in recent years (Table 3). These data and even the population-incidence data produced by such thorough studies as the MONICA project[44] do not represent the demand on A and E departments by cases of suspected myocardial infarction.

An illustration of this is from the city of Nottingham, which has been served by a single A and E department, University Hospital, for two decades and no other major A and E department in the vicinity has closed during that time. The numbers of patients assessed in the A and E department for the occurrence of acute myocardial infarction rose from 735 in 1982 to 1670 in 1992. The size of the catchment area population, 650 000, remained fairly constant and its demographic structure altered only in line with national demographic changes. Over the same period the numbers admitted for assessment directly to a ward or coronary care unit (CCU) also rose, from 555 to 1343. The rise in direct admissions was especially marked in the later part of the period (Table 4), presumably reflecting the perceived value of using fibrinolysis in the ward or coronary care unit as soon after the event as possible.

Table 4: Suspected acute myocardial infarction in Nottingham, 1982–92

Year	Assessed in A and E department		Admitted direct to ward/CCU		Total	
	no.[a]	rate	no.	rate	no.	rate
1982	735	113.1	555	85.4	1290	198.5
1986	1161	178.6	725	111.5	1886	290.1
1989	1696	278.0	948	145.8	2695	406.8
1992	1670	256.9	1343	206.6	3013	463.5

[a] Admissions to A and E department in University Hospital, numbers and rates per 100 000 catchment area population.

Source: *Nottingham Coronary Register* (Gray D, personal communication, 1994).

The rate of contact more than doubled among both A and E department and ward or CCU cases. The numbers of cases which, after full assessment, proved actually to have had infarctions rose less steeply, from 444 in 1982 (34% of those assessed) to 615 (20%) in 1992, irrespective of where the initial hospital assessment was carried out. For cases first assessed in the A and E department the number who proved to have had infarctions rose from 235 (32% of those assessed) in 1982, to 374 (22%) in 1992. By itself, therefore, an area's incidence rate for acute myocardial infarction is not necessarily a good indicator of the workload the condition will create for the local A and E department.

Asthma

Only the minority of asthma attacks result in the use of an A and E department. Recently in 218 general practices distributed around the UK there were an estimated 14.3 attacks per 1000 patients per year. Of these 86% were managed in general practice; 12% led to hospital admission (usually via the A and E department) and 2% were discharged from the A and E department.[45] At most two per 1000 population use the A and E department for asthma annually. Moreover reported management of these attacks was at variance with recommended guidelines, so the 'true' need for hospital services is unknown.

The increasing trend in asthma admissions observed before 1985 has not been continued in recent years,[46] although there was a sharp increase in 1993/94 (Table 3).

Psychiatric conditions

There are no recently published population-based estimates of the incidence of psychiatric emergencies in the UK population. Community-based care of these emergencies can result in better symptom control and patient satisfaction than hospital-based care and much less consumption of hospital resources.[47] However outside office hours A and E departments and hospital psychiatric wards are the most-used agencies for emergency assessments.[48]

Homeless people are characterized by an above average prevalence of psychiatric conditions and high levels of A and E department utilization. A one-day census in Sheffield (population 526 000) located 340 single homeless people, including 48 women, a ratio of 64.6 per 100 000 population; among whom 29% of the men and 64% of the women reported psychiatric illness; 30% of men and 9% of women reported alcoholism and 65 (19%) reported attending a general hospital in the previous month, 45 (13%) for A and E services.[49] Social conditions which produce homelessness may also raise the extent to which A and E services are used.

Substance abuse

While there is a large body of literature on the prevalence of alcohol and drug-related conditions among attenders at individual A and E departments and especially among specific groups of attenders, such as those injured in road traffic accidents, victims of assault, etc., there are no recent reports of population-based studies of utilization by substance abusers, nor of trends in utilization. It is difficult to forecast the impact of any changes in legislation or social policy in relation to these issues therefore.

Minor injury and illness

The picture with regard to minor injury or minor illness is more clouded, since they are managed through different forms of provision in different places. No representative local, regional or national data on the incidence of minor injuries could be found.

A major A and E department's caseload of minor conditions includes many cases where assessment of the undifferentiated problem is needed to establish that it is, indeed, minor in nature. This often involves using the type of diagnostic equipment available only in a major A and E department. For example, a person who collapses in the street may prove after investigation simply to have fainted and not to have had the suspected cerebro-vascular accident. A patient who limps in with a painful ankle may merely have sprained it and not fractured any bones.

Moreover minor ailments, with justification, often present to health care providers other than those in the NHS. For instance during exercise taken as a leisure activity in England and Wales there were an estimated 19.3 million new injury incidents in persons aged 16–45 years in England and Wales in the year July 1989 – June 1990, of which about half, 9.8 million, were not trivial. Only 20% were managed in A and E departments. The remainder was treated largely by GPs and sports clinic staff and physiotherapists and other professionals allied to medicine were also involved.[50]

Summary

The main determinant of changes in the nature or the volume of demand for A and E services over the next 20 years is likely to be the increase in the number of elderly people in the population. The progressively greater numbers of the elderly will yield more medical and surgical conditions needing urgent differentiation and treatment, though the bulk of A and E workload will be minor in nature. The increase in available leisure time and the resulting opportunities for pursuing energy-expending activities will result in more minor injuries, but the impact on major A and E departments will be relatively small. The introduction of even more safety measures in occupational and social settings is likely to maintain the reduction in the incidence of injury.

5 Services available and their utilization

In this section A and E departments are considered in terms of their number, location, facilities, medical staffing and utilization.

Number and type

The main source of statistical information about the structure and distribution of A and E departments is the Department of Health's annual return of outpatient attendances at each provider's unit(s) (DH KH09). On another return (DH KH03) A and E departments are classified according to whether they have medical staff on site and whether they are open continuously.

On the KH09 return for 1994/95 there were 264 provider units with A and E department outpatient activity in England on 30 September 1994, according to the type of A and E department (Table 5).

Table 5: Number of A and E departments in England, 1994/95

A and E type		Number of departments
1	Medical staff on site, intended to be open 168 hours per week	216
2	Medical staff on site, intended to be open less than 168 hours per week	21
3	Service covered by other than medical staff on site, intended to be open 168 hours per week	20
4	Service covered by other than medical staff on site, intended to be open less than 168 hours per week	7
	Total	264

Source: DH Statistical return (KH03).

Categorizing A and E departments as major or minor depends on how they are defined. 'Major' might include only the 216 Type 1 departments, or those together with some or all of the 21 Type 2 departments. According to the British Association for Accident and Emergency Medicine's (BAEM) Directory 1993, there were 237 major A and E units in England and 198 minor, or peripheral units. The major units included six A and E units in children's hospitals and four in ophthalmic hospitals or units.[51] In a 1995 survey the Audit Commission cited 228 major A and E departments in England and Wales, treating all types of injuries and medical emergencies and, with few exceptions, open 24 hours a day.[16] In the intervals between the BAEM survey, the 1994/95 statistical return and the Audit Commission Survey some departments will have closed and others may have merged. The comparison is not straightforward, however, in that the Department of Health collects and reports data on a provider basis so that an NHS trust covering more than one hospital site will provide only one return even if it has A and E services in more than one location.

Location

Using the BAEM source the locations of major A and E departments can be plotted according to health authority boundaries (Table 6). Four authorities each had four major units in their area. At the other extreme the population of nearly one million in Leicestershire is served by a single major unit, supported by a number of minor units countywide.

Table 6: Number of district health authority areas according to number of major A and E departments in England, 1993

No. of A and E departments	No. of authorities
0	1
1	102
2	43
3	11
4	4
Total	161

The Audit Commission compiled a 1995 atlas of major A and E departments in England and Wales. It located 19 major units (17 with less than 35 000 new attendances) which were more than 20 miles from the nearest alternative and concluded that there was little scope for closing such departments in small areas. In contrast 60% of major departments were within ten miles of another hospital with a full A and E service and a third, mostly in metropolitan areas, within five miles and serving less than 50 000 new patients a year.[16]

Facilities

There are no complete profiles available of the supporting specialties, units or equipment in hospitals with major A and E departments. A British Orthopaedic Association survey reported the on-site situation in 1992 in 217 hospitals with major A and E departments which claimed to be able to manage major fractures; 99% had a 24-hour radiology service; 98% pathology (24-hour transfusion service); 94% an intensive therapy unit; 51% computerized tomography (CT); 15% cardiovascular surgery and 12% a neurosurgery specialty on site.[52]

Accident and emergency wards

Around half the major A and E departments have associated short-stay, observation or initial inpatient treatment facilities.[53] The BAEM believes such a facility:

is an essential part of every Accident and Emergency (A&E) Department. The advantage of such a ward is that it provides expertise in the management of its typical patients. They stay in hospital for shorter periods than in other wards and are often better and more economically managed because of the use of social and other liaison services for crisis intervention. Such a ward provides a safety net for some patients who might otherwise be discharged injudiciously. Flexibility of use is also an important feature.

The BAEM recommends one bed in an accident and emergency ward for every 5000 new attenders.[54]

Computerized records systems

In 1992 the BAEM reported the prevalence of computerized registration systems, with or without a link-up to a patient administration system in 'the British Isles'. Of 268 A and E departments identified as having 25 000 or more new attendances annually, 165 (62%) responded to the enquiry. Fifty-two departments were computerized; another 70 planned to become computerized, 58 definitely and 12 hopefully. There were 15 commercial software systems in use and nine more developed 'in house'. No information was obtained about the respective data sets, nor the compatibility of their contents.[55]

Computerization is a requirement for providing the Contract Minimum Data Set for A and E departments, specified by the NHS Executive's Committee for Regulating Information Requirements (see section 9).

Staff

Doctors

In 1994 there were 2549 doctors in A and E medicine posts in England; an increase of 19.5% over 1980, but only 1.4% over 1990. However the number of consultants rose to a much greater extent – up by 70 (35%) over the period 1990–94. Moreover when translated into whole-time equivalents, the increase in the number of consultants, 1990 to 1994, was similar (34%). The staff grade also expanded appreciably – by 100 (98.5 whole-time equivalent (wtc)) over four years and there were 164 more doctors (158.5 wtc) in training grades (senior registrar, registrar, senior house officer) (Table 7).

Table 7: Numbers of doctors according to grade, A and E specialty in England

Grade of doctor	1980		1990		1994[a]	
	no.	wte	no.	wte	no.	wte
All grades	2133	1497.8	2514	1886.4	2549	2124.0
Consultants and senior hospital medical officer (SHMO) with allowance	123	122.3	199	196.4	269	263.4
Staff grade	–	–	43	41.6	143	140.1
Associate specialists	86	83.9	66	62.1	46	45.3
Senior registrars	16	16.0	56	54.6	81	78.6
Registrars	60	57.4	81	78.2	110	98.8
Senior house officers	1050	1047.3	1270	1262.2	1380	1376.1
House officers	6	6.0	6	6.0	1	1.0
Other staff with SHMO allowance	1	1.0	–	–	2	2.0
Hospital practitioners	44	9.3	35	5.9	41	6.9
Clinical assistants	747	154.6	758	179.4	476	111.8

[a]NHS Executive 1995 (personal communication).

Sources: Department of Health. *Health and Personal Social Services Statistics.*[56]

Surveying the management of skeletal trauma in the UK in 1991/92 the British Orthopaedic Association reported that 79% of the 228 departments with a major trauma service were administered by an A and E consultant; 49 (21%) had no A and E consultants; 141 (62%) had only one; 35 (15%) had two and three (1%) had three.[52] The ratio of A and E consultants to catchment area populations varied from one per 61 000 to one per 500 000, with an average of one to 223 000, which was little less than the average population of a health district. The total A and E medical staff of all grades in a hospital was broadly proportional to the size of the population served. 66% of the hospitals had no intermediate training grade doctors at all. Many hospital A and E departments function mainly through the services of junior medical staff, the majority at senior house officer level. It is not known what proportion of these doctors are trained in advanced life support.

There is scope, therefore, for exploring the most cost-effective mix of medical staff which A and E departments of various sizes need, taking into account the possibilities of role-sharing with nurses for the management of minor conditions.

Nurses

No collated data are available routinely on the levels of nurse staffing in A and E departments, nor on the range of activities which nurses undertake. In 9% of major A and E departments in 1990/91 there were nurses who were officially designated as nurse practitioners. Nurses who functioned in the same ways, but who were not designated as such, worked in 8% of major A and E departments; 48% of specialist A and E departments and 58% of minor injury units. Clinically they managed an estimated 3% of the new caseload in the year, mainly minor illnesses and injuries, but junior doctors working in the same departments managed even more cases with similar conditions.[5]

Again nothing is known of the proportion of nurses in A and E departments who are trained in advanced life support.

Minor injury units

A recent NHS Executive survey report defined a minor injury unit (MIU) as:

offering an open access, self-referral minor injury and ailments service for ambulatory patients but which may also see patients referred by GPs. It will provide a service more akin to that provided by an A and E department than by GPs in their surgeries, but there will be some overlap with the work of both A and E departments and GPs. A minor injury unit will not, however, fulfil the continuing care role undertaken by GPs. Minor injury units do not require in-patient facilities.[57]

The BAEM Directory in 1993 listed 198 minor or peripheral units.[51] The NHS Executive survey members visited seven such units and obtained information on three more. They found a number of different ways of staffing the units, which included nurse practitioners working alone or in combination with GPs and clinical assistants or staff-grade specialists working with nurses. Different units dealt with very different caseloads, with some in the more isolated areas accepting emergency ambulance cases within a given area.

Some units are in long-standing community (cottage) hospitals; a few, such as the units at Ancoats Hospital, Manchester[58] and St Charles Hospital, London[24] are on the sites of general hospitals which have closed, either totally or partially. At least one other is in specially converted premises in the community.[59]

A variant of the minor injury/illness unit is the King's College Hospital, GP-staffed facility located within its A and E department, to which patients are directed according to clear protocols and which offers treatment for minor injuries and ailments similar to that of a well-organized general practice, but also affording immediate access to X-ray and pathology facilities.[60]

Other settings for treating minor injuries are, as stated earlier, major A and E departments; primary care centres, such as the South Westminster Healthcare Centre which, as well as providing minor treatments during weekday office hours, also serves as a base for community nursing services, professions allied to medicine, and other community health services[61]; and traditionally, general practice premises.

The range of equipment available in MIUs varies according to their location. Units in community hospitals can utilize the resuscitation, pathology and radiographic services of the hospitals. There is however no source of information which can be used to profile the facilities for treating minor injury in England; nor is it usually possible to identify the discrete areas of expenditure which these units incur, because their particular functions are not disaggregated from those of the parent institution.

A and E department utilization

New attendances

There were 11 943 000 new A and E department attendances in England in 1994/95, a rate of 246 per 1000 population, or approximately one new attendance for every four persons. The new attendance rate ranged among regions from 188 per 1000 in the Oxford region to 295 per 1000 in the heavily urbanized Mersey and North Western regions (Table 8). Distance and the length of time expended in obtaining care are factors which are known to influence a decision to attend.[62] These new attendances include those of an unknown number of emergency patients who pass through A and E departments as arranged inpatient admissions (p. 21).

Table 8: A and E departments in England and in RHAs, 1994/95

	First attendances (thousands)	Rate per 1000	Attendances per new A and E outpatient
England	11 943	246	1.16
Northern	722	233	1.19
Yorkshire	916	247	1.17
Trent	1 006	211	1.21
East Anglia	466	222	1.11
NW Thames	772	219	1.12
NE Thames	1 062	279	1.09
SE Thames	1 067	287	1.13
SW Thames	719	240	1.13
Wessex	627	199	1.19
Oxford	487	188	1.11
South Western	756	227	1.25
West Midlands	1 432	271	1.15
Mersey	713	295	1.17
North Western	1 191	295	1.17
Special health authorities	8	–	

Numbers and rates per 1000 population, first attendances, and total attendances per new A and E outpatient

Source: Department of Health. *Outpatients and Ward Attenders, England, Financial Year 1994–95.* Government Statistical Service. OPCS. 1993-based sub-national population projections. Series PP3 No. 9.

The annual number of first attendances rose by approximately 17% over the decade to 1990/91. It then peaked in the period 1989–91 at 11.2 million; after that it fell slightly, but by 1994/95 it had risen again to nearly 12 million (Figure 2). The first-attendance rate rose from 202 per thousand population in 1981 to the highest level yet recorded; 246 per thousand in 1994/95.

Over the period 1984 to 1994/95 the number of first attendances rose by an annual average of 1.5%. Over the same period follow-up attendances fell annually by an average of 6.1%. By 1994/95 only one in seven first attendances yielded a follow-up attendance, compared with one in four a decade earlier.

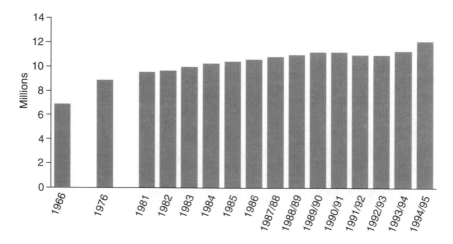

Figure 2: Number of new attendances at A and E departments annually 1966–1994/95 in England.

(Sources: Department of Health, *Health and Personal Services Statistics*, 1976–93. Department of Health, *Outpatients and Ward Attenders, England*, 1994–95.)

This increase in the use of A and E departments did not represent a shift of demand from general practice. Over the decade to 1993, according to the annual reports of the General Household Survey, consultation rates with GPs rose from four to five per 1000 population.[63] The 1990 GP Contract extended the hours for which GPs were to be personally available to qualify for the maximum practice allowance. It also provided incentives for extending the range of services offered.[7] This may have had the effect of actually diverting some of the demand away from A and E departments.

Aggregated regional data 'hide' wide inter-district differences in new attendance rates, however. They have varied among health district populations by as much as 18-fold[64] and the ratio of reattendances to new attendances has varied by as much as 26-fold.[65] The former is related to the proportions of males, young adults and non-marrieds in the population and only partly to the socio-economic diversity of the resident populations. The latter appears to reflect different departmental management policies.[66]

Emergency admissions through the A and E department

Emergency admissions of patients for inpatient care which are routed through the A and E department add considerably to the department's workload. This was the position in nearly one-third of the hospitals which were included in the Clinical Standards Advisory Group's 1992 survey of urgent and emergency admissions to hospital, particularly for patients en route to the orthopaedic specialty.[17] Moreover in an unknown number of major units they are logged as new A and E outpatients, inflating the numbers of first attendances. The number of emergency admissions rose by over 400 000 in the period 1989/90 to 1993/94, and by 4.2%, to 61.9%, of all admissions (Table 9).

Table 9: Emergency admissions as percentage of total ordinary admissions in England (and range for 14 RHAs)

Financial year	Number of admissions		% emergency
	Emergency	Total	
1989/90	3 418 623	5 923 799	57.7 (55.2–63.7)
1990/91	3 451 292	5 824 198	59.3 (55.8–64.2)
1991/92	3 454 746	5 960 935	58.0 (51.0–64.9)
1992/93	3 639 735	6 069 599	60.0 (55.9–65.6)
1993/94	3 825 994	6 184 144	61.9 (55.9–65.8)

Source: *Hospital Episodes Statistics.*

Patient activity

There is considerable variation in levels of patient activity in A and E departments in England.

Fewer than half the (major) Type 1 units had more than 50 000 new attendances, even allowing for the probably few cases where the activities of any minor units covered by the same provider Trusts were included in these numbers. Fifty-five providers had 65 000 or more first attendances, of which eight had 100 000 or more (Table 10).

Table 10: Number of providers according to type of main A and E department and number of first attendances in England, 1994/95

Type[a]	No. first attendances					Total
	0–	20 000–	35 000–	50 000–	65 000–	
1	18	36	59	48	55	216
2	11	3	4	3	0	21
3	17	1	1	1	0	20
4	6	1	0	0	0	7
0	4	0	1	0	0	5
All	56	41	56	52	55	269

[a] For description of types 1–4 see Table 5, p. 15. Type 0 indicates no A and E department.

Source: KH09 returns.

Data collected systematically in a research project from eight district general hospital A and E departments in various parts of England were used in a study of reattenders.[66] Another unpublished analysis of the data collected in this survey showed that young adults make up proportionately more of the clientele than other age groups; over 20% are children, a group for whom special arrangements are needed[67] (Figure 3).

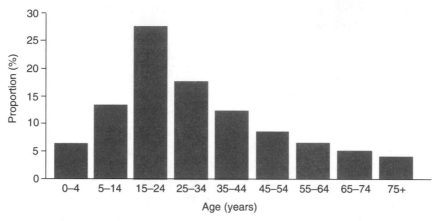

Figure 3: Percentages of new attenders at A and E departments in eight English hospitals in 1987.

A and E departments have proportionately more new attenders in the summer months than in winter (Figure 4), but there are generally no great differences from day to day (Figure 5).

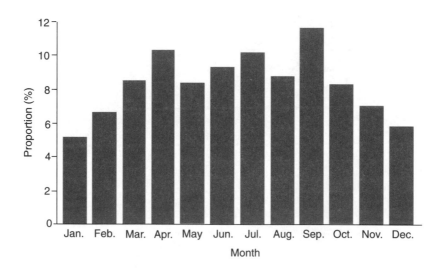

Figure 4: Percentage of new attenders according to month.

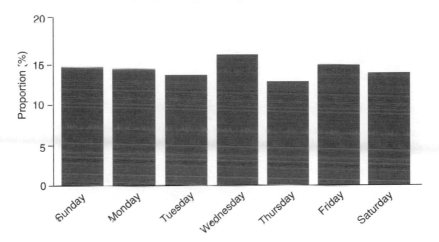

Figure 5: Percentage of new attenders according to day of the week.

Demand is high in the 12-hour period from 9.00 am, but very low after midnight. Demand from children (0–14 years) is high throughout the day but with a pre-bed-time peak, which is when most GP surgeries have closed for the day (Figure 6a). This is unlike the demand from adults, which is highest in the morning. Demand through the night is mainly from adults (Figure 6b).

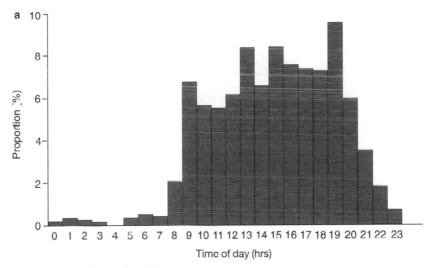

Figure 6a: Time of day of attendance for children.

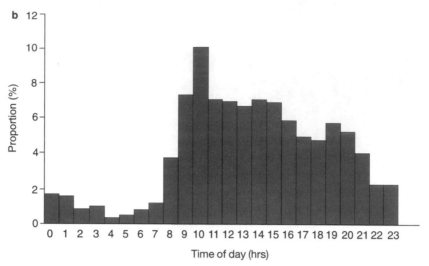

Figure 6b: Time of day of attendance for adults.

A study of major trauma in the Yorkshire region showed that only a minority of such cases reached hospital during 'office-hours', 9 am–5 pm. So most of the severely injured had to be dealt with when hospitals were staffed at the on-call level. One in seven arrived between 1 am and 9 am[21] (Figure 7).

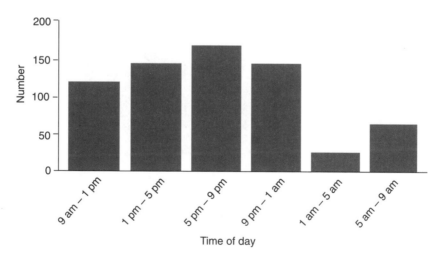

Figure 7: Time of day of attendance for new attenders with major trauma in A and E departments in Yorkshire region.

The patients

The age distribution of new attenders at A and E departments depends in part, of course, on the age structure of the population. In the combined inner and outer London electoral wards the estimated annual rates of new attendance in 1981 were consistently higher for males than for females and lowest for patients in the 35–64 years age groups[68] (Figure 8).

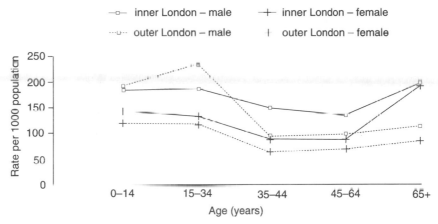

Figure 8: Attenders at A and E departments: estimated annual utilization rates by age and sex.
(Source: Chambers and Johnson.)

There was no consistent pattern of utilization rates by different social classes (Table 11). However from the table it is fairly clear that both in inner and outer London, the grouping of rates into a) social classes I and II; b) social classes IIINM, IIIM and IV and c) social class V reveals an upward trend in rates from the first group to the third.

Table 11: Estimated annual utilization rates per 1000 population by social class

Social class	Inner London		Outer London	
	(*n*)	Rate	(*n*)	Rate
I	(91.1)	200.2	(65.2)	110.8
II	(174.3)	102.4	(127.1)	65.5
IIINM	(258.2)	254.3	(230.5)	200.2
IIIM	(395.1)	223.1	(256.4)	155.0
IV	(205.0)	146.6	(143.1)	207.0
V	(185.1)	298.0	(71.1)	407.7

n = number in ward sample, adjusted pro rata for missing and unclassified data.

Source: Chambers and Johnson.[68]

Compared with a non-metropolitan urban environment, the clientele of an inner-city A and E department differs, in that there are more commuters and tourists, single people, people living alone and those who have moved recently or are homeless. Despite this in one recent study similar proportions of patients were admitted in the two settings and the distribution of diagnostic groupings of attenders was also similar.[69]

Deaths in the A and E department

Excluding patients who are brought in dead (b.i.d.), whose accompanying persons may nevertheless require comfort and advice; approximately one in 700 new patients dies while in the A and E department. This estimate is based on the observation of seven deaths among 5150 new patients attending A and E departments of a representative sample of 30 UK hospitals during one-week periods in 1992/93 during the course of the study of urgent and emergency admissions to hospital, commissioned by the Clinical Standards Advisory Group[17] (West RR, personal communication, 1995).

Comparisons with US

In contrast to the little we know clinically about patients attending A and E departments in this country, much more is known about attenders at hospital emergency rooms in the US. In the US in 1991 the National Hospital Ambulatory Medical Care Survey was inaugurated by the National Center for Health Statistics.[70] This annual sample survey of patients attending emergency rooms or outpatient clinics in short-stay or general hospitals uses a standard data collection form. On it are recorded data about the patient; the circumstances of the visit; the patient's diagnostic condition and the interventions undertaken. A copy of the form used is shown in Appendix I.

The estimated first attendance rate in 1992, 357 per 1000 population, was greater than the first attendance rate in A and E departments in England in 1991/92 (230 per 1000).[56] This no doubt reflected in part the absence of a generalized system of community-based, medical treatment services. In England many would probably be dubbed inappropriate attenders. The lower ratio of total attendances to first attendances (1.1 vs 1.2) also bears this out, although in the US financial issues may also affect decisions on whether or not to reattend.

As many as 45% of the patients were however categorized as 'urgent or emergent' by the staff treating them. Nevertheless only 14% of visits resulted in hospital admission. The proportion of new attenders at A and E departments in Central London who are admitted is around 18% and this is thought to under-represent the proportion nationally because a relatively high proportion of attenders in London present with minor injuries and ailments.[29] However this 18% probably includes some patients whose immediate admission had already been arranged and who were in transit to inpatient facilities.

In 17.5% of cases the patient did not see a physician, but in contrast to the assumed situation in England, 17.0% of cases did not see a registered nurse.

Summary

In summary the caseloads of major units in England vary greatly in size. In some instances this is understandable on account of the urban–rural differences in population density. It is in urban areas where there are major units with relatively small caseloads that the scope for merging units is greatest. Attendance rates are highest among males and among children and young adults. Contrary to expectations no consistent differences have been uncovered in the utilization rates of A and E departments according to the socio-economic classification of the populations they serve, but people in social class V have the highest rates.

6 Effectiveness and costs of A and E departments

Introduction

An important part of a needs assessment is to examine the cost-effectiveness of different service options. An option is cost-effective if it is found to be the cheapest way of achieving a given objective (e.g. a choice between different types of staff where they provide a service with equal outcome). A more difficult decision arises when a service option is both more expensive and more effective than the alternatives. The choice will then depend on the purchaser's priorities. Furthermore effectiveness has often been measured in terms of the processes of care, such as waiting times to see a doctor, rather than the health outcomes of that care. This raises further difficulties in making an assessment of cost-effectiveness in terms of health gain because improvements in processes will not necessarily translate directly into improved health outcomes.

Within these constraints, this section examines the effectiveness and costs of various characteristics of A and E departments and services which A and E departments could provide. The characteristics and services are listed in Table 13 on page 37, which also summarizes the evidence discussed in the text and offers tentative recommendations.

This section only considers options which A and E services could provide and the basic services and facilities available in a standard A and E department are assumed, without question, to be cost-effective.

First, general characteristics and service organization issues are discussed and second, issues relating specifically to the four categories of A and E patients referred to earlier – major trauma, minor trauma, major illness and minor illness.

Effectiveness

General services

Size and location of departments

The ideal size for A and E departments, which will depend on the sizes of the populations served and the distances involved amongst many other factors, is not known. Some studies have suggested that small hospitals can be as effective as larger hospitals in the management of both major[71] and minor[72] trauma, but others suggest that reducing the scale of the hospital leads to more frequent errors and avoidable deaths.[73] It is known that surgical procedures[74] and trauma management[75] supervised by senior medical staff have better outcomes than without such supervision and this implies that larger A and E departments, with more senior posts, may be preferable to smaller departments. There is some evidence that high-volume departments have better outcomes for severe trauma than low-volume departments[76] and the American College of Surgeons recommends that for optimal care 12–20 severe or urgent trauma cases should be seen each week in departments designated to manage major trauma.[77] Although such numbers are unlikely to occur in the UK setting even with triage of appropriate patients to such hospitals (since only approximately 0.1% of new attenders at A and E departments in England have sustained major trauma[21–23]) it does imply that large departments are preferable at least for the management of major trauma.

The distance to the nearest A and E department is another factor in the equation and while there is no evidence that, for example, the single major A and E departments serving Leicestershire[78] and Cornwall result in any worse outcomes for severe trauma than in other areas (for example in South Yorkshire where all of the population live within ten miles of their nearest A and E department) it is self-evident that there must be a penalty for too large a distance.

A North West Thames RHA Task Force suggested that A and E departments with fewer than 50 000 new patients per year did not have the necessary caseload or case-mix needed in order to provide the necessary experience to be able to provide the highest standards of care.[79] Where journey times from the scene to the nearest casualty hospital are frequently going to be excessive smaller departments might be more appropriate.

It should also be remembered that there are many major life-threatening conditions other than major trauma and these may benefit most from the earliest possible attention in departments of any size or complexity. The chances of resuscitating patients in cardiac arrest, for example, deteriorate rapidly within minutes of arrest; and chances of recovery from myocardial infarction improve with appropriate early treatment. Equally there is some non-major trauma such as drowning and poisoning from which early treatment in standard departments of any size and complexity will nearly always be preferable to later treatment. The arguments for larger, but inevitably more distant departments, cannot also be interpreted as arguments for the closure of smaller A and E departments.

Observation wards

Approximately 50% of A and E departments in England and Wales have associated short-stay observation wards[53] and although the value of these wards has not been universally established, short-stay wards are reported to be effective in improving the care of injured patients[80,81] particularly in the case of elderly patients[82,83] and patients with head injuries who might otherwise be discharged inappropriately.[84]

Hours-of-opening

As shown in section 5 demand for A and E services follows a very well characterized and distinct pattern, typically remaining high from about 0900 to 2100 hours but rapidly tailing off and remaining very low between 0100 and 0700 hours. During the out-of-hours period the nature of attendance at A and E department differs in some respects to that in-hours. For example 80% of asthma presentations occur between 1600 and 0800 hours[85] compared with 51% of all attenders and 72% of major trauma presents between 1700 and 0900 hours[21] compared with 48% of all attenders.[23] During the night time there is also considerable demand for radiographic services[86] and orthopaedic surgery[87], for example. Some of this out-of-hours activity has been shown to be essential. Furthermore where full A and E department services are available on two sites, with one or the other alternately not open for part of the 24-hour period, this has been reported to be unsatisfactory.[88]

Dedicated operating theatre services

There is good evidence that amongst many factors leading to poor outcomes in major trauma, delays in operation[3,89,90] which could be brought about by difficulties in access to operating theatres[91,92] are very important. There is evidence, for example, that early fixation of long bone fractures substantially increases chances of survival[93] and reduces morbidity.[94] Dedicated operating theatres are therefore assumed to be effective.

There is also some evidence that operations performed out-of-hours unsupervised by a consultant have comparatively poor outcomes[95] and it is presumed that the frequency of this happening might be reduced by dedicated emergency operating theatres which can enable the uninterrupted planned use of other theatres.

Triage

- **Pre-hospital** In order to help reduce the burden of untimely or inappropriate attendance, at least one hospital in the UK is encouraging patients with non-emergency conditions and their carers to telephone the A and E department about their problems first.[96] Although A and E staff are not usually trained to assess telephone enquiries,[97] telephone advice lines may provide a safe and low cost[98] means of controlling the number of inappropriate attenders.

For patients with severe trauma, triage to hospital A and E departments with appropriate expertise and services on the same hospital site may also be important and has been reported as improving outcomes over and above those found from taking patients to the nearest hospital[99] even if this results in a small increase in time to arrival at hospital.[100] Unfortunately there is no evidence from the UK about the effectiveness of triaging patients to the nearest appropriate hospital rather than the nearest hospital.

- **In hospital** Within hospitals the value in terms of patient outcomes of triage into priority categories remains undemonstrated as does its value in terms of the timing of care. Large numbers of patients triaged into an urgent (or 'see immediately') category may mean that no one is seen immediately; small numbers inevitably result in false negatives. One study concluded that nurse triage may impose additional delay for patient treatment, particularly among patients needing the most urgent attention.[101,102]

On the other hand triage of patients into types (suitable for GP care or attenders needing A and E care)[103] and the provision of appropriate care, has been found in one setting to improve the processes of care for those patients suitable for GP care.[60]

Services for children

Whilst benefits from separate children's facilities[104] and of observation wards for children[105] have been described, there is no conclusive evidence about whether children have better outcomes if they are treated in dedicated paediatric A and E departments rather than in general departments. It has been found that outcomes in major trauma generally are equally good for children and young adults treated in the same department,[106] but that in specific diagnostic groups children fare substantially better in dedicated facilities.[107]

Services for major trauma patients

In 1986 the American College of Surgeons reviewed the needs of the injured patient and issued guidelines on the services, facilities, training and experience which it is believed contribute to the care of major trauma.[77] Much of this remains plausible though knowledge of the effectiveness and cost-effectiveness of the various components is limited.

Specialties on site

Access to appropriate facilities and experienced personnel in such specialties as A and E medicine, anaesthetics, general surgery, neurosurgery and orthopaedic surgery, 24 hours per day in major A and E departments is presumed to be effective in improving outcomes in major trauma.[3,77] There is some evidence that secondary transfer of patients, particularly those with head injuries, should be avoided if possible,[108 111] that associated delays in treatment have adverse consequences,[112] that outcomes for patients with head injuries when neurosurgery is not available on site are not optimal[79] and that delays in orthopaedic treatment can lead to relatively poor long-term outcomes.[93] If neurosurgery is not available on site then it is suggested that detailed guidelines for the transfer of head injured patients need to be agreed locally to minimize the hazard of transfer.[113]

Trauma teams

The most common pattern of management of the seriously injured has been transportation to the nearest A and E department where the initial assessment and treatment are conducted by a casualty officer. Specialists are then called in to treat specific injuries.[114] Early management by a relatively junior doctor and late involvement of specialists can lead to inadequate resuscitation, missed diagnosis of injuries and delays in definitive treatment – all factors which have been judged to contribute to avoidable death in the trauma patient.[77] One response to this problem has been to develop the concept of the trauma team.[115] This involves the early mobilization of senior medical (accident and emergency, anaesthetics and surgical specialties) and nursing staff who can rapidly assess, resuscitate and prepare the patient for definitive treatment including transfer to another more appropriate hospital if necessary.[116]

Call out of the trauma team is usually initiated on the basis of the revised trauma score[75] (a measure of physiological compromise) or on the basis of physiological, anatomical and mechanism of injury criteria.[117] The latter criteria have been shown to have a very high sensitivity (> 95%) but poor specificity. However including mechanism of injury in the call-out criteria enables the trauma team to be alerted earlier than if this depends on the findings of the primary survey in the initial assessment.

Audit of trauma team performance has demonstrated several improvements in trauma management. Resuscitation times can be reduced although they vary from between 15 to 105 minutes.[118] It is also claimed that the trauma team approach results in more effective resuscitation, particularly volume replacement with intravenous fluids and fewer delays in treatment.[75] This is achieved by performing horizontal rather than vertical care,[119] where assessment, airway control and treatment are carried out concurrently rather than consecutively and by the early involvement of specialists.[75]

It is argued by some that the best way of managing major trauma is in trauma centres but until the issue of in which circumstances they are advantageous is resolved, the use of trauma teams provides a more efficient and organized approach to the care of the seriously injured in district general hospitals.[120]

ATLS training

Advanced trauma life support[121,122] is a highly structured protocol for the initial assessment, management and resuscitation of seriously injured patients, developed in the US during the 1980s for medical staff but now extending to other staff in the A and E department.[123]

Although there is considerable dispute about the effectiveness of the practice of advanced life support in the field,[124] in hospital the value of a casualty team trained in ATLS is accepted widely.[125,126]

Regional trauma systems

Whilst it seems self-evident that regional trauma centres, with 24-hour trauma teams led by senior, experienced medical staff and with all major specialties on site and with a high volume of major trauma activity, could be effective in improving the outcomes for multiply injured trauma patients admitted to the centres, the effectiveness of regional trauma systems is less clear cut.[127]

However evidence both from before and after studies[128] and from cross-sectional comparisons[129] has shown that regional trauma systems, based on designated trauma centres with pre-hospital triage to appropriately graded trauma centres, is effective in improving outcomes when the nature and volume of trauma is as seen in the typical US setting. The benefits of such systems depend not only on the performance of the trauma centres but also on the performance of the pre-hospital services and their ability to transfer patients to appropriate hospitals.

Preliminary indications from New South Wales, Australia also suggest that such systems may be effective outside the US (Lyall D, personal communication, 1994) although there is some doubt about the effectiveness of such systems in European settings.[130]

The regional trauma system set up in the North West Midlands to examine whether this concept would translate into the UK setting, showed little evidence of any benefit.[4] There were no statistically significant improvements in standardized major trauma mortality rates compared to two other regions and no improvement in the avoidable death rate. However the system had no method of triaging patients directly to the trauma centre in Stoke-on-Trent and the volume of major trauma seen in the centre was less than 20% of the volume recommended by the American College of Surgeons for a level 1 trauma centre. Furthermore although the North West Midlands system may have exemplified the performance of such systems in similar mixed urban and rural settings elsewhere in the UK, it is difficult to draw conclusions about their effectiveness in other settings such as densely populated conurbations like London.

Computerized tomography

Amongst patients with major trauma, the most common anatomical site of fatal injuries is the head[131] and it is widely recognized that CT scanning[132-135] and possibly on-site neurosurgery[79] are effective in improving the management and outcome of patients with severe head injuries. The value of CT scanning in less severe head injury patients (those with history of loss of consciousness, or post-traumatic amnesia and a Glasgow Coma Score greater than 12) is disputed. Some authors have claimed it is effective[136] and cost-effective,[137] partly because a normal neurological examination coupled with a normal scan may enable patients to be discharged from casualty without the need for a period of observation in hospital[138] and the use of CT scanning should be widened to include more patients with less severe injuries.[139] Others have suggested that if an initial neurological examination of blunt trauma patients is normal then CT scanning can be delayed safely.[140]

Computerized tomography scanning at sites other than the head is also common, but evidence is less clear cut. It has been shown, for example, that conventional diagnostic peritoneal lavage is more sensitive and specific than CT scanning in blunt abdominal trauma.[141] In the UK CT scanners are widely but not universally available[142] and some large hospitals were reported in 1990 not to have scanners[143] and to our knowledge as late as 1993 there were some hospitals in the UK receiving major trauma which did not have CT scanners. In many departments in the UK where there are scanning facilities but no neurosurgery services, CT scanning and the transference of the images to regional neurosurgery centres for assessment has been introduced, but such systems have not been formally demonstrated to be cost-effective.

24-hour radiographic services

The incidence of major trauma does not follow exactly the same pattern by time of day as other trauma. As has been mentioned one study, for example, showed that 72% of all major trauma occurred outside normal working hours (weekdays from 0900–1700).[21] Evidence about the reduced value of 24-hour radiographic services[87] may not apply therefore to 24-hour radiographic services for major trauma. However senior radiographic assessment has been shown to be important in the management of major trauma generally and the cost-effectiveness of 24-hour radiographic services for major trauma may therefore depend not only on the incidence of major trauma 'out-of-hours' but on whether there is a system in place for transferring or triaging major trauma to regional centres.

Minor trauma

Nurse practitioners

The primary function of a nurse practitioner in the A and E department is in the care of patients with minor trauma – although they also manage patients with other minor conditions.[5] A nurse practitioner is able to make diagnoses, decisions about patient management in some cases, including treatment and disposal and to administer and supply prescriptions for a limited range of drugs under standing orders/protocols. Ordering investigations may be a problematic area and nurse practitioners are not always empowered to order X-rays, for example.

Despite their patchy but widespread use there is no evidence yet from prospective randomized studies of the relative effectiveness, or cost-effectiveness of nurse practitioners and junior doctors. However if the use of nurse practitioners resulted in smaller costs, without affecting quality of care or patient outcomes, this would be one possible way of reducing junior doctors' hours without increasing expenditure.

Minor injury units

Special facilities for the care of patients with minor injuries have been established in several places in the UK, usually in the wake of the closure of A and E departments. Typically these minor injury units (MIUs) are GP supervised or have direct links to other local A and E departments and are staffed by appropriately trained nurse practitioners, have on site X-ray facilities, but are not usually open for 24 hours/day. They may be sited with community hospitals, or with community or primary health care facilities, or on DGH premises.

A number of uncontrolled audits[144–153] have shown that they see 5000–25 000 patients each year, nearly all of whom attend appropriately, that patient satisfaction is high and that MIUs adequately manage the processes of care for such patients with some patients being treated on site and others transferred to conventional A and E departments for further assessment or management.

A recent review of options for treating patients with minor injuries[154] concluded that for MIUs to be successful, a close relationship with the nearest major A and E department is desirable for clinical supervision, rotation of staff and continuing education, so that patients may be transferred without delay when necessary and that nurse practitioners working in MIUs need explicit and widely agreed working protocols or clinical guidelines which should include the authority to request X-rays.

However no formal studies of the effectiveness or cost-effectiveness of MIUs are known and their contribution to improving health as opposed to managing patient demand remains unclear.

Major illness

There are few special services which could be optionally purchased for the care of major illness patients, who include those with coronary emergencies, cerebro-vascular accidents and other conditions such as asthma, epilepsy and diabetes. For acute myocardial infarction, early thrombolysis[155] and resuscitation protocols[156] are known to be effective. Protocols and guidelines for the care of other patients with emergency medical conditions such as asthma[85] have also been shown to be effective and such protocols might form a valuable service.

Basic life support training involving skills in the resuscitation and management of the critically ill, non-trauma patient has also been demonstrated to be effective in improving survival chances for patients,[157] but other services such as coronary care ambulances[158] and other ways of integrating pre-hospital and in-hospital care, for example by direct transmission of electrocardiogram (ECG) recordings taken in an ambulance to coronary care units for assessment have yet to be shown to be effective.

Minor illness

Patients attending A and E departments with minor illnesses, which were assessed by GPs as capable of being managed in a general practice setting, make up approximately one quarter of the average caseload of a UK A and E department.[27] It does not follow that such patients should be managed in general practice. Some GPs may have little knowledge or interest in managing minor conditions, or if they do, they may lack the quantity and range of equipment needed. It has been shown that in the facility at King's College Hospital these patients, as well as those with minor injuries, are managed comparatively effectively and efficiently using on-site GP services rather than traditional junior casualty doctors.[60] For example primary care practitioners were less likely to utilize hospital resources and made fewer investigations and referrals to specialist teams or outpatient clinics, without any detrimental effect on clinical outcome. They were identified as practising more patient-centred care. This included broader assessment of patients' immediate health care needs and more concern about social and emotional factors. Their care was highly acceptable to patients. However these comparisons were between the care of junior casualty doctors and more experienced GPs and the differences could reflect the extent, rather than the nature, of their experience.

An alternative to the provision of GP services in A and E departments is an extension of GP-based services to cover minor, walk-in or book in medical emergencies for up to 24 hours/day,[9] although there is little evidence of the need for such a service between midnight and 0600. Such emergency care centres might typically be combined with a minor injuries service to create a polyclinic. Neither the effectiveness nor cost-effectiveness of such developments have yet been tested, but as they may become part of a common, alternative model in the future their cost-effectiveness needs to be evaluated.

Costs

The cost-effectiveness of alternative ways of delivering A and E services depends on the consequences for costs, as well as health.[159] The cost consequences of the A and E components identified in the previous section extend beyond the department itself. There are costs from the use of investigations, hospital admission, subsequent outpatient care and from the use of general practice, social services and ambulance services. A and E attendance also involves the time of patients and their friends and relatives. Studies undertaken in the US have found that the costs of care provided in emergency rooms represent only a fraction of the total costs of trauma care.[160] For minor trauma, costs incurred within an A and E department will be more important, but even for these cases it has been shown that investigations represent a substantial proportion of costs.[161] For major trauma cases a recent study of helicopter-transported cases found over 80% of NHS costs were related to the periods of inpatient admission.[162] There are few studies in the field of A and E medicine which examine costs in any way[160–166] and it is extremely rare for a study to examine all cost consequences. Therefore it has been necessary to look beyond what is published in academic journals and to include reports from academic and consultancy studies and use unpublished NHS statistics.

General services

Costs of A and E departments

All providers (trusts and directly managed units (DMUs)) are required to generate a financial return, which includes a code for expenditure on A and E services and attendance levels (THR and HFR21/22s). It includes all expenditure attributable to services provided within the A and E department and its associated overheads, but excludes the cost consequences of any treatment or investigative procedures provided outside the A and E department. These data have been used to examine expenditure on A and E services and whether they vary with the number of attendances by trust or DMU. The average costs per attendance for 250 trusts and district managed units are shown in Table 12.

Table 12: Average A and E costs per attendance by number of attendances in England 1992/93

Total number of attendances	No. of Trusts and DMUs with A and E departments	Mean cost per attendance (SD) £		Mean cost per new attendance (SD) £	
0–19 999	36	24.91	(13.34)	33.75	(18.85)
20–39 999	51	36.91	(14.55)	45.56	(16.45)
40–59 999	82	40.46	(11.06)	48.24	(12.81)
60–79 999	48	38.42	(13.22)	45.81	(14.80)
80–99 999	22	37.23	(10.73)	43.75	(11.47)
100 000+	11	39.76	(10.36)	45.95	(10.94)
Overall	250	36.28	(12.21)	43.84	(14.22)

Note: Data were not available on all providers with A and E departments.

Sources: NHS Financial Returns (DoH, 1993).

In 1992/93, the average cost of an attendance was £36.28 and £43.84 for a new attendance, but the range of costs was very wide. These data should be interpreted with caution, since the costings rely on apportionment procedures which permit considerable local discretion and returns for many trusts include satellite A and E departments such as minor injury units. Furthermore attendance levels are a poor measure of workload, since they take no account of the type and severity of the condition and these data should not be used to compare the efficiency of different departments.[16]

In addressing many of the cost-effectiveness questions it is necessary to estimate the marginal costs of treating the different types of trauma and to separate the costs of minor from major trauma and trauma from emergency medical cases. However in practice these are difficult to estimate. Currently there is no routine means of estimating the workload associated with each type of case. More fundamentally even if a valid measure of workload were available, cost allocation between these types of case is problematic due to the existence of joint costs within A and E departments. Large cost items are shared between all the types of attendance, including medical and nursing staff, administration, overheads and capital charges, which together may account for 78% of the total cost of an A and E department.[88] A consequence of these joint costs is that the marginal cost of a service depends on the context of the decision. For example the marginal costs of treating extra minor trauma in an existing A and E department could be limited to the cost of an additional nurse. Where the opening of an A and E department is required to manage minor trauma, then more of the costs would be included. Ultimately the marginal cost of a development in an A and E department depends on the local cost structure and standards of care and caution must be taken when extrapolating from studies conducted elsewhere.

Size and location of departments

In the NHS there have been moves to increase the size of A and E departments to improve the quality of care and to reduce costs. In the analysis of the costs of 250 providers presented in Table 12 there was no evidence to support the existence of cost economies, either for total or new attendances. The case-mix may have been more complex for the larger departments but this cannot be proven from this data set. In local studies it has been suggested that significant economies may occur at higher levels of attendance.[163] The amalgamation of two medium sized A and E departments was predicted to yield savings of around 15%, although this saving was substantially reduced by the additional costs for the ambulance service from the consequent increase in the number of patients transported between the two hospitals.[88] There have been no published follow-up studies of the cost consequences of any amalgamation or closure of A and E departments to see whether any of the expected cost savings were achieved.

Centralizing A and E services increases the average travel time for patients and their companions attending the A and E department. The private cost to patients of the time and inconvenience caused by the extra journey should be considered against any cost economics for the hospital. Reduced access may also deter some patients who, as a consequence, may decide to visit their GP or other locally-organized emergency treatment service.

Hours of opening

An important choice for A and E facilities is the hours of opening. Major A and E departments with consultant cover are usually open for 24 hours but minor injury units are often open between eight to 16 hours per day. Night-time opening is expensive because it involves employing extra staff at enhanced rates of pay when the number of attendances is low. In one study it was predicted that opening between 8.00 am and midnight for seven days a week would result in an average cost per attendance of 20% less than a 24-hour service[164] with little impact on the travel time of the 4% of cases attending A and E during these hours. Although this option retains the access advantages for the vast majority of patients of having an extra A and E department or minor injury unit, part-time opening may mean that patients are uncertain whether or not the department is open and this has been reported to be unsatisfactory.[88]

Observation wards and dedicated theatre services

Extra costs from providing these services might arise from the duplication of services and an increase in unused capacity. Nevertheless it reduces the disruption for other hospital departments and the transportation of patients. The overall cost consequence is not clear and has not been examined empirically.

Staffing

- **Senior house officers or GPs** Traditionally patients are first seen by a junior doctor. In the study at King's College Hospital in London, the cost-effectiveness of introducing GPs into an A and E department has been evaluated. For the NHS a GP's time is more expensive than a senior house officer (SHO) due to higher remuneration and GPs spend more time with each patient. However GPs were found consistently to use fewer investigations, particularly X-rays and refer fewer patients for specialist care.[60] The cost per case of patients seen by a GP, including the use of investigations, was 61% of the cost of patients seen by an SHO.[161] (The difference is considerably higher with admission costs included, but the authors were concerned about the reliability of these data.) This cost difference might be partly offset by the cost of a higher number of onward referrals to general practice by the GPs in the A and E department.
- **Nurses** Nurses are being used both to triage cases and as alternatives to junior doctors in the provision of services. The cost of having a triage nurse is the need to divert a trained nurse from other activities and this will depend on the grade of the nurse. The cost comparison between trained nurses and junior doctors is more complex since the cost of their time will depend not only on the grade of nurse and the scale points of the nurse and doctor, but whether they are working overtime, since junior doctors are paid only one-third of their normal hourly rate during this time. Furthermore the evidence from comparing GPs and SHOs in the King's College Hospital Study suggests it is also important to examine the consequences for the use of investigations, drugs and referrals to specialists.[161]

Services for minor trauma and illness

Minor injuries unit

Many of the facilities of an A and E department are regarded as inappropriate for minor trauma and therefore it might be more cost-effective to manage them in a minor injury unit (MIU). The average cost per attendance in a MIU is usually lower than in a full A and E department, but this is largely because of a higher proportion of low-cost reattenders. This is also a false comparison, since it should be between the marginal cost of treating minor trauma in MIU compared with A and E departments.[163] In A and E departments this is likely to be substantially less than the average since a minor case is less time consuming than major trauma and many of the facilities would be needed for the more major cases, with or without minor trauma. The appropriate question is whether the costs of the joint production of treating major trauma and minor trauma together is more than treating them in separate facilities[161] and to this there is no answer based on evidence. Within the MIU option there are many choices in terms of size, staffing, facilities and location, all of which may influence this cost comparison. (A MIU can vary in character from being in a hospital with an associate specialist and full X-ray facilities, to a small MIU, run by nurses with very limited access to X-ray.)

General practice

Patients with minor trauma could be encouraged to go to their local GP rather than the A and E department, either through education or by closing facilities. Both these options have been pursued, but again little is known about the cost consequences. The costs to the NHS depend partly on the marginal costs of using these two facilities and, where facilities are to be closed, the consequences for the number of attendances.

Services for major trauma patients

Trauma centre

The evaluation of the first UK trauma system based around a pilot trauma centre in Stoke included a detailed costing of the centre itself as well as a follow-up for six months of the use of hospital and other services.[4] There was a large investment in staff, including four extra consultants in A and E and anaesthetics to provide 24-hour consultant cover, 14 wte nurses and 10 wte ITU nurses and a dedicated theatre which accounted for around an extra £1 million per year on the costs of running the A and E department. Substantial variations in these costs are expected if trauma systems are established at other locations. The additional service requirements had only small additional consequences for costs elsewhere. There was little evidence that this investment significantly relieved pressure on the A and E departments in the surrounding area since the numbers of cases involved were small. Net of cost changes in A and E departments in the comparator regions it was estimated that the regional trauma system cost an additional £0.52 million per annum and because there was little evidence of any health benefits it was concluded that the system which developed around Stoke between 1990 and 1993 was not a cost-effective service for major trauma.

'Out-of-hours' radiography

A study of out-of-hours radiography in a major teaching hospital found that referrals from the A and E department accounted for 80% of utilization[86] and the total cost was approximately £250 000. The researchers estimated that the adoption of guidelines for the use of this service could yield savings of 18%.

Trauma teams and ATLS training

These are developments in trauma care appearing in conventional A and E departments as well as being a part of a trauma centre. Trauma teams have a cost in terms of a reduction in staff availability elsewhere, whilst they are active in A and E departments. Advanced trauma life support training has a cost in terms of staff hours. Published cost data are not available on either service development.

Cost-effectiveness

In a cost-effectiveness analysis costs of different investments in health care are compared with their effectiveness at the margin, where the beneficial effects are measured in comparable units.[159] This is rarely possible in practice and this is true, *a fortiori*, in the case of A and E services. Estimates of the size of the health effects and costs of the different components of A and E services are either unreliable, or non-existent. This makes any assessment of desirability or cost-effectiveness of the service components compared with other uses of NHS resources extremely difficult.

Recommendations have been made where possible and these are summarized in Table 13, using the system of grading of evidence which is common to all chapters in this series. They are usually based on very weak and incomplete evidence (grade III) or professional opinion or deduction (grade IV).

For some of the developments, costs and effects will be also determined by local factors, such as the availability of certain services and the geographical distribution of populations and the priorities of the local purchaser. Furthermore these components of an A and E service have been evaluated in isolation but, in practice, a purchaser will need to consider whole models of care in order to assess cost-effectiveness, and these are described in section 7.

Table 13: Summary of evidence on costs and effectiveness of A and E department components and recommendations

Component	Quality of research evidence[a]		Recommendation[b]	Strengths of recommendation[a]
	Effectiveness	Costs		
General characteristics and facilities				
Size of departments				
Adult A and E	III	III	35 000+	B
Children's A and E	not known	not known	uncertain	uncertain
MIU/MCC	III	III	5 000–25 000	B/C
Hours of opening				
Adult A and E	IV	III	24 hrs Unless two A and E	C
Children's A and E	IV	IV	24 hrs in one city	C
MIU/MCC	IV	III	16 hrs	B
Observation wards				
Adult A and E	III	IV	Yes ⎫ Subject to cost[c]	C
Children's A and E	III	IV	Yes ⎭	B
Triage: pre-hospital telephone				
Adult A and E	III	IV	Yes ⎫ Subject to cost	C
Children's A and E	IV	IV	Yes ⎭	C
MIU/MCC	not known	not known	Uncertain	
Triage: in-hospital				
Adult A and E	II–2	IV	Yes ⎫	B
Children's A and E	IV	IV	Yes ⎬ Subject to cost	B
MIU/MCC	III	IV	Yes ⎭	B

Table 13: Continued

Component	Quality of research evidence[a]		Recommendation[b]	Strengths of recommendation[a]
	Effectiveness	Costs		
Services for major trauma				
Neurosurgery on site				
Adult A and E	III	not known	Yes ⎫ Cost depends on	B
Children's A and E	III	not known	Yes ⎭ current disposition	B
Cardio-thoracic surgery on site				
Adult A and E	III	not known	Uncertain	C
Children's A and E	III	not known	Uncertain	C
Trauma teams				
Adult A and E	III	IV	Yes	B
Children's A and E	IV	IV	Yes	B
ATLS training				
Adult A and E	II–3	IV	Yes	B
Children's A and E	IV	IV	Yes	B
Dedicated operating theatre				
Adult A and E	II–2	IV	Uncertain ⎫ Depends on	B
Children's A and E	IV	IV	Uncertain ⎭ availability	C
24-hour consultant cover				
Adult A and E	IV	IV	Uncertain ⎫ Subject to	C
Children's A and E	IV	IV	Uncertain ⎭ costs	C
24-hour radiographic service				
Adult A and E	IV	IV	Depends on costs	C
Children's A and E	IV	IV		C
CT scanning				
Adult A and E	II–3	IV	Yes ⎫ Subject to	B
Children's A and E	IV	IV	Yes ⎭ availability	B
Minor injuries				
Nurse practitioners				
Adult A and E	III	not known	Yes Subject to costs	B
Children's A and E	IV	not known	No	B
Minor injury unit				
Adult A and E	III	not known	Yes Subject to costs	B
Children's A and E	IV	not known	No	C
Major illness				
ALS training				
Adult A and E	not known	IV	Yes	B
Children's A and E	not known	IV	Yes	B
Other protocols for management of specific conditions				
Adult A and E	various	not known	Yes	B
Children's A and E	various	not known	Yes	B
Other illness				
On site GP services				
Adult A and E	II–2	III	Yes	C
Children's A and E	IV	III	Yes	C

[a] See below for definition of grades I–III and A–E. Grade IV evidence also includes that which is deduced or derived from related research.

[b] Where the preferred option is more costly the decision must ultimately depend on purchasers' priorities.

[c] This is where costs are unknown.

Quality of the evidence

I   Evidence obtained from at least one properly randomized controlled trial

II–1   Evidence obtained from well-designed controlled trials without randomization

II–2   Evidence obtained from well-designed cohort or case controlled analytic studies, preferably from more than one centre or research group

II–3   Evidence obtained from multiple-timed series with or without the intervention, or from dramatic results in uncontrolled experiments

III   Opinions of respected authorities based on clinical experience, descriptive studies or reports of expert committees

IV   Evidence inadequate owing to problems of methodology, e.g. sample size, length or comprehensiveness of follow-up, or conflict in evidence.

Strength of recommendation

A   There is good evidence to support the use of the procedure

B   There is fair evidence to support the use of the procedure

C   There is poor evidence to support the use of the procedure

D   There is fair evidence to reject the use of the procedure

E   There is good evidence to support the rejection of the use of the procedure.

7 Models of care

Introduction

As we have seen no major changes in disease or injury patterns are anticipated in the near future which would radically alter the size of the demand for A and E services. There is no one model of provision of A and E services which can be applied in every locality, however. Different considerations apply to urban and rural populations and, within urban areas, to metropolitan populations and to smaller urban concentrations. The underlying principles are that levels of service should be provided which are appropriate in type and location to meet within an acceptable time limit the needs of presenting patients. This means, for example, that whilst the development of a regional trauma system might be considered appropriate in sparsely populated areas such as Scotland, or in large densely populated conurbations such as London, they may not be appropriate in other regions. There is no reason in terms of cost-effectiveness why any of the three models outlined on page 40 has to be taken up nationally; nor can we see any organizational or policy reasons why different regional developments are not possible.

Cases which are diagnostically less challenging and in which the treatment needed is technologically less complex (which includes the majority of cases currently presenting to major A and E departments) may be dealt with by different cadres of staff. These may be located in separate facilities, as well as in major A and E departments, bearing in mind that the marginal costs that major A and E departments incur for catering for minor injuries and ailments may, in fact be less than those incurred by establishing new, stand-alone facilities.

Purchasers who take a strategic view will consider an overall model of care and will not plan separate components of the system in isolation from each other. Three models are proposed, each envisaging a slightly different role for the major A and E departments.

Three model options

1 **Preservation of existing major A and E departments, with progressive development of alternative ways of dealing with part of the minor injury caseload – a near status-quo position**
In some rural areas with sparsely distributed populations, even where levels of new attendances are relatively low – 30 000 to 50 000 – there may be little alternative to adopting this model. Elsewhere where travelling times for ambulances and patients can be maintained at acceptable levels, a multiplicity of smaller, major A and E departments may imply duplication of resources and effort and inadequate numbers of cases of major trauma and major illness to allow professionals to acquire and maintain high levels of skill.

2 **Reduction in number of major A and E departments with simultaneous development of alternative facilities for minor injuries and illnesses treatment**
In this model, a major A and E department would rarely receive fewer than 50 000 new attendances per year and would more commonly receive 70 000–100 000 and serve 300 000–600 000 population. There is little information available on what happens to the streaming of patients and problems when certain types of facility are closed or changed in scale or scope. Among the principal issues are whether the remaining departments and their supporting diagnostic and inpatient services can support the diverted demand and what proportion of the demand actually materializes.

Cases of major illness and injury will continue to be taken or referred somewhere, and the size of this group can be predicted from pre-closure observation of the nature of the clientele. It seems from a review of what happened in North West London after A and E departments were closed or reduced in scope over the period 1960 to 1985 that the proximity of alternative A and E departments determined the extent to which the numbers of ambulant patients were reduced.[166] The closure of St Mary's, Harrow Road resulted in the first year in 68% of its first attenders being accommodated in the neighbouring (within two miles) hospitals of St Mary's Praed Street and St Charles Hospital. Nearly one-third of the attenders 'disappeared'.[24] The further effect of the subsequent down-grading of St Charles Hospital's A and E department to a nurse-practitioner-led, minor injuries unit in February 1993 is unknown, but it is conceivable that some of the previously 'lost' minor ailment cases in the area eventually reappeared.

The various ways in which alternative arrangements can be made for patients with minor injuries and ailments such as simple fractures, dislocations, sprains, cuts and abrasions are discussed in section 6. These alternatives all require a framework in which the scope of the services they offer is defined and where there is close collaboration and lines of communication with the major A and E department and clear guidelines for referral to it of relevant cases and also to the general medical and social services. All treatment providers need to agree among themselves and with the local ambulance service the arrangements for transferring cases. Effective systems of clinical audit will be needed by all the various providers, especially in view of the uncertain nature of the caseload with which they may be required to deal in the transitional period.

The marginal costs that major A and E departments incur for retaining such patients may, in fact, be less than those which purchasers might incur by establishing new, stand-alone facilities. But in any case these marginal costs have not been measured. We do know from the King's College Hospital study that the primary care element of an A and E department's caseload can be managed differently within the department to good effect and more cheaply, by employing GPs to manage it. This may be a sound option for inner-city hospitals, but whether it is a more cost-effective option overall than developing emergency treatment centres based on existing premises in the community the authors do not know.

Purchasers would be well advised not to make too many assumptions about the overall financial effects of measures introduced, prima facie, to produce savings. Costs may simply be transferred, not lost.

3 **Regionalizing trauma care services. Major trauma treatment concentrated on regional trauma centres, each serving 2.5 to 3.0 million people on average**

Clear protocols would govern the primary and secondary transfer of patients to these units. A smaller number of major A and E departments than at present, along with a variety of forms of provision for minor injuries, would continue to serve sub-regional localities and these would function along lines similar to present A and E departments (level 2) other than for cases of major trauma. There would thus be a three-tier system, with regional trauma centres, A and E departments and minor condition units. This is the system currently being proposed for Scotland.[167] The regional trauma centre would also act as the major A and E department for the surrounding population, catering for 70 000–100 000 new attendances per year. The regionalized trauma care system would probably involve the concentration of hospital specialties such as neurosurgery, which deal with complex effects of major trauma at the hospital designated as the regional trauma centre. It would also imply that a form of rotation of appointments between the trauma centre and other A and E departments would be needed for doctors and others receiving post-basic training in aspects of health care related to major injury.

Summary

There is as yet no evidence that outcomes for patients with life-threatening conditions have been significantly affected by the introduction of planned changes in the organization of A and E department services in recent years. This simply reflects the fact that little evidence has been systematically collected. It is not possible at this stage to perform convincing option appraisals which take into account evidence on cost changes and effects on patients. Clearly there is no one generally applicable model for an A and E department and its associated services.

8 Outcomes and targets

Outcomes

Reviewing the first volume of epidemiologically based needs assessments, the editors reflect that 'the costs of collecting the additional information required to monitor outcomes, whether directly or indirectly, need to be considered in setting priorities, and that it may only be worthwhile collecting outcome data when the effectiveness of particular services is questionable, or when outcome measures, or proxies thereof, are easy to collect'.[168]

Sufficient concerns have been expressed over the years about the management and effectiveness of A and E departments for the public and the professions to wish to know that standards are set and adhered to.

Outcomes of clinical management in A and E departments are usually stated simply in terms of avoiding mortality from survivable illness or injury and avoiding complications or recurrences through inadequate treatment. Ideally residual impairment of function or disability should be absent or minimal.

Processes of clinical audit are designed to deal with these issues, as are confidential enquiries into undesirable outcomes, such as perioperative deaths or deaths from major trauma. In these examples experts from relevant clinical fields reach a consensus on the appropriateness of, or lack of the various interventions. However if each institution or department sets its own standards for auditing clinical care there may be considerable differences of opinion on what are regarded as satisfactory outcomes.

There are very few outcomes which rely solely on clinical management received in A and E departments. Outcomes may depend also on what was done for patients before they reached and after they left the departments. Consequently there are very few inter-hospital comparators which purchasers might use to judge the clinical performance of their contracted providers. While every department is capable of reviewing the incidence of misdiagnoses, recurrences and complications of conditions treated, no reports have yet been found of the relative performance on these indicators over a representative range of providers, nor of definitive comparisons of the effects of interventions made by different grades and types of staff.

The exception to this general rule is the audit of the management of major trauma. The basis of this audit is the extent to which patients with injuries scored above a certain level of severity on a scoring system, which takes into account the degree of anatomical injury and physiological derangement, survive or die, and how a hospital compares in its associated risk of dying or surviving with other hospitals treating patients with comparable major trauma. The use of this system of audit, developed as part of a US major trauma outcomes study (MTOS) for comparing hospitals was reported for 33 hospitals in 1992.[169] Although major trauma forms only a minute proportion of caseload in an A and E department, the introduction of the MTOS system for auditing performance with major trauma is a commendable development and purchasers will probably wish to stipulate its use, despite its heavy reliance on clerical resources.

There are no similar, standardized ways of comparing the performance of A and E departments in the management of major illnesses of comparable severity.

The various intermediate 'outcomes' which can be measured include the intervals between the processes of assessment, treatment and discharge of patients. This calls for comprehensive management information systems in which timings can be recorded sequentially during a patient's career through the department.

Another measurement of process which will interest purchasers is the ratio of total attendances to new attendances in A and E departments. The ratio nationally is just under 1.2 : 1. Widely differing ratios from this would call into question the management policies of a department.

Targets

There is some scope for A and E department services to influence the incidence of illnesses and injuries though the identification of risk factors for occurrences and recurrences of various conditions,[170] patient education[171] and raising levels of immunity to infectious diseases.[172] However the departments do have more potential to reduce mortality rates from actual conditions. The caseload typically includes a significant amount of major illness, a relatively small amount of major trauma, and a great deal of minor illness and injury, of which a hard core is likely to remain, whatever alternative arrangements are made to cope with them.

Operationally targets may be set for the number, size and range of A and E services to be provided. It must be stressed again that owing to the dearth of information about costs and effectiveness of different configurations of service, it is not possible at this stage to perform convincing option appraisals. The following targets reflect the more convincing advice contained in the various reports reviewed in this needs assessment.

Major A and E departments

Size

There are advantages of economy of scale in having one, or relatively few large A and E departments in more densely populated areas. Departments with fewer than 60 000 new attendances per year are less well able to sustain the staffing levels needed to ensure that sufficient numbers of experienced staff can be deployed throughout the 24-hour period.

Bearing in mind the need for clinical back-up facilities, it is unlikely that a hospital could cope with more than 90–100 000 new attendances per year without causing patients to travel long distances for the other forms of secondary care which a hospital provides and unacceptably long primary transfer times for the ambulance services.

Volume

At present on average the 246 new attendances annually per thousand population include about 25% who do not require the facilities of a major A and E department. If some of the demand for the treatment of minor ailments is syphoned off to minor injuries units the average rate of new attendance could be reduced to 150–200 per 100 000. The numbers of patients presenting with major illnesses or injuries would not change, being simply the aggregate of the numbers hitherto presenting to any A and E departments merged to form the new department. With increasing severity of the case-mix it is unlikely that the total/first attendances ratio could be reduced below 1.1 : 1, a ratio which has already been achieved in at least one RHA in the UK.

Specialties

If hospital facilities are concentrated on fewer sites a wider range of specialist facilities will be needed to match the increased numbers and range of urgent and serious cases to be dealt with. There is no consensus of opinion about the range of specialties which should be on-site. The London Implementation Group A and E Reference Group considered that a policy of 'treat and transfer' for the majority of common emergencies is unacceptable and that the following specialties should be available as a minimum and readily accessible to all major A and E departments:

general medicine; paediatrics; acute psychiatry; general surgery (including vascular surgery) with 24-hour major theatre availability; trauma and orthopaedics; obstetrics and gynaecology; anaesthetics; intensive care; radiology (including CT scanning facilities) and pathology.

The specialties to which A and E departments would require access, but not necessarily on site were considered to include:

ENT; ophthalmology; geriatrics; neurosurgery and neurology; cardio-thoracic surgery; facio-maxillary surgery; plastic surgery; genito-urinary medicine; and any other forms of specialist surgery.[173]

The minimum mix of specialties needed is a target which most providers would aspire to. Hospitals designated as regional trauma centres would offer more than this, especially neurosurgery and neurology and cardiovascular surgery.

Staffing

The increased volume and complexity of the caseload inherent in reducing the number of major A and E departments and diverting patients with minor injury or illness calls for experienced medical, nursing and related professional staff to be available 24 hours a day and, in the opinion of the British Association of Emergency Medicine, actually present in the A and E department 16 hours a day, seven days a week.[6] Clinically in order to provide 24-hour cover at senior clinical level it would be difficult to oppose the BAEM's recommendation that a department seeing 100 000 new patients each year should have four consultants, eight middle grade doctors and 20 senior house officers. This is especially convincing if proportionately more of the caseload were to consist of serious illness or injury. It is difficult to see how any provider A and E department employing fewer than two consultants in A and E medicine can offer adequate training facilities to junior medical staff.

Similarly nurses and other non-medical staff will be required, appropriately trained for the clientele and range of clinical problems presenting and capable of filling extended roles.

Processes of care

Where established protocols for the effective management of serious illness and injury exist they should be adopted in A and E departments. While the widespread establishment of regional trauma centres cannot be recommended as cost-effective options, suitably skilled trauma teams should always be accessible. The levels of skill available should include proficiency in advanced resuscitation techniques and advanced trauma life support.

Minor injury services

Closure of some major A and E departments has uncovered the need for alternative modes of delivery of care for minor injuries and illnesses and this is being provided in a range of different settings including A and E departments, community hospitals, GP surgeries, primary care centres, community clinics, polyclinics and dedicated minor injury units. The principles governing the provision of these facilities are that the complex and expensive resources of major A and E departments should not be diverted to treating minor conditions and that the public should have easy access to facilities for treating minor conditions which are beyond the normal scope of general practice.

Purchasers will need to consider a variety of decentralized provider facilities, designed according to local opportunities, initiatives and preferences. The service specification for such minor injury services should accord with the example set out in the NHS Executive report on the subject.[57]

Such is the level of ignorance of the incidence of minor injury and illness and the proportions of occurrences which are currently dealt with respectively by major A and E departments, other institutional providers, or GPs, that no population-based quantitative targets can be suggested for the provision of facilities.

9 Information

The dearth of information about the ways in which A and E departments have been managed has already been indicated. A and E departments need systems which allow them to describe for purchasers the demographic and diagnostic mix of the clientele; the severity and urgency of their conditions; the setting in which injuries occurred; the origin of the demand according to GP practice or no practice; the mix and timing of procedures to which patients are subjected; the extent to which patients reattend and what characterizes the reattenders; and the administrative and clinical outcomes of attendance where valid means of measuring these exist.

There is already a variety of software for information systems in use in provider units.[55] These differ in their coverage. The NHS Executive has established a series of contract minimum data sets, including one related to A and E departments. The Executive's Committee for Regulating Information Requirements reviews the data set from time to time. The mandatory data set which was operative at April 1993 in A and E departments with computerized information systems was specified in the Executive's Data Set Change Notice (DSC Notice 19/92). Details of the data set are shown in Appendix II. They include patient details and logistic details of attendance.

Codes and classifications have been constructed for the A and E attendance category (first attendance, follow-up attendance planned, etc.), the patient group (deliberate self-harm, sports injury, etc.) and the incident location type (home, work, etc.). A national clinical classification and coding structure for A and E departments has also been developed. This is designed to reflect investigation and treatment activity relating to diagnosis.

The data set is accessible to the provider unit itself and also to the purchasing authority. The aggregated data which are presently accessed at regional and national levels are the numbers of first attendances and total attendances only. The conditions will soon exist however when national policy on the organization and utilization of A and E services may be informed by surveying the minimum data sets held by provider units, along the lines involved in the US National Hospital Ambulatory Medical Care Survey.[70] The data set also facilitates local clinical and administrative audit, including the Patient's Charter requirement for prompt assessment and will allow purchasers to compare performance across provider units. Universal adoption and exploitation of this minimum data set is urgently needed.

The inadequacy of the crude costing data produced on the functioning of major A and E departments and the failure to distinguish the costs of treating minor conditions in establishments which fulfil other clinical roles has already been mentioned. Developmental work is needed to increase the precision of cost information.

It is clear that comprehensive systems of information about morbidity relevant to the utilization of A and E departments are lacking. One area in which there is development is that of accident information. Data are available from a variety of sources on accident characteristics such as location, accident type (fall, poisoning, etc.), circumstances (adequacy of lighting, existence of smoke alarms, etc.), personal characteristics of the individual concerned, activity at the time (work, leisure, etc.) the consequences of the accident in terms of the nature and severity of the injury, the health service impact, and individual health outcomes. These sources include A and E department and ambulance records; hospital inpatient data, general practice records; Home Office fire statistics; the Department of Trade and Industry's Home and Leisure Accident Statistics (HASS and LASS); police records; the Department of Transport's Road Traffic Accident Statistics; the Health and Safety Executive's workplace injury reporting system (RIDDOR); the Office of Population Censuses and Surveys Mortality Statistics and coroners' records.

There are omissions and overlaps in the data coverage of accidents at present. To help overcome this the Department of Health's Public Health Information Strategy Group has drafted recommendations covering the standardization of data items and data linkage, based on a core minimum data set of accident characteristics and personal characteristics.[174] Read-coding of injuries is recommended for universal use and extensions to the present coding structure suggested to include codes for accident location, circumstances, activity, predisposing factors and individual health outcomes.

Benefits are likely to include enhanced means of monitoring injury severity and changes over time and the production of better quality information to assess prevention initiatives such as improvements in vehicle design and secondary prevention targets involving the organization of the health care services. There are cost consequences. Health commissions are encouraged to decide how the quality of information from local hospital A and E and inpatient service providers, associated health care agencies like the ambulance service and general practice records can be improved, with a view to requiring adoption of the standardized data set and linking arrangements when these have been piloted successfully.

10 Research needs

The NHS Executive priority areas of research and development include the evaluation of health technology and the primary–secondary care interface. Both embrace the needs for research into the organization and operation of A and E departments and related parts of the service.

This chapter has demonstrated to what little extent the methods of organizing, staffing and equipping and operating A and E departments have been evaluated clinically and economically. The added value of a regional trauma system has already been studied in one type of UK setting, but we do not know about the value of pre-hospital triage or high volume trauma units.

There is considerable scope for studying the costs and effects of having professions from different backgrounds perform similar functions in A and E departments. With so much effort being expended on the treatment of minor injuries and illness and attendance rates remaining high, the costs and effectiveness of different systems of provision in similar circumstances should be explored urgently. These include primary care emergency centres, free standing, alongside or within major A and E departments; and out of hours GP services administered by co-operatives or commercial deputizing services.

The impact of changes in the organization of pre-hospital care, such as the increased use of paramedical staff in the ambulance service and psychiatric crisis intervention services, should be measured. The consequences of closure and amalgamation of A and E departments for the organization of inpatient services, accessibility to the population served and health outcomes also need study.

Appendix I National hospital ambulatory medical care survey emergency department patient record

3. DATE OF VISIT	5. SEX	6. RACE	7. ETHNICITY	8. EXPECTED SOURCE(S) OF PAYMENT *(Check all that apply)*	9. MAJOR REASON FOR THIS VISIT *(Check one)*

3. DATE OF VISIT
___/___/___
Month Day Year

4. DATE OF BIRTH
___/___/___
Month Day Year

5. SEX
1 ☐ Female
2 ☐ Male

6. RACE
1 ☐ White
2 ☐ Black
3 ☐ Asian/Pacific Islander
4 ☐ American Indian/ Eskimo/ Aleut

7. ETHNICITY
1 ☐ Hispanic
2 ☐ Not Hispanic

8. EXPECTED SOURCE(S) OF PAYMENT *(Check all that apply)*
1 ☐ Medicare
2 ☐ Medicaid
3 ☐ Other government
4 ☐ Private/ Commercial
5 ☐ HMO/Other prepaid
6 ☐ Patient paid
7 ☐ No charge
8 ☐ Other

9. MAJOR REASON FOR THIS VISIT *(Check one)*
1 ☐ Injury, first visit
2 ☐ Injury, follow-up
3 ☐ Illness, first visit
4 ☐ Illness, follow-up
5 ☐ Other reason

10. CAUSE OF INJURY *(Complete if injury is marked in 9. Describe cause and place of injury.)*

11. PATIENT'S COMPLAINT(S), SYMPTOM(S), OR OTHER REASON(S) FOR THIS VISIT *(In patient's own words)*
a. Most important: _____
b. Other: _____
c. Other: _____

12. PHYSICIAN'S DIAGNOSES
a. Principal diagnosis/ problem associated with item 11a. _____
b. Other: _____
c. Other: _____

13. URGENCY OF THIS VISIT *(Check only one)*
1 ☐ Urgent/Emergent
2 ☐ Non-urgent

14. IS PROBLEM ALCOHOL- OR DRUG-RELATED?
1 ☐ Neither
2 ☐ Alcohol-related
3 ☐ Drug-related
4 ☐ Both

15. DIAGNOSTIC/SCREENING SERVICES *(Check all ordered or provided.)*
1 ☐ None
2 ☐ Blood pressure check
3 ☐ Urinalysis
4 ☐ HIV serology
5 ☐ Other blood test
6 ☐ EKG
7 ☐ Mental status exam
7 ☐ Chest x-ray
9 ☐ Extremity x-ray
10 ☐ CT scan/MRI
11 ☐ Other diagnostic imaging
12 ☐ Other *(Specify)*
_____
_____
_____

16. PROCEDURES *(Check all provided on this visit)*
1 ☐ None
2 ☐ Endotracheal intubation
3 ☐ CPR
4 ☐ IV fluids
5 ☐ NG tube/ gastric lavage
11 ☐ Other(s) *(Specify)* _____
6 ☐ Wound care
7 ☐ Eye/ENT care
8 ☐ Orthopedic care
9 ☐ Bladder catheter
10 ☐ Lumbar puncture
_____
_____

17. MEDICATION *(Record all new or continued medication ordered, administered, or provided at this visit. Use the same brand name or generic name entered on any Rx or medical record. Include immunizations and desensitizing agents.)*
☐ None
1. _____
2. _____
3. _____
4. _____
5. _____

18. DISPOSITION THIS VISIT *(Check all that apply)*
1 ☐ Return to ED PRN
2 ☐ Return to ED - appointment
3 ☐ Return to referring physician
4 ☐ Refer to other physician/clinic
5 ☐ Admit to hospital
6 ☐ Transfer to other facility
7 ☐ DOA/died in ED
8 ☐ Left AMA
9 ☐ No follow-up planned
10 ☐ Other *(Specify)*
_____

19. PROVIDERS SEEN THIS VISIT *(Check all that apply)*
1 ☐ Resident/Intern
2 ☐ Staff physician
3 ☐ Other physician
4 ☐ Physician assistant
5 ☐ Nurse practitioner
6 ☐ Registered nurse
7 ☐ Licensed practical nurse
8 ☐ Nurse's aide

Appendix II Provider minimum data set for A and E departments with computerized systems

Item	Field	
	Size	Type
Contract details		
Contract identifier	16	A/N
Patient details		
Patient's name	35	A/N
NHS number[a]	17	A/N
Marital status	1	
Sex	1	
Birth date	8	
Patient's usual address	105	A/N
Postcode of usual address	7	A/N
Health authority code (of residence)	3	A/N
Code of GP (registered)	8	A/N
Attendance details		
Code of GP practice	6	A/N
Local patient identifier	10	A/N
A and E attendance category[b]	1	
Date of attendance	6	
Source of referral[b]	2	A/N
Mode of arrival	1	
Arrival time (24-hour clock)	4	
A and E: patient group[b]	2	A/N
A and E: incident location type[b]	2	A/N
Time of initial assessment (24-hour clock)	4	
A and E: time seen for treatment[b]	4	
A and E: staff member code[b]	3	A/N
Investigations code		
– first	6	A/N
– second	6	A/N
Diagnostic code		
– first	6	A/N
– second	6	A/N
Treatment code		
– first	6	A/N
– second	6	A/N
A and E attendance conclusion time (24-hour clock)	4	
A and E: departure time[a]	4	A/N
A and E: attendance disposal[a]	2	

[a]Collection not mandatory at present.
[b]New/amended data item.
Field types are numeric unless otherwise shown.
Reference should also be made to the Minimum Data Set Model for the data needed to identify A and E episode, A and E department and lodged patient.
Enquiries about this DCS Notice should be addressed to the CRIR Secretariat, IMG ME(C), Room 5E28, Quarry House, Quarry Hill, LEEDS LS2 7UE. Tel: 01532 546012, or to the nominated enquiry point where this is given in the enclosure.

References

1 National Health Services Management Executive. *Report of the London Implementation Group. Overview of accident and emergency services in London*. London: NHSME, 1994.

2 National Audit Office. *NHS Accident and Emergency Departments in England*. London: HMSO, 1992.

3 Royal College of Surgeons. *The management of patients with major injuries*. Report of the Working Party of the Royal College of Surgeons. London: Royal College of Surgeons, 1988.

4 Nicholl, JP, Turner J, Dixon S. *Cost-effectiveness of a regional trauma system in the North West Midlands*. Report to the Department of Health. University of Sheffield: Medical Care Research Unit, 1995.

5 Read SM, Jones NMB, Williams BT. Nurse practitioners in accident and emergency departments: what do they do? *BMJ* 1992; **305**: 1466–70.

6 British Association for Accident and Emergency Medicine. *The Way Ahead. Accident and Emergency Services, 2001*. London: BAEM, 1992.

7 Secretaries of State for Health. *General Practice in the National Health Service*. London: Department of Health, 1989.

8 House of Commons. *National Health Service and Community Care Act*. London: HMSO, 1990.

9 Hallam L, Cragg D. Organisation of primary care services outside normal working hours. *BMJ* 1994; **309**: 1621–3.

10 Snooks H, Turner J. Countdown to Christmas. *Hlth Ser J*, 2 November 1995: 28–9.

11 Department of Health. *Review of ambulance performance standards. Interim report*. A discussion document. London: Department of Health, 1995.

12 NHS Executive. *Accident and Emergency Departments*. London: Department of Health, 1994.

13 Department of Health. *The Patient's Charter*. London: HMSO, 1991.

14 Krauss BS, Harakal T, Fleisher GR. The spectrum and frequency of illness presenting to a pediatric emergency department. *Ped Emerg Care* 1991; **7(2)**: 67–71.

15 Sacchetti A, Carracio C, Feder M. Pediatric EMS transport: are we treating children in a system designed for adults only? *Ped Emerg Care* 1992; **8(1)**: 4–8.

16 Audit Commission for Local Authorities in England and Wales. *By Accident or Design: improving emergency care in acute hospitals*. London: Audit Commission, 1996.

17 Department of Health. *Urgent and emergency admissions to hospital*. Report of a Clinical Standards Advisory Group Committee and the Government Response. London: HMSO, 1995.

18 Department of Health. *Health and Personal Social Services Statistics, 1991–*. London: Department of Health. 1991–.

19 Fitzgerald GJ, Robertson CE, Little K *et al*. The urgency distribution of an accident and emergency department's workload. *Arch Emerg Med* 1986; **3**: 225–30.

20 Burdett-Smith P. Estimating trauma centre workload. *J Roy Coll Surg* Edinburgh 1992; **37**: 128–30.

21 Airey CM, Franks AJ. *The epidemiology of major trauma in the Yorkshire Health Region*. Leeds: University of Leeds, 1992.

22 Gorman DF, Teanby DN, Sinha MP *et al*. The epidemiology of major injuries in Mersey Region and North Wales. *Injury* 1995; **26**: 51–4.

23 Phair I, Barton D, Barnes M *et al*. Deaths following trauma: an audit of performance. *Ann R C S Eng* 1991; **73**: 53–7.

24 McGinty P. *Accident and Emergency Services in London. An initial review of services*. Report to Inner London Purchasing Authorities, (unpublished), 1993.

25 Foroughi D, Chadwick L. Accident and emergency abusers. *Practitioner* 1982; **33**: 657–9.

26 Crombie DL. A casualty survey. *J Roy Coll Gen Pract* 1959; **2**: 346–56.

27 Lowy A, Nicholl JP, Kohler B. Attendance at accident and emergency departments: unnecessary or inappropriate? *J Pub Hlth Med* 1994; **16**: 134–40.

28 Bryce GM, Houghton JD. Out-of-district: the passing trade of an accident and emergency department. *Arch Emerg Medicine* 1993; **10**: 172–6.

29 Singh S. Self referral to accident and emergency department: patients' perceptions. *BMJ* 1986; **292**: 1179–80.

30 Davies T. Accident departments or general practice. *BMJ* 1986; **292**: 241–3.

31 Central Statistical Office. *Social Trends 25*. London: HMSO, 1995.

32 Health and Safety Commission. *Health and Safety Statistics 1994–95*. London: Government Statistical Service, 1995.

33 Department of Transport. *Road traffic accidents, Great Britain, 1993. The Casualty Report*. London: HMSO, 1994.

34 Department of Health and Social Security, Office of Population Censuses and Surveys. *Series MB4, No. 15. Hospital Inpatient Enquiry, Summary Tables 1980*. London: HMSO, 1983.

35 Department of Health and Social Security, Office of Population Censuses and Surveys. *Series MB4, No. 26. Hospital Inpatient Enquiry, Summary Tables 1985*. London: HMSO, 1987.

36 Department of Health. *Hospital Episodes Statistics Vol. I. England. Financial year 1989–90*. London: Government Statistical Service, 1993.

37 Department of Health. *Hospital Episodes Statistics Vol. 1. England: Financial year 1993–94*. London: Government Statistical Service, 1995.

38 Spestor TD, Cooper C, Fenton-Lewis A. Trends in admission for hip fracture in England and Wales, 1968–1985. *BMJ* 1990; **300**: 1173–4.

39 Larsen CF, Lauristen J. Epidemiology of acute wrist trauma. *Int J Epidemiol* 1993; **22**: 911–16.

40 Platts S, Hawton K, Kreitman N *et al*. Recent clinical and epidemiological trends in parasuicide in Edinburgh and Oxford: A tale of two cities. *Psychol Med* 1988; **18**: 405–18.

41 O'Dwyer FG, D'Alton A, Pearce JB. Adolescent self harm patients: audit of assessment in an accident and emergency department. *BMJ* 1991; **303**: 629–30.

42 Dennis M, Owens D, Jones S. Epidemiology of deliberate self-poisoning: trends in hospital attendances. *Hlth Trends* 1990; **3**: 125–6.

43 Garlick R, Home B. *Blue calls and the London Ambulance Service*. London: London Ambulance Service, 1992.

44 Tunstall-Pedoe H, Kuulasmaa K, Amouyel P. Myocardial infarction and coronary deaths in the World Health Organization MONICA Project. *Circulation* 1994; **90**: 583–612.

45 Neville RG, Clark RC, Hoskins G *et al*. National asthma attack audit 1991–2. General Practitioners in Asthma Group. *BMJ* 1993; **306**: 559–62.

46 Hyndman SJ, Williams DRR, Merrill SL *et al*. Rates of admission to hospital for asthma. *BMJ* 1994; **308**: 1596–600.

47 Merson S, Tyrer P, Onyett S *et al*. Early intervention in psychiatric emergencies: a controlled clinical trial. *Lancet* 1992; **339**: 1311–14.

48 Johnson S, Thornicroft G. Emergency psychiatric services in England and Wales. *BMJ* 1995; **311**: 287–8.

49 George SL, Shanks NJ, Westlake L. Census of single homeless people in Sheffield. *BMJ* 1991; **302**: 1387–9.

50 Nicholl JP, Coleman P, Williams BT. *Injuries in sport and exercise*. London: Sports Council, 1991.

51 British Association for Accident and Emergency Medicine. *Directory 1993*. London: Royal College of Surgeons, 1993.

52 British Orthopaedic Association. *The Management of Skeletal Trauma in the United Kingdom*. London: British Orthopaedic Association, 1992.

53 Beattie TF, Ferguson J, Moir PA. Short-stay facilities in accident and emergency departments for children. *Arch Emerg Med* 1993; **10**: 177–80.

54 British Association for Accident and Emergency Medicine. *Accident and Emergency Ward*. Report of Clinical Services Committee. London: Royal College of Surgeons, 1989.

55 British Association for Accident and Emergency Medicine. *Report of Clinical Services Committee*. Register of Computerised Accident and Emergency Reports Systems. London: Royal College of Surgeons, 1992.

56 Department of Health. *Health and Personal Social Services Statistics 1993*. London: HMSO, 1993.

57 NHS Management Executive. *A Study of Minor Injury Services*. London: NHSME, 1994.

58 Garnett SM, Elton PJ. A treatment service for minor injuries: maintaining equity of access. *J Pub Hlth Med* 1991; **13**: 260–6.

59 Jones G. Minor injury care in the community. *Nurs Stan* 1993; **7**: 35–6.

60 Dale J, Green J, Reid F *et al*. Primary care in the accident and emergency department: II. Comparison of general practitioners and hospital doctors. *BMJ* 1995; **311**: 427–30.

61 Newman P, Clarke S, Hanlon A. South Westminster Centre Appraisal: Options for the Way Ahead, *(Unpublished)*, (quoted in report to London Implementation Group), *The Closure of Accident and Emergency Services at St Bartholomew's Hospital. Needs Assessment and Option Appraisal*. London Health Economics Consortium, University of Sheffield and York Health Economics Consortium, 1993.

62 Ingram DR, Clarke DR, Murdic RA. Distance and the decision to visit an emergency department. *Soc Sci Med* 1978; **12**: 55–62.

63 Office of Population Censuses and Surveys. *General Household Survey. Report, 1991*. London: HMSO, 1993.

64 Milner PC, Nicholl JP, Williams BT. Variations in demand for accident and emergency departments in England from 1974 to 1985. *J Epidemiol Commun Hlth* 1988; **42**: 274–8.

65 Milner PC, Nicholl JP, Williams B . Variability in reviewing attenders at accident and emergency departments in England. *BMJ* 1988; **296**: 1645.

66 Milner PC, Beeby N, Nicholl JP. Who should review the walking wounded? Reattendance at accident and emergency departments. *Hlth Trends* 1991; **23**: 36–41.

67 Department of Health. *Welfare of Children and Young People in Hospital*. London: HMSO, 1991.

68 Chambers J, Johnson K. Predicting demand for accident and emergency services. *Comm Med* 1986; **8**: 93–103.

69 Jankowski RF, Mandalia S. Comparison of attendance and emergency admission patterns at accident and emergency departments in and out of London. *BMJ* 1993; **306**: 1241–3.

70 Centers for Disease Control and Prevention/National Center for Health Statistics. National Hospital Ambulatory Medical Care Survey: 1992. *Emergency Department Summary*. Hyattsville: US Department of Health and Human Services, 1994.

71 Waddell TK, Kalman PG, Goodman SJL *et al*. Is outcome worse in a small volume Canadian trauma centre? *J Trauma* 1991; **31(7)**: 958–61.

72 Hedges JR, Osterud HR, Mullins RJ. Adult minor trauma patients: good outcome in small hospitals. *Ann Emerg Med* 1992; **21(4)**: 402–6.

73 Draaisma JM Th, de Haan AFJ, Goris RJA. Preventable trauma deaths in the Netherlands – A prospective multicenter study. *J Trauma* 1989; **29(11)**: 1552–7.

74 Buck N, Derlin A, Lunn JN. *The report of a confidential enquiry into perioperative deaths*. London: Nuffield Provincial Hospitals/King's Fund, 1987.

75 Fischer RB, Dearden CH. Improving the care of patients with major trauma in the accident & emergency department. *BMJ* 1990; **300**: 1560–2.

76 Smith RF, Frateschi K, Sloan EP *et al*. The impact of volume on outcome in seriously injured trauma patients: Two years' experience of the Chicago trauma system. *J Trauma* 1990; **30(9)**: 1066–75.

77 Committee on Trauma of the American College of Surgeons. Hospital and pre-hospital resources for optimal care of the injured patient. *Am Coll Surg Bull* 1986; **71(10)**: 4–21.

78 Phair IC, Barton DJ, Allen MJ *et al.* Preventable deaths after head injury: a clinical audit of performance. *Injury* 1991; **22(5)**: 353–6.

79 North West Thames Regional Health Authority. *Primary and Community Care Task Force Report on the Tomlinson Enquiry.* NW Thames RHA, 1992.

80 Lewin W. Medical staffing and accident & emergency services. London: Joint Consultants Committee, 1978.

81 Nuffield Provincial Hospitals Trust. Casualty services and their setting: a study in medical care. London: NPHT, 1960.

82 Dallos V, Mouzas GL. An evaluation of the functions of the short stay observation ward in the Accident & Emergency Department. *BMJ* 1981; **282**: 37–40.

83 Harrop SN, Morgan WJ. Emergency care for the elderly in the short-stay ward of the Accident & Emergency Department. *Arch Emerg Med* 1985; **2**: 141–7.

84 MacLaren RE, Thoorahoo HI, Kirby NG. Use of an accident and emergency department observation ward in the management of head injury. *Brit J Surg* 1993; **80(2)**: 215–17.

85 Chidley KE, Wood-Baker R, Town GI *et al.* Reassessment of asthma management in an accident and emergency department. *Resp Med* 1991; **85(5)**: 373–7.

86 Clarke JA, Adams JE. A critical appraisal of 'out-of-hours' radiography in a major teaching hospital. *Brit J Radiol* 1988; **61**: 1100–5.

87 McKee M, Priest P, Ginzler M *et al.* What is the requirement for out-of-hours operating in orthopaedics? *Arch Emerg Med* 1993; **10**: 91–9.

88 Normand C, Hunter I *et al. Sheffield Health Authority Review of Accident and Emergency Services.* Health Services Research Units, Department of Public Health and Policy, London School of Hygiene and Tropical Medicine, 1991.

89 Campbell S, Watkins G, Kreis D. Preventable deaths in a self-designated trauma system. *Am Surg* 1989; **55**: 478–80.

90 Hoyt DB, Vbulger EM, Knudson MM *et al.* Death in the operating room. An analysis of a multi-center experience. *J Trauma* 1994; **37(3)**: 426–32.

91 McNicholl BP, Dearden CH. Delays in care of the critically injured. *Br J Surg* 1992; **79**: 171–3.

92 Rouse A. Study to examine the timeliness of care received by patients with open fractures of the lower limb. *J Pub Hlth Med* 1991; **13(4)**: 267–75.

93 Meek RN, Vivoda EE, Pirani S. Comparison of mortality of patients with multiple injuries according to type of fracture treatment: a retrospective age- and injury-matched service. *Injury* 1986; **17**: 2–4.

94 Rogers FB, Shackford SR, Keller MS. Early fixation reduces morbidity and mortality in elderly patients with hip fractures from low-impact falls. *J Trauma* 1995; **39(2)**: 261–5.

95 Campling EA, Devlin HB, Hoile RW *et al. The report of the national confidential enquiry into perioperative deaths, 1990.* London: NCEPOB, 1992.

96 Carew-McColl M, Buckles E. A workload shared. *Hlth Serv J* 4 January 1990; **100**: 27.

97 Evans RJ, McCale M, Allen H *et al.* Telephone advice in the accident and emergency department: a survey of current practice. *Arch Emerg Med* 1993; **10(3)**: 216–19.

98 Egleston CV, Kelly HC, Rope AR. Use of a telephone advice line in an accident and emergency department. *BMJ* 1994; **308**: 31.

99 Sampalis JS, Lavoie A, Williams JI *et al.* Impact of on-site care, pre-hospital time, and level of in-hospital care on survival in severely injured patients. *J Trauma* 1993; **34(2)**: 252–61.

100 Sloan EP, Callahan EP, Duda J *et al.* The effect of urban trauma system hospital bypass on pre-hospital transport times and level of trauma patient survival. *Ann Emerg Med* 1989; **18**: 1146–50.

101 George S, Read S, Westlake L *et al.* Evaluation of nurse triage in a British accident and emergency department. *BMJ* 1992; **304**: 876–8.

102 George S, Read S, Westlake L *et al.* Nurse triage in theory and in practice. *Arch Emerg Med* 1993; **10(3)**: 220–8.

103 Dale J, Green J, Reid F *et al.* Primary care in the accident and emergency department. 1. Prospective identification of patients. *BMJ* 1995; **311**: 423–6.

104 Richmond PW, Evans RC, Sibert JR. Improving facilities for children in an accident department. *Arch Dis Child* 1987; **62(3)**: 299–301.

105 Beattie TF, Moir PA. Paediatric accident and emergency short-stay ward: a 1-year audit. *Arch Em Med* 1993; **10(3)**: 181–6.

106 Bensard DD, McIntyre RC, Moore EE *et al.* A critical analysis of acutely injured children managed in an adult level 1 trauma center. *J Ped Surg* 1994; **29(1)**: 11–8.

107 Cooper A, Barlow B, DiScala C *et al.* Efficacy of pediatric trauma care: results of a population-based study. *J Ped Surg* 1993; **28(3)**: 299–303.

108 Lambert S, Willetts K. The transfer of multiply injured patients for neurosurgical opinion. *J Bone Joint Surg* 1992; **74-B**: Supplement 2.

109 Gentleman D, Jennett B. Hazards of inter-hospital transfer of comatose head-injured patients. *Lancet* 1981; **ii**: 853–5.

110 Andrews PJD, Piper IR, Dearden NM *et al.* Secondary insults during intrahospital transport of head-injured patients. *Lancet* 1990; **335**: 327–30.

111 Spence MT, Redmond AD, Edwards JD. Trauma audit – the use of TRISS. *Hlth Trends* 1988; **20**: 94–7.

112 Sharples PM, Storey A, Aynsly-Green A *et al.* Avoidable factors contributing to deaths of children with head injury. *BMJ* 1990; **300**: 87–91.

113 Gentleman D, Jennett B. Audit of transfer of unconscious head-injured patients to a neurosurgical unit. *Lancet* 1990; **335**: 330–4.

114 Spencer JD. Why do our hospitals not make more use of the concept of a trauma team? *BMJ* 1985; **290**: 136–8.

115 Deane SA, Gaudrey PL, Pearson I *et al.* Implementation of a trauma team. *Austral NZ J Surg* 1989; **59(5)**: 373–8.

116 Driscoll P, Skinner D. ABC of major trauma, initial assessment and management 1: Primary survey. *BMJ* 1990; **300**: 1265–7.

117 Deane SA, Gaudry PL, Pearson I *et al.* The hospital trauma team: a model for trauma management. *J Trauma* 1990; **30(7)**: 806–12.

118 Driscoll PA, Vincent CA. Variation in trauma resuscitation and its effect on patient outcome. *Injury* 1992; **23(2)**: 111–15.

119 Driscoll PA, Vincent CA. Organizing an efficient trauma team. *Injury* 1992; **23(2)**: 107–10.

120 Spencer JD, Golpali B. Audit of six months' activity of a trauma team. *Injury* 1990; **21(2)**: 68–70.

121 The American College of Surgeons. *Advanced Trauma Life Support*. Chicago: The American College of Surgeons, 1988.

122 Myers RA. Advanced trauma life support course (Ed). *J R Soc Med* 1990; **83**: 281–2.

123 Paynter M. Trauma support: revolution in care. *Emerg Nurse* Autumn 1993; 7–9.

124 Study design in prehospital trauma advanced life support – basic life support research: a critical review. *Ann Emerg Med* 1991; **20**: 857–60.

125 Ali J, Adam R, Butler AK *et al.* Trauma outcome improves following the advanced life support programme in a developing country. *J Trauma* 1993; **34(6)**: 890–8.

126 Collicott PE. Advanced trauma life support (ATLS): past, present, future. *J Trauma* 1992; **33(5)**: 749–53.

127 Nicholl JP, Brazier JE, Williams BT. Management of trauma. *BMJ* 1993; **307**: 683–4.

128 Guss DA, Neuman TS, Baxt WG *et al.* The impact of a regionalised trauma system on trauma care in San Diego county. *Ann Emerg Med* 1989; **18**: 1141–5.

129 Rutledge R, Messick J, Baker CC *et al.* Multivariate population-based analysis of the association of county trauma centres with per capita county trauma death rates. *J Trauma* 1992; **33(1)**: 29–38.

130 Ottosson A, Krantz P. Traffic fatalities in a system with decentralised trauma care. *JAMA* 1984; **251(20)**: 2668–71.

131 Gennarelli TA, Champion HR, Sacco WJ *et al.* Mortality of patients with head injury and extracranial injury treated in trauma centres. *J Trauma* 1989; **29(9)**: 1193–202.

132 Miller JD, Tocher JL, Jones PA. Extradural haematoma – earlier detection, better results. *Brain Injury* 1988; **2**: 83–6.

133 Bowers SA, Marshall LF. Outcome in 200 consecutive cases of severe head injury treated in San Diego county: a prospective analysis. *J Neurosurg* 1980; **6**: 237–42.

134 Cordobes F, Lobato RD, Rivas JJ *et al.* Observations on 82 patients with extradural haematoma. Comparison of results before and after the advent of computed tomography. *J Neurosurgery* 1981; **54**: 179–86.

135 Bricolo AP, Parker LM. Extradural haematoma: toward zero mortality. *J Neurosurgery* 1984; **14**: 8–12.

136 Shackford SR, Wald SL, Ross SE *et al.* The clinical utility of computed tomographic scanning and neurologic examination in the management of patients with minor head injuries. *J Trauma* 1992; **33(3)**: 385–94.

137 Stein SC, O'Mally KF, Ross SE. Is routine computed tomography scanning too expensive for mild head injury? *Ann Emerg Med* 1991; **20(12)**: 1286–9.

138 Livingston DH, Loder PA, Koziol J *et al.* The use of CT scanning to triage patients requiring admission following minimal head injury. *J Trauma* 1991; **31(4)**: 483–9.

139 Teasdale GM, Murray G, Anderson E *et al.* Risks of acute traumatic intracranial haematoma in children and adults: implications for managing head injuries. *BMJ* 1990; **300**: 363–7.

140 Nelson JB, Bresticker MA, Nahrwold DL. Computed tomography in the initial evaluation of patients with blunt trauma. *J Trauma* 1992; **33(5)**: 722–7.

141 Frame SB, Browder IW, Lay EK *et al.* Computed tomography versus diagnostic peritoneal lavage: usefulness in immediate diagnosis of blunt abdominal trauma. *Ann Emerg Med* 1989; **18(5)**: 513–16.

142 Hewer RL, Wood VA. Availability of computed tomography of the brain in the United Kingdom. *BMJ* 1989; **298**: 1219–20.

143 Wardrope J. Death of children with head injury. *BMJ* 1990; **300**: 534.

144 Jones G. Minor injury in the community. *Nurs Standard* 1993; **7:22**: 35–6.

145 Baker B. Model methods. *Nurs Times* 1993; **89:47**: 33–5.

146 Sykes P. Bridlington and District Hospital Minor Injuries Unit. Bridlington 1993 (internal report).

147 Garnett SM, Elton PJ. A treatment service for minor injuries: maintaining equity of access. *J Pub Hlth Med* 1991; **13:4**: 260–6.

148 Simon P. No doctor in the house. *Nurs Times* 1992; **88:28**: 16–17.

149 Dale J, Dolan B. *Health care in Gravesend: what future for the Minor Casualty Centre?* London: King's College A&E Primary Care Service and Kent FHSA, 1993.

150 Glasman D. Things that go bump in the night. *Hlth Serv J* 14 October 1993; **103**: 16.

151 Newman P. Evaluation of the St Albans Minor Injuries Unit. London: NW Thames RHA, 1994.

152 Newman P, Clarke S, Hanlon A. South Westminster Centre Appraisal. London: Kensington, Chelsea and Westminster Commissioning Agency, 1993.

153 Oerton J, Hanlon A, Newman P. *Evaluation of Outpatient Services at South Westminster Centre for Health.* London: Kensington, Chelsea and Westminster Department of Public Health, 1994.

154 Read S. Patients with minor injuries: a literature review of options for their treatment outside major accident and emergency departments or occupational health settings. *Discussion Paper No. 1*. Sheffield Centre for Health and Related Research, March 1994.

155 Joint Audit commission of the British Cardiac Society. Time delays in provision of thrombolytic treatment in six district hospitals. *BMJ* 1989; **305**: 445–8.

156 European Resuscitation Council Working Party. Adult advanced cardiac life support: the European Resuscitation Council guidelines 1992 (abridged). *BMJ* 1993; **306**: 1589–93.

157 European Resuscitation Council Basic Life Support Working Group. Guidelines for basic life support. *BMJ* 1993; **306**: 1587–9.

158 McLauchlan CA, Driscoll PA, Whimster F *et al*. Effectiveness of the call-out systems for a London Coronary Ambulance Service. *Arch Emerg Med* 1989; **6(3)**: 193–8.

159 Drummond MF. *Principles of economic appraisal in health care*. Oxford: Oxford Medical Publications, 1980.

160 Baraff LJ, Cameron JM, Sekhen R. Direct costs of emergency medical care: a diagnosis-based case-mix classification system. *Ann Emerg Med* 1991; **20**: 1–7.

161 Roberts JA, Dale J, Garcia de Ancos J *et al*. The provision of primary care in an accident and emergency department. An economic appraisal, 1993 (personal communication).

162 Nicholl JP, Brazier JE, Beeby NR. *Costs and health benefits of the Cornwall helicopter ambulance*. Final report to Department of Health. University of Sheffield: Medical Care Research Unit, 1993.

163 Brazier J, Jeavons R, Normand C. *The economics of accident and emergency services*. Paper presented to Health Economics Study Group, Brunel University, 1988.

164 Brazier J. *Study of accident and emergency services in East Yorkshire Health Authority*. York: University of York, 1988.

165 Steele R, Lees REM, Latchmann B *et al*. Cost of primary health care services in the emergency department and the family physician's office. *Can Med Assoc J* 1975; **112**: 1096.

166 Farmer RD *et al*. *Accident and emergency services in Riverside Health Authority*. Report to Riverside Health Authority, 1987.

167 Health Policy and Public Health Directorate. *Emergency health care in Scotland*. Report of a policy review. Scottish Home and Health Department: HMSO, 1994.

168 Raftery J, Stevens A (eds). Reflections and Conclusions. *Health Care Needs Assessment: the epidemiologically based needs assessment reviews. Vol. 2*. Oxford: Radcliffe Medical Press, 1994.

169 Yates DW, Woodford M, Hollis S. Preliminary analysis of the care of injured patients in 33 British hospitals: first report of the United Kingdom major trauma outcome study. *BMJ* 1992; **305**: 737–40.

170 Owens D, Dennis M, Read S *et al*. Outcome of deliberate self-poisoning. An examination of risk factors for repetition. *Br J Psych* 1994; **165**: 797–801.

171 McKenna G. The scope for health education in the accident and emergency department. *Accid Emerg Nurs* 1994; **2**: 94–9.

172 Murphy NM, Olney DB, Brakenbury PH. Objective verification of tetanus immune status in an apparently non-immune population. *Br J Clin Pract* 1994; **48**: 8–9.

173 London Implementation Group. *Overview of Accident and Emergency Services in London*. Report of Accident and Emergency Reference Group. London: NHSME, 1994.

174 Department of Health. *Public Health Information Strategy. Agreeing an Accident Information Structure*. Report of project 19B. London: Department of Health, 1995.

2 Child and Adolescent Mental Health

SA Wallace, JM Crown, M Berger, AD Cox

1 Summary

Introduction

This chapter reviews the need for care and services for children and young people with emotional and behavioural difficulties. Priority is given to considering those difficulties that give rise to substantial disruption of personal and social life. The emphasis throughout is on estimating need in populations, in order to make the data available in a form that will be of use to those professionals in health, social services and education who are responsible for care and service planning in child and adolescent mental health within a defined geographical area.

Health authorities are responsible for identifying the health needs of a geographically designated population and for ensuring that appropriate action is taken to meet them. Although health authorities co-ordinate child and adolescent mental health services (CAMHS), paediatric services and primary health care; other agencies provide complementary services. Social services departments are responsible for the care needs of children and adolescents and education departments provide appropriate educational facilities for all children, including those with special educational needs. Effective care in this field requires provision of services by all three major statutory agencies working in close collaboration with each other and the voluntary sector.

Child and adolescent mental health services aim to prevent, investigate, assess and treat child and adolescent mental health difficulties within the age range 0–16 years. Older adolescents who are still in full-time education may be included.

Some mental health difficulties may be dealt with effectively at the primary care level. However others, which are usually multi-factorial in aetiology and multi-faceted in their manifestations often require skilled assessment and the co-operation of different professionals and agencies for effective treatment. Child and adolescent mental health services therefore work in an interdisciplinary environment which includes professionals in the fields of psychiatry, psychology, psychotherapy, nursing, social work, education, occupational and speech and language therapy.

Epidemiological knowledge of many of the conditions has increased substantially over the past 25 years. From this it is apparent that there is a wide range of predisposing and precipitating factors which can result in an equally wide range of difficulties. Social factors are clearly implicated in the genesis and maintenance of these and in their extension into adulthood.[1] Such factors include characteristics of parents and care-givers; their mental and physical health and personalities; the quality of the parents' relationship; the style of child rearing and the contexts in which it occurs; relationships between the child and other family members; family structure and aspects of family function; life events, such as bereavements; relationships with peers; school experiences and broader environmental circumstances such as adequacy of housing.[2–7] There is also good evidence that childhood difficulties can be the precursors of adult criminality and mental disorder.[8,9]

Child and adolescent mental health is also directly and indirectly influenced by genetic factors, physical health, developmental status and educational ability. There is increasing evidence of interaction between all of these and other psychosocial factors in the genesis of mental health difficulties.[10,11]

2 Statement of the problem

Definitions

Children and young people who show patterns of behaviour, emotions or relationships that cause concern to themselves, parents, carers or teachers may be referred to CAMHS, other health services (primary care or paediatrics) or other agencies. The difficulties which precipitate such referral constitute the 'presenting problems', which may subsequently be assessed as 'clinical problems' requiring intervention. This assessment takes into account 'severity', which is a multi-dimensional concept, judged according to the criteria set out in Box 1. It may result in the diagnosis of 'disorder'. Both problems and disorders may exist in the presence of 'risk factors'.

Box 1: Dimensions used in assessing the severity of presenting problems

- Impairment: Impact on individual, carers, environment
- Age appropriateness: Departure from expected developmental course or common patterns
- Frequency
- Duration
- Persistence
- Intensity
- Extensiveness/pervasiveness
- Intrusiveness
- Manageability/controllability
- Multiple presenting problems

A **problem** is defined as a disturbance of function in one area of relationships, mood, behaviour or development of sufficient severity to require professional intervention (see Appendix II for a list of individual problems).

A **disorder** is defined either as a severe problem (commonly persistent), or the co-occurrence of a number of problems, usually in the presence of several risk factors.

Problems and disorders can include behaviour patterns and changes which are either quantitatively (e.g. tantrums or stealing) or qualitatively (e.g. autism or psychotic symptoms) different from normal, of which the latter is generally more serious. Both individual problems and disorders vary in severity.

A **risk factor** can relate to the individual child, family, environment, life events and school experience. Risk factors are such conditions, events or circumstances that are known to be associated with emotional and behavioural disorders and may increase the likelihood of such difficulties. (see Box 7 on page 70).

The association of risk factor(s) with problems or disorders implies increased severity. The prevalence of risk factors will vary from district to district (e.g. inner-city versus rural). High levels of any of the risk factors in a given population indicate the need for an increased level of provision of CAMHS.

The terms **care, service, need, demand, utilization,**[12-14] **professional** and **specialist** which are used in this chapter are defined in Appendix I.

Characterization and classification

Formal characterization and classification schemes for clinical problems and diagnoses in child and adolescent mental health have been developed for different purposes.

The proposed core data set for child and adolescent psychology and psychiatry services[17] is intended for use by professionals involved in direct patient care who are having to identify the characteristics of their patients for recording on computerized information systems. It provides a framework for detailing clinical features (problems), severity of the problems of patients and accompanying risk factors. Box 2 and Appendix II illustrate the data set.

Box 2: A clinically-based classification of child and adolescent mental health problems as derived from the Proposed Core Data Set for Child and Adolescent Psychology and Psychiatry Services

---

Problems

- Antisocial behaviour e.g. stealing, firesetting
- Problems related to school e.g. school refusal
- Problems of self-regulation e.g. tics, feeding problems
- Problems of social relationships e.g. with parents/sibs, attention seeking
- Self-harm/injury e.g. overdose
- Sexual and sex-related problems e.g. sexual offence, gender identity
- Autistic-type characteristics e.g. autism
- Psychosis-type characteristics e.g. confusion, psychotic symptoms
- Psychosomatic-related illness e.g. hypochondriasis, hysteria

Risk factors

Risk factors in the child

- Problems associated with cognition or academic abilities e.g. reading difficulty
- Personality/temperament e.g. shyness/social isolation
- Problems related to speech and language e.g. mutism, speech delay
- Physical e.g. epilepsy, head injury, chronic illness
- Sensory problems e.g. visual impairment, hearing difficulties
- Genetic condition e.g. chromosome anomaly

Risk factors in the family

- Relationship difficulty involving parent(s)/carer(s)
- Marital difficulties
- Family mental health problems
- Family physical health problems
- Abuse/neglect physical/emotional/sexual

Risk factors in social circumstances

- Adverse social circumstances
- Life events e.g. bereavement

The tenth revision of the International Classification of Diseases (ICD 10) summarized in Box 3[16] provides a diagnostic classification which concentrates almost solely on disorders and gives indications of probable aetiology, associated factors and prognosis. For a given child or adolescent, the ICD 10 diagnosis usually encompasses several of the problems listed in the Association for Child Psychology and Psychiatric Services (ACPP) core data set (for example 'conduct disorder' might encompass aggression, defiance and truancy) though a single pattern of behaviour such as persistent firesetting may also merit a diagnosis of 'conduct disorder' (F91).

Box 3: Child and adolescent mental health disorders: international classification of diseases (ICD 10) for child and adolescent mental health

---

F90–F98   Behavioural and emotional disorders with onset usually occurring in childhood and adolescence
F90   hyperkinetic disorders
F91   conduct disorders
F92   mixed disorders of conduct and emotions
F93   emotional disorders with onset specific to childhood
F94   disorders of social functioning with onset specific to childhood and adolescence
F95   tic disorders
F98   other behavioural and emotional disorders with onset usually occurring in childhood and adolescence
F99   mental disorder, not otherwise specified

F70–F79   Mental retardation
F70   mild mental retardation
F71   moderate mental retardation
F73   severe mental retardation
F74   profound mental retardation
F78   other mental retardation
F79   unspecified mental retardation

F80–F89   Disorders of psychological development
F80   specific developmental disorders of speech and language
F81   specific developmental disorders of scholastic skills
F82   specific developmental disorder of motor function
F83   mixed specific developmental disorders
F84   pervasive developmental disorders
F88   other disorders of psychological development
F89   unspecified disorder of psychological development

In addition, some adult mental health diagnoses can become apparent in adolescents and younger children. The major groupings for these are:

F10–F19   mental and behavioural disorders due to psychoactive substance use
F20–F29   schizophrenia, schizotypal and delusional disorders
F30–F39   mood (affective) disorders
F40–F48   neurotic, stress related and somatoform disorders
F50–F59   behavioural syndromes associated with physiological disturbances and physical factors
F60–F69   disorders of adult personality behaviour

Comparing the new ICD 10 codes with equivalent ICD 9 codes or the US DSM III – R classification can be difficult but epidemiology based on any of these classifications provides useful guidance for broad categories of disorder and some specific conditions. It should be noted that the US SDM IV has been produced recently and is more comparable to ICD 10

The ICD 10 incorporates findings from recent research and is needed when planning services for populations because epidemiological data are most commonly based on such higher-order diagnoses.

3 Context

There are several clinical and organizational issues which have led to an increase in demand for child and adolescent mental health services over recent years. In young people there has been an increase in the prevalence of mental health problems such as depression, self-injurious behaviour, delinquency and substance abuse.[17] In addition legislative changes affecting social services and education have led to an increased monitoring and assessment role for these authorities. Responsibilities for treatment have increasingly passed to health services.

Other issues include the increasing recognition of the importance of certain diagnoses in this age group (e.g. pervasive developmental disorders, hyperkinetic disorders, post-traumatic stress disorders) and the need to find effective interventions for uncommon and difficult conditions (e.g. self-injurious behaviour in children with severe learning difficulties). The role of prevention has become more important, particularly the recognition of precursors of severe conditions (e.g. psychosocial adversities).[18,19] All these issues have implications for service provision and should be considered when deriving appropriate models of care to meet the specific needs for this group of children and adolescents.

The Children Act 1989

Any review of child and adolescent mental health services must consider the major service implications of the changes resulting from the Children Act (1989). Essential principles of the act emphasize the welfare of the child, responsibilities of parents and the broad obligations of local authorities to ensure that children's needs are met. The requirements of the act place new, more complex and urgent demands on CAMHS for assessment, consultation and treatment of individuals and families, as well as greater involvement in the associated administrative and legal proceedings. The service implications of the act must therefore be given full consideration in service planning for child and adolescent mental health.

Child protection

Wider appreciation of the range and nature of child abuse and neglect has led to increased pressure on local authority services to carry out monitoring and co-ordinating functions relating to child protection. The Children Act (1989) has given a new range of statutory responsibilities to local authority social services departments and this has further reduced the capacity of those departments to do therapeutic work with individual families.

The increasing demands on social service resources have led to the withdrawal of social workers from collaborative multi-disciplinary work within child mental health services. This has diminished the efficacy of collaboration between child mental health services that is essential for the welfare of children.

The 1981 Education Act

The 1981 Education Act has led to educational psychologists within school psychological services being increasingly engaged in assessments of special educational need and this has been reinforced by the 1993 Education Act.

The integration of children with mental health problems into normal school and limitations on the number of children receiving special educational needs assessments has led to more children being referred to specialist child mental health services because of emotional and behavioural problems associated with educational failure, bullying and other school-related problems. Previously, educational psychologists were more often engaged in schools and clinics in direct therapeutic programmes for individual children. More recently the Department for Education has produced guidance on the assessment of children with special educational needs and the management of children with emotional and behavioural problems in the education system.[20]

Uncommon and difficult conditions

From time to time children or adolescents require complex, long term and expensive care for uncommon conditions such as severe behaviour disorders associated with epilepsy or challenging behaviour in association with learning difficulties, or autism. There is often confusion or even conflict about the type of service required and failure to agree on the responsible authority, resulting in unacceptable delays in placing the child.

Information

Demographic and related information required to develop services and effective contracts for child and adolescent mental health will need to be obtained from a variety of different sources (Table 1). The task of collecting such data will vary between districts and depends upon quality and accessibility of both computer and library-based information.

Table 1: Source of data for child and adolescent mental health needs assessment

Local data sources	Supplementary data sources
Demographic	Ethnic composition
Ethnic composition	Hospital activity
Mortality	Morbidity
Morbidity	Social Services data
Family and socio-economic data	Socio-economic information
Police and probation	Unemployment
	Family factors
	Criminality

Data are available from a number of written and computer-based sources to provide a background picture of need for services for child and adolescent mental health. This information is by no means comprehensive and will probably require a degree of extrapolation to be used effectively.

The sources of data available can be divided into local data and supplementary data collected at a national, regional or local authority level.

Further details of these data sources can be found in Appendix III. The problems associated with collection and reliability are also identified.

Conclusion

In summary CAMHS deal with a wide range of problems and disorders from minor and self-limiting difficulties through to conditions which result in major disability and may be life-threatening. These conditions occur within a background of individual, family and social risk factors, heightened by disadvantage. There are indications that such problems and disorders are increasing. Adequate management requires a network of multi-disciplinary and flexible services.

Recent legislative and policy changes have resulted in reduced involvement in therapy and care by some professional groups which have traditionally played a major part in this service.

Against this background we proceed to develop the framework for needs assessment for child and adolescent mental health.

4 Sub-categories of child and adolescent mental health problems and disorders

Introduction

There is no single sub-categorization in use in child and adolescent mental health which has been widely adopted and which would be universally accepted by all the professional groups contributing to services. In this chapter we have divided the areas of concern into:

- clinical problems
- disorders
- risk factors

These terms are defined on page 56.

The decision to seek help is often not taken by children or young people themselves but by parents, care givers or other adults. The type of service needed is indicated by the characteristics of the individual problems and disorders, their severity and the exact nature of the risk factors present. It should be re-emphasized that the relevant service may be required from any or all of the statutory agencies (health, social services and education).

This section describes in more detail the sub-categories of problems, disorders and risk factors. Diagnostic examples which may be of use to purchasers of CAMHS are set out with epidemiological evidence in section 5 (Boxes 5, 6 and 7 provide summaries).

Sub-categorization according to need for service

Child and adolescent mental health problems may be grouped according to whether the individual problem is likely to indicate the presence of a severe disorder. However it should be noted that severity depends not only on diagnostic classification but also on individual case characteristics (Box 1), complexity and risk factors.

Common problems with a low risk for a severe disorder

Disturbances of mood or behaviour which are quantitatively different from normal are not necessarily indicators of a severe disorder if they affect only one functional area (e.g. sleep problems or temper tantrums).

In this case they do not necessarily require management by specialist child mental health services. However if they persist or are associated with other problems such as school non-attendance, poor concentration, being bullied or teased, or multiple risk factors they may constitute a disorder and require specialist assessment or intervention.

Common disorders that are not necessarily severe

These relatively common mood and behaviour conditions usually incorporate problems that are quantitatively different from normal. They can be grouped broadly into:

- conduct disorders (e.g. problems of aggression, stealing, non-compliance)[a]
- emotional disorders (e.g. problems of anxiety, depression which do not meet adult diagnostic criteria for mood disorder)
- specific developmental disorders (e.g. problems of language and speech development). A proportion of these disorders are severe and require specialized resources, particularly those persisting beyond five years of age.

These and other disorders not infrequently co-occur in an individual and can often be dealt with satisfactorily by solo professional services. If they are persistent or there are several different risk factors present, multi-disciplinary management will be required.

Less common problems which indicate a severe disorder

Some problems are of particular importance because they point to the possibility of a severe disorder. They will usually require early, specialist CAMHS assessment. These include hallucinations, severe tics, pervasive hyperactivity, symptoms of autism and attempted suicide.

---

[a] Although some can be considered relatively mild, early onset conduct disorders and those associated with hyperactivity and poor peer relationships have a poor prognosis.

Potentially severe disorders

These comprise relatively uncommon disorders where the disturbances of mood and behaviour are qualitatively different from normal. They include:

- pervasive developmental disorders (e.g. autism)
- mental health disorders which meet diagnostic criteria for adult disorders (e.g. eating disorders, schizophrenia and mood disorders).

These disorders need multi-disciplinary specialist CAMHS assessment and may require multi-disciplinary treatment.

Risk factors

The presenting features of mental disorder in children can be associated with one or more risk factors. These add to the complexity of the condition, influence severity and so may determine the nature of the service required. Risk factors can relate to the following.

- **The child** Acute or chronic illness, specific or general learning difficulties, language and other developmental disorder.
- **The family** Parental discord, parental mental health, neglect, child abuse, criminality, economic circumstances.
- **The environment** Overcrowding, homelessness, discrimination
- **Life events** Parental separation, acute illness, bereavement and disasters.
- **School** Bullying, victimization, inappropriate curriculum.

Multiple risk factors point to the need for specialist assessment and treatment. This is of particular importance in places where the prevalence of risk factors such as unemployment, homelessness, single parenthood and drug misuse are high. Intervention to reduce risk factors (e.g. parental postnatal depression) is an important preventive measure. In the absence of child disorder, some risk factors, such as life events, can be dealt with by the family or in primary care.

When risk factors involve relationship dysfunction, or when they are multiple (e.g. abuse and parental mental illness), multi-disciplinary assessment and intervention are likely to be needed.

Relationship between sub-categories and the Children Act 1989

The Children Act 1989 distinguishes the following.

- General needs of children for the promotion of different aspects of their development (emotional, physical, intellectual, social, behavioural and educational).
- Children 'in need' whose development would be impaired without the provision of additional resources by the local authority or health services are thought to comprise some 20% of the population.
- Significant harm which constitutes a threshold for legal action. This comprises either maltreatment by parents or caregivers, or impairment or likelihood of impairment of physical, intellectual, emotional, social or behavioural development that is attributable to the care given to the child. The child may also be beyond parental control.

The act confirms the general need for the support for all children in their development. Any child with significant or long-standing problems or with a recognized mental health disorder is 'in need'. Recent research confirms that services should address children 'in need' and not just those experiencing significant harm.[21]

Relationship between sub-categories and primary, secondary and tertiary prevention

Primary prevention aims to reduce risk factors and prevent the development of problems. This is of potential benefit to all children.

Secondary prevention aims at early detection of problems, with a view to effective intervention and prevention of recurrence or escalation. This is of benefit to children with problems and disorders, or to those exposed to risk factors which are amenable to treatment.

Tertiary prevention seeks to alleviate or minimize the disability associated with a disorder. It is of benefit to children with more serious disorders which cannot be completely eliminated.

5 Prevalence

Introduction

This section reviews the prevalence of child and adolescent mental health problems, disorders and risk factors and is set out in three main groups consistent with the definitions and sub-categories described in sections 2 and 4; clinical problems (Box 5), disorders (Box 6) and risk factors (Box 7). It is important to understand that children and adolescents presenting to services in an average district will have a variety of problems but that the majority tend to fall into two broad groups of conduct or emotional difficulties. The severity of these problems and disorders and the extent to which they are associated with risk factors will determine the level of service required for each child.

General features

Among three year olds in an urban community the prevalence of moderate to severe mental health disorders is 7% and the prevalence of mild disorders is 15%.[22] In an older population the overall prevalence of child and adolescent mental health disorders has been estimated at 12% in children aged 9–11 in rural areas (Isle of Wight) and 25% in ten year olds in inner London.[23] Amongst adolescents higher rates have been found. Although these figures seem high, in practice only about 10% of those with disorders are seen by specialist services. Referral levels are influenced by society's and primary health care professionals' perceptions of mental health problems. They are also influenced by the availability of services. As would be expected the highest proportion of referrals are for children with more severe problems.

Differences in overall prevalence between these and other surveys are usually due to the characteristics of the target sample, the sampling method, case definition and assessment procedures.[24–26]

A broad indication of overall prevalence of symptoms, disorders and risk factors is shown in Box 4.[27,28] These figures include the full range of conditions from the very mild to severe, not all of which will need specialist care.

These wide ranges of prevalence also reflect differences among populations relating to characteristics such as age, sex, ethnic distribution and whether the population is from a rural or urban setting. Other important associated factors include social class distribution and levels of deprivation. The prevalences act as a broad indication which should be adapted to meet the characteristics of particular local populations.

Box 4: Overall prevalence of child and adolescent mental health problems, disorders and risk factors

Problems	5 – 40%
Disorders	5 – 25%
Risk Factors	5 – 40%

Age and sex

In general, the prevalence of disorders is lower in the younger age group than in the older group and higher in boys than girls, although girls begin to overtake during adolescence.[29]

Ethnic differences

Data from various studies show that the prevalence and presentation of child psychiatric disorder varies between ethnic groups.[30–32] The presence and pattern of variation is not constant across subgroups or across individual disorders.

Culture can influence the presentation of psychiatric disturbance in a number of ways. Idioms of distress appear to be culturally determined in adults, such as reactive excitation in Afro–Caribbean people[33] and somatization in people of Pakistani origin.[34] Culture may also affect the presentation of emotional disorders in children and influence the way parents interpret their children's behaviour and what action they take when they consider it abnormal.

Studies in the UK suggest that children of Asian origin appear to have comparable or slightly lower rates of psychiatric disorder than white children.[31,32,35,36] There are no recent studies giving adequate estimates of prevalence across all ages in the different ethnic groups in the UK.

Incidence

Assessing incidence in child and adolescent mental health is difficult as the majority of disorders that are sufficiently severe to be dealt with by specialist services are long standing and chronic. However there are some circumstances which require an acute response (e.g. attempted suicide, drug overdose, acute psychosis and reactions to life and traumatic events, and children refusing treatment on paediatric wards). Self-harm, anorexia and child abuse carry the greatest threat to life. As numbers for suicide, death from anorexia, abuse and undetermined death are small, mortality data are not particularly helpful as indicators of need for services.

Epidemiology of problems

This is summarized in Box 5.

Nocturnal enuresis

Rutter et al. found 6.7% of seven year old boys and 3.3% of girls were wet more than one night a week.[37] A study of seven year old children found that 8% of children experienced night wetting.[38] A study of 14 year olds found 1.1% of boys and 0.5% of girls to be wet at least one night a week.[37]

Box 5: Prevalence of specific child and adolescent mental health problems[a]

• Nocturnal enuresis	8% of seven year old children 1% of 14 year old children
• Sleep difficulties	13% of London three year olds have persistent difficulty settling at night 14% of London three year olds wake persistently during the night
• Feeding difficulties in children	12–34% among pre-school children
• Abdominal pain without organic cause	10% in five to ten year olds
• Severe tantrums	5% of three year olds in an urban community
• Simple phobias	2.3–9.2% of children
• Tic disorders	1–13% of boys and 1–11% of girls
• Educational difficulty	specific reading retardation – 3.9% (Isle of Wight) and 9.9% (London) of ten year olds general reading backwardness – 8.3% (Isle of Wight) and 19% (London) of ten year olds

[a]Greater detail can be found in the text. Not all specific problems are represented in this box

Sleep difficulties

A study of three year old London children found that 13% had difficulty settling at night with 14% waking during the night.[22]

Feeding difficulties in young children

The prevalence of feeding problems generally among pre-school children is estimated at between 12 and 34%.[39]

Abdominal pain without organic cause

This is a common complaint in children with one study finding it occurred in 10% of 5–10 year olds.[40] Another study reported symptoms in one-third of young children persisting into adulthood.[41]

Severe tantrums in young children

Severe temper tantrums have been found in 5% of three year olds in an urban community.[22]

Simple phobias

Persistent disabling fears of specific objects or situations such as dogs or the dark occur in 2.3–9.2% of children.[26]

Tic disorders

Transient tic behaviours are commonplace among children. Community surveys indicate that 1–13% of boys and 1–11% of girls manifest frequent 'tics, twitches, mannerisms or habit spasms'.[42] Children between the ages of seven and 11 years appear to have the highest prevalence rates (5%) with the male to female ratio less than 2 : 1 in most community surveys (see also page 68).

Educational difficulty

In the Isle of Wight study,[43] specific reading retardation (SRR) (i.e. reading performance significantly below what could be expected on the basis of both age and intelligence) was found to affect 3.9% of ten year olds. General reading backwardness (GRB) (i.e. performance specifically below what could be expected on the basis of age) affected 8.3%. In the comparable inner London study the respective rates were double; at 9.9% SRR and 19% GRB.[44]

Epidemiology of disorders

This is summarized in Box 6.

Emotional disorders with onset specific to childhood

These disorders include anxiety and other emotional disorders not fitting adult diagnostic criteria. The estimated prevalence of emotional disorders in population-based studies varies from 4.5% of ten year old children living in small town communities (estimated from Rutter *et al.*[23]) to 5.4%[45] or 8.7%[46] for anxiety disorders, with rates of 9.9% in inner-city areas.[23] They commonly represent 25–33% of clinic attenders.

Major depression

Uncertainties surrounding the concept of depression in young people and unstandardized methods of assessment led to huge variations in the reported rates of depressive disorder. However by using standard diagnostic criteria together with more comparable methods of data collection, it has been estimated that the point prevalence for major depression is 0.5–2.5% among children and 2–8% among adolescents.[9]

Conduct disorders

The overall prevalence of conduct disorder is 6.2% among ten year olds, with the rate in boys four times higher than that in girls.[23] When similar methods were used in a relatively poor area of London the rate of conduct disorder was 10.8%.[23] 33–50% of clinic attenders have oppositional, conduct or mixed conduct and emotional disorders.

More recently the Ontario Child Health Survey has provided a comprehensive picture of conduct disorder in the general population.[47,48] The overall rate of conduct disorder in a mixed urban and rural area (5.5%) was similar to the rate reported 25 years earlier in the Isle of Wight study. Although the male to female ratio was similar, no difference between urban and rural areas was found in this part of Canada. This was interpreted as showing the importance of socio-economic status with the effect of geographical area diminishing when the degree of poverty in the different contexts was taken into account.

Box 6: Prevalence of specific child and adolescent mental health disorders[a]

• Emotional disorders with onset in childhood	4.5–9.9% of ten year olds 25–33% amongst clinic attenders
• Major depression	0.5–2.5% among children 2–8% among adolescents
• Conduct disorders	6.2–10.8% among ten year olds 33–50% amongst clinic attenders
• Multiple tic disorders	1–2%
• Obsessive compulsive disorder	1.9% of adolescents
• Hyperkinetic disorder	1.7% of primary school boys 1 in 200 in the whole population suffer severe hyperkinetic disorders Up to 17% at least some hyperkinetic problems
• Encopresis (faecal soiling)	2.3% of boys and 0.7% of girls aged 7–8 years 1.3% of boys and 0.3% of girls aged 11–12 years
• Eating disorders – anorexia nervosa	0.2–1% of 12–19 year olds 8–11 times more common in girls
– bulimia nervosa	2.5% of 13–18 year old girls and boys
• Attempted suicide	2–4% of adolescents
• Suicide	7.6 per 100 000 15–19 year olds
• Substance misuse	no figures available for effect on mental health. See text for level of use

[a]Greater detail can be found in the text. Not all disorders are represented in this box

Multiple tic disorders

Many children have simple tics (page 67) although when they are multiple and persistent, they have a serious impact on the child's education and social life. The prevalence has been estimated as 1–2% of the general population.[49]

Obsessive compulsive disorders

Figures from recent studies suggest that the weighted prevalence of obsessive compulsive disorder among adolescents is 1.9%.[50,51]

Hyperkinetic disorders

The reported prevalence of hyperactivity varies greatly. This depends predominantly on whether the problem is confined to one setting such as school or is pervasive across settings. Surveys of teachers or parents suggest figures of 17% in primary school boys.[52] The International Classification of Diseases (ICD) definition for hyperkinetic disorder includes pervasiveness and for this the prevalence is 1.7% among primary school boys. After allowing for gender differences and geographical variation, these figures imply a prevalence of one in 200 in the whole population for severe hyperkinetic disorders, with situational hyperactivity which may be part of a conduct disorder, being much more common.

Encopresis

Encopresis (faecal soiling) is found in 1.5% of children between seven and eight years of age, (boys 2.3% and girls 0.7%).[53] Rutter *et al.* found that 1.3% of boys and 0.3% of girls aged 11–12 soil at least once a month.[43]

Eating disorders

Incidence and prevalence figures for anorexia nervosa and bulimia nervosa vary among studies due to different case definitions and diagnostic criteria, as well as a lack of homogeneity among the groups surveyed.[51]

For anorexia nervosa the majority of studies reporting prevalence figures suggest that 0.2–1% of the 12–19 year old population is affected. It is 8–11 times more common in females than males.[54]

For bulimia nervosa one study suggests a reported lifetime prevalence of 2.5% among 13–18 year old boys and girls. It is more common than anorexia nervosa, peaks at about 19 years of age and is far more common in girls than boys. Bulimic patients are under-represented in clinical samples of eating-disordered adolescent patients.[55]

Attempted suicide

In US studies reported lifetime suicide attempts have been estimated at 9% of adolescents and 1% of preadolescents.[56–58] The figure for French-Canadian 12–18 year olds is 3.5%, for Dutch 14–20 year olds 2.2% and Swedish 13–18 year olds 4%. The figure for adolescents in the UK is likely to be about 2–4%.

Suicide

Suicide in childhood and early adolescence (up to the age of 15) is uncommon[39] but it increases markedly in the late teens and early twenties. In 1989 in the UK the suicide rate for children aged 5–14 years was 0.8 per 100 000 and among 15–19 year olds, 7.6 per 100 000, with suicide being more common in boys.[60]

Substance misuse

There is little information on the effect of substance misuse on the mental health of children and adolescents. Figures are generally related to the level of use of different substances. In the UK just over one-fifth of 11–15 year old children said that they had an alcoholic drink in the previous week.[61] There are high levels of regular consumption and experimentation with solvents, cannabis and more recently hallucinogens. 16% of 16 year olds regularly use solvents and illegal drugs.[62] 3–5% of 11–16 year olds have used cannabis with this figure rising to 17% in older teenagers.[63,64] However very few have been involved in regular consumption of minor tranquillizers[65–67] with less than 1% having used heroin and cocaine.[68,69]

Epidemiology of risk factors

It should be noted that overall prevalence rates for disorder reflect the impact of risk factors in individual cases. Some of the risk factors are summarized in Box 7.

Box 7: Prevalence of specific child and adolescent mental health risk factors and impact on rate of mental disorder[a]

Risk factors in child	Impact on rate of disorder
• Physical illness – chronic health problems – brain damage	three times increase in rate 4–8 times increase in rate of disorder in youngsters with cerebral palsy, epilepsy or other disorder above the brainstem
• Sensory impairments – hearing impairment four per 1000 – visual impairment 0.6 per 1000	2.5–3 times more disorder no figures but rate of disorder thought to be raised
• Learning difficulties	2–3 times increase in rate, higher in severe than moderate learning difficulties
• Language and related problems – 2%, but better methods of identifying required	four times rate of disorder

Risk factors in the family	Impact on rate of disorder
• Family breakdown – divorce affects one in four children under 16 years of age – severe marital discord	associated with a significant increase in disorders e.g. depression and anxiety
• Family size	large family size associated with increased rate of conduct disorder and delinquency in boys
• Parental mental illness – schizophrenia – maternal psychiatric disorder	eight to ten times rate of schizophrenia 1.2 to four times the rate of disorder
• Parental criminality	two to three times rate of delinquency
• Physical and emotional abuse – of those on child protection registers, one in four suffer physical abuse and one in eight neglect	twice rate of disorder if physically abused and thrice if neglected
• Sexual abuse – 6–62% in girls and 3–31% in boys	twice rate of disorder if sexually abused

Environmental risk factors	Impact on rate of disorder
• Socio-economic circumstances	(see text)
• Unemployment	(see text)
• Housing and homelessness	(see text)
• School environment	9% in grades one to nine are victims of bullying 7–8% of children have self-reported bullying of other children

Life events	Impact on rate of disorder
• Traumatic events	three to five times rate of disorder. Rises with recurrent adversities

[a]Not all specific risk factors are represented in this box

Risk factors in the child

Physical illness

- **Chronic health problems** A consistent finding in general population surveys is the increased rate of mental health and adjustment problems in children with chronic health problems, as compared with their healthy peers.[70–72] Children with chronic medical conditions and associated disability (limitations of usual childhood activities) are at more than three-fold risk for disorders and at considerable risk for social adjustment problems. Children with chronic medical conditions but no disability are at considerably less risk.[73]

  Knowledge about the causal mechanisms involved in producing the association between chronic health problems and psychological and social morbidity is incomplete. Possible mediating factors include low self-esteem, poor peer relationships and poor school performance.[73]

- **Brain dysfunction** In the Isle of Wight study the rate of disorder was increased four to eight times in youngsters with cerebral palsy, epilepsy or some other disorder above the brainstem.[74,75] Several studies indicate that brain damage or dysfunction puts children at risk for disorder in general with some increased association with hyperkinetic and pervasive developmental disorders.[74,76,77]

Sensory impairments

- **Hearing impairment** Approximately one in 1000 children has moderate to profound congenital and bilateral early onset hearing impairment,[78] rising to four in 1000 if acquired losses are included.[79] The prevalence of disorder in this group is 2.5–3 times that seen in a control group.[80–82]

- **Visual impairment** 0.3 per 1000 blind and partially sighted children at six years and 0.6 per 1000 at 11 years have been recorded in the 1958 National Child Development study. This is often compounded with additional impairments such as cerebral palsy, epilepsy and hearing impairment.[83]

Specific and general learning difficulties

The needs of children with learning difficulties have been assessed in a separate report.[84]

Children who do poorly at school, whether because of low IQ or a specific learning disorder, are at increased risk of disorder. This may be as high as 40%.[85]

The increased risk applies for a wide range of conditions, including conduct disorder,[43] delinquency,[86] hyperactivity,[87,88] depressive symptoms in adolescents,[89–95] child-reported anxiety disorders, over-anxious disorder[96] and self-reported anxiety symptoms in 11 year old girls.[97] The mechanisms by which poor school performance leads to increased rates of disorder have been investigated most fully in conduct disorder.

Language and related problems

In a longitudinal study conducted by Fundulis *et al.* the prevalence of developmental language disorder was estimated at 2%.[81] They varied in complexity and severity, the most severe requiring specialist teaching and speech therapy during school years.

However better ways of identifying children whose language impairments are truly handicapping are required. In three year olds the prevalence of behaviour problems amongst those with language delay was four times that of the general population and predicted educational difficulty at age eight.[98] Other studies have produced comparable estimates across a wide age range.[99,100]

Risk factors in the family

Family breakdown

Poor parenting, marital discord and family dysfunction have all been associated with an increased rate of disorder in children.[101] For example harsh and inconsistent parenting,[102] coercive interchanges between parent and child[103] and marital discord[104–106] are all associated with antisocial behaviour in children.

Many different factors and processes contribute to higher rates of disorder among children whose parents have separated or divorced. These include exposure to parental discord both before and after the family break up, involvement in parental disagreement and changes in family circumstances. For example if the parent with custody is emotionally distressed following the separation, then the child's behaviour may lead to critical and hostile parental responses that only serve to make the child more disturbed. These processes contribute to a prevalence of disorders as high as 80% in the first year after divorce. A US national survey showed that adolescents whose parents separated and divorced by the time the children were seven years old were three times as likely to have received psychotherapy as those from an intact family.[107]

A recent community survey of 15–20 year old girls in London confirmed that parental separation/divorce was associated with increased risk of psychiatric disorder[108] and that the quality of a mother's marriage was associated with the presence of depression and anxiety disorders.[109]

According to the General Household Survey divorce rates in England and Wales have increased markedly in the last few decades, partly as a result of legislation changes.[110] The number of persons divorcing per 1000 married people per annum rose from 9.5 in 1971, to 12 in 1980, to 13 in 1990. Haskey has estimated that if the divorce rates stabilize at the current levels, 37% of marriages will end in divorce.[111] Kiernan and Wickes suggest that divorce now affects one in four children before the age of 16.[112]

Family size

Large family size (usually four or more children) has been associated with increased rates of conduct disorder and delinquency in boys,[80,102] but not in girls.[113] The results of the Farrington and West study of inner-city boys indicate that large family size is related to antisocial behaviour and delinquency, independent of sociodemographic and parental factors.[102]

Parental mental illness

Evidence suggests that mental disorder, particularly personality disorder in either parent, is associated with increased rates of child psychopathology.[114] There is emerging evidence that specific parental psychiatric disorders are associated with increased rates of particular childhood disorders. For instance parental alcoholism and antisocial behaviour are associated with increased rates of conduct disorder and depressive symptoms and disorder (especially in the adolescent age group). Also parental anxiety disorders are associated with increased rates of anxiety disorders, particularly separation anxiety disorder (SAD).[115,116]

From a genetic perspective, children born to a schizophrenic parent have an elevated and specific risk of approximately 8–10 times for developing the disorder during their lifetime.[117]

Children whose mothers suffer from a psychiatric disorder have a 1.2–4 times increased risk of mental health problems (estimated from Rutter et al.[23]).

Parental criminality

Evidence suggests that parental criminality is particularly associated with disorders of conduct and delinquency in children.[101,118] The strength of the association increases if both parents have a criminal record, if they are recidivist and if their crime record extends into the period of child rearing.[119,120]

The association may be contributed to by personality abnormalities in parents such as excessive drinking or persistent aggression, modelling of deviant behaviour and child rearing that is neglectful, lacking in supervision or includes cruelty or hostility towards children.[86,119,121,122] A genetic predisposition is considered to be at least a partial explanation.[123]

Rutter has estimated that children of parents involved with crime have a 2–3 times increased risk of delinquency.[j]

Abuse/neglect

- **Physical and emotional child abuse** 4% of children up to the age of 12 are brought to the attention of professional agencies (social services departments or the National Society for the Prevention of Cruelty to Children) because of suspected abuse each year. In England in 1988, 3.5 per 1000 children below the age of 18 years were on child protection registers and more than a quarter of these were in the care of local authorities.[124] There were 24 500 additions to the register in England in 1992.[21] About one in four of those on child protection registers had suffered physical abuse and one in eight neglect. The largest proportion – one third – were subjects of grave concern, a term that often indicates another child in the family is known to have been abused. Exact figures on mortality from child abuse are unknown in the UK; a figure of at least one in 100 000 may be an underestimate.

  Young children who have been exposed to physical abuse and those exposed to neglect have twice and three times the risk of mental health problems respectively.[125]

- **Sexual abuse** The incidence of child sexual abuse is defined as the proportion of a population that has experienced it at any time during childhood. There is wide variation – from 6 to 62% in females and 3 to 31% in males – in quoted rates.[126] Categorization of sexually abusive experiences according to their severity (e.g. whether involving sexual contact) indicates that severe abuse has been experienced by 5% of women and 2% of men.[127] Children who have suffered sexual abuse have twice the risk of mental health problems.[125]

Environmental risk factors

Socio-economic circumstances

The strength of the relationship between social class and child disorder is dependent on both the measurement of social class and the measurement of disorder. If occupational prestige is used to operationalize social class, then there is a weak or non-existent relationship between it and child disorder.[22,80,128,129,130] In contrast when social class is measured in terms of economic disadvantage, then there is a strong and consistent relationship between it and child disorder.[47,48,131,132]

Unemployment

Banks and Jackson have shown that in the years after leaving school, older teenagers who had failed to find a job showed more psychiatric symptoms than those in employment.[133] The specific risk in crimes involving material gain among the unemployed suggests that the relative poverty associated with unemployment is an important mediating factor.[134]

Housing and homelessness

The links between quality of housing and child mental health has been reviewed by Quinton.[135] Living in the upper floors of high-rise accommodation, where supervision of the child's play is inevitably more difficult, is associated with depression in the mothers of young children.[136]

The deleterious effects of homelessness in families with children have been reviewed by Alperstein and Arnstein.[137] Uncontrolled studies of children living in homeless families accommodation (hotels, hostels, etc.) have revealed very high rates of developmental delay as well as emotional and behavioural problems.[138] Parents have high rates of depression.

School environment

Children spend a minimum of some 15 000 hours in school. It is therefore not surprising that experiences in school, such as bullying and pressure for academic achievement together with overall school ethos can influence the rate of childhood disorder.

Wolkind and Rutter have summarized three major aspects of schools which influence behaviour: the composition of the student body; the qualities of the school as a social organization and the efficiency of classroom management techniques.[139] If many children in the school have poor behaviour and attainment this is likely to be a consequence of poor organization and unclear discipline, lack of recognition of children as individuals, high teacher turnover and low morale.

One problem faced by children at school is bullying. A study from Norway suggests that 9% of children in grades 1–9 are victims of regular bullying and that 7–8% self-reported bullying other children.[140]

Life events

The impact of certain life events on a child or adolescent can have a varied effect on psychological well-being. Not all life events are stressors. This depends on characteristics of the event such as the social context and on the child's previous experiences.

Single traumatic events

There is evidence that life events can play a significant part in precipitating a wide range of childhood disorders.[6,7] Studies of one-off disasters which are outside normal experience indicate that they can result in reactions which are the distinctive manifestations of post-traumatic stress disorder but other disorders such as depression may also be precipitated.[2,141–143] The risk of disorder may be increased 3–5 times and rise to 100 times if there have been three recent adversities.[144]

Other life events include bereavement. In 1984 it was estimated that 3.7% of US children under the age of 18 had lost a parent.[145] Adults bereaved as children approximately double their risk of developing depression, especially if they experience a subsequent loss.[146,147] Factors that modify the outcome are reviewed by Black and include age (younger is worse), sex (girls seem more vulnerable), mode of death (sudden deaths and violent ones such as suicide or murder are associated with worse outcome) and subsequent experiences (good care lessens the risk).[148] It was concluded that bereaved children are more likely to develop disorders in childhood and in adult life, although the risk is small. Children most at risk are those bereaved young and those whose surviving parent has a prolonged grief reaction.

6 Current child and adolescent mental health services

Introduction

In this section the current variety of services available for children and adolescents with mental health problems is described. This is quantified using information from a recent national survey and highlights the different types of services available and the present staffing levels of relevant professionals.[149] There is considerable variation in available CAHMS resources in different districts.

The main service activities involve assessment, treatment, consultation/liaison, training and research. These are undertaken in community clinics, child guidance, adolescent and 'drop-in' clinics, outpatient, day-patient and inpatient services. Five types of response to child and adolescent mental health problems are described. These are:

- informal care
- primary care
- the child and adolescent mental health service: care by solo professionals
- the child and adolescent mental health service: multi-disciplinary care
- supra-district specialist multi-disciplinary care.

The pattern of care is variable across the country and several extremely successful models exist. For example solo professional care may be delivered from a unidisciplinary service or from a multi-disciplinary team. It should be noted that it is usual for any one specialist child and adolescent mental health professional to contribute to several types of care, e.g. supporting primary health care, solo, multi-disciplinary and supra-district care.

All specialist CAMHS involve professional activity outside the main professional base. This includes home and school visits for assessment or treatment purposes, attendance at child protection case conferences convened by social services and attendance at court.

It must be remembered that most child and adolescent mental health difficulties are dealt with through informal or primary care. These two areas are not covered in the recent survey and there is little additional information available from other sources.

Informal care

Single problems which are short-lived, mild and produce minimal social impairment are often dealt with entirely informally by family, friends or teachers. Examples include emotional reactions to life events, such as school entry or minor illness.

Primary care

Single problems with a low risk for severe disorder (with or without minor risk factors, see page 62) are dealt with by primary care professionals. Such problems include uncomplicated nocturnal enuresis, some general behavioural problems, feeding and sleep problems. Risk factors include overcrowding, isolation, mild parental mental health or relationship difficulties. Some general practitioners (GPs), paediatricians and health visitors have had additional specialist training in child mental health and are able to provide a service intermediate between that generally available in primary health care and specialist child mental health services.

Current status of services in primary care

Existing services vary widely across the country. Primary health care services exist in all districts, but there are often unfilled posts amongst health visitors, school nurses or community medical officers, especially in inner-city areas. Health visitors or community paediatricians with additional training in assessment and treatment of child mental health problems are present in some districts. Pilot programmes, often supported by research funds, have not always been sustained following the cessation of start-up or research funding.[150] A child development programme from Bristol is being used by many health authorities in the UK.[151] It involves a training programme for health visitors to become more aware of mental health and social problems of families they see and to help parents find their own solutions to their child rearing problems. A booklet on child mental health problems has recently been made available to all GPs in England and Wales.[152]

The child and adolescent mental health service for a population of 250 000

Solo professional care

Children with common disorders that are not necessarily severe (page 62) occurring in association with one or two risk factors need specialist care. This is often dealt with by a specialist professional (who need not be a psychiatrist) acting alone or in collaboration with primary or general paediatric care, provided that the risk factors fall within the professional's specific expertise. Examples include some children with emotional and behavioural disorders or those associated with acute and chronic physical illness, feeding difficulties and specific educational difficulty. Services may be provided by child mental health service professionals, educational psychologists and social workers or by adult psychiatrists and paediatricians who have received additional relevant training, particularly those working in the community. Solo professional care may be provided by professionals based in a multi-disciplinary group or based on a unidisciplinary service that works in a co-ordinated fashion with the multi-disciplinary service.

A less common problem which indicates a severe disorder (page 62) and common disorders that are severe and/or with multiple risk factors (page 62) will require multi-disciplinary assessment.

Multi-disciplinary care

Children with disorders comprising particularly persistent single problems, or multiple problems with several aspects of dysfunction (page 62) commonly need multi-disciplinary specialist assessment and treatment (including a child and adolescent psychiatrist), with outpatient or sometimes day unit treatment provision. Such care is also needed for children and adolescents with less common problems which indicate a severe disorder and those with potentially severe disorders (page 62). These disorders will usually be associated with major risk factors and be of long duration (three months or more). They are likely to continue if there is no intervention. For example a child with a hyperkinetic conduct disorder, who is not compliant, shows aggression to peers, has educational problems and experiences family discord, would need such management. Other examples include children and adolescents with schizophrenia or obsessive-compulsive disorders, who will require such care at some stage.

Some services run by education and social services (special schools and family units) also aim to meet this type of need. They are usually supported by specialist child mental health professionals.

Range of child and adolescent mental health services: solo professional and multi-disciplinary care

Dedicated child and adolescent mental health services within districts can include the following.

- A full range of non-residential solo professional and multi-disciplinary assessment and treatment services, including emergency cover for self-harm and other urgent conditions.
- Health day-patient facilities for children with mental health problems to complement facilities provided by educational and social services.
- A service for adolescents which may include a more directly accessible and age-appropriate component, e.g. a walk-in facility.
- Consultation and liaison services for other agencies concerned with children and adolescents. Examples include:
  a) schools, including special schools
  b) social services, especially observation and assessment centres, day nurseries and child protection services
  c) primary health care, including general practice, health visitors and school nursing
  d) specialist health services: adult psychiatry, adult clinical psychology, paediatrics including community paediatrics, child development teams and learning difficulty services
  e) voluntary agencies, e.g. NSPCC, Newpin and Home-start, and in particular, any residential or day care establishment for children and adolescents.
- Facilitation, support and training for voluntary organizations, e.g. befriending schemes and self-help groups.
- Training and collaboration with agencies listed under consultation and liaison services (a)–e) above) and to the general public.
- Administration and monitoring of the service using appropriate secretarial staff and computing.
- Admission of some children and adolescents with mental health problems to health facilities for assessment and/or treatment, e.g. paediatric wards.
- Access to services appropriate to meet the need for specialist multi-disciplinary care for populations of around one million in national centres.

Multi-disciplinary services involve closely co-ordinated assessment and treatment by fully trained child and adolescent psychiatrists, child and adolescent clinical psychologists, child psychiatric nurses, social workers and child psychotherapists, with ready access to other professional colleagues such as paediatricians, speech and language therapists, occupational therapists and teachers.

Figures for these services and the present recommended staffing levels are described on pages 78, 95 and 113.

Supra-district specialist multi-disciplinary care

Children with major mental disorders such as schizophrenia, bi-polar affective disorder, obsessive compulsive disorder, anorexia nervosa, bulimia and complex cases of autism receive care in specialist inpatient units or tertiary outpatient referral centres, with moderate to close geographical accessibility.

Severe conduct disorders also receive this provision if there is an associated mood disorder or self-injurious behaviour or factors such as epilepsy, requiring inpatient assessment. However children with uncomplicated severe conduct disorders requiring residential provision may be placed in a residential school or social service units with education.

National centres

Highly specialized services based around multi-disciplinary assessment and treatment are used for a small number of children with complex neuropsychiatric problems associated with severe behavioural disturbance, those with severe behavioural disorders who require containment within secure units and those with certain rare conditions such as gender identity problems or profound sensory problems with associated psychiatric disorders.

Current service status for child and adolescent mental health services

The following information is a summary of the findings from a recent survey of services for the mental health of children and young people in the UK.[149] It looks at purchasing authorities and the various aspects of child and adolescent services, including community-based care, inpatient and special units, day treatment services, clinical psychology services, paediatric services, social services, education and the non-voluntary sector. Further details including figures from the survey are described in Appendix IV.

- The matching of provision to local needs has hardly begun and purchasers are still dependent on what the local units say they are providing.
- The specialist child and adolescent mental health services are largely delivered from a community base, by means of inter-disciplinary teams. Psychiatrists and psychiatric social workers are almost universally members of these teams, although the number of social workers has reduced in the past three years. In this period there has been both expansion and reduction of services in different parts of the country. However the overall provision of service has remained roughly the same. Changes appear to have been somewhat arbitrary, often based on local enthusiasm or on enforced reorganization in local authority services. Numbers of staff and the range of skills available vary widely. There is little input from the education sector.
- There is major variation in the distribution of child and adolescent psychiatrists across the country and in the type of work they undertake.
- Clinical psychology is a growing profession, working increasingly from an independent base. Clinical psychologists still work mainly with the child and adolescent mental health teams, but they also provide direct solo and consultative services to acute and community services in other parts of the NHS, to social services and other agencies.
- Almost two-thirds of mental health services for children now employ a psychiatric community nurse. However few nurses have training in children's and adolescents' psychiatric care and many seem to rely on skills acquired on short random courses.
- Many inpatient units, including former regional adolescent units, are experiencing problems particularly with respect to the new system of contracting for services.
- More children with emotional and behavioural disorder present to paediatricians than to any other profession. Paediatricians' training in the main does not prepare them for this and they would welcome further opportunities to gain relevant experience.
- Local education authorities are greatly concerned with emotional and behavioural difficulties in their pupils.
- Behaviour support services, as currently provided in three-quarters of local education authorities, include assessment of the educational needs of pupils with severe behaviour problems, but infrequently no relevant medical contribution is included. Special schools for children with emotional and behavioural difficulties report that few pupils have statements in which therapeutic help is specified, although the head teachers consider that nearly half of all pupils would benefit from such help.

- The educational psychology services state that part of their function is to work with individual children whose behaviour is causing concern, but most find that assessment activity takes up most of their time. Although all services agree that joint work should make a major contribution to the management of problems in children, education authorities limit their staff resources for collaborative work.
- Social services departments concentrate resources on children in need, many of whom have serious emotional and behavioural problems. They report unsatisfactory access to specialist expertise in children's mental health from the NHS.
- The voluntary sector plays a large part at primary care level, particularly in providing services such as counselling. They often take self-referrals. Voluntary organizations also act as a filter to specialist mental health and social services. Since the NHS mental health services accept self-referrals less and less, the voluntary services may be filling a gap in provision. Some voluntary services such as the NSPCC, Barnardos and NCH offer particular expertise of value also for secondary and tertiary provision.

Assessment, management and treatment procedures

To respond to the mental health needs of their patients, child and adult mental health services initiate a variety of assessment, management and treatment procedures. The diversity of these activities is illustrated in Box 8 which shows the broad categories of treatment, investigations and case management undertaken by services. Because of the complexity of needs dealt with, several of these investigative, treatment and care-related procedures will be implemented concurrently or sequentially during an individual care episode.

Box 8: Range of assessment, management and treatment procedures

```
Assessment
Limited involvement
Individual treatments – child/young person
Physical illness management
Group procedures – child/young person
Work with parents
Family/marital therapy
Community visits
Collaborative work (non-team/service member)
Referral out of team/unit for opinion/non collaborative management during episode
Tests and investigations
Reports
Attending meetings and formal procedures
Consultation
Status change/extension during episode (e.g. switch to inpatient care)
Clinical trial/experimental interventions
```

Source: [15]

The information in Box 8 does not detail many of the more specific forms of treatment, investigations and other procedures that have been developed, for instance the variety of medications to deal with anxiety or hyperactivity or the variants of family, psychotherapeutic and behaviourally-based therapies among others. Further it does not list the activities aimed at larger scale prevention or those aimed at the enhancement of practice and the quality of services through training of both service staff and the staffs of other agencies.

Finally services are also involved in the conduct of clinical and service-relevant research recognized as important activities for child and adolescent mental health services.

The activities listed in Box 8 can be grouped into a number of major forms of service which are undertaken in fully resourced and staffed services.

Assessment

Child and adolescent mental health services provide a number of specialist assessments as a basis for treatment or for other purposes:

- The establishment of 'caseness'. The referrer wishes to establish whether the individual has problems that constitute a mental health disorder, but does not request the assessor to undertake treatment.
- Second opinion requests. The referrer requests confirmation of a diagnosis and will deal with the ensuing needs.
- Conventional assessments to inform treatment and management within the service. Such assessments can be fairly rapid or may need to develop over time. Sometimes these include the clinical assessment of complex problems such as neuropsychiatric disorders.
- Complex assessments are those usually carried out for the courts, social services or other agencies. They require detailed information, usually culminating in a long report and consume substantial amounts of professional time. These assessments may not lead to treatment by the service. Most commonly requests for such assessments are from social services or the courts and arise because of proceedings under the Children Act. (Adequate assessment involves not just formal diagnostic categorization of the disorder, but full formulation of the problems including establishment of predisposing, precipitating and maintaining factors, prognosis and plans for intervention.)

Consultation/liaison

Parents, carers and agencies involved in looking after children and young people often need to discuss issues related to referral, diagnosis and management with specialist mental health services without wishing the case to be taken on by the child and adolescent mental health service. The processes of consultation are well-established.[153] In these instances the 'consultant' works with staff who have direct contact with the patient or patients. The individual patient may not be seen during the consultation, although he or she may be known to the service. Such work can be a more effective use of resources in dealing with the individual child or groups of children. In these instances the consultant works with staff (e.g. in schools or children's homes) who have direct contact.

Some services also provide psychiatric, psychological and psychotherapeutic input to paediatric and other wards to assist in diagnosis, management or treatment.[154]

Treatment and management

It is not always easy to differentiate assessment and treatment since the act of referral or even the recognition that a referral to specialist services is needed can initiate changes, as can the first meetings with clinic services even when no systematic attempt is made to produce change.

Interventions involve the use of recognized procedures aimed at removing, reducing or containing symptomatology and achieving a more constructive adaptation and healthy development. Since the symptomatology is invariably expressed in or influenced by the family or school, work with other family members and teachers is essential. Other adults and children may also be involved e.g. club leaders and class peers. There are several further goals of intervention as follows.

- To help clients and relevant responsible adults develop an understanding of the problems and the mechanisms of treatment so that they can anticipate and avert relapse.
- To deal with the symptomatology and contributing context in such a way that interference with the ordinary life and on-going functioning of patient, family or other carers is minimized.
- To prevent the emergence of other difficulties.
- To enhance the quality of psychosocial functioning, present and future.

Emergency services

Many child and adolescent psychiatrists and some multi-disciplinary teams provide emergency input to hospital A and E and paediatric departments dealing with psychiatric emergencies in children and young people. Most commonly these are instances of self-harm or attempted self-harm.

Training

Part of the skill and knowledge base of mental health professionals can be taught to individuals (for instance teachers, nursery staff and social workers) who have non-specialist responsibilities for dealing with mental health needs. Requests for training will sometimes emerge following consultation or may arise directly from other agencies such as day nurseries, social services or schools. Training has both a reactive and a proactive intent: to deal with current difficulties and to make those being trained better able to prevent the emergence or recurrence of problems and disorders.

Professional education and continuing professional development

In common with other professional groups, child and adolescent mental health professionals are responsible for training entrants to their and other disciplines through both formal academic teaching and supervised clinical practice. Training schemes are commonly linked with university academic departments.

Professionals with academic posts usually carry responsibility for training in conjunction with honorary NHS sessional contracts.

Research

Many services undertake research into treatment and other aspects of service delivery, both to enhance practice and improve organizational processes. Job descriptions commonly include provision for research.

Academic psychiatry and psychology departments also play a central role in supporting research carried out by NHS staff as well as initiating and undertaking clinical and academic research of direct relevance to NHS CAMHS.

7   Treatment effectiveness of mental health services for children and young people

Treatment and outcomes: an overview

Mental health services for children and young people provide a variety of assessments, treatments and other interventions for individuals, families and groups, as well as teaching, training and research. It is difficult to demonstrate conclusively a cause and effect relationship between interventions and changes, particularly with children and families with severe or long-standing difficulties.

In the introduction to a recent collection of papers on the topic of 'Psychosocial treatment research' in child and adolescent mental health, Hibbs states that:

... except in the instance of attention deficit hyperactivity disorder (ADHD), there is little research to corroborate the efficacy of well-defined treatments ... behavioural, cognitive-behavioural, and combined pharmacological/psychosocial/parent training... And there is even greater dearth of research for treatments such as psychodynamic, interpersonal, group, family therapy, and eclectic approaches, which are commonly used in clinical settings and by private practitioners. (page 2)[155]

The evaluation of treatments for children and young people with mental health needs is probably more complex than evaluations in other conditions. Some of the reasons for this are discussed later.

Evidence is accumulating for the efficacy of a range of treatments and clinicians working in mental health services for children, young people and their families will identify many clients who they feel have benefited enormously from the therapeutic interventions provided by the service. Likewise there will be teachers, social workers, health visitors and other professionals who will attest to the ways in which the advice and support provided by these services have been of benefit to them and their clients. There will also be others whose response will be less positive and yet others where the impact of the service has been negligible or who will report that intervention made things worse. In this respect child and adolescent mental health services are similar to many other clinical services.

The absence of a substantial body of information or strong evidence of the effectiveness of psychological and pharmacological treatments for children and young people is well recognized and of general concern. This has been of such importance as to have led, at the request of the Federal Government in the US, to the establishment of a task group by the National Institute of Mental Health with the brief to expand research on 'psychosocial treatments' of young people.[155] A need for similar action exists in this country.

Consequently what is possible at the present time is a limited evaluation of the effectiveness of the treatments that services offer although, even here it will be seen that while the conclusions provide good grounds for optimism, there is much that still has to be done to establish that treatments meet strong criteria for effectiveness.

This section focuses on treatment outcomes rather than the effectiveness of services. It examines some of the major reasons for the present uncertainty and provides an update of the evidence regarding the treatment of the major psychological and psychiatric disorders and an overview of the current state of treatment research.

Evaluating interventions

Research on the effectiveness of interventions for mental health needs in children and young people is complex. In order to undertake controlled studies with random assignment of cases – the standard methodology – potentially influential variables such as the severity of the condition, economic status of the family, ability, ethnicity, marital status of carers, mental ability of the child, age and sex, all need to be taken into account. Few researchers have the resources to assemble the very large samples of patients needed to achieve such control, so that research on treatment tends to involve small groups with resulting limitations on the generalizability of the findings.

Psychological treatments are also very difficult to standardize: the therapist follows a general approach but has to tailor this to the idiosyncrasies of the individual patient and family. In some cases treatment may be given by the parent on the instruction of the clinician so that procedural uniformity may be difficult to achieve. Added to this is the tendency for placebo and placebo-like effects to be very influential in research involving psychological or psychopharmacological treatments.[156] Given such complexity and the variety of human individual differences, it is also difficult to mount replication studies to check on initial findings.

These sorts of difficulties are not unique to mental health investigations but are particularly salient and intrusive in research involving multi-faceted social and psychological processes, especially with children and young people.

Consequently evidence for the efficacy of interventions is accumulated through a series of studies, each having some limitations, but each nevertheless contributing to an understanding of treatment effectiveness. Authoritative, independently assessed review articles which contain detailed methodological critiques of a large number of studies bring this together. Examples include the effects of child psychotherapy, as reported in 43 separate studies, and documented by Barnett, Docherty and Frommelt.[157] Pfeiffer and Strzelecki have reviewed the outcomes reported in 34 studies of residential and inpatient psychiatric treatment.[158] Graziano and Diament reviewed 155 empirical studies of the effects of training parents of children presenting with behaviour problems in behaviour management techniques.[159] Allen et al. examined 904 child behaviour therapy studies for evidence that the authors had attempted to check that effects generalized beyond the treatment programme.[160]

It is from reviews such as these that the emergent views of the effectiveness of different treatment procedures or treatments for particular conditions arise: that is, from publications that have taken due account of the methodological constraints of the contributing studies.[a]

Reviews of studies of clinical effectiveness then serve to inform and guide practice. They cannot however either determine what is done or even ensure favourable outcome in the individual case.

Treatment trials and service effectiveness

Controlled trials with random allocation of cases to different treatments require selection of cases, standard procedures and intensive monitoring of impact. Because of these and other special characteristics of the research it is difficult to extrapolate conclusions from such trials to likely outcomes in clinic populations or for clinic services: patients cannot be selected and the therapists are applying a wider range of treatment procedures to a symptomatically and otherwise heterogeneous client group.

Furthermore in clinical trials patients or their carers may be volunteers or agree to participation in research trials. In child and adolescent mental health services the identified patient and family may not have actively sought or even be willing participants in treatment. Children and young people are brought to the service, sometimes reluctantly, by family members or other carers. The family itself may have had to be persuaded or even, on occasion, coerced to attend because of a threat of expulsion from school or the concerns of social services or other agencies.

For these and other reasons, as Weisz and Weiss have suggested, it is difficult to generalize from research treatments to clinic service treatments.[161]

In a more recent analysis of the limited success of clinic services as contrasted with the outcomes of research treatments carried out in academic centres, Weisz et al. found only three of ten possible reasons were supported by their analysis of the research literature.[162] First research therapy that is structured is more successful than the unstructured approaches that tend to be used in clinics. Second the research treatments that are more successful tend to be focused and specific. As such treatments tend to be easier to implement

---

[a] In the main, the information on the effectiveness of mental health interventions in children and young people presented in later sections of this chapter is based on the conclusions drawn from such reviews. In those instances where this is not the case, conclusions are based on the views of clinicians who are themselves commonly involved in treatment research and who would in any event be taking account of the reviews and related literature.

and control for research purposes and may account for the better outcomes of controlled laboratory studies. Third behavioural treatments tend to have greater effect sizes than non-behavioural interventions.

These authors go on to note that if 'effect sizes are generally higher for behavioural methods... and if behavioural methods are more common in research therapy... then the superior effects of research therapy might be attributable to differences in methods of intervention.' (page 96)

Weisz *et al.* in trying to account for differences in effect sizes and noting the limitations of their approach, nevertheless found that the epoch of the study, severity of condition, the clinical setting, therapist experience, training and caseload and the length of therapy did not emerge as significant influences.[162]

Constraints on outcome

Apart from the efficacy of treatments the factors that influence outcome in the individual case are many, some facilitating and others constraining the effectiveness of services. Not all of these are under direct control of the service.

Procedures for management and treatment are in many cases not carried out by health professionals but others, particularly parents and teachers. The impact of interventions is therefore dependent on, among other factors, parent/carer compliance with the regimen. This can involve bringing the child to clinic appointments, sometimes on a weekly basis for therapy sessions; rigorous data collection (for instance on tantrum frequency); carrying out of precise procedures of monitoring and intervention at home. It may require the involvement of the whole family, sometimes over an extended period. The patient may also have several sibs so that the 'parent as therapist' is implementing the treatment in a family context of competing demands.

Apart from the critical role of parents as facilitators of the intervention processes for their children, parents have their own needs. These may require the attention of services and should also be taken into account in the evaluation of treatment outcomes as the unmet needs of parents may prevent effective interventions with their children.[163]

Participants in treatment (children and parents) may have firm ideas about the appropriateness of the treatment proposed which can limit compliance. Treatments that include medication may be resisted, even though there is increasing evidence of efficacy in specific conditions. Carers may have particular expectations, for instance that the child will be offered dynamic psychotherapy and so resist other treatment.

Many external factors confound treatment effectiveness. Concurrent factors such as inadequate housing can indirectly maintain and prolong the child's problems. In this case improvement may depend on external agencies over which health services have little if any control. Similar circumstances arise in the treatment of school phobia where the school for organizational or other reasons may not be able to participate actively in the treatment programme.

It is against this background that we proceed to examine the empirical evidence for treatment effectiveness.

Research and clinical findings

Reviews of treatment research can be major condition-centred (i.e. following ICD categories), problem-centred (e.g. the treatment of aggression), procedure-centred (e.g. analytical psychotherapy), event-centred (e.g. post-traumatic reactions) or quality of life centred (e.g. focusing on impact on family and others as well as the index individual).

As noted earlier there is as yet no evidence of high probability outcomes for the interventions provided by CAMHS. Instead there are individual case reports and a number of controlled studies in the literature on the effectiveness of psychosocial interventions, the conclusions of which support the use of some of the procedures. The ways in which they are used will be discussed at the end of this section.

While there are many case reports recording the success of specific interventions with children and young people, some of which incorporate methodologies such as single case designs, it is recognized that such studies are limited in terms of the generalizations they permit. For instance a recent report on the effectiveness of cognitive-behavioural interventions with and without pharmacotherapy, in cases of obsessional compulsive disorder supports the effectiveness of this approach but is based mainly on treatment reports of single cases.[164] Single-case studies and clinical reports will not be considered further here, even though they frequently provide an inspiration for clinicians, especially when treatment options are otherwise limited.

This section is based on reviews of empirical research on psychological and pharmacological treatments of child and adolescent mental health disorders, as these are the basis of much epidemiological research. It is intended to provide a broad perspective on psychosocial treatments rather than a detailed review of all studies or all types of intervention for specific conditions.

General evidence

Overviews of the controlled studies are at present analysed in terms of the effect sizes from meta-analyses. Taken overall the outcomes of psychological treatments (collectively called the psychotherapies, encompassing behavioural and psychodynamic, as well as other approaches) of children and adolescents 'indicate that psychotherapy is better than no treatment, that the magnitude of improvement in juveniles parallels the treatment gains reported in adults, and that differences between treatment tend to favour behaviour therapy', the latter including cognitive treatments.[163] These outcomes have however to be qualified. First according to Kovacs and Lohr, many of the studies did not include clinically referred children. Second they note that the positive outcomes for behavioural treatments may reflect a form of criterion contamination in that the treatment targets were similar to the outcome measures – when this effect is eliminated, the superiority of behavioural treatments no longer holds.

The meta-analysis studies also mask significant differences in outcomes between younger children (4–12 year olds) and teenagers (13–18 year olds).[163]

Conduct/antisocial disorders

Earls notes that chronic conduct disorders carry a high social cost and are among the most resistant to intervention.[165] Treatment needs to be focused on the individual, family or wider group depending on the outcome of assessment. Individual-only treatment is unlikely to have an impact.

Recent research is beginning to identify successful approaches to treatment.

According to Earls community-based approaches and those that involve social problem solving skills training have been shown to have beneficial effects.[165] Medication has yet to be demonstrated to have any specific value, apart from its use where other conditions coexist with the conduct disorder.

However in aggressive children who are hospitalized, treatment with lithium appears to have some beneficial effects according to the findings of a recent double-blind trial.[166] Alessi *et al.* suggest that there is increasing evidence for the usefulness of lithium in a number of childhood and adolescent disorders.[167]

Kazdin *et al.* have demonstrated the usefulness of parent training and problem solving skills training in the treatment of severe antisocial behaviour.[168]

Predictors of treatment drop-out have been described.[169] These include having a very severe form of the disorder, a mother undergoing severe stress and high levels of socio-economic disadvantage. This information enables procedures to be developed which reduce drop-out and so increase the chance of improved outcomes.

In their review Offord and Bennett also conclude that there is as yet little effective treatment for these disorders.[170] This is of major concern because of the associations with difficulties in later life.

Affective disorders

The treatment of affective disorders in children and young people tends to follow the pattern of treatment of such disorders in adults, but with greater emphasis on the involvement of the family and less frequent use of medication.

The outcome of treatment for depression has been recently reviewed.[171–174] Reynolds has also reviewed studies of depression in adolescents.[175] There is some, albeit weak, evidence that psychological approaches can have a beneficial effect on mild forms of depression, though the main thrust in treatment research has been in the use of anti-depressant medication. To date there is little firm evidence that such medication works better than placebo in children or adolescents with major depression.[171,175] As depression in children is a recently recognized condition, it is suggested that it is still too early to make firm judgements regarding all forms of treatment.[174]

Anxiety disorders

There have been a number of recent reviews and overviews of the treatment of anxiety disorders in children and young people.[176–180] One reviewer[176] recommends the use of pharmacological treatments for these disorders, while others are consistent in the conclusion that as yet, no approach to treatment is well substantiated, other than that for obsessional compulsive disorder (see below). Bernstein and Borchardt discuss treatments for anxiety.[177] They note a number of studies using different forms of medication and suggest the use of, as well as further research into the effectiveness of different medications. Klein believes that behavioural treatments are rational since rapid improvements are noted clinically in many children when such treatments are instituted.[180]

Post-traumatic stress disorder and attempted suicide

There is no research involving controlled trials but there are well documented and commonly applied management procedures. In the case of attempted suicide, for example, there needs to be a rapid response from the service in order to engage the young person and family and initiate treatment.

Anorexia nervosa and bulimia nervosa

Anorexia is a life threatening condition.[181] A variety of treatment approaches is available and should include family and individual psychotherapy, behavioural treatments, availability of inpatient treatment or occasionally medication.

Bulimia is a more recently studied condition.[181] Although there has been a substantial amount of treatment research the reported studies are methodologically inadequate so there is as yet no firm evidence of specific benefits.

Obsessive compulsive disorders

The treatment of obsessive-compulsive disorders in children closely follows that in adults. Although the efficacy of behavioural approaches is well documented in adult patients it has yet to be demonstrated through controlled studies with children.[182] Medication with clomipramine is effective, though it is likely to be needed for a prolonged period.[182,183] There are no systematic comparisons of drug versus behavioural approaches. As noted earlier the use of cognitive-behavioural treatments alone or in combination with medication in the treatment of obsessional compulsive disorder is supported by some.[164]

Attention deficit and overactivity

These syndromes are characterized by frequent co-morbidity and psychosocial adversity.[184] The most effective symptomatic treatment is stimulant medication,[184,185] though the benefits are lost on cessation of treatment.[186] Therefore medication should be accompanied by treatment of other difficulties, such as school learning, social relationships and self-esteem. DuPaul and Barkley reviewed the combined use of behavioural and pharmacological therapies and noted the added benefits for some children treated this way.[187]

Tic disorders

Psychosocial interventions involving education about the disorder as well as support, form the core of treatment, with pharmacological treatment being used in the more severe cases. While there is consistent evidence of response to medication in the majority of those treated, side-effects can be intrusive. Cognitive, behavioural and other psychotherapeutic treatments show some evidence of effectiveness, but the findings need to be replicated in further studies.[188]

Feeding and sleeping disorders in young children

There are well documented procedures for treating feeding difficulties in young children, but as Skuse notes, the main evidence on effectiveness derives from successfully treated single cases.[189]

Difficulties of getting to sleep and night waking are the most common forms and tend to be responsive to simple behavioural management.[189] There are well-tried treatments for other conditions that arise during sleep but as yet without documented controlled trials of their effectiveness.

Disorders of attachment

These problems, usually in the relationship between mother and infant or child, have been treated in various ways commonly involving the mother–child pair in the programme. There is however no systematic treatment research that provides a clear basis for specific interventions.[190]

Autism, learning difficulties and related developmental disorders

Although the core problems in these conditions are not modifiable to a major extent, they may require long-term intervention from mental health services. Of particular importance are programmes that deal with secondary behavioural or emotional disorders and training in social skills. The needs of individuals with autism and their families have been well documented and the overall management programme involves provision for medical care, appropriate education, family support and where necessary, focused treatment with speech and language, social skills or other therapies. Pharmacological treatments are as yet without major value but are seen as potentially helpful adjuncts to the overall treatment programme.[191]

Bed wetting and faecal soiling

Nocturnal enuresis has inspired a wide variety of treatments including surgery, medications, night waking and the use of a special alarm which is the only procedure known to cure the condition.[60] Cure rates average about 80% using the alarm, but it can be a difficult procedure to maintain. While relapses do occur, they do so with lesser frequency than when cessation of wetting is accomplished by other means. Medication has short-term benefits in nocturnal enuresis. Encopresis requires both medical and psychological management.

Schizophrenia

Schizophrenia is an appropriate diagnosis for a few older children and adolescents. As with the adult form, it is an incurable or recurrent condition, but persistent symptoms can be controlled with appropriate treatment. The major concerns relate to the consequences of the disorder for the child and family. As there is little evidence on the treatment and outcome in children and young people, Werry and Taylor propose that the efficacy of treatment is assumed to be much the same as for adults.[192] Pharmacotherapy is a major component of treatment and there is substantial evidence that it is 'very helpful in schizophrenia in adults'.[192] Work with the child's family may be important for prevention of relapse.

Some psychologically based approaches to management and treatment in adults appear to have value but their efficacy with this group still requires much stronger support from adequate research. Consequently there is little basis for generalizing to younger age groups.

Atypical psychosexual development

There are several treatment approaches for children and young people with atypical sexual development that report some successful results but there are no trials of treatment sufficient to enable firm conclusions to be drawn.[193]

Somatic diseases and disorders combined with chronic physical illness

The risk of psychological and psychiatric disorders is doubled in populations with major chronic illnesses.[194] The nature of the disorders is much the same as in individuals without the illness so treatment approaches follow those adopted for patients without physical illness. There are no controlled trials of treatment procedures for combined psychological and physical disorders. Specific approaches are available for pain management and to help children cope with medical procedures.

Physical and sexual abuse

The treatment of individuals who have been abused is complex and needs to take account of a multiplicity of factors. The aims are to deal with any current disorder resulting from the abuse and to prevent future mental ill-health. Removal of the child to a hospital, residential unit or other place of safety may be required. The treatment approach depends on the extent to which the factors that led to the abuse can be identified and the willingness of the individuals concerned to participate in treatment. Work with parents and families is essential if children are to remain at home. There are indications that successful behaviour modification, such as anger management in the abusers, can be beneficial for some children.[195] Individual dynamic psychotherapeutic approaches are also used.

O'Donohue and Elliott have reviewed reports of studies using psychotherapeutic procedures with sexually abused children.[196] Systematic studies have begun to delineate some of the characteristics of families which are not treatable, so that service resources can begin to be focused more efficiently.[197]

Smith and Bentovim note that an increasing number of treatments for sexual abuse are being investigated but there are insufficient controlled studies so that conclusions about the effectiveness of treatments are still premature.[198]

Prevention

Prevention of child and adolescent mental health difficulties is important because of the risk of problems continuing into adult life. Recent reviews of prevention are provided by Cox[18] and Graham.[19]

While much research has focused on treatment or other aspects of disorders, comparatively little attention has been given to prevention. There is, however, an increasing interest in prevention, particularly on a more 'macro', community level. Conceptual and methodological frameworks for the evaluation of preventive interventions have been elaborated.[199] Systematic studies in the US are also beginning to show that preventive interventions can have a beneficial impact on different aspects of the behaviour and mental health of children and young people. Interventions include helping them to resist drug taking and to deal with such stressful transitions as school transfer.[199] Recent reviews of research on the prevention of physical abuse and neglect[200] and sexual abuse[201] have also shown that some benefits can be achieved through focused prevention programmes. One major study in the UK provided encouraging results for a school-based psychotherapeutic intervention for children with behaviour problems.[202]

Preventive interventions are clearly possible and of great potential benefit, and given the assumption that such interventions can lead to the reduction in the prevalence and incidence of disorders, evaluative studies appear to be well worth supporting, particularly in communities or contexts where the risks for emotional and behavioural problems are known and high.

Criteria for judging treatment research in child and adolescent mental health services

Methodological difficulties are common in all clinical research.[203] Since the earlier reviews of treatment for children with emotional and behavioural disorders,[204] some of the major advances that have taken place involve methodological refinements and the consequent introduction of new criteria to be used in the evaluation of studies and outcomes.

Criteria for judging the efficacy of treatment have become increasingly sophisticated and complex. Although some of these criteria are condition specific – for instance in autism the underlying problem is not curable but change in major secondary symptoms is a realistic goal – there are general criteria that are now seen as core requirements.

Among the changes and improvements noted by Kovacs and Lohr has been the introduction of treatment manuals which are aimed at clearer specification of how the treatment should be implemented. Criteria to assess improvement 'have become more specific and multidimensional' and definitions solely in terms of clinicians' global judgements replaced by more objective measures involving direct observations and 'operationally defined scales' (pages 14–15).[163]

It is also recognized that it is now no longer sufficient to report statistical significance. Treatment research must also demonstrate that the changes have clinical significance, and that there is an impact on daily life, adaptation and relationships. There is also the need to demonstrate that treated clients move much closer to, or into the 'normal' range on assessment instruments. Other criteria include:

- a range of different methods for appraising outcome, rather than a single procedure (this includes evaluating process or relationships and not just symptomatology)
- a number of judges of outcome, each with a differing perspective
- assessments of functioning, both pre- and post-intervention which monitor 'internal changes' (both physiological – if appropriate – self-perceptions, and behaviours)
- statistical or other controls for co-morbidity

- assessments of stability of changes over time, since benefits are often not apparent for some time after the intervention
- monitoring of generalizability of improvements across situations (e.g. home and school)
- evidence that the intervention is better than no treatment
- evidence that the intervention is more cost-effective than other procedures
- evidence that there are minimal harmful side-effects.

Treatment research and service implications

The clinical and research literature on treatment, consisting of case reports, small-scale studies and controlled trials, constitutes the major resource for innovation and the modification of service interventions and practice. It is however not realistic to assume that favourable outcomes reported in the literature will invariably translate into positive outcomes in practice.

The nature of individual differences in the aetiology, presentation and external circumstances of children and young people, as well as the resources of services, militate against a simple formula for linking need, intervention and outcome in clinical practice. Even impressive interventions such as the use of medication in children with attention deficit and hyperactivity do not succeed in every case: an appreciable number of children are not helped by the treatment. Indeed, prediction of outcome in the individual case, given the complexity of aetiology, presentation and individual circumstance, is hazardous and a challenge for future research.

Furthermore it is necessary for findings to be replicated in independent studies. Much research emanates from the US and differences in the regulation of medication, the contexts of clinical practice, and the clinical populations studied make it hazardous to extrapolate the results to the UK population.

There can also be a major time lag between the identification of a psychological treatment procedure that shows promise and its systematic introduction in services. This is partly because suitable cases appear intermittently in services and the procedures, for instance cognitive-behavioural treatment, can require specialized training and a period of ongoing supervision.

Conclusion

At present there are few examples of child and adolescent mental health treatment that can unequivocally demonstrate their effectiveness. However substantial progress has been made in identifying the range of interventions that have the potential to benefit children and young people with mental health problems and disorders and their families. This range of treatments should be potentially available to all children and adolescents.

Klein has asserted that '...clinicians cannot await the scientific verdict to care for children who seek treatment.' (page 367).[180] The research underlines the importance of careful monitoring of progress in individual cases undergoing treatment. There should be a preparedness to change the approach where the current procedures are ineffective. The critical importance of controlled treatment trials lies in the inspiration, opportunities and direction they give to clinicians in selecting procedures likely to be the most efficacious. The effectiveness of services is then dependent on their having the resources and the skill to exploit the treatment research literature.

8 Models of care

Principles

There are several important principles which need to be accepted in developing models of care in child and adolescent mental health.

The majority of child and adolescent mental health problems can be dealt with in primary care

Many mental health problems in children and young people can be dealt with at the primary care level. As with other disciplines this can only be achieved if the health professionals at this level have adequate training in the subject and maintain their skills through continuing education. This will usually be provided by specialist child mental health professionals. Primary care teams may identify members who will develop particular expertise in this field, though all team members must be able to recognize mental health problems in children at an early stage.

The primary care team should have ready access to colleagues with additional training such as school nurses or community paediatricians, who may be team members.

The primary care team can only function satisfactorily if it is confident that specialist help is readily available when needed through local CAMHS. Primary care staff should recognize the limits of their competence and not retain responsibility for the care of children whose problems are beyond their experience.

Specialists should provide support to other groups

Specialist child and adolescent mental health professionals should support and promote the activities of primary health care, other professionals and of voluntary agencies concerned with the treatment and welfare of children with mental health problems. Support includes consultation and training and requires ready accessibility of the specialist services.

Service should be patient centred

There is inevitably a tension between accessibility and specialist services. When a child's problems cannot be adequately dealt with in primary care, specialist mental health professionals should be readily available. CAMHS require limited use of complex, hospital-based diagnostic facilities: most assessments and treatments can be adequately carried out in clinic or outpatient premises. When it is geographically desirable, the professional member of the solo professional or multi-disciplinary group should work on a sessional basis to cover more than one site. This will improve convenience for patients and relatives and enhance compliance with treatment. It is undesirable for families to travel long distances with disturbed children. Facilities should be convenient and appropriate for children and adolescents.

However if individual professionals work across several sites much time will be wasted in travel and there will be difficulty in forging good working links with other professional colleagues.

There should be patient choice

Wherever possible patients and carers should be informed about treatment possibilities and given a choice of the professions and services from which they would like advice and help.

Specialist services should accommodate the spectrum of need

Not all children and young people with mental health needs require multi-disciplinary resources. There should therefore be a solo professional service provided by child and adolescent psychiatrists, clinical psychologists specializing in work with children and young people, or child psychiatric nurses. This type of care facilitates the geographical spread of provision, whether organized as a uniprofessional service or as solo professionals doing outreach work from a multi-disciplinary base.

Multi-disciplinary resources should include psychiatrists, psychologists, psychotherapists, nurses and social workers, in order to provide for children and families with more complex needs. Speech and language and occupational therapists, and specialist teachers can make a contribution to such resources.

Where there are both unidisciplinary and multi-disciplinary groups, they should work in close liaison with each other and with social services and education colleagues to facilitate joint assessment and treatment. Multi-disciplinary resources may work as a team receiving referrals or as independent professional groups who collaborate on individual cases. Where a team organization is used professionals can also work in a solo or unidisciplinary mode. Team organization is needed for day and inpatient services. Inpatient services require educational provision.

Services should be concentrated in areas of greatest need

The prevalence of mental health problems in children and young people is high among those with special educational needs, those with developmental problems and physical illness, those with mental and physically ill parents and those in contact with social services and the law. Efforts should be made to ensure that services are distributed to provide maximum resource at points of greatest need.

Professional isolation should be avoided

It is unsatisfactory for professionals of any discipline to work in isolation. This can lead to undue work stress and idiosyncratic practice, as well as problems with the organization and continuity of service delivery. All services should therefore include at least two members of each professional group, one of whom should be of senior status.

Service organization

Services should have at least one senior member of each profession to organize and be responsible for intra-professional matters e.g. training, supervision, recruitment and service development. There should be clear management structures with lines of accountability for provision of services, incorporated by appropriate contracts or job plans.

Professional accountability

Professional accountability should be to an individual within the same discipline. There will need to be clear distinctions between the spheres of professional (clinical) and management responsibility.

Service isolation should be avoided

Solo professionals should have ready access to multi-disciplinary services, if staff are not also members of such services. There should be agreed procedures to prevent duplication of referrals to different services and mechanisms to distribute resources effectively and appropriately.

Good communication and collaboration are essential

If communication and collaboration are poor, resources will be wasted through duplication, there will be gaps in services and patients and carers will be confused.

Services can only be effective if there are easy and open channels of communication between all parties, independent of their management structure. This does not imply the need for a single management structure, but emphasizes the importance of a co-ordinating structure with shared strategies and policies.

The model of care

Localities

Each will have a primary care team, with a measure of specialist support from, for example, a school nurse or consultant community paediatrician who may work with several teams. Outreach services from child mental health professionals should be available in primary care as part of the solo professional specialist service.

Communities up to 250 000

Each should have both a solo professional and multi-disciplinary specialist service providing day and outpatient services. They should work closely with co-terminous local authority social services and education teams, preferably with some social workers and/or educational psychologists working from the same base. The model of co-ordination of solo and multi-disciplinary service can vary. What is essential is that the two components are co-ordinated. Two main models exist at the present time.

- Professionals collaborating in a multi-disciplinary service that also provides a solo service.
- Multi-disciplinary and solo professional services that are organizationally distinct but have mechanisms to collaborate effectively. In these circumstances the solo professional is usually a clinical psychology service.

The services will also work closely with the general paediatric and adult psychiatry services at the district general hospital. The specialist services will provide clinics at several sites, with the aim of ensuring that under-fives can be assessed reasonably close to their homes and that distance is not a barrier to care for older children. Intensive day treatment provision should be available for families of under-fives for parenting problems and for school age children. Day units need a range of dedicated staff similar to those in inpatient units. Local services for adolescents can be more concentrated, since this age group is likely to be more mobile and may be encouraged to attend by the availability of an environment which is sensitive to their interests and attitudes. Temporal as well as geographical access is important for this group: services should be available out of school hours. This also helps to ensure the attendance of parents who are working outside the home.

The specialist services should provide concentrated input in areas of high need, such as special schools, local authority family centres and residential homes and paediatric clinics. Joint approaches to funding of staff should be considered.

There should be access to hospital diagnostic facilities and inpatient paediatric beds on an occasional basis.

Communities of 750 000–1 000 000

Inpatient facilities for children and adolescents should be provided. An inpatient unit for younger children may be satisfactorily sited within a district general hospital, preferably close to outpatient and paediatric facilities. Adolescent units are best sited away from the district general hospital: access to investigatory, paediatric and adult mental health services is essential.

The Royal College of Psychiatrists has estimated that for a total population of 250 000 the inpatient provision should be 2–4 beds for children and 4–6 beds for adolescents up to the age of 16 in wards of a minimal size of 15 and 20–25 beds respectively.[205]

The inpatient facilities should be staffed by a dedicated, multi-disciplinary team which works closely with the community-based specialist services that will normally be the source of referrals. The inpatient team should include the following professional groups, as a minimum:

- child and adolescent psychiatrists
- clinical psychologists
- nurses
- occupational therapists
- social workers
- psychotherapists.

All inpatient units must have proper educational facilities (staffed by the local authority education department) and adequate recreational opportunities.

Adjacent outpatient and day care facilities can be helpful in managing the transition from inpatient to community-based care and eventual discharge.

Communities of 3 000 000

There are some rare and difficult-to-manage conditions for which highly specialist services are required. They can be divided into the following.

- Conditions needing complex assessment. For example:
  a) pervasive developmental disorders
  b) neuropsychiatric problems
  c) gender identity problems
  d) severe psychoses
  e) severe obsessional disorders
  f) complex child abuse
  g) sensory handicaps.
- Difficult treatment problems. For example:
  a) severe conduct disorders, including those needing secure accommodation
  b) other severe disorders not responsive to more local inpatient treatment (e.g. obsessional and mood disorders)
  c) neuropsychiatric disorders
  d) post-traumatic disorders
  e) severe epilepsy
  f) other brain dysfunction
  g) complex child abuse, including treatment of Münchausen Syndrome by Proxy and child/adolescent perpetrators of sexual abuse.

'Regional' centres are needed for these patients. These units are by definition dealing with highly demanding patients. It is essential that their staffing is maintained at a sufficiently high level to promote effective treatment and to prevent stress among staff.

Service targets

In a co-ordinated service for a population of 250 000 no professional should work in isolation. This means that both solo and multi-disciplinary services should have at least two professionals from any discipline, whether child psychiatry, clinical child psychology or community psychiatric nursing.

The targets for individual disciplines outlined below derive from recommendations from professional bodies where such recommendations exist. These recommendations do not take adequate account of the need for solo professional activity. Child psychiatrists and clinical psychologists will be expected to take a leading role in the development of solo and multi-disciplinary outpatient/day patient services, assessment, treatment, teaching and research. The involvement of senior nursing staff is vital for the planning of inpatient and most day patient services.

Psychiatrists

The Royal College of Psychiatrists recommends that there be 1.3 whole time equivalent (wte) consultants in child and adolescent psychiatry per 100 000 total population (for uni- and multi-disciplinary care). In addition to this there should be consultant provision for regional or supra-district services. In centres with a major teaching responsibility, consultant numbers should be increased to take account of teaching and research responsibilities.[205] Bridges over Troubled Waters has recommended that there should be 0.8 wte consultants per 200 000 population with a special responsibility for adolescent mental health services.[206] Child psychiatrists will usually be based in multi-disciplinary groups although some of their activity will be as a solo professional. All inpatient units need a child psychiatrist who carries appropriate responsibility for leadership and organization in collaboration with senior nursing staff.

Clinical psychologists

The Division of Clinical Psychology of the British Psychological Society recommends that there should be at least one full-time clinical psychologist working with children and families per 75 000 population. A child clinical psychologist at Grade B level with relevant skills and experience should head the psychology services for a given population. There should be at least one child clinical psychologist in all major service segments (e.g. under-fives, adolescents) provided by the unit or hospital trust. In a population of 250 000 a minimum of 3.5 wte posts are required. Additional posts will also be needed to provide specific services to specialist units for children and young people in primary health care.

Solo professional activity (page 76) is often appropriately conducted by clinical psychologists. This solo professional activity may be provided by clinical psychologists working from a multi-disciplinary base or a uniprofessional service.

Nurses

Nurses will usually be based within a multi-disciplinary group or team. They make an essential contribution to inpatient services but require additional training to work in an outpatient service. There are no specific recommendations for the expected levels of staffing for nurses working with multi-disciplinary outpatient groups. It is suggested that there should be a minimum of two community child psychiatric nurses for every consultant child psychiatrist. A day unit working intensively with between 50 and 80 children and their families per annum will require at least three full-time nursing staff of whom one should be at least Grade H. Inpatient units should maintain safe levels of staffing with trained nurses at all times. This may require a nurse: patient ratio of 1 : 1, depending on organizational arrangements in the unit.

Child psychotherapy

Psychotherapists perform a valuable role in both direct work with children and parents and in supporting and supervising intensive individual and group psychotherapy by other professionals. One child psychotherapist is required per 100 000 population with an additional child psychotherapist for every inpatient unit. The Child Psychotherapy Trust has proposed a target of one child psychotherapist for every child mental health team (a total of 660) with additional senior child psychotherapists who can take teaching responsibility.

Occupational therapy

Occupational therapists with specific training and expertise in working with children contribute towards day and inpatient treatment services. A minimum of one occupational therapist is needed per 100 000 population to work in day unit facilities. An additional occupational therapist will be required for every inpatient unit.

Social workers, educational psychologists and specialist teachers

Many children referred to child and adolescent mental health services are involved with social services or have special educational needs. Closely co-ordinated work is required in matters relating to child care, child abuse and educational difficulty. Ideally there should be three whole-time social workers per 100 000 population doing regular joint work with child and adolescent mental health services. There need to be arrangements to co-ordinate assessment and joint work with the school psychological service (educational psychologists). This is sometimes facilitated by co-location of educational psychologists with child and adolescent mental health services. As many children attending these services have specific educational difficulties, there can be significant benefit if some teachers with relevant specialist skills are co-located with the child and adolescent mental health services.

Support staff

Secretarial/administrative support staff are required: a ratio of one per three wte health professionals has been suggested, but this depends on organizational arrangements and office systems.

Range of services

The following range of non-residential services should be available in each district.

Assessment

- child and adolescent psychiatric, including neuro-psychiatric
- psychological including psychometry
- physical
- developmental
- educational
- social, including child protection.

Specific treatments

- cognitive and behavioural therapy
- individual child psychotherapy, including play therapy and art psychotherapy
- family therapy
- parental counselling, including marital therapy and advice on child management
- physical methods of treatment, including drug treatment
- social skills training
- special educational treatment
- day unit services
- consultation.

Group therapies should also be available (e.g. for social skills training or in the treatment of sexual abuse of child perpetrators of sexual abuse).

In addition resources should be available throughout the services for training (including continuing education).

Research

Service-related research is necessary to promote and monitor service developments and sustain the quality of staff activity. Appropriate resources are required.

Physical facilities

Within any district there should be at least one hospital and one community base for specialist child mental health professionals. The hospital base should be within a district general hospital or general teaching hospital, situated to enable satisfactory collaboration with paediatric and adult mental health and A and E services. All services should work in collaboration with community health services. Hospital and community clinic premises need to be dedicated and have:

- furnishing and equipment congenial for children and families
- toys and play equipment
- rooms suitable for the full range of assessments and treatments including physical examination, psychometry, individual psychotherapy, family therapy. Video facilities should be available
- an appropriate reception and waiting area
- clinic premises sympathetic to local culture to promote accessibility
- services for adolescents geared to their sub-culture with easy, direct access.

Contracts for care

Each commissioning authority will wish to ensure access for its population to the following.

- **Locally based specialist CAMHS** Provide regular, accessible solo and multi-professional assessment and treatment services, in liaison with other relevant professional groups. These are the 'core' services.
- **Inpatient units** Clear admission and discharge policies are needed and work in close co-operation with the local community-based specialist team is also needed. Commissioners should consider setting standards for waiting lists for admission to these units.
- **Specialist inpatient units for rare conditions** The patients requiring these services are often 'difficult-to-place' and their care is expensive. Purchasing authorities should decide how such cases will be dealt with and arrangements should be explicit in contracts. This may be done by requiring providers to deal with the matter, or by retaining contingency funds for such cases or by agreements on risk-sharing between purchasers and providers. In all cases a time limit for resolution of difficulties and appropriate placement of the child should be set. Clear arrangements also need to be agreed with local authorities about mechanisms for resolving problems relating to responsibility for care, with explicit systems for ensuring that children and families are not passed from one agency to another with unacceptable delays and deficiencies in care.

9 Outcome measures

Introduction

The general aim of child and adolescent mental health services is to relieve suffering in children with mental health problems, to support their families and promote their development into stable adults who fulfil their potential.

The assessment of outcome for specific problems can address:

- symptomatology
- general development
- impact on others
- long-term personal functioning.

It is nevertheless valuable to consider interim measures of structure and process as well as clinical outcomes.

Structure

Although the level of investment in a service is not in itself a measure of quality, it is clear that a seriously under-resourced service will not be able to provide acceptable care. Commissioners should bear in mind the manpower standards outlined in section 8 when specifying service requirements.

- Each commissioner should ensure that community-based specialist services are available to appropriate population groups (see section 8) and that there are clear systems of access to the service and from the service to inpatient and other specialist units when required.

- Specialist services should be set up in such a way that there are no isolated professionals.
- Services should have appropriate administrative and secretarial support to ensure efficient service provision.
- The level of provision should reflect local needs and take account of factors such as social disadvantage.
- Staffing and facilities should take account of local ethnic diversity.
- All premises should be appropriately equipped and furnished for the service age group (children or adolescents) to maximize acceptability and attendance.
- There should be a realistic quality standards framework and systems for service monitoring.

Process

Accessibility

- Clinics should be held at times which are convenient to school-age children and working parents.
- Clinics should be located in places accessible to parents of young children and individuals with disabilities.
- Clinics should be organized so that referrals are seen promptly for assessment, while the individuals are still motivated.
- Clinics should be organized so that there is minimal delay between assessment and the start of a treatment programme.
- Child and adolescent mental health staff should have regular, mutually agreed meetings with paediatric staff and there should be an on-call service for paediatric inpatients requiring urgent assessment (e.g. deliberate self-harm, abuse, psychosis).
- Specialist advice should be readily available to paediatricians, local authority social services, adult mental health, education and primary care services.

Communications

Explicit arrangements should be established for communications between the following.

- **Specialist professional staff** Especially for the multi-disciplinary assessment and monitoring of patients and co-ordination between solo and multi-disciplinary services.
- **Specialist professional staff and other health professionals** All those with responsibility for the health and welfare of children and adolescents with mental health problems and their families should be kept informed of treatment initiation, programmes and progress, subject where necessary to the normal constraints of confidentiality.
- **Services and clients** All those requiring treatment or support should be given a clear explanation of the nature of the problem, as assessed by specialist services, be informed about possible choices of management and be encouraged to participate actively in treatment. Where possible and in particular where this does not prejudice the welfare of the child assessment reports should be available to parents and care-givers.

Professional standards

The maintenance of professional standards of practice is an important, if indirect, consideration in ensuring satisfactory outcomes of care.

Purchasers should require that:

- all professional staff are qualified and registered with the appropriate body
- all professional staff have access to the time and resources needed for continuing education and professional development. There should be particular attention to training and treatment procedures where effectiveness has been demonstrated
- all professional staff participate in clinical audit, which is reported to the district or trust audit committee in accordance with local arrangements. An example of multi-disciplinary audit has recently been described[207]
- professional training taking place in the service is monitored by the appropriate professional body
- opportunities are available for research.

Outcomes

Clinical

Symptomatic

Some specific conditions allow direct measurement of outcomes. For example:

- specific phobias – proportion of those treated who overcome phobia
- enuresis – proportion of those treated who remain 'dry' for a specific time
- school refusal and truancy – proportion of children attending school regularly
- eating disorders – proportion of those treated who maintain a target weight and normal eating habits.

Goal attainment

In many cases progress cannot be assessed by symptomatic improvement and is measured by attainment of diverse treatment goals which are specific for each patient and include qualitative indicators. These goals should be identified for each referral and monitored at specified intervals. They should take into account the goals of parents, referrers and professionals and should be operationally defined.

Quality of life

The impact of treatment on the child and others can also be assessed by measures such as:

- school progress
- friendships
- family discord
- evidence of repeated abuse
- enjoyment of activity.

In all cases objective measures should be used. The C-GAS has been used in a number of services as a measure of impairment and its reduction.[208]

Adverse events

There are some adverse events which, though from time to time unavoidable, may require specific investigation through a confidential enquiry. This ensures that there were no service failures and allows procedures to be improved where necessary. These include:

- suicides under the age of 18 (whether or not under the care of mental health professionals)
- death or serious self-harm while under the care of child mental health services
- abuse while under the care of child mental health services
- pregnancy under the age of 16.

There are many other events or circumstances which may give rise to significant concern and could be used as a monitoring tool e.g. running away from home.

The clinical outcome of the treatment of child mental health problems may only become clear in later life. In many instances it is never known whether an apparently mildly successful intervention in reality prevented serious deterioration.

User satisfaction

The views of service users are an important aspect of outcome assessment. If users are unhappy with the service, they are likely to discontinue treatment and hence will not be able to benefit. It is particularly difficult to assess the satisfaction of users of child and adolescent mental health services since the designated patient may not be in a position to give an opinion and the interests and satisfaction of the carer or parent may not be concordant with those of the child. However many services have carried out evaluations of both client and referrer satisfaction. Purchasers should, however, encourage providers to develop approaches to this subject and report regularly on findings.

10 Targets

Introduction

Purchasers should aim for the provision of services and staff as set out in section 8. This would include:

- an adequately staffed solo professional and multi-disciplinary service for each 250 000 population
- geographically and temporally convenient services
- appropriate child-centred accommodation that facilitates the full range of assessment and treatment
- ready access to more specialist services, on a larger population base
- no isolated professional staff.

Specific targets

Specific service targets might include:

- no child or young person should wait more than four weeks after referral for specialist assessment by a local solo professional or multi-disciplinary team (a multi-disciplinary assessment is not necessary for every case)
- no child or young person should wait more than two weeks for the start of a treatment programme, following assessment
- a child who might require inpatient care should be assessed within 24 hours if the referring professional considers the case urgent
- a child who following assessment is considered in need of urgent inpatient care should be admitted within 24 hours
- a child requiring inpatient care that is not urgent should be admitted at an appropriate time, as advised by the clinician responsible for the case, and the family should be given at least one week's notice
- no child or young person should be admitted to an adult psychiatric inpatient unit unless there is a positive indication. If this is not considered an appropriate setting, the child or young person should be transferred to appropriate accommodation within one week
- in 'difficult-to-place' cases, senior staff in the authorities concerned (usually health and social services) should meet and decide which agency will take responsibility and set a timetable for placing the child in appropriate care
- all children or young people admitted to hospital or seen in A and E departments as a result of actual or suspected physical, sexual or emotional abuse should be referred for assessment. Local child protection procedures should clearly explain the correct mechanism. Social services will normally be the first line of assessment
- all children or young people admitted to hospital or seen in A and E departments as a result of deliberate self-harm should be seen by a child and adolescent psychiatrist before discharge or by a professional with appropriate training and ready access to a psychiatrist
- all provider units should have explicit procedures, copies of which are available to purchasers, for the two situations set out above.

11 Information

Introduction

Though there is considerable epidemiological information on child and adolescent mental health, clinical and management information is inadequate at present, although some services have produced local needs based assessments.[209] The situation is, of course, common to many other health services. It is particularly difficult in this service, however, because of the complex nature of some of the problems, the dependence of many of the designated patients on carers or other adults for referral to services, for participation in treatment and the multi-sectoral range of services. Information availability is variable and commissioners should check with professionals and other agencies on their local situation.

Areas for improvement

In order to improve needs assessment for child and adolescent mental health services, better information is needed on the following.

- **Mental health status in the community** This may require the development of instruments or other measures which can be realistically used in particular populations, though several standardized instruments are already available and screening for major disorders is possible.
- **Information on the number and location of high risk groups** These include relatively easy-to-identify groups, such as those in special schools, those in local authority care, or those with serious physical illness. It is also necessary however, to obtain better information on 'hidden' groups – poor achievers at school, children recently bereaved, children suffering following family break-ups, so as to intervene, if necessary, at an early stage and try to prevent the development of possible serious sequelae.
- **Information on the relationships between mental health and various environmental, social and economic factors** These may be useful proxies for health care needs (section 12).
- **Information from other providers** For example voluntary agencies.

Child and adolescent mental health services are essentially interdisciplinary: they involve different levels of health care and different agencies. Information should ideally be available to all professionals involved in care and integrated records of service use and care should be developed. Advances in information technology should enable more sophisticated systems to be used which could meet operational needs as well as service planning, research and monitoring requirements.

A coding framework such as the 'proposed core data set for child and adolescent mental health services' provides one example of the core data requirements for services.[15] In the medium term the read codes are likely to form the basis of an integrated health record of patient characteristics and core events, which will also cover child and adolescent mental health. At present there are very few operational systems that meet the full spectrum of information needs for these services.

12 Research priorities

Introduction

Child and adolescent mental health services share with most other clinical specialties serious omissions in knowledge about the effectiveness of interventions and the optimal organization of care. It is indeed to the credit of the specialty that so much has been achieved in areas fraught with methodological problems which are not encountered in, for example, surgical specialties with relatively clear cut outcome measures and a short time frame. The evidence available at present is sufficient to support purchasing decisions but there are important areas where further research would be valuable. Both the Medical Research Council and the Royal College of Psychiatrists have made recommendations for research priorities which have been taken into account in the development of these proposals.[210,211]

Research infrastructure

It is vital that appropriate staff and facilities are available within each population of 750 000 if there is to be satisfactory assessment of local needs and evaluated development of treatment and services. Both the Royal College of Psychiatrists and the British Psychological Society require trainees to undertake research. It is difficult for this to be achieved satisfactorily unless senior staff in academic departments engaged in research are available to provide support.

Normal and abnormal development

Research in this field is inevitably long term. Retrospective studies can produce useful and valid data. However prospective and follow-up studies are likely to be more reliable since they are not dependent upon retrospective recall but use information that has been collected for the purpose. The following areas of enquiry would merit further investigation.

Links between child and adult mental disorders

Which developmental characteristics and which mental problems in childhood predispose to which adult disorders? What is the strength and nature of the relationship? How do risk and protective factors during development influence outcome?[212]

The development of personality disorders in adolescence needs to be better understood.

Cross-generational influences

How do childrens' experiences of parent care at different stages of development affect their present mental health and subsequent psychological and emotional development?[213] It is particularly important to understand the influence of the contemporary changing patterns of family life and child care on child and adolescent mental health.

Genetic influences: interaction between genetic and environmental influences

Genetic influences on development and behaviour are increasingly recognized. The interaction between these and environmental influences need to be better understood. Certain conditions are particularly appropriate for genetic research. These include autism, learning difficulties and hyperkinetic disorders.

Differential response to environmental influences

Children within the same family vary in their mental health. Is this due to differences in individual resilience or vulnerability or in detailed family interactions? Can these be measured and does the evidence provide clues for prevention?[211]

Influence of brain dysfunction on mental health, including the interaction between brain function and environment

This is of particular importance for understanding the influence of different types of brain dysfunction on mental health. Increased collaboration between neuropsychiatry, paediatric neurology and child neuropsychology is required in studies of the psychological, social and educational consequences and management of neurological disorders and acquired dysfunction. Biological studies, including brain imaging, are likely to be of particular value.

Socio-economic relationships

The role of socio-economic factors in the genesis and maintenance of mental health problems is unclear. Research should examine the factors and mechanisms which determine why some children survive in conditions of psychosocial adversity while others do not.

Organization and standards of clinical practice

Development and evaluation of treatments

More research is needed across the range of treatments on effectiveness, with particular emphasis on longer term outcomes and the management of specific problems, including management in primary care.[212,213]

Development and evaluation of services

Studies are particularly needed of the relative merits of different service delivery settings (primary care, special care, special clinic, school) as well as modes of service delivery (direct intervention versus parent training and responsiveness to the needs of different communities and ethnic groups). Studies to improve recognition of mental health problems such as depression in primary care are needed.[213]

Developmental evaluation of preventive interventions

Examples of such research could include the prevention of conduct disorders and of psychiatric disorders in children with mental handicap.[213]

Developmental evaluation of specific treatments/interventions

Examples will include treatments for depression and difficulties arising from development characterized by Asperger's Syndrome and drug treatments.

Skill mix

What is the balance of uni- and multi-disciplinary service delivery? What are the costs and benefits of specific service delivery by different professional groups: to what extent is substitution feasible and desirable? Which problems are appropriately dealt with by voluntary agencies or primary health care?

Development of outcome measures

Since the ultimate outcome of child and adolescent mental health services is the child's success as an adult, valid interim measures need to be established. These should include clinical and quality of life measures.

Specific studies of special groups

Evidence on the effectiveness of care of specific groups of children and young people needs to be co-ordinated through broadly based research studies.

Examples are:

- 'hard-to-place' adolescents
- children in social services care
- children who have been abused[213]
- children and adolescents with challenging and/or persistent self-injurious behaviour
- childhood hyperactivity.[213]

Epidemiological studies

There would be particular value in local epidemiological studies to clarify service priorities by evaluating need for the different types of care. Some basic epidemiological work remains to be done.[212] In particular detailed studies are needed of those conditions which are, according to current evidence, increasing in incidence. These include:

- anorexia nervosa
- suicide
- juvenile delinquency
- depression.

Research in the field of child and adolescent mental health should normally be conducted by multi-disciplinary and multi-sectoral groups.

Attention also needs to be paid to the development and dissemination of research findings across the very broad range of professionals involved in the care of children. Research into this field, and the determinants of change in clinical practice would benefit both child and adolescent mental health services and other clinical specialties.

Priorities

Each of these areas for research is important for a number of reasons. There needs to be an overall balance between the more theoretical and academic studies and health services research. Both are needed to inform each other. However in terms of personal and social consequences, the aetiology, development and persistence of conduct disorders as well as their management and treatment in service settings should be given high priority.

Appendix I Definition of terms

- The term **care** is used to cover treatment, rehabilitation, counselling and social welfare.
- The term **service** covers **service agents** (formal and informal carers) and the **service settings**, varying from the domestic home to secure units.
- A **need** for care exists when an individual has an illness or impairment for which there is an effective and acceptable intervention. In this context an 'effective' intervention is one which achieves the treatment objective. It does not necessarily imply 'cure'. There will usually be a hierarchy of methods, from those which produce a complete and rapid recovery with no side-effects to those which achieve amelioration and/or secondary or tertiary prevention.

  The fact that needs are defined does not mean that they will be met. Some may remain unmet because other problems must be dealt with first, or because the more effective method is not available locally or availability is limited by rationing, or because the person in need or the carer objects. There are also 'potential' needs for forms of care that do not at the moment exist but which research may eventually provide.
- A **demand** for care exists when the individuals consider that they have a need and wish to receive care.
- **Utilization** occurs when an individual actually receives care.

  Need may not be expressed as demand; demand may not be followed by utilization; there can be demand and/or utilization without any need.
- **Professional** is a term used to encompass individuals such as GPs, nurses, health visitors, paediatricians, teachers and social workers who have a recognized professional qualification.
- **Specialist** is a term used to describe someone who has had specific training to work with individuals who have mental health needs. Child psychiatrists, clinical psychologists, psychiatric nurses, child psychotherapists and some social workers and teachers are the main groups with such specialist knowledge and skills.

Appendix II Core data set for child and adolescent psychology and psychiatric services

This list includes both problems and risk factors.

Anti-social (FA)
1   Tantrums/outbursts
2   Non-compliance at home
3   Stealing from home
4   Stealing other
5   Aggressive behaviour
6   Cruelty/violent brutality
7   Firesetting/destruction of property
8   Bullying/fighting
9   Substance abuse
10   Running away/wandering
11   Lying

School (FB)
1   School refusal/phobia
2   School non-attendance – other
3   School discipline problem

Cognition/abilities (FC)
1   Gifted
2   General learning disability
3   General academic under-achievement
4   Specific reading difficulty
5   Specific number difficulty
6   Specific spelling difficulty
7   Writing difficulty
8   Unusual cognitive pattern
9   Memory problems
10   Attention abnormality
11   Poor self-care skills

Self (FD)
1   Self-deprecation
2   Self-aggrandizement
3   Disability/disfigurement awareness

Mood (FE)
1   Irritability/moodiness
2   Fatigue/lassitude
3   Depression/misery
4   Euphoria/expansive disinhibition
5   Mood swings

Anxiety-related (FF)
1   General anxiety
2   Phobias
3   Separation anxiety

Self-regulation (FG)
1   Tics/habits/stereotypes
2   Obsessions/rituals
3   Overactivity
4   Enuresis/wetting
5   Soiling/constipation
6   Sleep/wake pattern problems
7   Problems during sleep
8   Subjective insomnia
9   Feeding problems/fads
10   Anorexia
11   Bulimia
12   Obesity/overeating

Social/relationships (FH)
1   Relationship difficulty parent/s/carers
2   Relationship difficulty other adults
3   Relationship difficulty siblings
4   General family relationships problems
5   Relationship difficulty peers
6   Harassment/persecution victim
7   'Attention seeking' behaviour
8   Social disinhibition
9   Social withdrawal
10   Social sensitivity

Context (FI)
1   Marital difficulties
2   Family mental health problems
3   Family physical health problems
4   Adverse social circumstances

Life event (FJ)
1   Bereavement/loss
2   Stress reaction/adjustment reaction
3   PTSD/at risk for
4   Emergency/crisis during episode

Abuse/neglect (FK)
1   Failure to thrive
2   Neglect
3   Physical abuse
4   Emotional abuse
5   Sexual abuse

Self-harm/injury (FL)
1   Self-harm/overdose
2   Self-injurious behaviour
3   Risk-taking

Sexual and sex related (FM)
1   Inappropriately sexualized behaviour
2   Sexual misdemeanour/offence
3   Promiscuity/prostitution
4   Unusual/excessive solitary sexual activity
5   Concern about sexuality
6   Gender identity problem
7   Pregnancy

Personality/temperament (FN)
1   Shyness/social isolation
2   Personality/temperament extreme
3   Inappropriate immature behaviour

Speech and language (FO)
1   Mutism
2   Speech delay/disorder
3   Language delay/disorder

Autistic type characteristics (FP)
1   Autism/autistic features

Psychosis type characteristics (FQ)
1   Confusion/disorientation
2   Psychotic symptoms
3   Unusual/bizarre behaviour

'Psychosomatic' (FR)
1   Hypochondriasis
2   Factitious illness
3   Hysteria/conversion
4   Pain/discomfort non-organic origin
5   Headache

Physical illness/general paediatric (FS)
1   Non-neurological physical illness
2   Pain organic origin
3   Physical disability/deformity
4   HIV/AIDS
5   Other deteriorating organic condition
6   Terminal illness
7   Anxiety about physical medical procedures
8   Poor compliance with medical management

Physical/neurological (FT)
1   Physical slowness
2   Clumsiness/co-ordination difficulty
3   Epilepsy/turns/fits
4   Head injury

Sensory (FU)
1   Visual impairment
2   Blind
3   Hearing difficulties
4   Deaf

Genetic condition (FV)
1   Chromosome anomaly
2   Dysmorphic features
3   Behavioural phenotype

Normal limits (FW)
1   Parental concern but no clinical abnormality
2   Referrer concern but no clinical abnormality

Local other (FX)
1   *n* (Clinical problems locally specified)

Clinical features residual (FZ)
1   Other
2   Not known
3   Not coded

Appendix III Official statistics

Local data sources

Demographic

Basic demographic data covering the age and sex breakdown of a district population can be obtained from either the Public Health Common Data Set or the 1991 Census. These can be used to calculate the numbers within the 0–16 age group and to estimate the potential numbers of children with mental health problems. However the age bands used in the Common Data Set do not fully match those required to cover the 0–16 year olds as it uses the bands 0–4, 5–15 and 15–24 years. The Census, on the other hand, will allow analysis for single years of age. The Census also provides data on residence at ward level.

Ethnic

Both the Common Data Set and the Census provide data on the ethnic composition of district health authorities. The Common Data Set provides the percentage of heads of households born in the New Commonwealth or Pakistan. The 1991 Census provides data on the proportions of different minority groups within a district. The census also provides data on ethnic group by age categories (0–4, 5–15, 16–29).

Mortality

Deaths as a result of mental disorders classified under the ICD 9 codes for mental illness and suicide are classified by age and sex as part of a district's VS3 mortality statistics from OPCS.

Morbidity

Morbidity data can be obtained from a variety of sources. Hospital activity data on parasuicide and ICD codes for mental disorders can be obtained from the regional information system (RIS) or other relevant hospital administration systems (e.g. PAS). Hospital activity data provide a record of existing hospital service provision using the ICD codes for diagnosis. From this data it is possible to identify the age, admission method, postcode of patient, length of stay, etc. This data source will not include patients who are treated outside a district health authority area and will include patients from other districts who are treated in the provider unit. The RIS data will need to be interrogated by district code and data from the Mersey tapes (data on patients treated outside the relevant district health authority) added to this.

Hospital admission rates are as much a reflection of bed availability, referral rates and admission procedures as an indicator of need, but they can provide a useful guide on how need is currently being met. Hospital admission data also require care with interpretation as it is likely that an individual patient will be admitted more than once in a year and the data available are by admission episode and not by individual patient. This can result in an over-counting of some cases.

Some provider units have good data on attenders of psychiatric services as outpatients, inpatients or day care patients. The availability of data is not uniform or compulsory, however.

As an indicator of potential morbidity in the area of mental illness, disability and long-standing illness can be of relevance. Some health authorities and some local authorities keep a handicap register which holds details of children with either mental or physical disabilities. These are not compulsory and their completeness varies from place to place.

The Common Data Set contains details of selected congenital malformations; however, this only covers those malformations identified at or shortly after birth.

Details of limiting long-term illness can be obtained from the 1991 Census. The relevant age bands are 0–15 and 16–29. These data are divided into those resident in communal establishments and those resident in households.

Numbers of children with special educational needs and learning disabilities can be obtained from local education authorities. The Education Act of 1981 requires that children with special educational needs are statemented and their special need documented. This provides a source of information on intellectual and physical disability in an area but can be incomplete. Where a local education authority runs special schools, the number of children attending will be relatively easy to obtain.

Family and socio-economic data

Social class, unemployment rate, numbers receiving housing benefit, car ownership level, proportion of homes with basic amenities and housing tenure type can all indicate levels of social deprivation.

Details of housing tenure, dwelling type, access to cars, overcrowding and economic position can be obtained at ward level from the 1991 Census. Composite deprivation scores include the Jarman index and Townsend, both of which are available at ward level. The Common Data Set provides an underprivileged area score based on the 1981 Census; this may be of limited value because the data from the 1981 Census is now out of date. Local town councils can provide regular data on unemployment figures at ward level.

Criminality

Information on levels of crime among young people may be obtained from local police and probation services; however, this would involve requests in writing detailing exactly what data are required and permission will need to be obtained from the Chief Constable. However soft information can often be obtained informally by discussions with officers from these services.

Secondary data – based on national, regional and local authority areas

The following list provides a number of sources of data that provide a background picture of need and may be of value in determining service requirements for child and adolescent mental health.

Ethnic

Details of the percentage population in each ethnic group for 1983, 1989, 1990 and 1991 – *GHS 1991*, OPCS. Available from public or academic libraries.

Detailed information about the ethnic data provided by the 1991 Census and information on the use of the Labour Force Survey to estimate Britain's ethnic minority population – *Population Trends No. 72*, Summer 1993, pp. 12–17, OPCS. Available from public and academic libraries.

Hospital activity

Admissions to NHS hospitals for mental illness and mental handicap by age group (under ten, 10–14, 15–19) for 1978–1990 including age-specific rates per 100 000 population – *Health and Personal Social Statistics for England*, 1992 edition, HMSO. Tables 9.2 and 9.4. Available from public and academic libraries.

Morbidity

Physical illness – percentages of children reported as having long-standing illness by age bands (0–4, 5–15) – *Regional Trends No. 27*, 1992, p. 69, Table 6.3. Available from public and academic libraries.

Self-reported sickness by age (0–4, 5–15) and sex and economic status for 1972–91. Percentage reporting: a long-standing illness; b limiting long-standing illness; c restricted activity in last 14 days. *GHS 1991*, Tables 8.1–8.4. Available from public and academic libraries.

Social services information

Children and young people on child protection register 1993 – *DoH Personal Social Services (A/ F92/ 13)*. Data on children included in child protection registers for different regions of England by abuse category. Available from public and academic libraries, or from: The Statistician, SD3A Room 454, Skipton House, 80 London Road, Elephant and Castle, London SE1 6LW.

Children accommodated in secure units 1993 – *DoH Personal Social Statistics (A/ F92/ 21)*. Data on children accommodated in secure units both within and outside child's care authority, lists of secure units, etc. Available from public and academic libraries, or from: The Statistician, SD3A Room 454, Skipton House, 80 London Road, Elephant and Castle, London SE1 6LW.

Children in care in local authorities 1993 – *DoH Personal Social Statistics (A/ F91/ 12)*. Information on the numbers of children in each different region of England, reasons for admission to care, etc. Available from public and academic libraries, or from: The Statistician, SD3A Room 454, Skipton House, 80 London Road, Elephant and Castle, London SE1 6LW.

Socio-economic information

Usual gross weekly household income by family type for married couples, lone mothers and lone fathers – *GHS 1991*, Table 2.30, p. 28. Unemployment rates by socio-economic group and sex, Tables 5.7 and 5.8. Available from public and academic libraries.

Unemployment

Percentage of unemployed by age and sex for 1992 – Table 7.15. Unemployment rates for years 1981–91 for regional areas of England – Table 7.16, and households by economic status of head for 1991 – Table 7.5. *Regional Trends No. 27*, 1992. Available from public and academic libraries.

One parent families – trends in the number of one parent families in Great Britain – *Population Trends No. 71*, Spring 1993. Demographic characteristics of one parent families in Great Britain – *Population Trends No. 65*, Autumn 1991.

Children in families broken by divorce – *Population Trends No. 61*, Autumn 1990. Available from public and academic libraries.

Details of the number of dependent children by family type and marital status of lone mothers – *GHS 1991*, Table 2.20. Available from public and academic libraries.

Criminality

Young offenders found guilty or cautioned by type of offence and age (10–13, 14–16, 17–20) in 1981 and 1991 – data covers different regions of England – *Regional Trends No. 28*, 1993, Table 9.6. Available from public and academic libraries.

Supervision orders and intermediate treatment year ending March 1991. *DoH Personal Social Statistics (A/ F9/ 16)*. Available from: The Statistician, SD3A Room 454, Skipton House, 80 London Road, Elephant and Castle, London SE1 6LW.

Appendix IV Current service status for child and adolescent mental health services

Much of the following information has been derived from a recent survey of services for the mental health of children and young people in the UK.[149] It looks at purchasing authorities and the various aspects of child and adolescent services, including community-based care, inpatient and special units, day treatment services, clinical psychology services, paediatric services, social services, education and the non-voluntary sector.

Purchasing authorities

69 of 121 (57%) purchasing authorities were included in the survey. 52% (36 authorities) had done developmental work on a specific strategy for mental health services for young people and 28% (19) had such a strategy in use. A third had consulted with at least four departments or agencies in developing this strategy. The remaining 33 authorities (48%) reported that they had no specific strategy.

In 62% (43) of authorities included in the study, the current specification was separate from that of adult mental health services. Only nine (13%) purchasing authorities had a basis for their specification that was related to the needs of their population i.e. either a formal needs assessment or at least three other indicators of need.

In 55% (38) of authorities, the current contract was separate from that of adult mental health services. In a fifth of cases a single contract was in place covering community, day and inpatient care for children and for adolescents. Every purchasing authority had contracts with named provider units for inpatient care, or else mentioned that they used extra-contractual referrals (8%), or either a block regional contract or a subscription system (7%).

In 28% of authorities, older adolescents (aged 16 to 18 years) were included in the same contract as younger age groups; in 16% they were included by design in the contracts for adult mental health; in 17% they were included with adults, by default.

In most cases the work of clinical psychologists was included within wider contracts, but separate contracts with clinical psychology were specified by 7% of authorities. In 13% of authorities the main contract included services to be provided in education and/or social services.

Plans for evaluation of the service were largely undeveloped.

Child and adolescent mental health services

The specialist child and adolescent mental health services are largely delivered from a community base, by means of multi-disciplinary teams. Within these teams psychiatrists and social workers are almost universal members, although the number of social workers has reduced in the past three years, mainly as a result of local authority reorganization. Numbers of staff and the range of skills available vary widely between different units. There is little regular input to the service from the education sector.

Community-based care

Of the 151 (81%) departments of child and adolescent mental health included in the survey, 94% provided a service in community clinics; 19% were an integral part of units also providing inpatient care and also 11% provided care on a day basis. 70% provided a community service only. There was a designated budget for child and adolescent psychiatry in 56% of services.

There is major variation in the distribution of numbers of child and adolescent psychiatrists across the country and in the type of work they undertake. 15% of services had less than one wte consultant, 40% between one and two, and 44% more than two. The number of children (aged 0–18 years) per one wte consultant ranged from 6 403 to 244 135. The number of wte consultants per 100 000 child population ranged from 0.41 to 15.62. Child and adolescent psychiatrists provided emergency cover in 69% of districts.

Other professional staff included:

- 58% had junior medical staff in training positions
- 69% had clinical psychologists
- 44% had a psychotherapist
- 17% had a family therapist
- 11% had an educational psychologist
- 63% had a psychiatric community nurse
- 81% had a social worker.

Provision to other professional groups included:

- 36% of departments provided five or more sessions (half-day duration) per month to paediatrics. 27% provided no services to paediatrics
- 11% provided sessions in general practice (majority were one session per week)
- 35% provided more than five regular sessions a month for social services departments
- 28% provided five or more regular sessions a month to schools
- 18% provided occasional sessions for the police and 8% for the probation service
- 37% did sessions for voluntary sector agencies.

Overall 15% provided no, or very limited, services to any other department.

Inpatient and special units

Many inpatient units, including former regional adolescent units, are experiencing problems particularly with respect to the new system of contracting for services.

Of the 37 NHS inpatient units (60%) who replied, 32% had contracts with a single purchasing authority, 22% with two authorities and 41% had multiple contracts.

Staffing revealed:

- consultants – 8% of units had less than one wte while 51% had two or more
- 95% had junior medical staff
- 76% had clinical psychology input
- 65% had an occupational therapist
- all but one had teachers
- 32% of units had psychotherapy
- 70% of units had social work input.

65% had a distinct and separate budget, but only 23% held it themselves within child and adolescent psychiatry.

25% of units catered for both children and adolescents, a further 25% for children only and 50% for adolescents only.

60% functioned on a seven-day basis, while 40% closed at the weekend. 80% provided 24- hour cover for emergencies.

33% provided care entirely in one location.

Innovative or specialist clinics and other services most frequently mentioned included child sexual abuse/post-abuse therapy, parenting and early intervention, eating disorders, early onset psychoses, severe enuresis, communication disorders/neuropsychiatry and autism.

Day treatment services

A quarter of all units (37) replied that they provided treatment on a day basis. Of these 59% also provided inpatient care.

Of these units:

- 95% had at least one wte consultant
- 89% had junior medical staff
- 78% had a clinical psychologist
- 84% had a social worker
- the median number of psychiatric community nurses was four.

33% of units stated that treatment on a day basis was available somewhere within the district. A further 10% used education authority facilities, such as emotional and behavioural difficulty (EBD) units or social services day centres as a base from which to provide day treatment. Facilities in neighbouring districts were often otherwise available.

Clinical psychology services

Clinical psychology is a growing profession, working increasingly from an independent base. Clinical psychologists still work mainly with child and adolescent mental health teams, but they also provide direct and consultative services to acute and community services in other sectors of the NHS, to social services and to other agencies.

Of the 168 (90%, covering 88% of districts) clinical psychology services who replied, 67% provided some care on a unidisciplinary basis and 25% had separate contracts with GP fundholders.

The responses covered 513 clinical psychologists, comprising 156 grade B and 357 grade A. There were 277 trainees and 18% of responses stated that their work was essential to maintain the present level of service. In 13% of services other professional staff were employed, including counsellors.

In the past three years, 44% of the services had seen no change in the numbers of clinical psychologists; in 36% there had been an increase and in 12% a reduction. 30% reported that an increase was planned for next year.

42% received referrals from child and family or child guidance clinics. Many clinical psychologists worked regular sessions with acute paediatrics, on the wards (36% of services) and in outpatients (46%). Sessions were provided as required by 27% in cases of deliberate self-harm and by 29% in cases of emergency admissions for abuse. Even more (61%) did sessions in child development clinics and in 20% of services this amounted to more than 20 sessions a month (the equivalent of a half-time post).

The third most important area of work was for social services, with regular commitment from 57% of clinical psychology departments.

Only 8% of services gave more than the occasional sessions in mainstream schools, but 18% provided regular sessions in special schools for children with learning difficulties, physical disabilities or sensory impairment.

On a smaller scale, sessions were provided for the police and probation services by 10% of services, largely on an occasional basis. Similarly 10% of services provided a small input to drug and alcohol services. 32% worked with the voluntary sector, helping particularly with training and management.

22% of clinical psychology departments were members of a multi-disciplinary group that gave advice to the purchasing authority.

Paediatric services

Data from this survey suggest that more children with emotional and behavioural disorder present to paediatricians than to any other profession. Paediatric training in the main does not prepare them for this and they would welcome further opportunities to gain relevant experience.

Hospital paediatrics

It is estimated that 5–15% of children referred to paediatric departments is due primarily to emotional and behavioural problems. The main conditions were: constipation/encopresis/soiling (54% of directorates), enuresis (42%), headaches/abdominal pain/psychosomatic conditions (34%), sleep problems (34%) and feeding problems (27%).

Paediatricians estimated that 15% (median) of their patients had an underlying or additional emotional or behavioural disorder in addition to the main presenting condition, although 42% of departments suggested a lower proportion (between 3% and 10%).

29% of hospital-based paediatric consultants felt that their training had adequately prepared them for dealing with emotional and behavioural problems, although 46% stated that training was still inadequate in this respect. Junior staff needed regular placements or an opportunity to participate in clinics in child and adolescent psychiatry.

Psychological training and support for nurses and junior doctors was regularly provided in 37% of departments. 70% of departments said they needed more support and training for staff in these types of problem.

48% of paediatric departments held formal planning sessions together with the child and adolescent psychiatry department; 32% were part of a multi-agency group, advising the purchasing authority on children's needs, including those for mental health services.

Community paediatrics

20% of children referred to community paediatricians were referred primarily for emotional and behavioural problems. The main sources of referral were health visitors (reported by 83% of departments), GPs (64%) and educational authority staff such as teachers and educational psychologists (53%).

22% of community paediatricians said that they referred between 40% and 50% of cases for further opinion. The main emotional and behavioural conditions treated were largely the same as those treated by hospital paediatricians.

Community paediatricians, even more so than hospital paediatricians, felt that the resources for child and adolescent psychiatry in their district were quite inadequate. Long waiting lists and frequent personnel changes were described by 75%.

Community paediatricians were involved formally in planning provision with the child and adolescent psychiatry teams in 56% of districts. They were represented on a multi-agency group advising the purchasing authority for these services in 40%.

Social services

Social services departments concentrate resources on children in need, many of whom have serious emotional and behavioural problems. They report unsatisfactory access to NHS specialist expertise in children's mental health.

Social service departments contribute to mental health services by providing social work input to the multi-disciplinary team in 81% of services. Of the 59 (56% covering 62% of health authorities) social services departments who replied, 17% had no formal or written policy on assessment and therapeutic services for children and young people with emotional and behavioural problems. All others had some sort of policy, though often part of a general policy for children in need, based on the Children Act. 46% were either working on, or had already developed, joint policies or joint commissioning with the health service. A further 9% had firm plans to start negotiations in this particular field with the NHS in the coming year. Five departments had also included the local education authority in policy making.

Assessment and therapeutic services for children and young people were mostly provided in social services family or day centres (in 29% of departments), though in 17% child guidance centres were used. 20% negotiated provision of part of the service by the NHS; a very small number stated that they purchased these services.

49% of social services departments were represented on a multi-agency group to advise the NHS purchaser. A large proportion (75%) had representation on a multi-agency group to plan services with the NHS providers.

61% of respondents stated that they had had no staff losses in the last three years and 56% said they had had staff increases during that time. Other changes that might have had an effect on services for this client group included the establishment of new team structures (mentioned by 20%) and this was frequently linked with the need to meet the requirements of the Children Act.

64% of the departments stated that they ran services or programmes specifically for children with emotional and behavioural difficulties, providing group, family and individual sessions. The social services department had a direct input into schools in 54% of authorities. 86% of departments contributed on a regular or occasional basis to health services, with half providing sessions in at least five different health settings. The most common contribution was to child and family (psychiatric) outpatient or community-based clinics (58% of the responses), followed quite closely by work in child development clinics (51%), paediatric inpatient wards (49%) and children's outpatient clinics (42%).

Work with the police and the probation service was carried out by a number of authorities, although 30% did not do anything in this respect.

61% of social services departments had direct input into voluntary or joint SSD/voluntary facilities. 12% stated that they had firm plans to increase work with the voluntary sector in the coming year.

The education sector

Local education authorities are greatly concerned with emotional and behavioural difficulties in their pupils. Behaviour support services, as currently provided in three-quarters of local education authorities, include assessment of the educational needs of pupils with severe behaviour problems, but frequently no relevant medical contribution is included. Special schools for children with emotional and behavioural difficulties report that few pupils have statements in which therapeutic help is specified, although the head teachers consider that nearly half of all pupils would benefit from such help.

Local education authorities

Of the 29 (27%) local education authorities who replied, 59% had developed a policy for pupils in mainstream education who had, or were at risk of, emotional and behavioural problems. A further 17% were currently reviewing their policy.

Educational psychology services

Of the 47 (44% covering 45% of health districts) educational psychology services who replied, work in this field was specifically included in the job descriptions of 55% of services.

Special schools for children with emotional and behavioural problems

Of the 165 (approximately 55%) special schools who replied, 80% felt that help from the referring agency was token in that children were rarely visited by specialists from home and that the resources available from the referring agencies were inadequate. Similarly 86% did not feel that the NHS provided resources that the children needed.

90% of schools had provided in-service training for teaching staff on emotional and behavioural problems or related issues in the past year.

Non-teaching specialists with a particular role in therapeutic support were not widely or regularly available.

64% of EBD schools had not been visited by child and adolescent psychiatrists in the past year. 36% had been, 68% of them on a regular basis.

The non-statutory sector

The voluntary sector plays a large part at primary care level, particularly in providing services such as counselling, and taking many self-referrals. Voluntary organizations also act as a filter to specialist mental health and social services. Since the NHS mental health services accept self-referrals less and less, the voluntary services may be filling a gap in provision. They offer particular expertise for secondary and tertiary provision.

15% of the child and adolescent psychiatry services stated that they had used private hospitals for inpatients. Several responses mentioned that the major and sole use was for eating disorders, such as anorexia nervosa.

In planning (including health needs assessment), 42% of NHS purchasing authorities said that they had included voluntary organizations in their discussions and several had involved particular organizations in a substantial way.

A detailed study of data for one region (Yorkshire) revealed 154 independent or semi-independent organizations, covering all cities and towns in the region. 42% were classified as providing a service for a range of general problems that were of concern to young people. 18% provided services to help people misusing drugs, alcohol or other substances. 12% provided services for children and young people who had been abused sexually, physically or emotionally. About 8% of organizations helped children or their families with problems related to serious physical illness or disability. Another 8% specialized in problems surrounding homelessness.

25% specifically provided for the 16 to 25 age group and 14% for the under 16s.

The sources of funding were varied and few relied entirely on one source. 51% received some local authority funding, including grants from social services, education and housing departments. 6% specifically mentioned joint funding from health and social services. 8% received some funding from central government. 46% raised at least part of their costs by general fundraising, through appeals, corporate fundraising, grants from trusts and subscriptions. 6% charged for their services, either directly or through contracts.

Psychiatric community nurses

There were 260 wte nurses working in community-based units, of whom 47% had been specifically trained in children's and adolescent's psychiatric care (ENB 603). Of the 87 units who employed a community psychiatric nurse (CPN) only one-third (34%) had a nurse with this qualification. Of nurses working within inpatient units less than one-fifth (18%) had undertaken the ENB course, though there were only four units with no nurse with this qualification.

Child psychotherapy

Child psychotherapists working in community-based units were unevenly distributed across the country with 92% employed in the four Thames regions, Wessex, Oxford and South Western.

References

1 Rutter M. Pathways from childhood to adult life. *J Child Psychol Psych* 1989; **30**: 23–51.

2 Garmezy N, Rutter M. Acute reactions to stress. In *Child.and Adolescent Psychiatry: Modern Approaches* (eds M Rutter and L Herzov). Oxford: Blackwell Scientific Publications, 1985, pp. 152–76.

3 Rutter M, Cox A. Other family influences. In *Child and Adolescent Psychiatry: Modern Approaches* (eds M Rutter and L Herzov). Oxford: Blackwell Scientific Publications, 1985, pp. 58–81.

4 Wolkind S, Rutter M. Separation, loss and family relationships. In *Child and Adolescent Psychiatry: Modern Approaches* (eds M Rutter and L Herzov). Oxford: Blackwell Scientific Publications, 1985, pp. 34–57.

5 Shaw D, Emery R. Chronic family adversity and school age children's adjustment. *J Am Ac Child Adol Psych* 1988; **27**: 200–6.

6 Goodyer I. Family relationships, life events and child psychopathology. *J Child Psychol Psych* 1990; **31**: 161–92.

7 Goodyer I. Life events and psychiatric disorder. *J Child Psych Psych* 1990; **31**: 839–48.

8 Farrington DP, Loeber RG, van Kammen WB. Long-term criminal outcomes of hyperactivity-impulsivity-attention deficit and conduct in childhood. In *Straight and Devious Pathways from Childhood to Adulthood* (eds LN Robins and M Rutter). Cambridge: Cambridge University Press, 1990, pp. 62–81.

9 Harrington R. *Depression disorder in childhood and adolescence*. Chichester: Wiley, 1993.

10 Brown GW, Harris TO, Bifulco A. Long-term effects of early loss of parent. In *Depression in young people: developmental and clinical perspectives* (eds M Rutter, CE Izard, PB Read). New York: Guilford Press, 1985, pp. 251–96.

11 Rutter M (ed.). *Studies of Psychosocial Risk*. Cambridge: Cambridge University Press, 1988.

12 Brewin CR, Wing JK. *The MRC Needs for Care Assessment Manual*. London: Institute of Psychiatry, 1988.

13 Mathew GK. Measuring need and evaluating services. In *Problems and progress in medical care* (ed. G McLachlan). Sixth series. Oxford: Oxford University Press, 1971.

14 Wing JK, Brewin C, Thornicroft G. Defining mental health needs. In *Measuring Mental Health Needs* (eds G Thornicroft, C Brewin, Wing JK). London: HMSO, 1993, chapter 1.

15 Berger M, Hill P, Sein E *et al*. *A proposed core data set for child and adolescent psychology and psychiatry services*. Association for Child Psychology and Psychiatry, 1993.

16 World Health Organization. *International Statistical Classification of Diseases and Related Health Problems*. Tenth Revision. Geneva: WHO, 1992.

17 Rutter M, Smith DJ. *Psychological Disorders in Young People. Time trends and their causes*. Chichester: Wiley, 1995.

18 Cox AD. Preventive aspects of child psychiatry. *Arch Dis Child* 1993; **68**: 691–701.

19 Graham PJ. Prevention. In *Child and Adolescent Psychiatry: Modern Perspectives* (eds M Rutter, E Taylor, L Hersov). 3rd edn. Oxford: Blackwell Scientific Publications, 1994, pp. 815–28.

20 Department for Education. *Pupils with Problems: Circulars 8–13/94*. London: Department for Education, 1994.

21 Department of Health. *Child Protection: Message from Research*. London: HMSO, 1995.

22 Richman N, Stevenson JE, Graham PJ. Prevalence of behaviour problems in 3 year old children: an epidemiological study in a London borough. *J Child Psych Psych* 1975; **16**: 277.

23 Rutter M, Cox A, Tupling C *et al*. Attainment and adjustment in two geographical areas. I: The prevalence of psychiatric disorder. *Brit J Psych* 1975; **126**: 493.

24 Rutter M, Graham P. The reliability and validity of the psychiatric assessment of the child. *Brit J Psych* 1968; **114**: 563.

25 Verhulst FC, Berden GFG, Sanders-Woudstra JAR. Mental health in Dutch children. II. *Act Psych Scan* 1985; **72**: 1.

26 Costello EJ. Developments in child psychiatric epidemiology. *J Am Ac Child Adol Pysch* 1988; **28**: 836.

27 Graham P, Rutter M. Psychiatric disorder in the young and adolescent. *J Roy Soc Med* 1973; **66**: 1226–9.

28 Rutter M, Graham P, Chadwick O *et al*. Adolescent turmoil: fact or fiction? *J Child Psychol Pysch* 1976; **17**: 35–56.

29 Offor DR, Boyle MH, Szatmari P *et al*. Ontario Child Health Study. II. Six month prevalence of disorder and rates of service utilisation. *Arch Gen Psych* 1987; **44**: 832.

30 Rutter M, Yule W, Berger M *et al*. Children of West Indian immigrants. 1. Rates of behavioural deviance and psychiatric disorder. *J Child Psychol Psych* 1974; **15**: 241–62.

31 Cochrane R. Psychological and behavioural disturbance in West Indians, Indians and Pakistanis in Britain. A comparison of rates among children and adults. *Brit J Psych* 1979; **134**: 201.

32 Hackett L, Hackett R, Taylor DC. Psychological disturbance and its association in the children of the Gujarati community. *J Child Psychol Psych* 1991; **32**: 851–6.

33 Rack P. Psychiatric disorder in immigrants. In *Readings in Psychiatry 3*. Oxford: Medical Education Sevices, 1984, pp. 53–7.

34 Rack P. *Race, culture and mental disorder*. London: Tavistock, 1982.

35 Kallarackal AM, Herbert M. The happiness of Indian immigrant children. *New Soc* 1976; **35**: 422.

36 Hackett L, Hackett R. Parental ideas of normal and deviant child behaviour. A comparison of two ethnic groups. *Brit J Psych* 1993; **162**: 353–7.

37 Rutter M, Yule W, Graham P. Enuresis and Behavioural Deviance: some epidemiological considerations. In *Bladder Control and Enuresis* (eds I Kolvin, R MacKeith, SR Meadow). Clinics in Developmental Medicine, nos 48/49. London: Heinemann/Spastics International Medical Publications, 1973.

38 Jarvelin MR, Vikevainen Tervonen L, Moilanen I *et al*. Enuresis in seven year old children. *Acta Paed Scand* 1988; **77**: 148–53.

39 Minde K, Minde R. *Infant psychiatry: an introductory text*. London: Sage Publications, 1986.

40 Apley J, Nalsh N. Recurrent abdominal pains: a field study of 1000 children. *Arch Dis Child* 1958; **33**: 165–70.

41 Apley J. *The Child with Abdominal Pains*. 2nd edn. Oxford: Blackwell Scientific Publications, 1975.

42 Zahner GEP, Clubb MM, Leckman JF *et al*. The epidemiology of Tourette's Syndrome. In *Tourette's Syndrome and Tic Disorders* (eds DJ Cohen, RD Bruun, JF Leckmann). New York: Wiley, 1988, p.79.

43 Rutter M, Tizard J, Whitmore K. *Education, Health and Behaviour*. London: Longmann, 1970

44 Berger M, Yule W, Rutter M. Attainment and adjustment in two geographical areas II: the prevalence of specific reading retardation. *Brit J Psych* 1975; **126**: 510–19.

45 Benjamin RS, Costello EJ, Warren M. Anxiety disorders in a paediatric sample. *J Anx Dis* 1990; **4**: 293–316.

46 Kashani JH, Orvaschel H. Anxiety disorders in mid-adolescence: a community sample. *Am J Psychiatry* 1988; **145**: 960–4.

47 Offord DR, Boyle MH, Jones BA. Psychiatric disorder and poor school performance among welfare children in Ontario. *Can J Psych* 1987; **32**: 518.

48 Offord DR, Boyle MH, Racine YH. *Ontario Child Health Study: Children at risk*. Toronto: Queen's Printer for Ontario, 1990.

49 Shapiro AK, Shapiro ES, Young JG *et al*. (eds) *Gilles de la Tourette Syndrome*. 2nd edn. New York: Raven, 1988.

50 Flament MF, Whitacker A, Rapoport J *et al*. Obsessive compulsive disorder in adolescence. *J Am Ac Child Adol Psych* 1988; **27**: 764–77.

51 Whitacker A, Johnson J, Shaffer D *et al.* Uncommon troubles in young people: prevalence estimates of selected psychiatric disorders in a non-referred adolescent population. *Arch Gen Psych* 1990; **47**: 487–96.

52 Taylor E, Sandburg S, Thorley G *et al. The Epidemiology of Childhood Hyperactivity. Maudsley Monographs no. 33.* Oxford: Oxford University Press, 1991.

53 Bellman M. Studies on encopresis. *Acta Paed Scand* 1966; suppl: 170.

54 Nielson S. The epidemiology of anorexia nervosa in Denmark from 1973 to 1987: a nationwide register study of psychiatric admission. *Acta Psych Scand* 1990; **81**: 507-14.

55 Steinhausen H-C, Seidal R. A prospective follow-up study in early-onset eating disorders. In *The Course of Eating Disorders: Long-Term Follow-Up Studies of Anorexia and Bulimia Nervosa Course* (eds W Herzog, HC Deter, W Vandereycken). Berlin: Springer, 1992.

56 Freidman JM, Asnis GM, Boeck M *et al.* Prevalence of specific suicidal behaviour in high school samples. *Am J Psych* 1987; **144**: 1203–6.

57 Smith K, Crawford S. Suicidal behaviours among 'normal' high school students. *Suicide Life Threat Behav* 1986; **16**: 313–25.

58 Pfeffer CR, Newcorn J, Kaplan G *et al.* Suicidal behaviour in adolescent psychiatric patients. *J Am Acad Child Adol Psych* 1988; **27**: 357–61.

59 Shaffer D, Fisher P. The epidemiology of suicide in children and young adolescents. *J Am Acad Child Psych* 1981; **20**: 545–65.

60 Shaffer D, Piacentini J. Suicide and Attempted Suicide. In *Child Psychiatry: Modern Approaches* (eds M Rutter, L Hersov, E Taylor). 3rd edn. Oxford: Blackwell Scientific Publications, 1994.

61 Office of Population Censuses and Surveys. *Adolescent Drinking.* London: HMSO, 1992.

62 Swadi H. Drug and Substance Use Among 3333 London Adolescents. *Brit J Add* 1988; **83**: 935–42.

63 Health Education Authority. *Tomorrow's Young Adults. 9–15 Year Olds Look at Alcohol, Drugs, Exercise and Smoking.* London: Health Education Authority, 1992.

64 Mott J. Self-reported cannabis use on Great Britain in 1981. *Brit J Add* 1985; **80**: 37–43.

65 Miller JD, Cisin IH, Gardenere-Keaton H *et al. National Survey on Drug Abuse: Main Findings. National Institute on Drug Abuse Research Monograph.* Rockville, MD: National Institute on Drug Abuse, 1983.

66 Johnson LD, O'Malley PM, Bachman JG. *Drug Use among American High School Students, College Students and other Young Adults: National Trends Through 1985. National Institute on Drug Abuse Research Monograph.* Rockville, MD: National Institute on Drug Abuse, 1986.

67 Coggans S, Davies J. *National Evaluation of Drug Education in Scotland: Final Report.* Strathclyde: University of Strathclyde, 1989.

68 Farrell M. Ecstasy and the oxygen of publicity. *Brit J Add* 1989; **84**: 943.

69 Ashton M. *Drug Misuse in Britain: National Audit of Drug Misuse Statistics.* London: ISDD, 1991.

70 Breslau N. Psychiatric disorder in children with disabilities. *J Am Acad Child Psych* 1985; **24**: 87.

71 Pless IB. Clinical assessment. Physical and psychological functioning. *Ped Clin North Am* 1984; **32**: 33.

72 Satter-White B. Impact of chronic illness on child and family. An over-view based on five surveys. *Int J Rehab Res* 1978; **1**: 7.

73 Cadman D, Boyle M, Szatmari P *et al.* Chronic illness, disability and mental and social well-being. Findings of the Ontario Child Health Study. *Paed* 1987; **79**: 805.

74 Rutter M. Brain damage syndrome in childhood. Concepts and findings. *J Child Psychol Psych* 1977; **18**: 1.

75 Goodman R. Brain disorders. In *Child Psychiatry: Modern Approaches* (eds M Rutter, L Hersov, E Taylor). 3rd edn. Oxford: Blackwell Scientific Publications, 1994.

76 Brown G, Chadwick O, Shaffer D *et al.* A prospective study of children with head injuries, III. Psychiatric sequalae. *Pyschol Med* 1981; **11**: 63.

77 Goodman R. Brain development. In *Development Through Life: A Handbook for Clinicians* (eds M Rutter, DF Hay). Oxford: Blackwell Scientific Publications, 1994.

78 Martin JAM. Aetiological factors relating childhood deafness in the European Community. *Audiol* 1982; **21**: 149–58.

79 Bamford J, Saunders E. *Hearing impairment, auditory perception and language disability*. 2nd edn. London: Whurr, 1991.

80 Rutter M, Graham P, Berger M. *A neuropsychiatric study in childhood. Clinics in Developmental Medicine. Nos 35/36*. London: Spastics International Medical Publications, 1970.

81 Fundulis T, Kolvin I, Garside RF. *Speech retarded and deaf children: Their Psychological Development*. London: Academic Press, 1979.

82 Schlesinger H, Meadow KP. *Sound and Sign*. Cambridge: University of California, 1972.

83 Hill AE, McKendrick P, Poole JJ *et al*. The Liverpool Visual Assessment Team: 10 Years Experience. *Child: Care, Hlth Develop* 1986; **12**: 37–51.

84 Felce D, Taylor D, Wright K. *People with learning difficulties. Project 12. Epidemiologically based needs assessment*. DHA Project: Research programme, 1992.

85 Graham PJ. Behavioural and Intellectual Development in Childhood Epidemiology. *Brit Med Bull* 1986; **42(2)**: 155–62.

86 West DJ, Farrington DP. *Who becomes delinquent?* London: Heinemann, 1973.

87 Hoy E, Weiss G, Minde K *et al*. The hyperactive child at adolescence: Cognitive, emotional and social functioning. *J Abnormal Child Psychol* 1978; **6**: 311.

88 Minde K, Lewin D, Weiss G *et al*. The hyperactive child in elementary school: A five-year controlled follow-up. *Exceptional Child* 1971; **38**: 215.

89 Emslie G, Rush AJ, Weinberg W *et al*. *Self-report of depressive symptoms in adolescents. Ethnic and sex differences*. Paper presented at the annual meeting of the American Academy of Child and Adolescent Psychiatry. Washington, DC, 1987.

90 Fleming JE, Offord DR, Boyle MH. Prevalence of childhood and adolescent depression in the community: Ontario Child Health Study. *Brit J Psych* 1989; **155**: 647.

91 Friedrich WN, Reams R, Jacobs JH. Sex differences in depression in early adolescents. *Psychol Reports* 1988; **62**: 475.

92 Garrison CZ, Schoenbach VJ, Kaplan BH. Depressive symptoms in early adolescence. In *Depression in multidisciplinary perspective*. New York: Brunner-Mazel, 1985, pp. 60–82.

93 Hoberman HM, Garfinkel BD, Parsons JH *et al*. Depression in a community sample of adolescents. Paper presented at the annual meeting of the American Academy of Child and Adolescent Psychiatry. Los Angeles, 1986.

94 Reynolds WM, Coats KI. Depression in adolescence: incidence, depth and correlates. Paper presented at the 10th International Association of Child and Adolescent Psychiatry and Allied Professions. Dublin, 1982.

95 Terr LC. The use of the Beck Depression Inventory with Adolescents. *J Abnormal Child Psychol* 1982; **10**: 277.

96 Costello EJ, Costello AJ, Edelbrock C *et al*. Psychiatric disorders in paediatric primary care. *Arch Gen Psych* 1988; **45**: 1107.

97 Williams S, McGee RO, Anderson J *et al*. The structure and correlates of self-reported symptoms in 11 year old children. *J Abnorm Child Psychol* 1989; **17**: 55.

98 Richman N, Stevenson JE, Graham PJ. *Pre-school to school: a behaviour study*. London and New York: Academic Press, 1982.

99 Baker L, Cantwell DP. Psychiatric disorder in children with different types of communication disorder. *J Commun Dis* 1982; **15**: 113–26.

100 Beitchman JH, Nair R, Clegg M *et al.* Prevalence of psychiatric disorders in children with speech and language disorders. *J Am Acad Child Adol Psych* 1986; **25**: 528–35.

101 Frick PJ. Family dysfunction and the disruptive behaviour disorders. In *Advances in Clinical and Child Psychology* (eds TH Ollendick, RJ Prinz). Vol. 16. New York: Plenum Press, 1994.

102 Farrington DP, West DJ. The Cambridge study in delinquent development (United Kingdom). In *Prospective Longitudinal Research: An empirical basis for the primary prevention of psychological disorders* (eds SA Mednick, AE Baert). Oxford: Oxford University Press, 1981, pp. 133–45.

103 Patterson GR. *Coercive Family Process.* Eugene, Oregon: Castalia Publishing Company, 1982.

104 Earls F, Yung KG. Temperament and home environment characteristics as causal factors in the early development of childhood psychopathology. *J Am Acad Child Adol Psych* 1987; **26**: 491.

105 Emery RE, O'Leary KD. Children's perceptions of marital discord and behavioural problems of boys and girls. *J Abnorm Child Psychol* 1982; **10**: 11.

106 Rutter M. Epidemiological-longitudinal strategies and causal research in child psychiatry. *J Am Acad Child Psych* 1981; **20**: 513.

107 Zill N. Divorce, marital conflict and children's mental health: Research findings and policy recommendations. Testimony before the Subcommittee on Family and Human Services, US Senate Committee on Labour and Human Resources Senate Hearing 98–195. Washington, DC: US Government Printing Office, 1983, pp. 90–106.

108 Monck E, Graham P, Richman N *et al.* Adolescent girls I: Background factors in anxiety and depressive states. *Brit J Psych* 1994; **165**: 760–9.

109 Monck E, Graham P, Richman N *et al.* Adolescent girls II: Background factors in anxiety and depressive states. *Brit J Psych* 1994; **165**: 770–80.

110 Office of Population Censuses and Surveys. *General Household Survey.* Series GHS. No. 22. London: HMSO, 1992.

111 Haskey J. Patterns of marriage, divorce and cohabitation in the different countries of Europe. *Europ Pop Trends* 1992; **69**: 27–36.

112 Kiernan K, Wickes M. *Family Change and Future Policy.* Family Policies Study Centre, 231 Baker Street, London NW1 6XE, 1990.

113 Jones MB, Offord DR, Abrams N. Brothers, sisters and anti-social behaviour. *Brit J Psych* 1980; **136**: 139.

114 Offord DR, Fleming JE. *Child and Adolescent Psychiatry. A Comprehensive Textbook* (ed. M Lewis). Baltimore: Williams and Wilkins, 1989.

115 Leckman JF, Weissman MM, Merikangas KR *et al.* Major depression and panic disorder. *Psychopharmacol Bull* 1985; **21**: 543.

116 Weissman MM, Merikangas KR, Gammon GD *et al.* Depression and anxiety disorders in parents and children. Results from the Yale Family Study. *Arch Gen Psych* 1984; **41**: 845.

117 Gottesman II, Shields J. *Schizophrenia: The Epigenic Puzzle.* Cambridge: Cambridge University Press, 1982.

118 Rutter M, Giller H. *Juvenile Delinquency: Trends and Perspectives.* New York: Penguin Books, 1983.

119 Robins LN, West PA, Herjanic BL. Arrests and delinquency in two generations: a study of black urban families and their children. *J Child Psychol Psych* 1975; **3**: 241.

120 Osborn SG, West DJ. Conviction records of fathers and sons compared. *Brit J Criminol* 1979; **19**: 120–33.

121 McCord W, McCord J. *Origins of Crime.* New York: Columbia University Press, 1959.

122 Rutter M. Family and school influences: meanings, mechanisms and implications. In *Longitudinal studies in child psychology and psychiatry* (ed. AR Nicol). Chichester: Wiley, 1985.

123 Dilalla LF, Gottesman I. Heterogeneity of causes for delinquency and criminality: life-span perspectives. *Develop Psychopathol* 1989; **1**: 339–49.

124 Brown K, Saqui S. Parent–child interaction in abusing families and its possible causes and consequences. In *Child Abuse: The Educational Perspective* (ed. P Maher). Oxford: Basil Blackwell, 1987.

125 Erickson MF, Egeland B, Pianta R. The effects of maltreatment on the development of young children (eds D Cicchetti, V Carlson). In *Child Maltreatment*. Cambridge: Cambridge University Press, 1989.

126 Finkelhor D. *A Sourcebook on Child Sexual Abuse*. Beverly Hills: Sage, 1986.

127 Kelly L, Regan L, Burton S. *An exploratory study of the prevalence of sexual abuse in a sample of 16–21 year olds*. London: University of London, 1991.

128 Earls F. Prevalence of behaviour problems in 3 year old children: a cross-sectional replication. *Arch Gen Psych*, 1980; **37**: 1153.

129 Achenbach TM, Edelbrook CS. Behavioural problems and competences by parents of normal and disturbed children aged four through to sixteen. *Monograph Society Res Child Develop* 1981; **46**: 1.

130 Lapouse R, Monk MA. Behaviour deviations in a representative sample of children: variation by sex, race, social class and family size. *Am J Orthopsych* 1964; **34**: 346.

131 Anderson J, Williams S, McGee R *et al*. Cognitive and social correlates of DSM-III disorders in preadolescent children. *J Am Acad Child Adol Psych* 1989; **28**: 842.

132 Offord DR. Social factors in the aetiology of childhood disorders. In *Handbook of studies on child psychiatry* (eds B Tonge, G Burrows, J Werry). Amsterdam: Elsevier, 1990, pp. 56–68.

133 Banks M, Jackson P. Unemployment and risk of minor psychiatric disorder in young people: cross-sectional and longitudinal evidence. *Psychol Med* 1982; **12**: 786–98.

134 Farrington DP, Gallagher B, Morley L *et al*. Unemployment, school leaving and crimes. *Brit J Criminol* 1986; **26**: 335–56.

135 Quinton D. Urbanisation and child mental health. *J Child Psychol Psych* 1988; **29**: 11–20.

136 Richman N. The effects of housing on pre-school children and their mothers. *Develop Med Child Neurol* 1974; **16**: 53–8.

137 Alperstein G, Arnstein E. Homeless children – a challenge for pediatricians. *Ped Clin North Am* 1988; **35**: 1413–25.

138 Fox SJ, Barrnett J, Davies M *et al*. Psychopathology and developmental delay in homeless children. *J Am Acad Child Adol Psych* 1990; **29**: 732–5.

139 Wolkind S, Rutter M. Socio-cultural factors. In *Child and Adolescent Psychiatry: Modern Approaches* (eds M Rutter, L Hersov). 2nd edn. Oxford: Blackwell Scientific Publications, 1985.

140 Olweus D. Bully/victim problems among school children: basic facts and effects of a school based intervention program. In *The Development and Treatment of Child Aggression*. Erlbaum, Hillsdale, New Jersey, 1991.

141 Pynoos RS, Frederick C, Nader K *et al*. Life threat and post-traumatic stress in school-age children. *Arch Gen Psych* 1987; **47**: 1057–63.

142 Yule W. The effects of disasters in children. *Ass Child Psychol Psych News* 1989; **11**: 3–6.

143 Yule W. Children in shipping disasters. *J Roy Soc Med* 1991; **84**: 12–15.

144 Goodyer IM. Development psycholpathology: the impact of recurrent life events in anxious and depressed school age children. *J Roy Soc Med* 1994; **87**: 327–9.

145 Masterman SH, Reams R. Support groups for bereaved preschool and school-age children. *Am J Orthopsych* 1988; **58**: 562–70.

146 Birtchnell J. Early parent death and mental illness. *Brit J Psych* 1970; **116**: 281–8.

147 Brown GW, Harris T, Copeland JR. Depression and loss. *Brit J Psych* 1971; **130**: 1–18.

148 Black D. Annotation: The bereaved child. *J Child Psychol Psych* 1978; **19**: 287–92.

149 Kurtz Z, Thornes R, Wolkind S. *Services for the Mental Health of Children and Young People in England A National Review*. London: Maudsley Hospital and South Thames (West) Regional Health Authority, 1994.

150 Stevenson J. Health visitor-based services for pre-school children with behaviour problems. Association for Child Psychology and Psychiatry. *Occasional papers No. 2.* London: ACPP, 1990.

151 Barker W, Anderson R. The Child Develoment Programme: an evaluation of process and outcomes. Evaluation Document 9. Manuscript. Early Child Development Unit. Bristol: University of Bristol, 1988.

152 Hughes T, Garralda ME, Tylee A. *Child Mental Health Problems: A Booklet on Child Psychiatry for General Practitioners.* London: St Mary's CAP, 1994.

153 Steinberg D, Yule W. Consultative work. In *Child and Adolescent Psychiatry: Modern Approaches* (eds M Rutter, L Hersov). 2nd edn. Oxford, Blackwell Scientific Publications, 1985, pp. 914–26.

154 Lask B. Paediatric liaison work. In *Child and Adolescent Psychiatry: Modern Approaches* (eds M Rutter, L Hersov, E Taylor). 3rd edn. Oxford: Blackwell Scientific Publications, 1994, pp. 996–1005.

155 Hibbs ED. Child and adolescent disorders: issues for psychological treatment research. *J Abnorm Child Psychol* 1995; **23**: 1–10.

156 Gadow KD. Pediatric psychopharmacotherapy: a review of recent research. *J Child Psychol Psych* 1992; **33**: 153–95.

157 Barnett RJ, Docherty JP, Frommelt GM. A review of child psychotherapy research since 1963. *J Am Acad Child Adol Psych* 1991; **30**: 1–14.

158 Pfeiffer SI, Strzelecki SC. Inpatient psychiatric treatment of children and adolescents: a review of outcome studies. *J Am Acad Child Adol Psych* 1990; **29**: 847–53.

159 Graziano AM, Diament DM. Parental behaviour training: an examination of the paradigm. *Behav Mod* 1992; **16**: 3–38.

160 Allen JS, Tarnowski KJ, Simonian SJ *et al.* The generalization map revisited: Assessment of generalized treatment effects in child and adolescent behavior therapy. *Behav Therap* 1991; **22**: 393–405.

161 Weisz JR, Weiss B. Assessing the effects of clinic-based psychotherapy with children and adolescents. *J Consult Clin Psychol* 1989; **57**: 741–6.

162 Weisz JR, Donenberg GR, Hann SS *et al.* Child and adolescent psychotherapy outcomes in experiments versus clinics: why the disparity? *J Abnorm Child Psychol* 1995; **23**: 83–106.

163 Kovacs M, Lohr WD. Research on psychotherapy with children and adolescents: an overview of evolving trends and current issues. *J Abnorm Child Psychol* 1995; **23**: 11–30.

164 March JS. Cognitive-behavioural psychotherapy for children and adolescents with OCD: a review and recommendations for treatment. *J Am Child Adol Psych* 1995; **34**: 7–16.

165 Earls F. Oppositional-defiant and conduct disorders. In *Child and Adolescent Psychiatry: Modern Approaches* (eds M Rutter, L Hersov, E Taylor). 3rd edn. Oxford: Blackwell Scientific Publications, 1994, pp. 308–29.

166 Campbell M, Adams PB, Small AM *et al.* Lithium in hospitalized aggressive children with conduct disorder: a double-blind trial and placebo-controlled study. *J Am Acad Child Adol Psych* 1995; **34**: 445.

167 Alessi N, Naylor MW, Ghaziuddin M *et al.* Update on lithium carbonate therapy in children and adolescents. *J Am Acad Child Adol Psych* 1994; **33**: 291–304.

168 Kazdin AE, Siegal TC, Bass D. Cognitive problem-solving skills training and parent management training in the treatment of anti-social behavior in children. *J Consult Clin Psychol* 1992; **60**: 733–47.

169 Kazdin AE. The effectiveness of psychotherapy with children and adults. *J Consult Clin Psychol* 1991; **59**: 785–98.

170 Offord DR, Bennett KJ. Conduct disorder: long-term outcomes and intervention effectiveness. *J Am Acad Child Adol Psych* 1994; **33**: 1069–78.

171 Ryan ND. The pharmacologic treatment of child and adolescent depression. *Psych Clinic North Am* 1992; **15**: 29–40.

172 Ambrosini PJ, Bianchi MD, Rabinovich H *et al.* Anti-depressant treatment in children and adolescents. I. Affective disorders. *J Am Acad Child Adol Psych* 1993; **32**: 1–6.

173 Ambrosini PJ, Bianchi MD, Rabinovitch H *et al.* Antidepressant treatments in children and adolescents. II. Anxiety, physical and behavioral disorders. *J Am Acad Child Adol Psych* 1993; **32**: 483–93.

174 Harrington R. Affective disorders. In *Child and Adolescent Psychiatry: Modern Approaches* (eds M Rutter, L Hersov, E Taylor). 3rd edn. Oxford: Blackwell Scientific Publications, 1994, pp. 330–50.

175 Reynolds WM. Depression in Adolescents: Contemporary Issues and Perspectives. In *Advances in Clinical and Child Psychiatry* (eds TH Ollendick, RJ Prinz). Vol. 16. New York: Plenum Press, 1994, pp. 261–316.

176 Coffey BJ. Anxiolytics for children and adolescents: traditional and new drugs. *J Child Adoles Psychopharmacol* 1990; **1**: 57–83.

177 Bernstein GA, Borchardt CM. Anxiety disorders of childhood and adolescence: a critical review. *J Am Acad Child Adol Psych* 1991; **30**: 519–32.

178 Dadds M, Heard PM, Rapee RM. Anxiety disorders in children. *Int Rev Psych* 1991; **3**: 231–41.

179 King N, Tong BJ. Treatment of childhood anxiety disorders using behaviour therapy and pharmacotherapy. *Austr NZ J Psych* 1992; **26**: 644–51.

180 Klein RG. Anxiety disorders. In *Child and Adolescent Psychiatry: Modern Approaches* (eds M Rutter, L Hersov, E Taylor). 3rd edn. Oxford: Blackwell Scientific Publications, 1994, pp. 351–74.

181 Steinhausen H. Anorexia and bulimia nervosa. In *Child and Adolescent Psychiatry: Modern Approaches* (eds M Rutter, L Hersov, E Taylor). 3rd edn. Oxford: Blackwell Scientific Publications, 1994, pp. 425–41.

182 Rapaport J, Swedo SH, Leonard H. Obsessive-compulsive disorders. In *Child and Adolescent Psychiatry* (eds M Rutter, L Hersov, E Taylor). 3rd edn. Oxford: Blackwell Scientific Publications, 1994, pp. 441–54.

183 Piacentini J, Jaffer M, Graae F. The psychopharmacologic treatment of child and adolescent obsessive compulsive disorder. *Psych Clin North Am* 1992; **15**: 87–107.

184 Taylor E. Syndromes of attentional deficit and hyperactivity. In *Child and Adolescent Psychiatry: Modern Approaches* (eds M Rutter, L Hersov, E Taylor). 3rd edn. Oxford: Blackwell Scientific Publications, 1994, pp. 285–307.

185 Jacobvitz D, Sroufe AL, Stewart M *et al.* Treatment of attentional and hyperactivity problems in children with sympathomimetic drugs: a comprehensive review. *J Am Acad Child Adol Psych* 1990; **29**: 677–88.

186 Greenhill LL. Pharmacologic treatment of attention deficit hyperactivity disorder. *Psych Clin North Am* 1992; **15**: 1–27.

187 DuPaul GJ, Barkley R. Behavioural contributions to pharmacotherapy: the utility of behavioural methodology in medication treatment of children with attention deficit hyperactivity disorder. *Behav Therap* 1993; **24**: 47–65.

188 Leckman JF, Cohen DJ. Tic disorders. In *Child and Adolescent Psychiatry: Modern Approaches* (eds M Rutter, L Hersov, E Taylor). 3rd edn. Oxford: Blackwell Scientific Publications, 1994, pp. 455–66.

189 Skuse D. Feeding and sleeping disorders. In *Child and Adolescent Psychiatry: Modern Approaches* (eds M Rutter, L Hersov, E Taylor). 3rd edn. Oxford: Blackwell Scientific Publications, 1994, pp. 467–89.

190 Zeanah CH, Emde RN. Attachment disorders in infancy and early childhood. In *Child and Adolescent Psychiatry: Modern Approaches* (eds M Rutter, L Hersov, E Taylor). 3rd edn. Oxford: Blackwell Scientific Publications, 1994, pp. 490–504.

191 Lord C, Rutter M. Autism and pervasive developmental disorders. In *Child and Adolescent Psychiatry: Modern Approaches* (eds M Rutter, L Hersov, E Taylor). 3rd edn. Oxford: Blackwell Scientific Publications, 1994, pp. 569–93.

192 Werry JS, Taylor E. Schizophrenic and allied disorders. In *Child and Adolescent Psychiatry: Modern Approaches* (eds M Rutter, L Hersov, E Taylor). 3rd edn. Oxford: Blackwell Scientific Publications, 1994, pp. 594–646.

193 Green R. Atypical psychosexual development. In *Child and Adolescent Psychiatry: Modern Approaches* (eds M Rutter, L Hersov, E Taylor). 3rd edn. Blackwell Scientific Publications, 1994, pp. 749–58

194 Mrazek DA. Psychiatric aspects of somatic disease and disorders. In *Child and Adolescent Psychiatry: Modern Approaches* (eds M Rutter, L Hersov, E Taylor). 3rd edn. Oxford: Blackwell Scientific Publications, 1994, pp. 697–710.

195 Skuse D, Bentovim A. Physical and emotional maltreatment. In *Child and Adolescent Psychiatry: Modern Approaches* (eds M Rutter, L Hersov, E Taylor). 3rd edn. Oxford: Blackwell Scientific Publications, 1994, pp. 209–29.

196 O'Donohue WT, Elliott AN. Treatment of the sexually abused child: a review. *J Clin Child Psychol* 1992; **21**: 218–28.

197 Jones DP. The untreatable family. *Child Abuse Neglect* 1987; **11**: 409–20.

198 Smith M, Bentovim A. Sexual abuse. In *Child and Adolescent Psychiatry: Modern Approaches* (eds M Rutter, L Hersov, E Taylor). 3rd edn. Oxford: Blackwell Scientific Publications, 1994, pp. 230–51.

199 Lorion RP, Myers TG, Bartels C *et al.* Preventive intervention research. In *Advances in Clinical and Child Psychology* (eds TH Ollendick, RJ Prinz). Vol. 16. New York, Plenum Press, 1994, pp. 19–39.

200 McMillan HL, McMillan JL, Offord DR *et al.* Primary prevention of child physical abuse and neglect: a critical review. Part I. *J Child Psychol Psych* 1994; **35**: 835–56.

201 McMillan HL, McMillan JL, Offord DR *et al.* Primary prevention of child sexual abuse: a critical review. Part II. *J Child Psychol Psych* 1994; **35**: 857–76.

202 Kolvin I, Garside RF, Nicol AR *et al. Help starts here: The Maladjusted Child in Ordinary School.* London, New York: Tavistock, 1981.

203 St Leger AS, Schneiden H, Walsworth-Bell JP. *Evaluating Health Service Effectiveness.* Milton Keynes: Open University Press, 1992.

204 Levitt EE. Psychotherapy with children: an evaluation. *J Consult Psychol* 1957; **21**: 189–96.

205 Royal College of Psychiatrists. *Mental Health of the Nation: the contribution of psychiatry: a report of the President's Working Group.* London: Royal College of Psychiatrists, 1992.

206 Health Advisory Service. *Bridges over Troubled Waters: A Report from the NHS Health Advisory Service on Services for the Disturbed Adolescents.* London: Department of Health, 1986.

207 Leahy A, Thambirajah MS, Winkley LM. Multidisciplinary audit in child and adolescent psychiatry. *Psych Bull* 1992; **16**: 214–5.

208 Shaffer D, Gould MS, Brasie J *et al.* Children's Global Assessment Scale. *Arch Gen Psych* 1983; **40**: 1228–31.

209 Light D, Bailey V. *A Needs-Based Purchasing Plan for Child Based Mental Health Services.* London: North West Thames Regional Health Authority, 1992.

210 Research Committee of the Royal College of Psychiatrists. Future directions for research in child and adolescent psychiatry. *Psych Bull* 1991; **15**: 308–10.

211 Medical Research Council. *Field Review of Biological Psychiatry.* London: Medical Research Council, 1993.

212 McGuffin P. *Mental Health: Priorities in Research for the 1990s.* London: Mental Health Foundation, 1989.

213 Department of Health. *Central Research and Development Committee: Mental Health Research and Developmental Priorities.* London: Department of Health, 1992.

3 Low Back Pain

P Croft, A Papageorgious, R McNally

1 Summary

Low back pain is common. Both orthodox and complementary practitioners have traditionally regarded it as a mechanical problem of the spine and a wide range of therapies is claimed to relieve symptoms of presumed spinal disease. Despite this the incidence of work-related disability attributed to low back pain has soared in the past two decades. Research during that time has indicated that the symptom represents a complex social and psychological problem as well as a biological one. Low back pain can no longer be simply equated with spinal disease.

The assessment of the needs of people suffering from back pain is here based on the results of surveys in the general population. These rely on self-report of low back pain. The conclusion is that the critical dimensions for categorizing low back pain are:

- total days in pain over a period of one year
- extent to which it restricts activities of daily living.

The small but distinct subgroup of patients who have potentially serious pathology of the spine are dealt with as a separate category.

Overviews of trials of therapy in low back pain have emphasized their lack of rigorous methodology. However there have been randomized controlled trials on which a crude assessment of efficacy and cost-effectiveness can be based. The conclusion is that there is a reasonable basis for selection of treatments which are beneficial in the short term and for rejection of a number of regimens which do not have any basis in good scientific evidence.

The key question which the trials do not answer is whether these interventions have an impact on the prevention of recurrence and chronicity of low back pain. In the absence of good evidence for the efficacy of primary prevention, the potential cost-effectiveness of delivering effective care for new or recurrent episodes must rest on the optimistic assumption that what is effective in the short term will also be effective in the long term.

On this basis the models for care propose a shift of resources towards early intervention in an attempt to treat more actively a less disabled and chronic case-mix and to reduce the reliance on investigation. This may imply a change of philosophy among general practitioners (GPs), physical therapists, clinical psychologists and hospital specialists towards:

- positive but brief programmes of treatment in patients with new and recurrent episodes
- a more organized approach to the intensive therapy offered to those with long-term problems.

This proposal is in line with the recommendations of the Clinical Standards Advisory Group (CSAG) and its epidemiological implications are investigated.

2 Introduction

Back pain is common, whether it is measured as a symptom in the general population, as a source of disability, as a reason for seeking health care, or as a cause of both short- and long-term work loss. In any one year 38% of adults experience at least one day of low back pain – a figure which does not include menstrual pain or pain accompanying a feverish illness.[1,2] Some 10% of adults in any one month experience restriction of work or other activities as a result of low back pain. The course of low back pain in an individual's lifetime is often recurrent, intermittent, and episodic[3] and for 5% of adults it becomes a more persistently disabling condition.

3 Statement of the problem

It is helpful to distinguish three ways in which back pain may arise. The first two concern the direct results of disease or injury.[4]

1   Disease or injury (physical or chemical) involving spinal tissues (vertebral bone, muscle, ligament, joints, or the cartilaginous disc) can:
- irritate local nerve receptors, giving rise to pain located in the back. Terms such as lumbago are synonyms for such pain
- put pressure on the spinal cord, on the nerve roots arising from the cord or on the nerves tracking away from the cord. Such pressure might give rise to pain located in the back or to pain distant from the site of pressure. Sciatica refers to such pain in the leg or foot, radiating to areas served by the sciatic nerve.
2   Disease or injury of tissues and organs outside the spine can cause pain which is perceived as coming from the back (referred pain). Pain located in the back can thus result from disease elsewhere in the body.

An underlying disease or injury however can be identified in only a minority of patients with back pain and lumbago and sciatica are more often applied to pain which has no clear pathophysiology. There is much controversy and disagreement about the basis of such pain. The third mechanism of pain offers an insight into how back pain might arise and persist in the absence of continuing disease or injury.[5]

3   The biology of pain is more complex than the simple 'mind–body' model which depicts the brain receiving pain messages from irritated peripheral tissues. The central nervous system (CNS) has the ability to remember, reproduce and elaborate pain, even in the absence of continuing peripheral irritation and may be more prone to do so in the context of stimuli from elsewhere in the CNS, such as depression or fear.

Causes of back pain

The aetiology of most individual episodes of back pain is not understood. A small proportion of cases can be attributed to specific problems such as infection, inflammation, vertebral fracture or cancer. However most episodes of back pain can only be classed as non-specific – no convincing underlying explanation of the episode.[6] This has not discouraged the publication of many schemes of classification of back pain based on unproven theories of causation.

The small number of cases where a specific cause can be identified is important in the assessment of health care needs. From the point of view of purchasing health care they provide the rationale for a classification based on pragmatic clinical questions, such as those outlined by Waddell[7] and taken up by the CSAG in its clinical triage approach.[8]

- Is there an underlying diagnosis which is potentially serious? If so, is it a spinal problem or a problem causing pain to be referred to the back?
- Is there evidence of pressure on a spinal nerve root and, if so, is it getting worse?

The answers to these questions guide important early clinical decisions and inform the need for urgent referral to a specialist and to diagnostic services. They will only identify and address the needs of a small group of back pain sufferers however. An alternative to classification by cause is required for the majority of back pain cases.

In considering the health care needs related to back pain, the potential for prevention in the general population should not be obscured. Investigation of factors which increase the risk of back pain in populations has shed some light on this preventive potential. Manual handling of heavy weights, sedentary work in poor positions, smoking, psychological status and job satisfaction may all contribute to back pain risks.[9–12] Since most back pain cannot be attributed to such factors however, strategies for prevention cannot be isolated from the wider need for effective treatment and care.

Classification of back pain

To address the needs of back pain sufferers in general requires a less traditionally clinical approach. On page 135 it is argued that measures of symptom duration and severity and of disability provide the best basis for subgrouping patients in terms of their needs. The dimensions measured must be broad enough to incorporate restriction of physical, psychological and social functions in everyday life.[13]

In our current state of knowledge, back pain cannot be equated to spinal disease. Abnormalities in the spine can give rise to back pain, but they frequently do not; and most back pain cannot be clearly attributed to a known spinal condition.[14,15] The most disabling and life-threatening spinal problems may not even present with back pain as a main clinical feature.

Many authorities, including leading orthopaedic surgeons from Europe and the US, have stressed that back pain is as much a problem of an individual's response to pain, as it is a problem related to the back itself.[16–18] Psychosocial, cultural, economic and political influences on the experience of pain are crucial to an understanding of the back pain phenomenon in its broadest sense. In biological terms this view clearly concords with the broader theory of pain mechanisms outlined previously as mechanism 3.[5]

The issue is relevant to needs assessment because current medical care has had little discernible impact on the occurrence of back pain in the population. On the contrary the economic impact of back pain in industrialized countries has accelerated in recent years because of the increasing number of lost working days attributed to the problem and the accompanying rise in sickness and invalidity benefit payments.[19] A recent estimate of the economic cost of back pain in Britain was £3.8 billion in lost production in one year. In addition social security expenditure due to low back pain was estimated at £1.4 billion per year.[19] Such figures dwarf the costs associated with health care of back pain sufferers. Yet the prevalence of back pain symptoms in the population appears to have changed little during this time. The 'epidemic' of back pain is as much to do with the politics, economics and culture of industrialized society as it is with inadequacies of health care.

However if health care were more effective in meeting the needs of back pain sufferers, then it might also influence these broader costs to society by:

- preventing the onset or recurrence of back pain
- limiting its effect on job status
- reducing its severity and duration.

The broader social and economic outcomes of effective interventions need to be kept in view.

Theoretical framework

The issues raised so far highlight one area of agreement in the back pain literature of the last decade: that back pain cannot be viewed simply in terms of the back or of pain. There have been two important contributions to conceptualizing this: the biopsychosocial model and the impairment, disability, handicap model.

Biopsychosocial model

This framework was applied to low back pain by Gordon Waddell, an orthopaedic surgeon.[13] Despite its catch-all title, it provides a simple encapsulation of the multiple influences on the symptom and its persistence.

Its premise is that pain cannot be divided artificially into physical or psychogenic, organic or non-organic, real or imaginary: physical disorders are inextricably linked to their emotional context and effect. The vast majority of backache starts with a physical source of pain. However distress (the emotional reaction to pain and disability) and illness behaviour (the presentation of distress to the carer) may come to dominate the picture, which in turn both affects and is affected by the patient's social interactions.

This model has expanded our view of low back pain from a narrow medical view (back pain as only a mechanical problem of the spine) to an emphasis on the crucial contributions which distress and accompanying illness behaviour make to the problem and on the relevance of the social world in which the patient lives and works.

Impairment, disability and handicap (IDH) model

This is the framework adopted by the World Health Organization in its international classification of the consequences of disease (ICIDH).[20] The system as a whole is not a particularly useful tool for classifying low back pain, but the underlying concepts are helpful. They expand the focus from pain and pathology to embrace an individual's ability to function in everyday life.

Impairment

This is the disturbance of normal structure or function which results from disease or injury. The term covers symptoms and signs and is concerned with both physical and mental functions. Back pain is an impairment. It can be categorized without reference to underlying pathophysiology: for example, by its intensity, radiation, duration, periodicity and the presence of other impairments. Such grouping can be done without implying that the different categories represent particular 'diseases'.

The traditional medical approach to impairments is to move backwards from symptoms and signs to causes and pathology. The IDH model, by contrast, moves to the consequences which impairments may have for an individual's life. This is an advantage when characterizing a symptom such as low back pain, the underlying cause of which is usually not clear.

Disability

This is any restriction of everyday activity (physical or psychological) which results from an impairment. It represents the effect which specific impairments may have on general functioning. The presence of back pain for example might mean that a person is unable to lift a suitcase or has difficulty in walking to the bus-stop or cannot sit for too long in one chair. These are all disabilities. They can be graded and classified, for example by their severity or their number.

Handicap

This refers to the actual impact of disability on any individual's social functioning. It concerns the context of each individual's impairment and disability. If a person never has to catch a bus, their inability to do this anyway (disability) because of low back pain (impairment) is not a handicap to them. The commuter who has caught a bus for years and suddenly finds back pain makes this difficult, will find it a handicap. Although this is a highly individual assessment, it is useful to view general restrictions on social functioning, such as inability to do a job, as handicaps.

One way in which this model expands our traditional medical view of low back pain is that it encourages the use of different options for tackling the problem. For low back pain with a clear-cut cause, a primary preventive or curative approach might be possible. Methods of treatment which alleviate pain, but do not address its cause, might still reduce the consequent disability and handicap. If pain persists, treatment can still reduce disability by improving everyday psychological and physical functioning. Even if the latter remain restricted rehabilitation into a new job or adaptations of the home environment might mean that persistent disabilities cease to be handicaps.

Care of the back pain sufferer

It is clear that the attention of healers, both orthodox and heterodox, has a beneficial effect on the symptoms of many back pain sufferers. First this section considers which approaches might have the largest effects and when, how, by whom and to whom they should be delivered. Two issues addressed are:

- How long does any benefit last?
- Do any of the approaches reduce the disability and handicap as well as the pain of back sufferers?

Second this section considers the potential for prevention of back pain. There are two key questions for the public health which remain unresolved:

- Would more effective delivery of appropriate health care for individuals with back pain reduce the population prevalence of low back pain by preventing recurrence and chronicity?
- Are measures directed at the primary prevention of new episodes of low back pain likely to reduce the rising 'epidemic' of work loss attributed to back pain?

Clinical and epidemiological evidence supports the notion that health care for back pain sufferers could be more effectively delivered than at present. Whether more effective care set in the context of a primary prevention programme could reduce the occurrence and burden of back pain can only be answered by further studies.

Available sources of care

One manifestation of the size and complexity of the back pain problem and the lack of broadly effective treatment, is that the range of individuals, professions and agencies involved in the care of back pain is vast. This symptom impinges on most of the health care industry.

In any one year four out of five people with back pain will tackle their problem without seeing a GP, although the GP is the most sought after source of professional help for back pain in the UK.[2] In addition a variety of self-care activity – based on advice from family, friends, media, self-help literature and the local chemist – is reported by back pain sufferers in the community.[2,21]

However most of the population will consult their doctor about low back pain at some time in their lives and back pain is the commonest musculoskeletal symptom presented in primary care.[22] General practitioners have access to a bewildering variety of options, although they manage most back pain episodes without further referral.[21] Access to secondary services varies from place to place. Open access to lumbar spine radiography is common but utilization varies greatly. Practice-based physiotherapy or open access to hospital physiotherapy is not universal – where it is available, back pain tends to dominate reasons for referral.[19]

Patients may refer themselves to various forms of physical therapy, notably physiotherapy, chiropractic and osteopathy. Parliamentary assent is now in the process of ensuring official recognition of chiropractors and osteopaths.[23] Some referrals to them are already made from primary care and there are medical practitioners who hold qualifications in these modalities.

Other complementary therapies are popular for back pain treatment, including acupuncture, homeopathy, aromatherapy and the Alexander technique. Again health service practitioners may practise some of these techniques.

Back pain is the main reason for using complementary therapies in America, where as a whole they command more out-of-pocket payments than health service treatments.[24] In the UK the demand continues to rise for such approaches to back pain, the limiting factors being cost and availability.[25]

Although there are regional variations, the dominant hospital specialty to which back pain sufferers are referred is orthopaedics, although only a minority undergo surgery.[21] Neurosurgery occupies a distinct, albeit small, niche for the management of back pain associated with nerve compression. Back pain is the most common problem dealt with by outpatient pain services, whether urgent or routine. Some hospitals now employ orthopaedic physicians, skilled in manipulation and injection techniques, who have a specific remit to concentrate on back problems.

The extent of rheumatological involvement in back pain varies from hospital to hospital, depending on the workload and interest of the specialist and on local referral preferences.[26] Where the cause is suspected to be an inflammatory disease, such as ankylosing spondylitis, most rheumatologists will be involved. Rehabilitation specialists or rheumatologists with a rehabilitation interest have chronic back pain as a major part of their workload.

Accident and emergency (A and E) departments are involved in the management of back pain for two main reasons:

- back injuries – isolated or part of multiple trauma such as road traffic accidents
- acute back pain episodes presenting to A and E departments.

Many hospital specialists' involvement in back pain is because they are the point of access to other services – physiotherapy, orthotics (notably lumbar supports), rehabilitation and occupational therapy.

Plain radiography of the lumbar spine is commonly an open access service and represents an estimated 15% of outpatient radiography requests.[27] Imaging, particularly the newer non-invasive techniques of computerized tomography and magnetic resonance imaging, is increasingly popular in the investigation of back pain patients referred to hospital and some GPs are beginning to request direct access to such specialized investigations.

Psychologists are important members of a multi-disciplinary approach to rehabilitation and are also involved in the assessment of back pain problems at earlier stages.[28,29] In the community occupational health services, both in the manual industries and in sedentary occupations, have back pain and back injuries as a major part of their workload.[30] Such work involves surveillance, prevention, education, treatment and rehabilitation. Industrial rehabilitation services and social services for the chronically disabled are actively involved in the care of chronic back pain sufferers. Health education units, the unions, and the Health and Safety Executive provide ergonomic advice and education. The voluntary sector will clearly contribute locally, but national organizations, such as the National Back Pain Association, Arthritis Care and more disease-specific groups such as the National Osteoporosis Society and the National Ankylosing Spondylitis Society, provide sources of support, advice and education for back pain sufferers.

4 Sub-categories of back pain

Back pain can be classified into pain in the neck, the upper back and the low back (cervical, thoracic and lumbo-sacral). Low back pain is the commonest back problem, it is the most heavily researched and findings related to low back pain are likely to apply in more general terms to pain higher in the back. The assumption will be made that low back pain in general means pain in the lumbo-sacral area. A more precise definition which has been used in population surveys and in clinical research is given in section 9.

Classification stage I: Is there a serious disease?

The simplest clinical approach is a pragmatic classification, designed to separate serious from less serious reasons for low back pain. A number of authors have proposed broadly similar systems[7,31,32] and the same principles form the basis for the triage approach to classification of low back pain in primary care adopted by the CSAG of the Department of Health.[8]

The relevance of this classification to needs assessment and purchasers is three-fold:

- it is simple and pragmatic and recognized as such by GPs
- it clarifies the important areas for which specialist and urgent care must be provided
- it highlights the fact that the vast majority of cases of low back pain fall into the non-specific category, for which there is no good evidence that hospital specialist care and investigation are required, although a minority will require specialist pain relief and rehabilitation services.

Pragmatic classification of low back pain

- Low back pain arising from potentially serious or life-threatening spinal disease:
  a) cancer (including metastases)
  b) infection
  c) inflammation and metabolic disease (particularly ankylosing spondylitis and osteoporosis).
- Low back pain accompanied by cord or root compression. (Such compression may also occur in the absence of low back pain):
  a) cancer, infection, inflammation
  b) disc prolapse (including cauda equina lesions)
  c) spinal and root canal stenosis.

- Low back pain arising as a result of systemic disease outside the spine – this is essentially a problem of referred pain.
- 'Non-specific' or 'mechanical' low back pain: the vast majority of low back pain in our current state of knowledge falls into this category.

Other clinical or spinal disease classifications of low back pain are used by clinicians, surgeons or therapists to justify therapy or to link assumed structural or functional abnormalities of the spine to low back pain. The approach taken in this chapter is that none of these classifications is of proven general use or help in the broad sub-categorizing of low back pain, although this does not imply a judgement on the therapies associated with them. The treatment of spinal disorders such as scoliosis is particularly problematic in this regard because the treatment of the spinal deformity *per se* is an issue separate to the management of low back pain. The links between low back pain and scoliosis and between low back pain and many other structural abnormalities of the spine are weak and unclear.[33,34]

Classification stage II: Categorizing non-specific low back pain

How is it best to classify the rest of low back pain for the purpose of needs assessment and purchasing of health care? The needs of patients with long-term problems are different to those presenting with new episodes. In the face of the sheer size of the problem, health service practice has tended to focus on delivery of care (diagnosis and treatment) to patients whose symptoms have become persistent, and this has meant a traditional sub-categorizing of low back pain to acute and chronic. We present an alternative to this.

The argument adopted by the CSAG[8] is considered here in an epidemiological context: namely that effective intervention early in an episode of low back pain may reduce the impact and burden of persistent problems. For this a simple classification which covers the spectrum of low back pain in the general population is required. A proposed scheme is shown in Box 1.

Impairment: time-course

The traditional classification is into acute and chronic. This is helpful only in part. The recurrent, fluctuating, intermittent, variable course of low back pain does not accommodate easily to such a simple dichotomy. The most useful distinctions follow.

- **New episode** Onset or recurrence of low back pain after a pain-free period.
- **Exacerbation** An episode which represents more severe pain in the context of persistent background pain.
- **New episode, recurrence or exacerbation lasting more than four weeks** A commonly used cut-off for an episode which is beyond the acute stage.
- **New episode, recurrence or exacerbation lasting more than three months** Another arbitrary point used to define a persistent low back problem.
- **Chronic low back pain** Low back pain in which the notion of episode has been lost and it is seen as a long-term problem, regardless of current severity.

Box 1: Sub-categorizing low back pain

Category 1 Low back pain due to serious spinal disease

- cancer
- infection
- inflammation

Category 2 Low back pain with cord or root compression

- cancer, infection, inflammation
- disc prolapse (including cauda equina)
- spinal and root canal stenosis

Category 3 Non-specific low back pain

- Total days in pain during past 12 months

  a)   < 1 week
  b)   1-1 weeks
  c)   5+ weeks
  d)   13+ weeks
  e)   whole year

- Restriction of daily activities due to low back pain

  a)   none
  b)   moderate
  c)   severe

In this scheme, pain referred to the back because of disease in other systems has been omitted.
Categories 1 and 2 are small but important because of the need for early diagnosis and appropriate treatment.
The majority of patients who have clinical signs of root or nerve compression will not have progressive damage and they can be classified with category 3 because the same sub-categorizing criteria (total days in pain and extent of disability) are relevant to the assessment of health care needs.
Patients in severe pain form a small but important sub-category of those with severe restriction of their daily activities, particularly when it is a feature of a short duration problem.

However the concept of most importance is that low back pain encompasses an individual's life history. Four observations are relevant to this:

- between 60 and 80% of the population experience low back pain during their lives[35]
- by the age of 30 years 45% of the population recall an episode of low back pain which lasted for more than 24 hours[36]
- the strongest known risk for developing a low back pain episode is a history of a previous episode[37]
- most acute episodes of pain presented to the GP improve rapidly.[38]

Figure 1a (after Deyo[3]) better represents the experience of low back pain than the acute–chronic dichotomy. Low back pain, once started, is potentially chronic. Individuals with this chronic problem can experience episodic exacerbations of pain, as well as periods of freedom from pain. However each exacerbation will increase that person's overall experience of back pain and the likelihood of a further episode is thus increased. Over time the cumulative experience may become more persistent and more disabling.

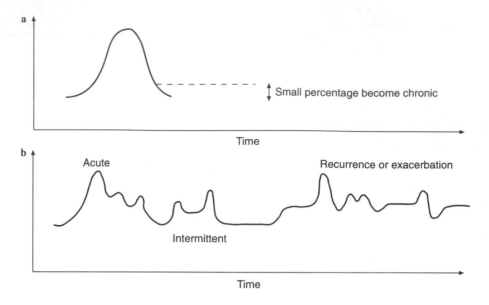

Figure 1a: Assumed course of acute low back pain;   **b:** real course of low back pain.[3]

This means that the best sub-categorizing for needs assessment is likely to be a summary of experience over a period of time and across episodes or exacerbations.[39] This might be a sub-categorizing based on categories of duration (less than seven days, seven days to six weeks, seven weeks or more and so on) which does not assume a particular definition of what is, or is not, acute and chronic.

More useful however is the total number of days on which back pain has been experienced during a defined period (the past six months; the past 12 months) putting aside assumptions about the nature or length of the current episode.

The other dimensions of low back pain which have been used to sub-categorize impairment are:

- pain severity, usually on a visual analogue or numerical scale
- presence of pain in areas other than the low back.

These are less amenable to simple summary over time.

Disability and handicap: restricted activities of daily living

The impact of low back pain on daily living – physical, psychological and social – has emerged as the other important way to classify non-specific low back pain in the general population. There are a number of measures available and these are considered in section 9 (outcome measures).

Combined scales for sub-categorizing the back pain population

Workers in the US and Germany have begun investigations in the general population and in primary care, using scales which combine days in pain with scores of physical and psychological disability.[39,40] This pooling of different dimensions of the back pain experience provides the most promising basis for classifying non-specific low back pain for needs assessment.

There is an urgent need for population and practice-based studies which utilize these schemes, but they have not yet been carried out in Britain. The most recent population surveys in this country have used some of these dimensions and these will be considered in section 5.[1,2,36]

5 Prevalence and incidence

Introduction

The argument is now further developed that, for an intermittent, recurrent, episodic problem such as low back pain, prevalence needs to be measured across a defined period of time.

The one year period prevalence (the proportion of people in the general population who experience the problem in the course of one year) is a useful measure of occurrence, for which there are now national published data.

The incidence of new episodes or recurrences of back pain is estimated in relation to the background prevalence in the previous year.

The most useful measure of need is based on sub-categorizing low back pain according to severity, in particular the total days in pain during a one year period and the extent of any restriction of daily activities which the symptom imposes. The prevalence of these sub-categories is estimated from population survey data.

Low back pain

Population surveys rely on self-report of low back pain. The intermittent, recurrent, episodic nature of low back pain means that traditional measures of prevalence in the community such as 'point prevalence' are less appropriate as a basis for needs assessment than measures which summarize experience over time.

Lifetime prevalence: do not use for needs assessment

In two separate UK surveys[1,36] the proportion of adults aged 18 years and over who had ever experienced low back pain was reported as 59%. A similar figure was reported from a Belgian population study.[41]

The age distribution of lifetime prevalence of back pain which has lasted for more than 24 hours in the adult population is shown in Figure 2. By the age of 30 years, 45% report ever having had this symptom; by the age of 60 years and above, this has risen to 63%, a paradoxically lower figure than for the 45–59 years age group. There may be a number of subtle explanations of this paradox, such as selective survival of generally fitter people or a cohort effect in which the older generation has experienced less back pain. However it is more likely that recall is influenced by age and circumstance: recalled 'back pain ever' is likely to be dominated by more recent symptoms.[42]

The observation that low back pain is established as a common experience before the age of 30 years is an important one. However this 'lifetime' measure is a confusing and difficult summary of prevalence for the purpose of needs assessment. Measures related to a defined period of recalled time, regardless of age, are more appropriate.

Period prevalence and episode incidence: general principles

Because the symptom of low back pain is already a common experience by early adulthood, the traditional meanings of incidence as the first ever occurrence and of prevalence as the product of incidence and disease duration are difficult to apply.

The resolution adopted here is to treat the population as containing a dynamic prevalence pool. During their lives most people will at some point move in and out of this pool. Helpful measures of prevalence can be identified by taking a defined period of time (a period of 12 months which is referred to as the prevalence

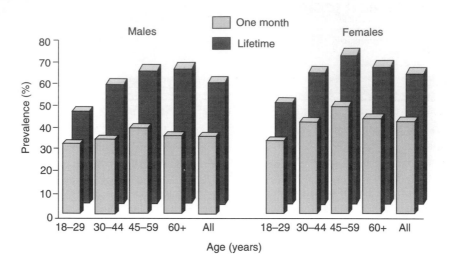

Figure 2: Age distribution of lifetime prevalence of 'back pain that has lasted for more than 24 hours' in the UK adult population. Taken from the South Manchester population survey.[36]

year), estimating how many people are in the pool during that time and classifying them by the sub-categories in Box 1.

Incidence can then be measured by identifying episodes during the 12-month period following the prevalence year. (This second year can be called the incidence year.) These are counted separately for:

- people who were in the prevalence pool in the previous year (the episodes will be recurrences or exacerbations)
- people who were free of low back pain during the previous year (new episodes).

The choice of one year as the window is arbitrary. However a number of population studies have adopted a year as the period for recall of symptoms in questionnaire schedules.[1,2] Subjects whose back trouble has persisted continuously for more than one year present a very different set of needs to those whose episode or recurrence or exacerbation has a more recent onset.

One year period prevalence

Low back pain during the past year has been reported in two different UK surveys.[1,2] In each study the one-year adult population prevalence of low back pain lasting for more than one day was 38%. Peak prevalence was in the 45–59 year age group, but variation overall with age was small. There was little difference between men and women. Basic prevalence and incidence data can thus be summarized crudely across age and gender categories. (Figures throughout this section refer to the adult population aged 18 years and over.)

Table 1: Low back pain in the adult general population: prevalence and incidence

Year 1: period prevalence pool	Year 2: cumulative incidence (new episode or recurrence)		
	% of whole population	% within group	% of whole population
Group I: no low back pain	62	31	19
Group II: low back pain for part of year	32	46	15
Group III: low back pain all year	6		

The assumption about the pool of continuous low back pain is that, in year 2, approximately one-third (2% of the whole population) leaves that pool and becomes intermittent or recurrent, but is replaced by a similar number coming into this pool from the new or recurrent groups. The proportion of long-standing low back pain in the population thus remains constant at about 6%.

The overall period prevalence in year 2 thus remains at 38%.

Figures have been calculated from the OPCS study and the Manchester prospective studies [2, 21, 36]

Episode incidence

The figures for incidence and prevalence are summarized in Table 1. At the start of any twelve-month period the adult population can be separated into three groups by prevalence in the previous prevalence year:

- **Group I** Those who have been free of low back pain for the previous 12 months (62% of the adult population).
- **Group II** Those who have had intermittent or moderately disabling pain during the previous 12 months (32% of the adult population).
- **Group III** Those who have had long-standing or serious disabling low back pain during the previous 12 months (6% of the adult population).

New episodes

Among people free of low back pain at the start of the incidence year (group I) the estimated proportion who develop a new episode of low back pain in the year is 31%.[21,36] Since group I forms 62% of the whole adult population at baseline, the cumulative incidence of new episodes is 19% per annum for the adult population as a whole. Only a small minority of them are experiencing their first ever episode of low back pain.

Recurrences

The proportion of people in group II who report a further episode of low back pain during the following incidence year is 46%. Since group II forms 32% of the whole adult population at the start of the incidence year, this represents an annual cumulative incidence of recurrent low back pain episodes in 15% of the population as a whole.

Persistent problems

In group III the assumption is that pain continues in the majority of those who have had serious disabling or long-standing low back pain during the prevalence year, but that one-third of them (i.e. 2% of the whole adult population) will have less severe problems during the incidence year. They will be replaced by a comparable number of people from groups I and III who develop severe or disabling problems during the incidence year and enter group III. The result of this is that the prevalence pool of chronic disabling low back pain is maintained at around 6% of the population.

Overall the incidence figures are such that the annual period prevalence of low back pain in the adult population as a whole at the end of the incidence year is 38% – as it was at the start of the year.

Summary

These figures are derived from prospective and retrospective studies and the two sources produce surprisingly consistent figures, although both methods do rely on patients recalling episodes of low back pain.

The message from the figures is that, in any one year, recurrences, exacerbations and persistence dominate the experience of low back pain in the community. Even among those classified above as having new episodes, most will recall having had low back pain at some time in the past.

Low back pain by sub-category

The basic period prevalence figures illustrate just how common is the symptom of low back pain. In order to quantify potential health care need, the one year prevalence must be further sub-categorized. Summaries of the prevalence according to the pragmatic and the severity sub-categorizing are shown in Tables 2 and 3.

Low back pain due to serious spinal disease

There are no straightforward data on the occurrence of malignancy and infection presenting as back pain. It can be assumed that all such patients will be among the 7% of the adult population who present to their GP with low back pain in one year.[22] The Royal College of Radiologists estimates that one in 2500 plain lumbar spine films carried out in general practice would detect a serious problem.[43] This leads to an estimate of three cases per year per 100 000 adult population. However these figures will underestimate the numbers because of lesions which are not detectable initially by X-ray. Deyo's US-based figures give ten cases per 100 000 adults per year.[31]

The prevalence of ankylosing spondylitis in the population is approximately 100 per 100 000,[44] higher in men than in women.

Low back pain with cord or root compression

Population studies from the UK,[1,2] Finland,[45] Denmark[35] and the US[45] are in broad agreement. The one year period prevalence of low back pain which radiates to the legs below the knees is 12 to 15% of all adults. However as Waddell has described,[46] the majority of such cases do not indicate 'true' sciatica or nerve root compression.

Heliovaara has estimated the prevalence of true sciatica at 5%,[46] whilst Deyo puts the prevalence of surgically important disc herniation, the commonest cause of root compression, at 2%.[31] The prevalence of other conditions causing root compression – notably spinal stenosis – is simply not known to any degree of accuracy.

Most prevalent cases with cord or root compression are treated non-surgically in the same way as all other low back pain, depending on persistence and the degree of disability. Many cases will be associated with chronic or persistent problems and represent the health care needs associated with these problems rather than the need for surgical intervention. We have thus chosen the more conservative Deyo figures to indicate new episodes of low back pain with potentially serious cord or root compression.[31]

Cauda equina lesions – centrally prolapsing discs with progressive and potentially catastrophic damage to the spinal cord – represent the real emergencies and are rare. From Deyo's figures the annual cumulative incidence might be three per 100 000.

Total days in pain

The prevalence of low back pain which has occurred on more than four weeks in the past year is 16%; 10% of adults report that they have experienced it for more than three months in the previous year; 6% of the adult population state that they have had low back pain continuously throughout the past year.[2]

Disabling low back pain

In the OPCS survey, 11% of the population had restricted their activities in the month prior to the survey because of low back pain; 3% had spent at least one day in the past month lying down.[2] It is likely the proportions of people affected by low back pain in this way are higher during the course of a whole year, but Scandinavian studies[46,48] confirm the broad estimate that 25 to 30% of subjects who report low back problems have impairment of daily activities: i.e. 10 to 12% of the adult population as a whole.

Another UK study attempted to define more significant disability.[1] Their figures suggest that during the course of a year 5% of the adult population experience considerable difficulties with mobility or extreme difficulty with putting on socks, stockings or tights because of low back pain.

None of these studies showed major contrasts between men and women. There was greater disability attributed to low back pain above 45 years compared with younger ages but no further increase in the older age groups. However this may ignore the problem of co-morbidity. In a careful German population study of back pain,[40] restriction of physical activity increased linearly with age and on a score which combined pain severity and physical and psychological restrictions on daily life, there was a higher proportion of severe problems in the elderly.

An estimate of the population prevalence of low back pain for needs assessment combining total days in pain during the past year with clinical and restriction of daily activity gradings is shown in Table 2.

Other groupings not included in the 'needs' classification scheme

Low back pain causing work loss

In the OPCS survey it was estimated that the employment of 4% of the population aged 16 to 64 years was affected by low back pain in the course of a four-week period: one-third because of time off sick and two-thirds because low back pain was given as one reason for not being in current employment. Figures were similar for men and women.[2]

The effect over a period of 12 months was estimated by the Southampton group to be 10% of men and 7% of women, aged 20 to 59, who had low back pain which had led to time off work.[1]

Table 2: One year period prevalence of low back pain by sub-category

	In whole population	By total days in pain in past year				
		<7	7–28	29–84	85+, but <1 year	All year
Prevalence of low back pain (%)	38	7	15	6	4	6
Prevalence of low back pain with leg pain (%)	11		4	1	2	4
Prevalence of severe sciatica (%)	2		0.1	0.1	0.3	1.5
Prevalence of moderate and severe disability (%)	10	0	0	2	3	5
Prevalence of severe disability (%)	6	0	0	1	2	3

The category 'low back pain with leg pain' includes severe sciatica

Chronic low back pain

The prevalence of low back pain during the past year which had started long before the year in question was 30% in the OPCS survey.[2] Such a definition of chronicity for health needs purposes is clearly unhelpful, since it constitutes the majority of low back pain in the population and affects almost a third of all adults. This emphasizes the need to get away from traditional notions of chronicity – most people with low back pain have experienced it before in some form. The smaller pool of chronic low back pain with specific needs is best defined by a combination of disability and days in pain during the previous year.[39,40]

Pyramids of need

The two broad classifications for estimating prevalence with respect to need, namely the pragmatic and the severity sub-categories, can be translated into numbers.

In a population of 100 000 adults, the likely number presenting with potentially serious problems for urgent investigation is ten to 50 in one year. The number with ankylosing spondylitis of varying severity, but posing mostly long-term problems, will be 100.

The number of patients with radiating leg pain which might represent cord compression from a disc lesion or spinal stenosis is summarized in the 'surgical pyramid' in Box 2.

The numbers of low back pain patients can be summarized separately in a 'severity pyramid', using total days in pain and disability as the classifying features (Table 3).

Box 2: The 'surgical pyramid'

*	Need surgery
2 000	Serious sciatica
11 000	Radiating back pain
38 000	Low back pain during one year
100 000	Total adult population

These are inclusive categories. *The proportion of severe sciatica cases who need surgery is not known

Table 3: The 'severity pyramid'

Number of days with low back pain in past year	Number of people in each category	Number of people with moderate and severe disability	Number of people with severe disability
All year	6 000	5 000	3 000
85+	10 000	8 000	5 000
29+	16 000	10 000	6 000
1+	38 000		
	Population base 100 000		

These are inclusive categories

6 Current service use

Introduction: case-mix and service use

The pragmatic classification highlights small but important groups who will present to the hospital services. In the following sections some ideas about the likely relation between back pain sub-categories and general practice consultations are discussed.

It is difficult however to relate current levels of care to the sub-categories of 'need' in any comprehensive way. The evidence on the case-mix of patients seeking or referred to different sources of health care is not available.

One piece of evidence does give an indication of what is going on. In studies in Manchester the total days in pain during the past year were estimated in three separate groups of people:[21]

- those with low back pain in the general population who had not consulted their GP about the symptom during the previous year
- those who had consulted their GP in the past year
- a group referred to a district general hospital for specialist opinion.

The results of this comparison are shown in Table 4.

The table provides evidence of some differences between consulters and non-consulters in the community, mainly with respect to working days lost through the previous year. However the main contrasts are between back pain sufferers in the community or primary care and those attending hospital outpatient

Table 4: Back pain sufferers in the community/primary care/hospital

	Population base		
	Non-consulters in general population (%)	GP consulters (%)	District hospital attenders (%)
Continuous pain	17.6	30.5	59.0
Pain down leg	46.1	35.6	75.6
>3/12 pain in past year	36.7	37.7	65.4
Need bed rest all day	18.1	20.0	39.7
Restricted activity	43.5	55.0	62.8
Lost days from work	8.3	23.0	33.3

clinics. The latter are more likely to have had more than three months of pain during the previous year or to have been in continuous pain throughout the year.

So the circumstantial evidence points to the conclusion that hospital consultations for low back pain (most of which are with orthopaedic surgeons) are mainly for patients who have persistent problems and whose total days in pain and disability levels are highest. In section 7 (effectiveness) the question of whether this is a reasonable match of need to care is discussed.

Consultations for low back pain

Prospective studies of consultations in primary care indicate that approximately 7.2% of adults in the UK population will consult their GP at least once in the course of a 12-month period because of low back pain.[22] About two-thirds of these consultations will be for new episodes, which may be first ever episodes or recurrences; whilst one-third is for more long-term problems: exacerbations or repeat visits about persisting symptoms.

Surveys of the general population which ask subjects to recall whether they have visited the GP during the past year because of low back problems give higher estimates of consulting levels.[1,2] Waddell has considered this in detail in the Annex to the CSAG report.[8] It is likely that subjects focus their recall on a period which is in reality longer than one year, whilst GPs may not identify low back pain as a specific reason for consultation in the context of multiple complaints. An additional explanation is that patients are probably expressing in their recall a measure of perceived severity of their problem.

One other aspect of relevance to health needs assessment which has not been investigated fully is the observation from one study[1] that there is considerable regional variation in consultation rates for low back pain, as measured by patient recall. In Peterlee and Arbroath for example, patients with low back pain during the previous 12 months were more than three times more likely to have consulted their doctor as those living in St Austell and Dorking, an effect not explained by social class or severity of symptoms.

Consultation incidence according to baseline period prevalence

The following groups are taken from the definitions given on page 141.

- **Group I** Among adults free of low back pain at the start of the incidence year, the proportion who consult at least once for low back pain during the year has been estimated as 4.2%.[21] Since this group is 62% of the total adult population, this means a cumulative incidence of 2.4% new episode consulters in the adult population as a whole.

- **Group II** The proportion of people who consult at least once during the incidence year in this group (those who reported episodic low back pain during the previous prevalence year) is 7.1%, i.e. 2.5% of the total adult population.
- **Group III** The OPCS survey suggests that about 50% of those with persistent problems causing appreciable disability will consult their GP in the course of a year.[2] The prevalence of such continuous problems in the adult population is estimated on page 142 to be 6%, so the expected proportion who consult at least once in the incidence year would be approximately 3% of the adult population.

In summary, in one year in primary care:

- one-third of all people who consult during the year because of low back pain will be attending with a new episode after at least 12 months free of low back pain
- one-third will be coming with recurrences of a problem which they had suffered for some part of the previous year
- one-third will be coming with a persistent disabling problem.

Prescribed medication

Studies from UK general practice suggest that 67% of those who attend with low back pain are prescribed medication. This figure is remarkably consistent, but it is also the figure for the average percentage of consultations which result in a prescription for whatever reason. Among low back pain sufferers in the general population during a 12-month period who did not attend the GP, 19% reported taking medication and this presumably represents the prevalence of over-the-counter medication.

The duration of therapy will be dictated by case-mix. The evidence from US studies is that a high percentage of those with persistent low back pain continue to take prescribed medication.[49] A conservative assumption might be that rather more than half of those consulting with persistent, disabling problems (i.e. 1.5% of the adult population) will take prescribed drugs for three months of the year in total.

In the CSAG document, the assumption was made of an average two or three week prescription per consultation. An audit in a single general practice confirmed an average of two weeks at maximum dosage for an initial prescription.[50] We have applied this figure to those patients who receive a prescription but who do not return after a single consultation for low back pain (3.8% of the population).

Fitton's study of the costs of prescribing for low back pain in general practice[51] suggested that compound analgesics were more popular than nonsteroidal anti-inflammatory agents for low back pain but this may have changed in the decade since the study was published. More recent work suggests that these drugs are now prescribed about equally as frequently for low back pain.[19,52] Based on current NHS costing in MIMS, a two-week course could cost from £2 to £15. An average of £7 will be assumed here.

Summary

In one year, one in five of subjects who experience low back pain in the population will present to the GP. This is one estimate of demand for health care. It is in these patients that initial estimates of the impact of treatment on the natural history of low back pain must be made.

The likelihood of consultation is higher among those with a recent history of problems. Hence roughly equal numbers of consulters each year will come from the three groups in the prevalence pool. Most (two-thirds) will be new episodes or recurrences or clear exacerbations.

In a population of 100 000 adults, during a 12 month period, approximately 5000 receive at least one prescription for low back pain, with analgesics and nonsteroidal anti-inflammatory tablets dominating. Of these 1500 are on prescribed drugs for their low back pain for a minimum of 12 weeks in the year, whilst 3500 receive a single short course of therapy for an average of two weeks.

A further 6000 take over-the-counter tablets for low back pain.

Repeat consultations for low back pain

In the Royal College of General Practitioners' Morbidity Survey the annual rate of total consultations for low back problems was twice as high as the figure for the annual proportion of people who consult. This means that each patient who consults with low back pain has on average one further consultation within a year about the same symptom.[22] In a study of two group practices, three month follow-up of all patients who consulted at least once with low back pain revealed a skewed picture:[21] 60% of consulters did not return, but some people had returned more than twice within the three-month period.

Hospital referral

Specialists

During one year 10 to 20% of low back sufferers seen in primary care are referred to a hospital specialist. The majority see an orthopaedic surgeon, although there are likely to be regional variations, with the others being seen mainly by rheumatologists, neurosurgeons and pain specialists. A study of two hospital groups in Manchester[21] produced estimates of the annual rate of referral from local GPs which were similar to those reported by the National Morbidity Survey in General Practice.[22]

In a population of 100 000 adults, an estimated 800 will be seen in the course of a year by a specialist because of low back pain as the main presenting problem; a further 800 will be seen in A and E departments with low back pain as a presenting problem.

Radiology

During one year 15 to 20% of general practice attenders are referred for a lumbar spine X-ray, with wide variation between practices. In addition 40% of new hospital attenders with low back pain will be X-rayed and most A and E attenders with low back pain will have an X-ray.[21] There will in addition be X-rays carried out in private practice, and by chiropractors and osteopaths.

In a population of 100 000 adults, 3000 lumbar spine X-rays will be carried out in one year to investigate low back pain.

Physical therapists

Based on Waddell's summary of available evidence from surveys of the practitioners themselves or from their professional bodies,[19] the following estimates apply to new referrals for physical treatments of low back pain in a population of 100 000 adults during one year:

- 2000 (2.0%) to NHS physiotherapy
- 600 (0.6%) to private physiotherapy
- 1500 (1.5%) to osteopathy
- 600 (0.6%) to chiropractic

This however will range widely from region to region depending on socio-economic mix and availability. In one population survey in Manchester, 1.9% had seen a physiotherapist, 1% an osteopath, 0.6% a chiropractor.[21] In a national sample studied by the OPCS, the figures were 3%, 2% and 1% respectively.[2]

The case-mix poses an interesting problem. European evidence is emerging that osteopaths and chiropractors tend to see sufferers early in their episode, who are in work and remain in work during their episode and who tend to be from better-off social classes as measured by low smoking, low levels of obesity and non-manual jobs. Those people at higher risk of low back pain are under-represented, as is the pool of persistent, more severely disabled back sufferers.[53,54]

Physiotherapists in hospitals by contrast will tend to receive specialist referrals which will reflect the dominance of persistent problems in this group. Direct referrals from GPs to physiotherapists in their surgeries, in community clinics, or in hospital will inevitably produce a different case-mix for the physiotherapist. Private physiotherapy practice presents another referral picture.

A crucial issue is the number of treatments offered. This is a major influence on the number of patients seen and on the costs per patient. In the US chiropractors have a higher number of visits per episode than other practitioners.[55] In the UK the average number of visits within an episode of low back pain appears to be similar for all physical therapists: six, five and six for physiotherapists, osteopaths and chiropractors respectively[19] and the proportion of back patients who see a chiropractor or osteopath is also much lower here than it is in the US. There is no clear scientific basis for specifying the length of a set of treatments.

The possible role of fee for service in determining the number of treatments cannot be ignored. In a recent US study[55] patients presenting with new episodes of low back pain to primary care physicians were compared to patients presenting with similar problems to chiropractors and to orthopaedic surgeons. Clinical outcomes were similar in the different groups and charges for each radiograph and each visit were lower in the chiropractic group. However the latter had a far higher number of treatments (and hence visits) per episode. This high volume made chiropractic a far more expensive option than the physicians and surgeons.

Inpatient care

The most detailed review of hospital admissions for low back pain appears in Waddell's Annex to the CSAG Report,[19] which is based on Hospital Episodes Statistics for England and Wales and Scottish Health Service Statistics. His considered estimate of the total number of patients in England and Wales admitted to hospital in 1989–90 for back problems is in excess of 100 000. In a population of 100 000 adults, the equivalent number would be more than 200. This figure excludes ankylosing spondylitis and combines ordinary and day case admissions. However it includes cervical and thoracic problems, which on the basis of surgical procedures would constitute some 20% of all back admissions.

Admissions for low back problems would thus total 160 patients in one year in a population of 100 000 adults: 115 ordinary admissions and 45 day cases.

In a survey of low back pain in one Manchester hospital 10% of new clinic referrals with low back pain were admitted for inpatient care within three months and a further 4% were admitted as day cases. This would represent some 112 patients in a population of 100 000: 80 ordinary and 32 day cases. This is an underestimate of ordinary admissions, since some patients will be admitted later than three months after their initial visit. So these figures are compatible with Waddell's estimate. They are however about one-quarter of the numbers as calculated from the OPCS population survey using recall of 'treatment on a hospital ward' during the past year.[2] Waddell, working from hospital discharge statistics, estimated a figure for inpatient treatment which was also one-quarter of that in the population survey. This suggests the estimates of current workload given above are reasonable.

From the Hospital Episodes Statistics 1989–90 there is also a breakdown of surgical procedures for the low back.[19] The operations are dominated by lumbosacral disc procedures, but the majority of procedures were paraspinal injections.

In a population of 100 000 adults, there are approximately 84 procedures performed on the lumbosacral spine each year: 28 disc operations and 56 other procedures, mostly paraspinal injections.

Some of these may be on the same people so they are not directly comparable to the admission data, but we will assume that for a one year period these represent people rather than events.

There is no evidence about the exact number and nature of admissions for non-surgical inpatient care of low back pain, such as bed rest, traction and plaster jackets. In the Manchester studies, 13% of hospital attenders and 1% of the general population reported receiving lumbar traction during the previous 12 months.[21] These figures do not distinguish between inpatient admissions for treatment and treatment provided for physiotherapy outpatients. If it is assumed that recalled figures are again approximately a four-fold inflation of the true prevalence of such treatment, this gives a figure of 30 patients receiving traction annually in a population of 100 000.

Ankylosing spondylitis accounts for 1% of the hospital admissions for back pain. Since the estimated prevalence of this condition in the general population is one per 1000, this suggests that approximately 1% of people with ankylosing spondylitis in the general population are admitted to hospital in any one year.

Apart from ankylosing spondylitis and the small number of emergency admissions, the problem in assessing these figures against subgroup prevalence figures is that there are no details about the case-mix of hospitalizations. If we assume that the majority are for low back pain with cord or root compression, this suggests that about 10% of potentially serious sciatica in the community is hospitalized in any one year, of whom rather less than half have surgery. In Weber's carefully followed group of 208 acute lumbar radiculopathies, four underwent surgery during a 12 month follow-up.[56] It seems unlikely that there is a large unmet need for lumbosacral disc surgery, although it is not known whether those who have the need are receiving the operations. Against this has to be placed the finding that the US and Holland have four to five times the spinal surgery rate of the UK.[57] Once again the possible influence of fee for service and of cultural views about surgical intervention must be taken into account when interpreting such comparisons.

Other services available

Occupational health services

In the OPCS and Manchester population surveys, approximately 1% of low back pain sufferers reported a contact with the occupational health services (doctor or nurse) during a one year period.

The most recent information from the Health and Safety Executive suggests that 75% of all employees in England and Wales are in establishments where there is coverage by occupational health services of some sort.[58] The high figure reflects wide coverage in large firms and in the public sector. Approximately 50% of all employees have access to a health professional of some sort through the workplace.

This indicates that there is less use made of occupational health services compared with attendance in primary care, but that a back pain service in the workplace could be available to approximately 20% of low back sufferers (i.e. 50% of the low back pain sufferers who remain in work).

In a population of 100 000 adults during one year 7500 people who experience low back pain have potential access to an occupational health professional but only 400 will utilize this service.

Occupational therapy

In the OPCS survey 1% of subjects reported having seen an occupational therapist because of low back pain during the previous year, but in the Manchester study no one recalled using this service.

Corsets

These remain a popular treatment for low back pain: reported by 10% of low back patients attending their GP and 25% of new attenders with low back pain in hospital clinics.

Self-care

This may follow the advice of professionals or may be gleaned from other sources. Sources of general information include:

- **National Back Pain Association** Individual access to advice and information. Educational material, information pack, local group membership.
- **Arthritis Care** Telephone help-line, comprehensive information sheets on pain management and back pain.

In the Manchester studies bed rest as a therapeutic approach to low back pain was reported by 25% of individuals who had had low back pain during the past year; 17% had tried exercises; 50% had avoided heavy lifting; 40% had tried cream or sprays. In each case those who had consulted their GP were more likely to have tried these approaches than those who had not.

Summary and estimated costs of current care for low back pain

The summary of main sources of health service care is shown in Table 5. Total costs are slightly lower than the CSAG estimate when applied to a population of 100 000. The figure here should be regarded as a probable minimum because:

- the prescription figure is likely to be higher if more patients with persistent pain are on medication for longer than three months in a year

- costs of hospital treatment do not include emergency admissions for pain relief; secondary referrals to other specialist services such as psychology and psychiatry; orthotics; or multi-disciplinary treatments where these are available. The inpatient estimates are dominated by surgical admissions.

So the costs might be as high as £800 000 per year in an adult population of 100 000. The CSAG costings[a] used different approaches to reach their figure, although we have used a number of their quoted item costs as the basis for our calculations (for example, the average cost of a GP consultation, of a hospital outpatient visit, and an A and E department attendance). The CSAG figure was £880 000 for a population of this size, the main difference being that they assumed an average of four consultations per patient consulting with low back pain in primary care.[19] Figures from the National Morbidity Surveys in primary care suggest this is an overestimate.[22] However the possibility that consultation data underestimate what the patient perceives as back pain consultations (page 146) underlines that such costs could be higher.

Table 5: Main sources of health care for patients with low back pain with approximate costs (1993 prices)

	Number seen	Total contacts	Cost (£)
Primary care consultations	7 500	15 000	165 000
Prescribed medication[*]	5 250	3 700 single	26 000
		1 500 multiple (persistent and severe)	63 000
A and E attendances	800	800	28 000
Specialist referrals	800	2 400	72 000
Hospital episodes	170	138 inpatient admissions 32 day cases	200 000
Physical therapy	2 000	10 000	100 000
Plain lumbar radiographs	3 000	3 000	90 000
Specialist imaging	160	160	16 000
Total estimated costs			670 000

[*] Based on estimates from MIMS. Unit cost of single contact = £7 and multiple contacts = £42. Estimated unit costs are as follows (source in brackets): GP consultations £11.00 (CSAG); Outpatient consultations £30.00 (CSAG); Physical therapy £9.00 (CSAG); Inpatient day £133.00 (CSAG); A and E £35.00 (CSAG); X-ray £30.00 (CSAG); Imaging £100.00 (NHS Trust).
Hospital episodes have assumed an average of ten days per episode.

---

[a] Since this section was compiled, a fuller version of the CSAG economic analysis has been published by the University of York: Klaber Moffett et al.[120] This has used a number of other sources and provides a detailed and valuable estimate of the costs of back pain. Its range for total costs to the NHS, at 1993 prices, was £270–380 million per annum. This range is close to the estimates in the previous paragraph when applied to the adult population of the UK.

7 Effectiveness and cost-effectiveness of treatments

This will be considered in two parts:

1   Short-term relief of symptoms: important, but always to be put in the context that symptom relief will occur in the majority of patients seeking health care for low back pain, regardless of the treatment given.
2   Long-term relief of symptoms and improvement in mobility, functioning, work capacity and psychological well-being among patients whose problems are established and persistent and in whom spontaneous improvement is less likely to occur.

The following question is rarely addressed but it is crucial to the public health perspective: does early treatment of new episodes help to prevent long-term problems of pain and disability?

In general overviews of randomized controlled trials of treatment of low back pain reach the pessimistic conclusion that their quality is poor.[59,60]

Our approach is that, despite their flaws, these studies can be used to inform judgements on the efficacy and effectiveness of different interventions. The real gap in the literature is in trials of longer term outcome among study populations sufficiently unselected to be generalizable to the health care requirements of all low back pain sufferers.

Current efficacy of primary care

The diagnostic triage

The CSAG report made clear that the small proportion of potentially serious cases could best be sorted out by general practice diagnostic triage followed by appropriate referral, investigation and hospital treatment, using the pragmatic classification outlined on page 135. This includes those with severe nerve root pain, who may not require referral but for whom extended bed rest for example is a recommended option.

The efficacy of diagnostic triage remains to be tested, despite the enthusiasm of the CSAG for it. It has strong expert recommendation and is potentially cost-effective because it should keep unnecessary investigation and referral to a minimum. However it may demand initial investment to support a full hospital emergency back pain service.

From a strictly epidemiological point of view, it remains possible that the diagnostic triage could increase referrals if it were to have a poor specificity for serious pathology in the primary care setting (i.e. many patients referred with possible serious pathology, who turn out to have non-specific low back pain). Good clinical epidemiological studies of the outcome of triage in the aftermath of the CSAG report are needed.

Management of non-specific low back pain

The presumed benign outcome of low back pain seen in primary care is based on a restricted view of the problem.

Among subjects with localized low back pain (i.e. no radiation to the leg) who attend their GP within 48 hours of its onset, there is rapid recovery in 90%.[38] These are a minority of cases attending primary care.

Overall 55% of primary care attenders will have completely recovered (25%) or improved (30%) from their presenting symptoms within three months.[21] The proportion of those who are the same or worse will vary according to the status of the episode as new, recurrent, or an exacerbation – i.e. the point in the patient's whole back pain history at which this particular episode is occurring.

There is evidence that some general practice interventions can affect the natural history of low back pain in the short term (see below). It is GPs in the main who apply the pragmatic classification of low back pain and refer potentially serious problems for investigation and management. Patients who require sickness certification for more than one week will also attend.

The question of overall efficacy has been circular however. Since the impression given by the clinical medical literature is that, left alone, most low back pain will get better, then the question of whether GPs or members of their team could actively improve the short- and long-term outcomes has been by-passed.

Patient advice and education

The idea that educational approaches to the low back pain patient will improve outcome is an attractive one. In an interesting and important study in UK primary care, consecutive surgery attenders with low back pain were randomized to receive or not to receive an information booklet.[61] After 12 months the booklet group had reduced consultations and referrals, although there was no impact on working days lost. A study in a Dutch general practice suggested that the 'information/simple analgesics' approach was as good as physiotherapy in influencing recovery.[62]

In a Finnish study workers presenting to an occupational health service with acute low back pain were randomized to receiving bed rest, or to specific back-mobilizing exercises or to simple advice to 'avoid bed rest, not to engage in specific back exercises and to continue normal activity to the extent that they were able to tolerate it'.[63] The simple advice group showed better recovery at three and 12 weeks than the first two groups (see also page 158, psychological approaches).

More intensive educational approaches have received attention: particularly 'back schools'. Swedish in origin, these are group educational programmes, of variable length and content broadly designed to educate low back sufferers in pain management, ergonomics and general measures to improve back 'fitness'.[64] There have been a number of randomized controlled trials of this approach and several overviews of the trials[65,66] – most recently the detailed and careful review by Cohen.[66] The conclusions were that the case for back schools remains unproven. Some short-term benefits in reducing pain intensity in both acute and chronic episodes have been observed, but there are no convincing long-term effects on function, symptom recurrence or work loss. Where there is reported benefit, it seems to be in the short term and to be non-specific. The case for choosing group educational methods to achieve this is doubtful. The difficulty lies in identifying the important therapeutic features of the programmes given the wide variation in content and approach detailed in the literature.

One of the better trials of the group educational approach did note other benefits when it was linked with visits to and liaison with the workplace.[67] As part of secondary prevention approaches in industry there is a stronger case for the back school.[66]

Tablets and injections

Simple analgesia, narcotic analgesia, nonsteroidal anti-inflammatory drugs, muscle relaxants, sedatives – all are used in the treatment of low back pain. Patients in severe acute pain need pain relief, so the use of appropriate short-term analgesia is not in doubt. The question is whether other therapies offer any additional advantage over simple analgesia.

In the very short term (i.e. seven days or less) some active therapies appear to do better than their placebo in terms of the proportion of patients who recover or of the degree of pain relief achieved (nonsteroidals and muscle relaxants). In one careful trial of treatment of acute low back pain within 48 hours of the onset of an episode piroxicam offered no advantages over placebo in terms of reported pain relief by seven days, although it had reduced the need for simple analgesia and had resulted in more subjects returning to work. However there seemed little advantage in the active tablets over placebo for outcomes after one week.[68]

An overview of injection therapy concluded that there was little good trial evidence to recommend it.[60] The possible options include steroid or local anaesthetic injections (or both) into tender soft tissue points, discs, ligaments, facet joints or the epidural space. The most positive trial evidence suggests some effect beyond placebo, but in one careful trial (of methylprednisolone to facet joints) the effect was entirely explained by concurrent medication.[69] Likewise with acupuncture, there is little firm evidence to support its use as a specific treatment for low back pain.[70]

The same pattern of evidence appears in most trials of analgesia: considerable improvement is seen in 60 to 70% of all participants regardless of therapy. The active therapy under investigation is attributed with the benefit in one-third of the patients who improve. The difficulty of interpretation is that such additional improvement might be important but not specific to the particular treatment under investigation.

Bed rest or early activity?

Two randomized controlled trials, one in primary care and the other in a 'walk-in' US clinic, have provided evidence that bed rest interferes with return to full activity in acute back pain.[71,72] Early mobilization (after a maximum of two days in bed in one of the studies) resulted in a reduction in total days lost from work up to three months later; the second study however found no difference 12 months later between groups treated with and without early activity. The Finnish trial discussed on page 154 has provided new evidence that patients with acute low back pain who are advised to rest in bed for as little as two days do not do as well as those who are encouraged to continue ordinary activity.[63]

Up to two weeks bed-rest still seems to be the advised conservative approach for severe radicular pain; however one study has found that early mobilization is beneficial even in this group.[72] Since it is agreed that patients with progressive neurological problems should be referred, it seems only a very few patients need to remain in bed for any length of time.

Physical therapy

Physiotherapists offer three general approaches in addition to education and information:

- **Back exercises** These can be active (taught to the patient) or passive (aided by the therapist). Flexion, extension and physical strengthening exercises form three of the main group of exercises. Different 'schools' of physiotherapy place different emphasis on these: the McKenzie method for example stresses extension, the Williams school favours flexion.
- **Manipulation and mobilization** These are discussed on page 157, together with osteopathy and chiropractic.
- **Technology** Various pieces of equipment have been introduced to the physiotherapists' approach to low back pain, including trans-cutaneous electrical nerve stimulation (TENS), ultrasound and laser therapy.

Exercise

If bed rest is bad and early activity is good, the next question is whether specific exercises can achieve anything which general encouragement to stay active cannot.

Early intervention

In a review of randomized controlled trials of exercise therapy from physiotherapists most trials which compared specific exercises in acute low back pain with no exercise or with placebo were negative.[73] There is some evidence of an early effect on pain relief but it does not appear any better to other methods of treating pain. In one important general practice study, 512 patients presenting with localized low back pain of three weeks duration or less were randomized. Exercise sessions (for five weeks, twice a week, at 20 minutes per session) were no better at preventing recurrences during a 12 month follow-up period compared with usual care and standardized information given by the GP.[62] There were some symptomatic benefits from physiotherapy attention in the first three months (decreased tiredness and emotional problems) but exercise sessions were no better than parallel placebo ultrasound sessions in achieving this. Disability was unaffected but repeat consultations were reduced in the physiotherapy groups, whilst some physiotherapy referrals occurred in the usual care group.

Later intervention

In chronic back pain, there is evidence that exercises do improve symptoms. In a US study designed mainly to evaluate TENS therapy, subjects with at least three months of low back pain recruited through newspaper adverts were randomized.[74] Exercises (taught for home use and coupled with three physiotherapy sessions over one month) had a clear benefit during three months follow-up in increasing activity and reducing pain. Once again there was no effect on disability. By three months, only half the patients were still performing the exercises regularly and the overall effect in the treated groups was diminishing. Since these were well-motivated patients, not at the severe end of the disability scale, it seems unlikely that the observed effects would persist in practice without further visits and reinforcement.

A controlled trial of an exercise, education and behavioural programme run by a physical therapist involved subjects who had been off work for six weeks because of a persistent episode of low back pain. There was an earlier return to work (average eight weeks earlier) and improvement in mobility and fitness 12 months later in the actively treated group.[75] The evidence points to exercise in such patients being as much about improving confidence and managing pain as about direct effects of exercises on physical capacity.

A similar result was found when chronic sufferers of more than six months duration were followed for 12 months: here disability score was improved as well as physical performance.[76] The estimate was that 50% of such people under the age of 50 years could be safely involved in a vigorous multi-disciplinary rehabilitation programme.

A recent UK study has provided important new evidence, which suggests a more cost-effective approach is possible.[77] Patients with at least six months of low back pain were randomized to a fitness class where eight group exercise sessions were carried out over a four-week period by a physiotherapist who used psychological principles as an integral part of the intervention. This meant that attention was diverted from the back and the pain and on to a more positive 'sports exercise' approach, focused on what the individual could do in terms of general fitness exercising. Both the intervention and the control groups were also taught specific back exercises and were referred to a back school. Six months later the fitness group had lower disability than the control group. In summary, there is evidence that, in those who have been off work for some weeks or months because of low back pain, exercise programmes confer benefit for up to 12 months.[74–77] The interventions however have ranged from simple advice sessions to involvement of multiple disciplines and range widely in complexity, cost and duration. Supervised group fitness programmes which emphasize positive psychological approaches to pain seem to offer a promising cost-effective option.

Manipulation and mobilization

Although individual practitioners emphasize the importance of tailoring treatment to the individual patient, overviews of studies of 'hands-on' approaches to manipulation or mobilization of the spine have tended to group different methods together in an attempt to judge their efficacy. In the absence of a clear justification for treating them separately, the same approach was adopted in the CSAG report, in which manipulation and mobilization by physiotherapists were bracketed with treatments given by osteopaths and chiropractors and these three groups were referred to collectively as 'physical therapists'. Manipulation is taken here to mean high-velocity thrusts to the spine beyond the patient's restricted range of movement and mobilization to mean low-velocity passive or assisted movements within or at the limit of the patient's range of movement.

In general the evidence supports a short-term benefit of manipulation or mobilization in patients with a short duration of the current episode, particularly with respect to reduction in pain intensity measured by either self-report or a reduced need for analgesia.[78,79] The effect was less in those seen very early on in their episode – hardly surprising given the increased likelihood that such patients settle rapidly anyway. Studies which include longer term follow-up provide no convincing data to suppose that these therapy approaches do alter the long-term course and there is insufficient evidence yet to reach a conclusion about their contribution to secondary prevention of recurrent and persistent low back pain.

Two interesting studies stand out. Hadler's study, although small, showed an advantage of a single treatment involving a high velocity thrust compared with mobilization omitting the thrust. This was seen in patients with less than one month of pain in the current episode, who were attending a primary care rheumatology clinic in the US.[80] Follow-up was for two weeks only. The study is important because:

- it demonstrated the efficacy of a single treatment (much of the concern about the cost-effectiveness of physical therapy relates to the seemingly open-ended number of sessions provided for any one case)
- it began to tackle whether one form of manipulation or mobilization was superior to another – the general absence of data on this makes it difficult to make recommendations about specific forms of physical therapy.

The second was a controversial pragmatic randomized comparison of patients referred to chiropractors or to hospital physiotherapists.[81] Although interpreted as an unfair assessment of physiotherapy undertaken under usual NHS conditions, its importance lay in demonstrating that a physical therapy can have an effect on disability in the longer term, i.e. after two years. A recent follow-up has suggested that the effects persist for even longer.[82] What aspect of the chiropractic intervention was important is not clear, but it is one of the few studies to suggest that intervention might alter the future natural history and therefore contribute to secondary prevention.

In general the available overviews are agreed that in early treatment manipulation–mobilization hastens short-term recovery, but the long-term benefits are unknown. From available studies the average size of the effect 2–4 weeks after treatment averages 20%. The problem is that half of the patients are going to get better anyway. The additional effect seems worth achieving, but it might not be specific to the particular treatment studied and the costs of extending it to all who might benefit in the short term could be prohibitive.

It is here that the lack of evidence about long-term effects is frustrating. If manipulation and mobilization were an intervention with secondary prevention benefits, the case for providing it on a wide scale would be stronger. As it is, one argument states that there has to be some selection to identify which patients presenting with low back pain should receive such intervention. The conclusion of the CSAG was that persistence of an episode for two weeks was a suitable criterion for referral.[8] This has not been put to the test and it is quite plausible, given the known occurrence of low back pain in primary care, that even this sift would result in an overload on the system. There is an urgent need for evidence about the results of introducing such a policy in terms of the rates of referral to physical therapists, of actual attendance and of follow-up visits generated, as well as the overall costs.

The lack of evidence about costs and benefits of early physical therapy means that these must be conjectural. However it seems reasonable to suppose that it would have other benefits (reduced emphasis on diagnosis in the majority of low back pain patients, reduced medication costs as an alternative symptomatic treatment, improved education and information for individuals). Against these points there are likely to be costs, such as needless treatment and multiple visits to the therapist.

The empirical evidence suggests that the likelihood of major side-effects of routine manipulation and mobilization is extremely low,[83] but acute progression of cord or root compression can occur very rarely. There is little evidence on which to recommend courses of manipulation for more chronic low back pain.

Cost-effectiveness of physical therapy

In studies which have compared manipulation with other forms of physiotherapy, one feature was that manipulation courses were shorter than therapy courses. Clearly this is dependent on local conditions, trial protocols and therapist variation but does suggest that short courses of manipulation in the treatment of acute pain are potentially cost-effective.

The cost-effectiveness of exercise programmes in more chronic low back pain is difficult to judge, since the content of the programme has varied enormously in published studies. In one study, the authors state that the intervention was simple and inexpensive; in another, a multi-disciplinary team of a physician, psychologist, social worker, physiotherapists, occupational therapist and work trainee were involved. However the simple group exercise programme for moderately disabled patients with chronic low back pain outlined in the Frost *et al.* study discussed previously was less costly than providing individual therapy sessions.[77]

Technology

Good randomized controlled trials have provided no evidence of the superiority of these interventions over placebo in acute or chronic low back pain; nor do they offer advantages over other methods of pain relief.[84,85]

Psychological interventions

There is a large body of evidence that psychological factors are important predictors of the progress and outcome of episodes of low back pain.[86] These embrace emotional factors, such as depression and anxiety; cognitive factors, which concern elements of the individual's appraisal of their pain, such as catastrophizing thoughts; and pain-related behaviour, such as previous propensity to seek health care for painful symptoms. There is now strong observational evidence about the influence which such factors have on the course and outcome of episodes of low back pain.[87-90]

Trials of psychological interventions have been carried out, although many have tended to concentrate on patients with long-standing problems and on the psychological component of multi-disciplinary interventions. The trials have ranged from programmes which have concentrated on behaviour change, such as the 'operant conditioning' methods pioneered by Fordyce and colleagues,[91] to those which have tackled thoughts and feelings about pain and its consequences, the cognitive-behavioural approach.[92] For chronic back pain sufferers the message seems clear: combining behavioural or cognitive-behavioural approaches with physical rehabilitation is more successful than a physical regime alone. There is evidence that such multi-disciplinary approaches are effective in improving the ability of some patients with long-standing disability and handicap to function in the world.[90]

However there is very limited evidence about the benefits of psychological interventions early on in a back pain career when the population impact could potentially be enormous. In particular the nature of an effective psychological intervention for primary care attenders is an urgent area for investigation. There is some evidence that it is worthwhile. Fordyce for example reported on a trial of behavioural versus traditional management of acute back pain, which showed some differences in favour of the behavioural group up to 12 months later.[93] In multi-disciplinary treatment of chronic cases this would mean expensive specialist time. However brief interventions at an earlier stage might be cost-effective if they enhanced the secondary prevention component of other treatments.

It is likely that the emerging case for active management of new episodes or recurrences rests on it having a 'cognitive–behavioural' element. The randomized controlled trial evidence for simple encouragement to keep active in acute episodes[63] or for a 'general fitness approach' in those with more persistent problems[77] suggests that reduction of fear and improving confidence are beneficial. In addition Symonds and colleagues have recently shown that the inclusion of material which tackles emotions and beliefs about low back pain in an educational leaflet for factory workers was associated with a reduced number of subsequent work absences due to low back pain.[94]

Efficacy of diagnosis

How important is diagnosis in low back pain? Since most cases of low back pain cannot have a label attached (or only one for which there is no good or consistent clinical epidemiological evidence of validity or utility), then the rationale of 'needing' a diagnosis must be questioned.

Imaging

The role of imaging in the management of low back pain focuses on the relationship between the 'low back pain' syndrome and spinal abnormality. Requests for lumbar spine films are the most frequent referral by GPs in their management of low back pain (10–20% of low back consulters but with wide variation between practitioners); in hospital, one-third of new attenders were referred for an X-ray in a district teaching hospital despite the fact that 80% of them had already had one previously.[21]

The evidence points strongly to the inappropriateness of lumbar spine films in the early management of low back pain. There are two main reasons as follows.

- In population studies, the prevalence of abnormalities on X-ray are common in those with and without low back pain.[95,96] Disc degeneration, spondylolisthesis and scoliosis are only weakly associated with pain.
- There is no clear evidence that treating these abnormalities, even if they were responsible for some of the pain, is beneficial.

Imaging is needed for two reasons as follows.

- To investigate the possibility of a serious diagnosis – i.e. malignancy, fracture or infection. These are so rare as causes for low back pain that the use of a routine lumbar spine film to screen for them is not justified – the 'yield' in one series of 2500 adults aged under 50 years was one. The low yield and the unnecessary radiation argue against routine use of such plain films in the assessment of uncomplicated low back pain.

  The need for an X-ray can be based on clear clinical indications: the CSAG report gives a list of 'red flag' symptoms and signs. Even the usual caveat (pain for more than six weeks) does not justify a routine

X-ray in the absence of other clinical indications, since simple persistence of low back pain for more than six weeks will apply to a majority of patients presenting in primary care.

Consultation behaviour, anxiety, the cultural perception of the importance of the X-ray, doctor variation – all these cannot be ignored in judging the current place of lumbar films, and yet there is little or no research-based evidence of their importance. They need to be weighed against the lack of evidence that lumbar spine films contribute to diagnosis and management in patients other than those in whom clinical suspicion of a serious problem is strong.

- To justify surgical procedures. The diagnoses of disc herniation and spinal stenosis do not depend on plain lumbar radiography, and so the lumbar film is unlikely to influence management in cases being considered for invasive procedures in hospital. Whether myelography, CT or MRI should be used as the diagnostic procedure of choice for these two conditions is unclear.[96] The popular move is towards MRI because it can identify other pathologies also (such as tumours), but there is no good evidence comparing these three approaches with respect to utility and cost benefits.

There is strong evidence against routine use of these procedures in low back pain management. The MRI has revealed how common disc bulging, protrusion and extrusion are in the human population, regardless of symptoms.[97] The implication of this is that imaging should only be undertaken when clinical suspicion is high. Since the prognosis of root pain is good, investigation of persistent sciatic root symptoms after conservative therapy is one indication for imaging.

Other forms of imaging are controversial. An example is discography, in which discs are injected under imaging control to investigate whether pain is reproduced, on the basis that discs may cause pain even when not herniating. There is no clear evidence that such procedures lead to more effective treatment.

Imaging in primary and secondary prevention

The observation that disc abnormalities are common in teenagers and in asymptomatic adults suggests that there may be fruitful lines of research into early influences on spinal health. Despite the lack of a cross-sectional relationship between structural abnormalities and low back pain, it is possible that altering the early natural history of spinal problems may have a later influence on symptoms.

However there is no evidence that screening for spinal abnormalities contributes to secondary prevention of low back pain, either in childhood or for example in industrial placement. The debate on the value of two-stage childhood screening (clinical plus imaging) for scoliosis of the spine continues, but its value is debated in terms of preventing progressive structural deformity rather than preventing low back pain.

Surgery

In an international study comparing spine surgery rates, the most dramatic difference was the five times higher rate in the US compared with England and Scotland.[57] Within the US rates also vary,[98] and during the past decade operation rates there have dramatically increased whilst non-surgical hospitalization rates for low back pain have fallen.

Open disc surgery, chemonucleolysis and microdiscectomy each have their advocates as treatment for herniated discs; laminectomy for spinal stenosis and lumbar fusion for degenerative disease with spinal instability are the other major procedures.

There seems to be a consensus that open disc surgery for herniated lumbar discs is a reasonable option. The small minority of patients with a cauda equina lesion or progressive neurological signs constitute surgical emergencies. However it is not clear whether surgery should be advocated for herniated discs which are not in these serious categories.

Conservative therapy for radicular pain is a reasonable approach, as discussed earlier. In Weber's randomized controlled trial, there were clear short-term benefits for surgery compared with conservative therapy, but at long-term follow-up the differences had disappeared.[56] In Hoffman's overview he stated that 'most studies had design flaws and omitted important clinical data' but reached the conclusion that short-term relief of sciatica was better in those who had undergone surgery.[99]

Against this must be placed the following points.

- Weber's studies also showed that 70% of patients with sciatica of less than 14 days duration (i.e. acute) were pain-free one year later after conservative treatment only.[56] This is broadly similar to the improvement seen in trials and studies of many active therapies. It supports the clinical view that surgery is not usually indicated for uncomplicated early sciatica.
- The faster pain relief obtained by surgery has to be put beside the admittedly rare rate of serious complications of open disc surgery (estimated at less than 1% of cases) and the consistent finding that disc surgery confers a risk of further surgery – 10% re-operation at one year, 18% by five years. Such figures could of course reflect patient selection, but there is no evidence that conservative therapy leads to a similarly high rate of subsequent operation. In many randomized trials of intervention in low back pain, an important predictor of poor outcome is a previous history of back surgery.
- Randomized trial evidence offers little support for newer procedures in disc surgery. Chemonucleolysis carries a consistently higher rate of subsequent operation than conventional surgery, together with problems of post-operative pain, and no evidence of symptomatic superiority over conventional surgery one year later.[100] Because of the subsequent operation rates it costs more. Microsurgical techniques in one randomized trial also carried a high rate of re-operation.[101]

Overviews of fusion and surgery for spinal stenosis have concluded that there is no clear evidence yet available concerning the efficacy of these procedures.[102,103] In three out of four randomized controlled trials of fusion identified by Turner, there was no advantage of surgery with fusion compared with surgery without; there appeared to be unacceptably high rates of complications. It would thus seem likely that there are only very select populations for whom fusion is an advantage; one randomized controlled trial has indicated that fusion added to laminectomy for spinal stenosis with spondylolisthesis had a better outcome in terms of pain relief two years later, although there were design flaws in this study.

Inpatient traction remains a popular choice of treatment in some centres. There has been good randomized controlled trial evidence available for some years now that shows no effect in the short- or long-term, although these same studies did suggest that manual traction provides short-term relief of pain.[104,105]

Summary and tables of evidence

The critical reviewer of evidence must exercise caution and humility. For many interventions used in low back pain treatment there is simply insufficient good evidence to either support or refute their effectiveness. Forms of evidence other than the randomized controlled trial are important to the clinician in making judgements about treating individual patients. 'No scientific evidence' should not be interpreted as 'strong evidence against'. With this caveat, the following summary represents a personal view of the evidence reviews published to date.

New or recurrent episodes

The evidence is summarized in Table 6.

Quality of evidence

This applies to short-term outcome only. Some trials have given results for 12 months or longer, but we do not have clear evidence of the potential for these interventions to prevent subsequent low back pain.

Cost-effectiveness

This is coded as follows. 'Yes' means that the intervention is almost certain to be cost-effective in primary care, even if demand increased. 'No' means that the intervention could not be applied to the generality of patients without major cost implications. 'Possible' means that cost-effectiveness is likely to depend on the demand and the actual process involved in implementing it: a single visit to a physical therapist for example could be highly cost-effective even if it was applied to a lot of patients. If that visit were to become a 'course' of six visits per patient, then it could not be applied to everyone without major cost implications. 'X' means that it is cost-effective to reduce or phase out such treatments.[a]

Persistent and disabling low back pain

The summary of evidence on efficacy is shown in Table 7. Again it is focused on relatively short-term questions of efficacy. The difficult question is how to relate this to the severity of the sub-categorizing. Most trials have taken place in long-term patients; the maximum efficacy might be achieved in patients who have accumulated, for example, six weeks of low back pain. This is addressed in the 'models of care' section. The cost-effectiveness column reflects this uncertainty: most of the interventions, if applied to all those with a total of 12 weeks or more of pain in a year, would have to prevent long-term or recurrent problems to be cost-effective.

---

[a] The system of grading evidence and strength of recommendation is common to all the reports in this series and is explained in the introduction to *Health Care Needs Assessment Volume 1*. Edited by A Stevens and J Raftery (1994). In summary:

Quality of evidence

I	at least one properly randomized controlled trial
II-1	well-designed controlled trials without randomization
II-2	well-designed cohort or case controlled analytic studies
II-3	multiple timed series with or without the intervention
III	opinion of respected authorities based on clinical experience etc.
IV	inadequate owing to problems of methodology.

Strength of recommendation

A	good evidence for acceptance
B	fair evidence for acceptance
C	poor evidence for acceptance
D	good evidence for rejection.

Table 6: Efficacy table: new and recurrent episodes

	Quality of evidence	Recommendation	Cost-effectiveness
Use of the pragmatic classification by GPs	III	B	Possible
Information and educational leaflets	I	A	Yes
Encourage normal activity within pain	I	A	Yes
Simple analgesia or cheapest nonsteroidals[a]	I	A	Possible
Single manipulation or mobilization	I	B	Possible
Cognitive–behavioural approaches	I	B	No[b]
Specific back exercise regimens	I	C	X
'Back schools'	I	C	X
Orthoses	II-1	C	X
Bed rest (excluding root pain)	I	D	X
Non-surgical hospitalization	I	D	X
TENS; ultrasound; laser therapy	I	D	X
Plain lumbar radiography in non-specific low back pain	II-2	D	X
Other imaging for non-specific low back pain	II-2	D	X
Injection therapy	II-1	C	X

All treatments assume that the GP has classified the episode as non-specific.

[a] The implication of this restriction is that blanket use of expensive nonsteroidals or of combined analgesia would not be cost-effective. However prescribing for pain is a complex issue and clearly there will be individuals who will benefit – but that statement applies to all the other therapies listed. In population terms there is no strong evidence in favour of one type of analgesic.

[b] This is a problem of process. Behavioural therapy has worked in some trials. The uncertainty is how best to put this into practice in an efficacious and cost-effective way. It could be taken as part of the primary care or physical therapy 'package', but this has yet to be tested in trials set in primary care.

Table 7: Efficacy tables: low back pain persisting for 12 weeks or more

Fitness programmes, supervised by physical therapist:		Quality of evidence	Recommend-ation	Cost-effectiveness
	group	I	A	Yes
	individual	I	B	Possible
'Back school':				
	community	I	C	X
	workplace	I	B	Possible
Multi-disciplinary rehabilitation including psychological treatments		I	B	Possible
Manipulation		I	C	No
Surgery for non-specific low back pain		III	D	X
Disc surgery for persistent sciatica with accompanying clinical evidence of nerve root compression		I	A	Yes

8 Models of care and their consequences

Introduction

In this section some alternative models of care will be considered on the basis that the current situation reflects a probable mismatch of needs and management. The main proposal will examine the consequences if more active early therapy was offered and was made available to the community in general and not only to those who visit the GP. Less radical options will also be explored.

Model I: Shift in emphasis from the search for a diagnosis to active treatment of episodes and to secondary prevention of recurrence and persistence

Diagnosis

Early in an episode

For this we will assume that the number of people in the population who delay seeking health care, when the need is for urgent diagnosis, is very small. Evidence from surveys of patients attending osteopaths and chiropracters suggest that most of them have already consulted their GP.

The proposed model of care assumes that the need for early referral for imaging or further assessment can be restricted to:

- patients with clear clinical indications that systemic disease is a possible diagnosis
- patients in whom neurological signs of cord compression are progressive.

There appears to be no rationale for plain lumbar radiography as a 'screening' procedure for patients in whom there are no clinical indications of a serious diagnosis ('red flags' in the terminology of the CSAG report).

The estimated requirement for lumbar films for diagnosis in one year would be one per 1000 primary care attenders with low back pain, i.e. ten patients in a population of 100 000 adults. This however ignores the function of the X-ray as reassurance and the question of whether more positive approaches to therapy might provide alternative reassurance – an urgent topic for research.

The estimated requirement for urgent referral for investigation of progressive neurological impairment in one year is one per 2000 attenders with low back pain. This will underestimate all such referrals because a number will occur in patients who do not present with low back pain.

Later in an episode

Apart from small numbers of subjects for whom investigation of persistent low back pain is indicated (suspicion of inflammatory disease such as ankylosing spondylitis, or of osteoporosis in the elderly) the main epidemiological question is: how many patients with radicular pain suggestive of a prolapsed disc (and to a limited extent, spinal stenosis) require referral to an orthopaedic or neurosurgeon for diagnosis and assessment of need for operation?

The number of patients in primary care who present with persisting radicular pain needing further assessment is estimated at 200 per 100 000 adult population per year. At present 800 low back referrals are seen in specialist outpatients, the vast majority by surgeons, most of whom are not followed up.

The conclusion from this is that the need to assess patients for possible surgical intervention is probably being met. The lack of evidence for the efficacy of many surgical procedures other than conventional disc surgery and laminectomy (and possibly fusion) for spinal stenosis suggests that the use of these should remain restricted and the subject of research on carefully selected patients.

The crucial point is that specialists see many patients at present in whom there is no indication of a need for a diagnosis or for specialist involvement in their management. This is presumably why 70% are not followed up.

There is evidence to support investment in measures designed to organize referrals to hospital back pain services and specialists. One example, practical and popular with patients,[106] is to institute a gate-keeper for hospital referrals: in one study a physiotherapist[106] and in another a trained nurse practitioner.[107] Waiting lists were reduced and services used appropriately. Such measures should only be needed in the short term if referrals are ultimately reduced by adequate community management. They should therefore prove neutral in cost terms, but they do depend on a strong multi-disciplinary service in support and this may require additional investment.

Early symptomatic care

The CSAG report has drawn attention to the need to provide a service for immediate treatment of very severe pain.[8] There are no epidemiological data on which to base an estimate of the need for such a service, but numbers are likely to be low.

Otherwise there are three broad issues.

Improvement in care

Could there be improvements in the care of patients who present in primary care with new episodes or exacerbations of low back pain and who will recover within six weeks regardless of the type of intervention?

The answer is a cautious 'yes'. Putting the evidence of efficacy beside the picture of current treatment suggests that the following changes could have an impact on the length and costs of the episode:

- reduce bed rest to a minimum, unless there is true radicular pain
- encourage activity and an early return to work
- choose simple analgesia
- early manipulation or mobilization procedure from a trained therapist as a single or short-term programme.

Early treatment changes

Much more important is the question, unanswerable at present, as to whether changes in early treatment would:

- prevent recurrence of pain and disability in those whose immediate problems settle in the short term
- prevent the persistence of symptoms and disability in patients whose low back pain is not going to recover spontaneously within six weeks.

The issue is whether early treatment would carry the bonus of secondary prevention by altering the long-term course of low back pain and thereby reducing the prevalence of low back pain.

There is some evidence from the review of efficacy for such an effect from the following interventions:

- information: ensuring that all patients consulting in primary care have adequate access to information and explanation about low back pain and that fears about the consequences of the symptom are addressed
- manipulation and mobilization: very limited evidence suggests that there may be longer term benefits from early manipulation–mobilization
- exercises taught under supervision for the patient to continue at home: the evidence from studies in patients whose pain has become persistent is hopeful that this may have an effect beyond immediate relief of symptoms
- involvement of the workplace: the apparent efficacy in some trials of physical therapy and back school interventions which involved visits to the workplace suggest added benefit when the intervention is linked with early return to suitable work and liaison with occupational health service
- early use of psychological approaches.

The model would require a reorientation of haphazard services into a true community back pain service in which primary care, hospitals and the private sector were all involved. The purpose would be to make early physical therapy and education available for primary care consulters; the implication is that the need for diagnostic referrals would be lowered and streamlined and that the delivery of therapy (physical and psychological) would be standardized within certain limits, notably the number of treatment sessions.

The CSAG suggests that this type of intervention be considered if the primary care attender has persistent problems after two weeks. The delay is to allow for the expected improvement in many patients and thus to act as a 'sieve' for further referral. The conundrum however is that already by the time of their first consultation in an episode, the length of time since the onset of the episode is already a key predictor of early outcome. Also for many attenders the precise onset will not be clear: the background will be of vague exacerbation.

Implications

Assume that early physical therapy which emphasized a 'positive' approach to low back problems was offered to all people who experience more than four weeks of moderate or disabling low back pain during a 12 month period, excluding those with long-term persistent pain. From the prevalence figures this would be some 5% of the adult population. In a population of 100 000 adults this would mean 5000 requests in one year. This is not too far from the current total of new physical therapy referrals for a population of this size (4700, see page 149).

However this ignores:

- the figure for physical therapists' current workload includes a majority of patients who are currently seen outside the health service
- the demand for such a service from those who have shorter periods in pain.

But it does include people who at present do not attend their GP with the pain.

This model might therefore mean the purchase of more new patient contacts with physical therapists. Against this can be balanced the following points:

- traditional physiotherapy for low back pain tends to have a high number of treatment sessions per patient. The evidence from randomized controlled trials suggests that the emphasis in the early treatment should be on short treatment courses with manipulation and mobilization, education and training in exercises and active rehabilitation with a positive approach, away from the emphasis on machinery and technology. The cost of the increased throughput of patients and additional therapists could be balanced by a reduction in numbers of sessions per patient.
- the unknown potential of such a service for secondary prevention – the crucial question in the longer term.

Care of prevalent problems: persistent disabling low back pain

The previous section viewed low back pain as an 'episodic' phenomenon, regardless of the background time-course of any one individual's episode. However there is also the patient with a more persistent history of low back pain, perhaps already treated in multiple ways, including operations.

The review of efficacy of controlled trials of management approaches to the chronic low back pain patient suggested that, although complete recovery is not the norm, short-term improvement certainly appears to be. As with interventions in 'episodes' there is no good evidence of a long-term effect and so the potential impact of rehabilitation programmes on the prevalence of chronic low back pain is difficult to gauge.

The CSAG recommends multi-disciplinary rehabilitation for patients with low back pain which persists for three months or longer. This is a crucial aspect of this model of care. Resources cannot suddenly be shifted to early low back pain management in the community, without at the same time ensuring an adequate service for those who do emerge with more persistent problems.

The estimate of the need for such a service in an adult population of 100 000 would be as many as 10 000 patients in a year. However if only patients with severe disability were included, the number would be 5000. Furthermore 3000 of these represent a long-term pool, some of whom would already have received such treatments. The rising numbers of those receiving long-term invalidity suggest that this prevalence pool may now be losing fewer than it gains each year, so demands on a rehabilitation service may well increase each year.

On present evidence it is likely that this 'prevalence pool' would continue to make demands on any dedicated service of rehabilitation for low back sufferers.

Balanced against the increased costs of providing such a service are the following:

- much health care expenditure goes on this group anyway: among patients attending as 'new' referrals to a hospital with a tertiary referral centre for back problems, 90% had experienced more than three months of low back pain during the 12 months prior to the outpatient visit
- the enormous costs of sickness and invalidity benefit. There is randomized controlled trial evidence to suggest that a dedicated back pain service could reduce the numbers of working days lost, although the pragmatic question of whether this could be achieved in the current employment climate has not been answered.

Model II: Evidence for secondary prevention is limited: services should be concentrated on those at high risk for persistent problems

This assumes arguments from the first model apply about a) reducing the emphasis on diagnosis and b) the need for an integrated service for those with longer term disability from low back pain.

However the approach in the second model would be that there is no good evidence that anything other than simple pain relief can alter the natural history of episodic low back pain. No resources therefore, other than encouragement to self-care and reassurance and information from the GP are required.

Can individuals be identified who are at unusually high risk that their back pain will not settle in the short term or will recur at an early stage? A whole body of research work now points to psychosocial distress, illness behaviour and pain cognitions as major influences on the course of low back pain.[28,29] However there is no available evidence on the therapeutic implications of this to make a judgement on how it could contribute to the provision of health care. There are a number of possibilities:

Psychological treatments for low back pain

Some of the randomized controlled trial evidence supports the incorporation of cognitive and behavioural therapies into multi-disciplinary treatment of chronic low back pain. Unfortunately there is little evidence on which to base a model of care in which these therapies were offered to those who are distressed on first presentation with low back pain. It is clearly an area worth exploring, given the following:

- the success of non-specific 'encouragement' and group fitness programmes in recent trials suggest that the cognitive and behavioural aspects of primary care interventions and physical therapies may be critical to their superiority over 'back-centred' approaches[63,77]
- the failure of current therapies to prevent the increase in sickness absence and disability payments
- the accumulating observational evidence that psychological measures are the strongest predictors of outcome in low back pain patients consulting GPs or community physical therapists[29]
- the evidence of effectiveness of psychological approaches in patients with longstanding low back problems[90] – in these patients it is negative cognitions and illness behaviours that are being tackled and, by extrapolation, tackling them earlier on in the low back history may carry even more potential for benefit.

The other major difficulty, apart from lack of evidence of efficacy in early low back pain, is that if psychological approaches were to be generally applied earlier in low back pain, then the need to develop 'brief' intervention packages would be essential. Even if efficacy were compromised the higher volume of patients treated should prove cost-effective and carry a potential impact on the total occurrence of persistent low back problems.

Preferential treatment service

An alternative is that a service which provided a range of the measures which seem to improve symptoms in the short term (education, physical therapies, exercise programmes, and psychological approaches) should be offered preferentially to those who are distressed and depressed. This would focus the type of acute back pain service discussed previously on to those who might gain most in terms of later secondary prevention.

Despite the evidence that psychological measures are the best predictors of the course of low back pain, there is a need for evidence that selectively intervening on the basis of these measures would have an impact on low back pain occurrence and outcome.

Workplace screening

Screening for suitability for jobs does not appear to be a viable option for those who have no low back pain. Job selection as part of a rehabilitation programme for low back sufferers has more evidence to commend it.[66]

Compensation procedures

The difficult problem of compensation procedures has been extensively written about in the US and Australian literature. The influence of compensation on the total occurrence of low back pain in the UK is probably small.

Model III: The course of low back pain episodes at any point is dictated by previous experience of low back pain: reducing the incidence of 'episodic' low back pain

There is epidemiological evidence about risk factors for low back pain episodes. There is very little empirical evidence that programmes of primary prevention reduce the impact of low back pain.

In theory the following should contribute (i.e. there is observational and analytic epidemiological evidence for an association between these factors and low back pain).

Workplace

- better employment and wage opportunities
- improved job satisfaction: this incorporates both physical and psychological environments at work
- improved manual handling regulations and their application
- reduction of injury incidence
- education about back problems
- use of orthoses (such as belts) in high risk jobs.

In a review of the controlled trial evidence for prevention, the authors' conclusion was that exercise programmes in industry had some evidence to commend them, but to date untargeted programmes for education and use of orthoses had no proven value.[108]

Lifestyle

- reduction in smoking
- improved physical activity levels throughout life
- postural education, better seating, less constant driving
- specific back strengthening programmes.

To the extent that certain factors, such as smoking and physical activity, are the targets of health promotion programmes in general, then there will be potential benefits of such programmes in reducing the occurrence of low back pain. Lahad *et al.* concluded that this was indeed the main hope for primary prevention, since current evidence did not point to large benefits from prevention programmes tailored specifically to prevent low back pain.[108]

Co-morbidity

- primary prevention and treatment of depression
- improved management of common symptoms, particularly pain, throughout life.

Society

Employment opportunities, income differences, benefit systems and the cultural propensity to somatize distress all influence low back pain occurrence in a powerful way. The difficulty in assessing needs is that, as Nachemson and Waddell have emphasized,[70,89] health care has created as many of the problems of low back pain as it has solved. The politics and economics of low back pain require political and economic solutions; throwing health care at the complex problem of low back pain is unlikely to make it go away.

9 Measuring outcome

The ICIDH provides a conceptual framework for classifying a problem like back pain with respect to its clinical features and its consequences.[20]

Grading impairments

Pain in the back and other areas

An arbitrary definition of the low back is the area between the lower costal margins and the gluteal folds. This definition standardizes what is meant by low back, has appeared in many epidemiological studies and has been used in the three most recent population surveys in the UK.[1,2,36]

Location

- pain drawings using a pre-shaded low back area
- the number of sites of pain, analysed from pain drawings or from simple lists in questionnaires or interviews.

Intensity

- visual analogue, numerical rating or verbal rating scales.

Duration

- current episode if the onset can be defined
- number of days on which pain has been experienced during a defined period such as the last 12 months ('every day in the past year' may be a useful subgroup)
- period of time for recall: 'pain today' does not reflect the intermittent, fluctuating nature of low back pain, low back pain experienced during the past month or the past year appears to be the most useful definition for prevalence
- time course: acute, intermittent, persistent. (A recurrence is assumed to be a new episode in the context that pain has been experienced at some time in the previous 12 months.)

Symptoms other than pain

There are instruments available which provide scales of severity for bodily symptoms, psychological distress and dysfunctional cognitions and behaviours.[29] These are emerging as useful predictors of outcome, although their relevance as measures of the outcome of intervention is not established.

Clinical measures

Many clinical measures can be categorized or ranked to provide a grading of severity, such as Schober's test, the fingertip to floor test, lateral flexion and straight leg raising. They appear to be useful as outcome measures of spinal mobility but do not necessarily correlate with symptom measures.

Summary

Available evidence suggests that grading symptoms and signs of low back pain fails to measure all important consequences of back pain. Impairments are followed by disabilities and handicaps but do not fully predict them.

Grading back pain related disabilities and handicaps

Restriction of activities of daily living (disability) and impact on social life (handicap)

Questionnaires

Roland and Morris' scale is a short back pain specific version of the Functional Limitations Profile, a large general interview about disability.[109] It was developed in primary care and has been used in other settings and is well validated.

The Oswestry Disability Index was developed in a hospital setting, and its utility in primary care is not as well established as the Roland and Morris questionnaire.[110] However it has been used in many studies, including two important intervention trials of physical therapy among patients selected from primary care referrals.[77,83]

A short set of questions suitable for use in population surveys and with good general population figures of prevalence is to be found in the scheme developed by Walsh et al.[1]

More recently, the Aberdeen Low Back Pain Scale was published, accompanied by a comprehensive account of its methodological development.[111] Its roots are more heavily clinical and impairment-orientated than the Roland and Morris scale, but it has been validated in primary care populations. Curiously the paper made no reference to the Roland and Morris questionnaire. The latter has been the measure of choice in recent US studies and would be our recommendation, until the Aberdeen scale has been compared with it in clinical trials and follow-up studies.

Single measures

Simple quantifying measures are the number of days during a specified period:

- spent in bed
- of restricted activity attributed to low back pain.

These were used in the OPCS survey.[2]

Work loss

Days off work, days in receipt of disability pensions, or the time to work resumption have been promoted as the most meaningful end-points for low back pain. There are problems with their use, even though they are the measures which describe the so-called back pain epidemic. Application to patients who are not working anyway is difficult, whilst return to work is contaminated by other factors such as local unemployment rates.

However in terms of public policy and the overall impact of back pain on society, many commentators regard this as by far the most important way to classify back pain (see the CSAG Annex for example). In addition it is an attempt to measure handicap directly. This contrasts with the restriction of daily activity questionnaires where the actual impact on the individual's life is not necessarily measured. For needs assessment in the general population however it is problematic to use work loss as the main measure of impact or severity.

Composite grading schemes

The Pain Grade of von Korff and colleagues combines pain intensity, disability score and disability days.[39] The authors demonstrate its association with 12-month outcome in a series of back pain patients who had presented in US primary care, although the information was gathered by telephone. Kohlmann et al. in Germany have similarly combined elements of disability and pain intensity in a general population sample and shown this to predict subsequent outcome.[112] Such a grading shows potential as a measure of outcome of health care, although it has not been put to the test in this form yet.

The Distress and Risk Assessment Method[29] provides a four-point classification of the psychological distress associated with low back pain (normal, at risk, distressed depressive, distressed somatic) based on two scales which quantify emotional factors and the extent of awareness of bodily symptoms other than pain (the Modified Zung Depression Index and the Modified Somatic Perception Questionnaire). In preliminary studies of patients presenting to osteopaths and in primary care, this was a strong predictor of outcome. As with other psychological measures, its exact place as a measure of outcome of treatment of low back pain is not clear and needs to be established.

An alternative to these specific schemes is to use validated measures of general functional status; the SF 36[111] and Nottingham Health Profile[113] are the two most popular examples. They are not specific for back pain but have been used in back pain research.

In general more empirical data are needed for many of these instruments with respect to their population-based distribution, their application in selecting individuals for specific treatments and their use as relevant measures of the outcome of health care.

Health care consumption

Utilization of health care appears as a category in some low back pain classifications. The Quebec Task Force scheme,[111] for example, includes surgery to the back as a classifying feature.

Attendance in primary care and referral to secondary and tertiary care (imaging, surgery, complementary medicine, physiotherapy, psychological intervention, comprehensive pain treatment) have been used to measure outcome of back pain episodes, as well as being measures of health care provision and demand among back pain sufferers.

Patient satisfaction with health care

Methods for measuring this in low back pain patients appear to be in their infancy, although a number of studies of back pain treatments have used a scale derived from a general questionnaire about satisfaction with treatment.[115–117]

Summary

The best way to summarize the low back pain experience and to measure outcome is by quantifying the following.

- **Impairment** Pain severity and total days in pain during a specified time period
- **Disability and handicap** Restriction of daily activity and for some purposes, days off work.

10 Targets

Potential outcome targets abound in the field of low back pain. Two examples are:

- to slow and reverse the exponential rise in number of working days lost
- to reduce the period prevalence of severely disabling, persistent low back trouble in the population.

The problem with these targets is that it is not known whether the effective treatments discussed previously would actually influence them (given, for example, the employment situation, or the nature of long-term disability).

It seems to be more practical to take some process measures as the targets, so that the extent to which the results of randomized controlled trials are actually put into practice can be judged. The nature of their impact on the period prevalence of low back pain, in particular severely disabling and persistent pain, and on work loss and benefit payments could be measured subsequently.

Proposed targets

- In any one year, for a brief physical therapy, education, exercise and cognitive–behavioural 'package' to be available for all people who develop moderate or severely disabling low back pain of more than four weeks duration.
- Single manipulation or mobilization available for general practice attenders with a new or recurrent episode.
- Provision of a hospital-based back pain service which can support the introduction of the CSAG 'diagnostic triage' approach in primary care. This would incorporate adequate urgent specialist availability and offer a multi-disciplinary course of rehabilitation to all patients in the community who have had severely disabling low back pain of more than three months duration. A supplementary short-term target would be the appointment of an appropriate person to co-ordinate the response to referrals to such a service.

The costs of these targets should theoretically be kept close to current costs if there are concomitant targets for reduction of services and interventions.

Proposed targets for reduction

- Lengthy courses of physical therapy and the use of technology in physical therapy departments.
- Expensive analgesia.
- The numbers of outpatient attendances and non-surgical inpatient admissions.
- The number of diagnostic investigations in the absence of clear clinical indications.
- A limitation on further growth in surgical operation rates would seem desirable in the face of limited evidence that high rates in the US have reduced disability or that new techniques are achieving anything. This must take account of the need to support good trials of promising treatments where evidence is lacking (to avoid the assumption that 'no evidence' is equivalent to 'evidence of no efficacy').

11 Information

Local

There are two main areas where easily available local information would greatly enhance the needs assessment exercise.

First reliable outpatient data, which can be related to GP referral, would include the specialist's diagnosis and management plan, and would link to A and E, radiology, physiotherapy, day case admissions and inpatients. Many areas are moving towards this type of information system. In particular the use by GPs of computers for morbidity recording should enable links with outpatient records systems to be initiated and for demands to be made on consultants to participate in morbidity recording also.

The reason for this is that a condition such as low back pain is a classically difficult problem to pin down – it does not cause many people to die, inpatient admissions are a very small proportion of the problem, many different parts of the health care system are likely to be involved and mapping the health care being provided in a district is like hunting the haystack needle.

The second point is related. The full range of community therapy which is available for back pain sufferers and the throughput of their patients should be known at a local level. This would include not only the orthodox services, such as community physiotherapy, occupational therapy and social services, but alternatives as well. Such is the popularity of alternative treatments that information about them should be available at a local level. In particular the regional availability of osteopathy and chiropractic, in the light of their now official status, would be helpful information. There seems to be no reason why such practitioners should not also be involved in local morbidity returns.

National

Once good systems of outpatient record linkage are in place they should be co-ordinated nationally in order to compare referral rates between regions. Again it is important that information on the context of regional variations should be available. To this end national registers of practitioners offering back pain treatment will be a useful addition; sentinel practitioners (physiotherapists, chiropractors, osteopaths) who took part in periodic morbidity recording would be worthwhile supporting.

A major national contribution should be through surveys, such as the one carried out by OPCS, [2] and this is addressed in the research section. In particular we need more detailed information on the health care provided by different sectors: what physiotherapists are actually doing around the country for low back pain patients for example; how many GPs can manipulate spines and how many would want to; what patient groups are being seen by psychologists.

12 Research priorities

The main priorities with respect to needs assessment research are:

- Population-based prevalence studies which assess disability levels, pain severity and total days in pain, using explicit measures. This chapter has discussed studies that were not designed to measure need and the figures in the tables need to be given more substance. There is no purpose in doing further studies of how much back pain there is in any local community – there is sufficient agreement on this. It is the subgroups which need more investigation – nationally and in smaller scale local studies.
- There is a need to combine such traditional quantitative surveys with in-depth qualitative interviewing of subjects from within the subgroups to establish the patient's perspective on need. The data on patient satisfaction suggests that hospital attenders in particular are a dissatisfied group, reflecting perhaps the mismatch of care and need which is apparent even from currently available data. This needs more investigation in relation to available care and current levels of pain and disability.

Pragmatic trials are also required, particularly primary care based interventions which examine the potential for using the principles of cognitive–behavioural therapy and brief physical therapy to produce generalizable treatment packages. Ideally these should be large and long term to address the crucial issue of secondary prevention of recurrence and persistence.

Appendix I Note on source materials

During writing, two systematic and thorough overviews of the evidence concerning treatment appeared[118] or were about to appear.[119] The view of the evidence presented here is based on a mixture of original articles and published reviews of individual topics and has not used the new overviews directly. The interested reader should consult both these publications for a more detailed review of all published evidence.

Some items from the United States Agency for Health Care Policy and Research (AHCPR) review[118] were available in the form that they were presented as evidence for the British Clinical Standards Advisory Group on Back Pain, and in this form have been used here.

Another useful publication *The costs of low back pain* from the University of York Health Economics Group has been published,[120] which updates and expands the analysis in the Annex to the CSAG Report. It is the CSAG version which has been used here.

The CSAG evidence summaries (which in turn reflected the AHCPR work) have been broadly adhered to in order to preserve some consistency, but overviews of specific topics and new trial evidence which appeared in the literature 1994–95 have been added. The interpretation and rating of the evidence referenced here is the author's responsibility alone.

Finally this needs assessment was not based on the formal system of systematic reviewing which is the hallmark of the Cochrane Collaboration. There is an obvious need in the field of low back pain for such collaborative reviewing of new evidence. The greatest need however is for a better supply of evidence.

References

1 Walsh K, Cruddas M, Coggon D. Low back pain in eight areas of Britain. *J Epid Comm Hlth* 1992; **46**: 227–30.

2 Mason V. *The prevalence of back pain in Great Britain*. Office of Population Censuses and Surveys. Social Survey Division. London: HMSO, 1994.

3 Deyo RA. Practice variations, treatment fads, rising disability. *Spine* 1993; **18**: 2153–62.

4 Bogduk N. The sources of low back pain. In *The Lumbar Spine and Back Pain* (ed. MIV Jayson). Edinburgh: Churchill Livingstone, 1992.

5 Wall PD. *Textbook of pain* (eds R Melzack, PD Wall). 3rd edn. Edinburgh: Churchill Livingstone, 1994

6 Jayson MIV. The problem of backache. *Practitioner* 1970; **205**: 615–21.

7 Waddell G. An approach to backache. *Br J Hos Med* 1982; **28**: 187–219.

8 Clinical Standards Advisory Group on Back Pain. *Back pain*. London: HMSO, 1994.

9 Deyo RA, Bass JE. Lifestyle and low back pain. The influence of smoking and obesity. *Spine* 1989; **14**: 501–6.

10 Heliovaara M, Makela M, Knekt P *et al*. Determinants of sciatica and low back pain. *Spine* 1991; **16**: 608–14.

11 Magni G, Caldieron C, Rigatti-Luchini S *et al*. Chronic musculoskeletal pain and depressive symptoms in the general population. An analysis of the first National Health and Nutrition Examination Survey data. *Pain* 1990; **43**: 299–307.

12 Leino PI, Hanninen V. Psychosocial factors at work in relation to back and limb disorders. *Scand J Work Environ Health* 1995; **21**: 134–42.

13 Waddell G. A new clinical model for the treatment of low back pain. *Spine* 1987; **12**: 632–44.

14 Fairbank JCT, Pynsent PB. Syndromes of back pain and their classification. In *The Lumbar Spine and Back Pain* (ed. MIV Jayson). Edinburgh: Churchill Livingstone, 1992.

15 Barker ME. A practical classification of spinal pains. In *Back pain: classification of syndromes* (eds PB Pynsent, JCT Fairbank). Manchester: Manchester University Press, 1990.

16 Raspe H. Back pain. In *Epidemiology of the Rheumatic Diseases* (eds AJ Silman, MC Hochberg). Oxford: Oxford University Press, 1993.

17 Dworkin SF, Von Korff M, LeResche L. Multiple pains and psychiatric disturbance. *Arch Gen Psych* 1990; **47**: 239–44.

18 Von Korff M, Ormel J, Keefe F *et al*. Grading the severity of chronic pain. *Pain* 1992; **50**: 133–49.

19 Clinical Standards Advisory Group on Back Pain. *Back pain: epidemiology and costs*. London: HMSO, 1994.

20 World Health Organization. *International classification of impairments, disabilities and handicaps*. Geneva: WHO, 1980.

21 Croft P, Papageorgiou A *et al*. *Report to the Clinical Standards Advisory Group on Back Pain*. ARC Epidemiology Research Unit, University of Manchester, 1994.

22 McCormick A, Fleming D, Charlton J. Morbidity statistics from general practice. Fourth national study 1991–1992. Office of Population Censuses and Surveys. *Series MB5 No. 3*. London: HMSO, 1995.

23 Maxwell RJ. The osteopaths' bill. *BMJ* 1993; **306**: 1556–7.

24 Eisenberg DM, Kessler RC, Foster C *et al*. Unconventional medicine in the United States. *NEJM* 1993; **328**: 246–52.

25 Ernst E. Complementary therapies: Working paper for NHS group on primary and community care. Unpublished draft.

26 Bamji AN, Dieppe PA, Haslock DI *et al*. What do rheumatologists do? A pilot audit study. *Br J Rheumatol* 1990; **29**: 295.

27 Royal College of Radiologists Working Party. A multicentre audit of hospital referral for radiological investigation in England and Wales. *BMJ* 1991; **303**: 809–12.

28 Nordin M, Vischer TL (eds). Common low back pain: prevention of chronicity. *Bailliere's Clinical Rheum* 1992; **6**.

29 Main CJ, Wood PLR, Hollis S *et al.* The distress risk and assessment method. *Spine* 1991; **17**: 42–52.

30 Personal communication from Health and Safety Executive, Bootle, 1994.

31 Deyo RA, Rainville J, Kent DL. What can the history and examination tell us about low back pain? *JAMA* 1992; **268**: 760–5.

32 Katz JN. The assessment and management of low back pain: a critical review. *Arthr Care Res* 1993; **6**: 104–14.

33 Virta L, Ronnemaa T. The association of mild-moderate isthmic lumbar spondylolisthesis and low back pain in middle-aged patients is weak and it only occurs in women. *Spine* 1993; **18**: 1496–503.

34 Lawrence JS. Disc degeneration: its frequency and relationship to symptoms. *Ann Rheum Dis* 1969; **28**: 121–37.

35 Biering-Sorensen F. Low back trouble in a general population of 30 to 60 year old men and women. *Danish Med Bull* 1982; **29**: 289–99.

36 Papageorgiou A, Croft P, Ferry S *et al.* Estimating the prevalence of low back pain in the general population. South Manchester Low Back Pain Survey. *Spine* 1995; **20(17)**: 1889–94.

37 Roland MO, Morrell DC, Morris RW. Can general practitioners predict the outcome of episodes of back pain? *BMJ* 1983; **286**: 523–5.

38 Coste J, Delecoeuillerie G, Cohen de Lara A *et al.* Clinical course and prognostic factors in acute low back pain: an inception cohort study in primary care practice. *BMJ* 1994; **308**: 577–80.

39 von Korff M, Deyo RA, Cherkin D *et al.* Back pain in primary care: outcomes at 1 year. *Spine* 1993; **18**: 855–62.

40 Raspe H, Kohlmann T, Deck R. Back pain as a chronic systemic disorder: results of two population surveys (abstract). *Arth Rheum* 1993; **(suppl.)**: S234.

41 Skovron ML, Szpalski M, Nordin M *et al.* Sociocultural factors and back pain. *Spine* 1994; **19**: 129–37.

42 Walsh K, Coggon D. Reproducibility of histories of low back pain obtained by self-administered questionnaire. *Spine* 1991; **16**: 1075–7.

43 Halpin SFS, Yeoman L, Dundas DD. Radiographic examination of the lumbar spine in a community hospital: an audit of current practice. *BMJ* 1991; **303**: 813–5.

44 Rigby AS. Ankylosing spondylitis. In *Epidemiology of the Rheumatic Diseases* (eds AJ Silman, MC Hochberg). Oxford: Oxford University Press, 1993.

45 Deyo RA, Tsui-Wu YJ. Descriptive epidemiology of low back pain and its related medical care in the United States. *Spine* 1987; **12**: 264–8.

46 Heliovaara M, Impivaara O, Sievers K *et al.* Lumbar disc syndrome in Finland. *J Epidemiol Comm Hlth* 1987; **41**: 251–8.

47 Waddell G, Main CJ, Morris EW *et al.* Normality and reliability in the clinical assessment of backache. *BMJ* 1982; **284**: 1519–23.

48 Svensson HO *et al.* A retrospective study of low back pain in women. *Spine* 1988; **13**: 548–52.

49 Hart LG, Deyo RA, Cherkin D. Physician office visits for low back pain. *Spine* 1995; **20**: 11–19.

50 Shapley M. Unpublished audit of low back pain in fund-holding practice. Personal communication, 1994.

51 Fitton F, Temple B, Acheson HWK. The cost of prescribing in general practice. *Soc Sci Med.* 1985; **21**: 1097–105.

52 Basmajian JV. Acute back pain and spasm. A controlled multicenter trial. *Spine* 1989; **14**: 438–9.

53 Gillies JH, Breen A, Ellis RM *et al.* Disability from back pain among four groups: a working population and patients attending chiropractic, osteopathy and rheumatology clinics. *Phys Med Rehab* 1993; **3**: 74–8.

54 Pedersen P. A survey of chiropractic practice in Europe. *Eur J Chiropractic* 1994; **42**: 1.

55 Carey TS, Garrett J, Jackman A *et al*. North Carolina Back Pain Project. Outcomes and costs of care for acute low back pain. *New England J Med* 1995; **333(14)**: 913–17.

56 Weber H. Lumbar disc herniation. A controlled trial with ten years of observation. *Spine* 1983; **8**: 131–40.

57 Cherkin DC, Deyo RA, Loeser JD *et al*. An international comparison of back surgery rates. *Spine* 1994; **19**: 1201–6.

58 Bunt K. Occupational Health Provision at Work. *Health and Safety Executive Report 57/1993*. London: HMSO, 1993.

59 Koes BW, Bouter LM, van der Heijden GJMG. Methodological quality of randomised clinical trials on treatment efficacy in low back pain. *Spine* 1995; **20**: 228–35.

60 Kepes ER, Duncalf D. Treatment of backache with spinal injections of local anaesthetics, spinal and systemic steroids. A review. *Pain* 1985; **22**: 33–47.

61 Roland M, Dixon M. Randomised controlled trial of an educational booklet for patients presenting with back pain in general practice. *J Royal Coll Gen Prac* 1989; **39**: 244–6.

62 Faas A, Chavannes AW, van Eijk JTM *et al*. A randomised placebo-controlled trial of exercise therapy in patients with acute low back pain. *Spine* 1993; **18**: 1388–95.

63 Malmivaara A, Hakkinen U, Aro T *et al*. The treatment of acute low back pain — bed rest, exercises, or ordinary activity? *New England J Med* 1995; **332(6)**: 351–5.

64 Nordin M, Cedraschi C, Balague F *et al*. Back schools in prevention of chronicity. *Bailliere's Clinical Rheum* 1992; **6**: 685–704.

65 Koes BW, van Tulder MW, van der Windt DAWM *et al*. The efficacy of back schools: a review of randomised clinical trials. *J Clin Epidemiol* 1994; **47**: 851–62.

66 Cohen JE, Goel V, Frank JW *et al*. Group education interventions for people with low back pain. An overview of the literature. *Spine* 1994; **19(11)**: 1214–22.

67 Gundewall B, Liljeqvist M, Hansson T. Primary prevention of back symptoms and absence from work. *Spine* 1993; **18**: 587–94.

68 Amlie E, Weber H, Holme I. Treatment of acute low back pain with piroxicam : results of a double-blind placebo-controlled trial. *Spine* 1987; **12**: 473–6.

69 Carette S, Marcoux S, Truchon R *et al*. A controlled trial of corticosteroid injections into facet joints for chronic low back pain. *NEJM* 1991; **325**: 1002–7.

70 Nachemson A. Newest knowledge of low back pain. *Clin Orth* 1992; **279**: 3–8.

71 Gilbert JR, Taylor DW, Hildebrand A *et al*. Clinical trial of common treatments for low back pain in family practice. *BMJ* 1985; **291**: 791–4.

72 Deyo RA, Diehl AK, Rosenthal M. How many days of bed rest for acute low back pain? A randomised clinical trial. *NEJM* 1986; **315**: 1064–70.

73 Koes BW, Bouter LM, Beckerman H *et al*. Physiotherapy exercises and back pain: a blinded review. *BMJ* 1991; **302**: 1572–6.

74 Deyo RA, Walsh NE, Martin DC *et al*. A controlled trial of transcutaneous electrical nerve stimulation (TENS) and exercise for chronic low back pain. *New Engl J Med* 1990; **322**: 1627–34.

75 Lindstrom I, Ohlund C, Eek C *et al*. Mobility, strength and fitness after a graded activity program for patients with subacute low back pain. *Spine* 1992; **17**: 641–9.

76 Alaranta H, Rytokoski U, Rissanen A *et al*. Intensive physical and psychosocial training program for patients with chronic low back pain. A controlled clinical trial. *Spine* 1994; **19**: 1339–49

77 Frost H, Klaber Moffett JA, Moser JS *et al*. Randomised controlled trial for evaluation of fitness programme for patients with chronic low back pain. *BMJ* 1995; **310**: 151–4.

78 Koes BW, Assendelft WJJ, van der Heijden GJMG *et al*. Spinal manipulation and mobilisation for back and neck pain: a blinded review. *BMJ* 1991; **303**: 1298–303.

79 Shekelle PG, Adams AH, Chassin MR *et al.* Spinal manipulation for low back pain. *Ann Int Med* 1992; **117**: 590–8.

80 Hadler NM, Curtis P, Gillings DB *et al.* A benefit of spinal manipulation as adjunctive therapy for acute low back pain: a stratified controlled trial. *Spine* 1987; **12**: 702–6.

81 Meade TW, Dyer S, Browne W *et al.* Low back pain of mechanical origin: randomised comparison of chiropractic and hospital outpatient treatment. *BMJ* 1990; **300**: 1431–7.

82 Meade TW, Dyer S, Browne W *et al.* Randomised comparison of chiropractic and hospital outpatient management for low back pain: results from extended follow up. *BMJ* 1995; **311**: 349–51.

83 Powell FC, Hanigan WC, Olivero WC. A risk/benefit analysis of spinal manipulation therapy for relief of lumbar or cervical pain. *Neurosurg* 1993; **33**: 73–8.

84 Marchand S, Charest J, Li J *et al.* Is TENS purely a placebo effect? A contolled study on chronic low back pain. *Pain* 1993; **54**: 99–106.

85 Herman E, Williams R, Stratford P *et al.* A randomised controlled trial of transcutaneous electrical nerve stimulation (CODETRON) to determine its benefits in a rehabilitation program for acute occupational low back pain. *Spine* 1994; **19(5)**: 561–8.

86 Weiser S, Cedraschi C. Psychosocial issues in the prevention of chronic low back pain – a literature review. *Bailliere's Clinical Rheum* 1992; **6**: 657–84.

87 Troup JDG, Videman T. Inactivity and the aetiogenesis of musculoskeletal disorders. *Clin Biomech* 1989; **4**: 173–8.

88 Klenerman L, Slade PD, Stanley IM *et al.* The prediction of chronicity in patients with an acute attack of low back pain in a general practice setting. *Spine* 1995; **20(4)**: 478–84.

89 Waddell G. Biopsychosocial analysis of low back pain. *Bailliere's Clinical Rheum* 1992; **6**: 523–58.

90 Lanes TC, Gauron EF, Spratt KF *et al.* Long-term follow-up of patients with chronic back pain treated in a multidisciplinary rehabilitation program. *Spine* 1995; **20(7)**: 801–6.

91 Fordyce WE, Fowler RS, Lehman JF *et al.* Operant conditioning in the treatment of chronic pain. *Arch Phys Med Rehab* 1973; **54**: 399–408.

92 Turner JA, Romano JM. Cognitive-behavioural therapy. In *The management of pain* (ed. J Bonica). Philadelphia: Lea and Febiger, 1990.

93 Fordyce WE, Brockway JA, Bergman JA *et al.* Acute back pain: a control-group comparison of behavioural vs traditional management methods. *J Behavioural Med* 1986; **9**: 127–40.

94 Symonds TL, Burton AK, Tillotson KM *et al.* Absence resulting from low back pain trouble can be reduced by psycho-social intervention at the workplace. *Spine* 1995; **20(24)**: 2738–45.

95 Quintet RJ, Hadler NM. Diagnosis and treatment of back pain. *Semin Arth Rheum* 1979; **8**: 261–87.

96 Deyo RA. Magnetic resonance imaging of the spine. Editorial. *N Engl J Med* 1994; **331**: 115–16.

97 Jensen MC, Brant-Zawadske MN, Obuchowski N *et al.* Magnetic Resonance imaging of the lumbar spine in people without back pain. *NEJM* 1994; **331**: 69–73.

98 Taylor VM, Deyo RA, Cherkin DC *et al.* Low back pain hospitalisation. Recent United States trends and regional variations. *Spine* 1994; **19**: 1207–12.

99 Hoffman RM, Wheeler KJ, Deyo RA. Surgery for herniated lumbar discs: A literature synthesis. *J Gen Int Med* 1993; **8**: 487–96.

100 Muralikuttan KP, Hamilton A, Kernohan WG *et al.* A prospective randomised trial of chemonucleolysis and conventional disc surgery in single level lumbar disc herniation. *Spine.* 1992; **17**: 381–7.

101 Ciol MA, Deyo RA, Kreuter W *et al.* Characteristics in Medicare beneficiaries associated with reoperation after lumbar spine surgery. *Spine* 1994; **19(12)**: 1329–34.

102 Turner JA, Ersek M, Herron L *et al.* Surgery for lumbar spinal stenosis. Attempted meta-analysis of the literature. *Spine* 1992; **17(1)**: 1–8.

103 Turner JA, Ersek M, Herron L *et al.* Patient outcomes after lumbar spinal fusion. *JAMA* 1992, **268**: 907–11.

104 Weber H. Traction therapy in sciatica due to disc prolapse. *J Oslo City Hosp* 1973; **23**: 167–76.

105 Weber H, Ljunggren AE, Walker L. Traction therapy in patients with herniated lumbar intervertebral discs. *J Oslo City Hosp* 1984; **34**: 61–70.

106 Hockin J, Bannister G. The extended role of a physiotherapist in an outpatient orthopaedic clinic. *Physio* 1994; **80**: 281–4.

107 Murray MM, Greenough CG. *Implementation of a nurse-led spinal assessment clinic.* Abstract presented to European Spine Society. 6th Annual Meeting. Netherlands, 1995.

108 Lahad A, Malter AD, Berg AO *et al.* The effectiveness of four interventions for the prevention of low back pain. *JAMA* 1994; **272**: 1286–91.

109 Roland M, Morris R. A study of the natural history of back pain: Part 1: Development of a reliable and sensitive measure of disability in low back pain. *Spine* 1983; **8**: 141–4.

110 Fairbank JCT, Davies J, Coupar J *et al.* The Oswestry low back pain disability questionnaire. *Physio* 1980; **66**: 271–3.

111 Ruta DA, Garratt AM, Wardlaw D *et al.* Developing a valid and reliable measure of health outcome for patients with low back pain. *Spine* 1994; **19**: 1887–96.

112 Kohlmann T, Deck R, Raspe H. Prävalenz und Schweregrad von Rückenschmerzen in der Lübecker Bevolkerung. *Akt Rheumatol* 1995; **20**: 99–104.

113 Hunt S, McKenna S, McEwan J. *The Nottingham Health Profile User's Manual.* Galen Research and Consultancy, Manchester, 1989.

114 Spitzer WO, LeBlanc FE, Dupuis M *et al.* Scientific approach to the assessment and management of activity related spinal disorders. *Spine* 1987; **12 (Suppl. 1)**: S1–S59.

115 Linn JS, Greenfield MD. Patient satisfaction among the chronically ill. *Med Care* 1982; **20**: 425–31.

116 Bowman SJ, Wedderbrun L, Whaley A *et al.* Outcome assessment after epidural corticosteroid injection for low back pain and sciatica. *Spine* 1993; **18**: 1345–50.

117 Hazard RG, Haugh LD, Green PA *et al.* Chronic low back pain. The relationship between patient satisfaction and pain, impairment and disability outcomes. *Spine* 1994; **19**: 881–7.

118 Bigos S, Bowyer O, Braen G *et al. Acute Low Back Problems in Adults.* Clinical Practice Guideline. Quick Reference Guide Number 14, Rockville, MD: US Department of Health and Human Services, Public Health Service, Agency for Health Care Policy and Research, AHCPR Pub. No. 95-0643, December 1994.

119 Evans G, Richards S. *Low back pain: an evaluation of therapeutic interventions.* Health Care Evaluation Unit, Department of Epidemiology and Public Health Medicine, University of Bristol, 1996.

120 Klaber Moffett J, Richardson G, Sheldon TA *et al. Back pain: its management and cost to society.* Discussion Paper 129. Centre for Health Economics, University of York, 1995.

4 Palliative and Terminal Care

I Higginson

1 Summary

This chapter provides assistance for those purchasing palliative care services. The analysis is based on current research evidence and national and local population and health services utilization data.

- Palliative care is the active total care of patients whose disease is not responsive to curative treatment. Control of pain, of other symptoms, and of psychological, social and spiritual problems is paramount. The goal of palliative care is achievement of the best possible quality of life for patients and their families.
- Modern approaches to palliative care have evolved since the 1960s. Hospices, domiciliary and home palliative care teams have evolved rapidly, to provide specialist palliative care, particularly for patients with advanced cancer.
- General palliative care approaches and attitudes such as good pain control and holistic care are needed by all health care professionals caring for people with advanced disease, particularly when curative measures are unhelpful or inappropriate. The specialist palliative care services such as hospices and home care teams are immediately concerned with only one segment of care.
- Funding arrangements between the NHS and specialist palliative care services vary. 75% of hospices are voluntary or charitable units, although many have contracts with health authorities.
- National and local data on the incidence and prevalence can be used to calculate the likely numbers of patients and families needing palliative care. The absolute numbers of patients dying from cancer and other diseases likely to have a palliative period are available from OPCS records. Applying the prevalence of symptoms to this population gives estimates of the range of problems and the size of population needing care.

    Within a population of 1 000 000 there are approximately 2800 cancer deaths per year and of these 2400 people will experience pain, 1300 will have trouble with breathing and 1400 will have symptoms of vomiting or nausea in their last year of life. There will be approximately 6900 deaths, due to progressive non-malignant disease and some of these will have had a period of advancing progressive disease when palliative care would have been appropriate. 4600 people will have suffered pain, 3400 will have had trouble with breathing and 1900 will have had symptoms of vomiting or nausea in the last year of life.
- A wide range of services is available. These include specialist palliative care services, such as hospices and mobile palliative care teams and general services, including primary and hospital care. Voluntary organizations, support groups and local authority services also play a significant role.
- Studies of the effectiveness of care have tended to demonstrate weaknesses in conventional care alone and support the use of inpatient hospices and mobile support teams, especially those operating in the community. Cost-effectiveness studies suggest that these services are not more expensive than conventional care and in some instances may be cheaper.

    However these evaluations have usually been confined to cancer patients and have been based on services where only a proportion of eligible patients and families received care. Therefore the proportion of patients that should most cost-effectively receive specialist care is not known. Furthermore services vary in their structure and methods of working, although a multi-professional approach appears to be that most recommended, further comparisons are needed to identify the most cost-effective models of specialist service provision.

- Evaluations of day care, hospice at home and services for children are limited and further work is needed in these areas.
- Examples of models of care for health districts, outcome measures, targets and service specifications are given. Many of the measures and service specifications are being tested in populations and services.
- The chapter concludes with recommendations for future research, including evaluation of those services currently unevaluated, cost-effectiveness studies and comparison of outcome measures, and recommendations for information, including the agreement of standard data sets based on those currently being piloted by various organizations.

2 Introduction

This chapter assists purchasing authorities in developing their needs assessments and setting service specifications for palliative care.

Development of palliative care

Uncontrolled symptoms or severe patient and family distress while a patient has a progressive illness severely inhibits the patient's quality of life and is believed to impact on the carers' or family members' subsequent resolution of their grief.[1,2] Palliative care seeks to control the symptoms and support the patient and family.[2,3] It aims to improve the quality of life and therefore offers health gain, in terms of adding health and life to years rather than extending life expectancy, for patients and their family members and carers. Death is an inevitable companion of life and therefore the appropriate care for people who are dying is a concern for all health districts. Changes in the nature of diseases during this last century have led to many more people dying from chronic diseases in later life rather than suddenly from acute infection.[2] Patients are increasingly likely to experience a palliative period during their illness.[2]

Modern approaches to palliative care are usually thought to have commenced in the 1950s and 60s with the development of the hospice movement. Dame Cicely Saunders worked in early hospices and in 1967 founded St Christopher's Hospice in Sydenham.[4] The Marie Curie Foundation was created in 1948 and, following a survey of 7000 cancer patients in their own homes in 1952, established a programme of a day and night home nursing service and nursing homes.[5] These developments were strongly supported by research evidence based on the reports of bereaved relatives or occasionally from patients. This indicated that existing care for patients with advanced disease, whether in hospital or at home, failed to meet patients' needs for pain and symptom control, psychosocial care, spiritual care, communication and information and care for the family.[2,4] Although many patients with advanced disease continued to be cared for by conventional health and social services, specialist palliative care services developed either to directly provide care or to provide education and support for the existing services.

During the 1970s, inpatient hospices were the principal type of specialist palliative services to be developed. Many of these operated from voluntary or charity run units, although some were created within the NHS. They concentrated on care for cancer patients and some, mainly the larger hospices, developed educational programmes for doctors, nurses and other health and social professionals. These programmes recognized that a great many patients were cared for by their primary care team in the community or by hospital staff, and sought to educate and support those working in these settings, providing updates in the most recent methods of symptom control and patient and family care.[2-6]

Although the number of inpatient hospices continued to grow, more and more emphasis was placed on the development of home care teams working from hospices and multi-professional palliative care teams in hospitals or the community. In 1980 a working group on terminal care advised that efforts should concentrate on educating and training hospital and community staff and supporting them in their work.[1] It was suggested that support teams, either in the hospital or community, could fulfil this need. The advice of the working group was partly ignored – hospices continued to grow as quickly as support teams – but support teams began to rapidly increase in numbers.[2] Recently the number of support teams has overtaken the number of inpatient hospices.

Support teams comprised specialist staff who would offer advice and support to health workers in the community or in hospitals. Teams were usually centred specifically on trained nurses (often initially funded by the Cancer Relief Macmillan Fund with an agreement that the health authority or Trust would take over funding after three to five years and called Macmillan nurses). Medical, social work and sometimes other professional support were usually provided, and in larger teams doctors, social workers and occasionally physiotherapists or occupational therapists were members of the team. Some teams worked specifically in the hospital while others worked exclusively in the community and in some instances the team would carry out both roles. Teams usually worked within geographically defined areas and did not take over from existing hospital or community nurses, or provide hands-on care.[2–7]

The most recent developments of specialist services have been in the areas of:

- **Day care** This can be operated by an inpatient hospice or a palliative care team.[2,3]
- **Hospice at home** Builds on existing community services and support teams but can also provide 24-hour nursing or sitting care at home, in a similar way to or by collaboration with Marie Curie day and night home nurses.
- **Specialist outpatient clinics** May be medical, or for lymphoedema or for families requiring intensive social work input.

These services encompass the hospice or palliative care philosophy (see the definitions of palliative care on page 187 and in Appendix II).

Philosophies of palliative care: home, hospital, hospice

Different philosophies regarding the most appropriate mix of services and the balance between home and institutional care have developed. Cartwright demonstrated, from random samples of deaths in England, that the proportions of patients who died in institutions increased between 1969 and 1987 from 46% to 50% (hospitals) and 5% to 18% (hospices and other institutions), while the proportion who died at home reduced from 42% to 24%.[8] In 1993 in England and Wales, 23% of all deaths and 26% of cancer deaths occurred at home.[9] Bowling argued against the 'institutionalisation' of death on the grounds that home death was more natural and that a person would have more chance to influence their quality of life.[10]

The development of domiciliary palliative care teams, home nursing services and, more recently, hospice at home and day care, sought to reverse this shift towards institutional care, by increasing the support for patients, their families and other community services. But hospitals, hospices and the increasing role of residential and nursing homes cannot be overlooked – because the majority of patients are cared for in these settings for at least part of their illness. Thus in many areas a wide range of palliative services has developed to attempt to meet needs and to provide choice. Development was often piecemeal and followed varying inputs, including planned need, response to inadequacies, local interest, active voluntary groups, concern within the NHS and champions of a particular approach.[2] However in 1987 a Department of Health circular required health authorities to examine their arrangements for terminal care;[11] this was followed by some funding.[12–16]

Funding arrangements

Financial relationships between palliative services and the NHS vary. The voluntary sector was responsible for the development of many of the specialist palliative care services, particularly inpatient hospices. Usually local groups who were committed to the idea were responsible for raising funds and establishing the hospice. During the 1970s and 1980s only a few of the inpatient hospices were funded or developed entirely by the NHS. In 1995 a large proportion (75%) of hospice inpatient care was provided by voluntary or independent hospice units. These are registered charities most of which have firm links in policy and practice with the NHS from whom they receive varying amounts of funding to supplement funds raised in their local community.[17] Three national charities are also involved in the provision of inpatient care: Marie Curie Cancer Care, the Cancer Relief Macmillan Fund and the Sue Ryder Foundation. Other charities also provide funding for hospices or specialist palliative care services, such as Help the Hospices.

In 1988 the Department of Health began to allocate money, top sliced from the NHS budget and distributed by regional health authorities, specifically for voluntary hospices and specialist palliative care services.[12] During the early 1990s the allocation rose rapidly – from £8 million in 1989 to £17 million in 1991 and £37 million in 1992.[2,13,14] In 1994/95 funding was: £35.7 million for specialist palliative care services (the regional allocations are shown in Appendix I), £5.7 million DSS transfer for voluntary hospices and £6.3 million for drugs for voluntary hospices.[15] This was built into recurrent baselines for health authorities and ceased to be separately identified from 1995/96.[16] Health authorities were encouraged to enter into three-year contracts. Other inpatient care was already funded and managed by the NHS in designated wards specifically for palliative care.[17]

The NHS was more active in the development of home and hospital support teams and was either responsible for the development of many services or took over funding from the Cancer Relief Macmillan Fund after an initial period of 3–5 years of funding. EL(94)14 stated that many authorities already fund NHS specialist palliative provision and that these existing levels of support, wherever possible, should be maintained. The separately identified funding was not intended to be used to take over the funding of nursing services provided within the three year pump priming from the Cancer Relief Macmillan Fund and the NHS contribution already committed to Marie Curie Cancer Care Nursing Services.[15] Many independent or voluntary hospices also provide home care teams and day care services.[17]

Key issues

Appropriate care for people with advanced disease is generally a high priority among patients and consumers. This is evidenced by the development of hospices within the voluntary sector. After public consultation in the Oregon Priority Setting exercise in the US, 'comfort care', such as palliative treatment, was ranked the seventh highest priority (and in some versions, the fifth) out of 17 categories of care.[18] In the UK health districts have also found that palliative care or care for people who were dying came usually in the top 8–15 priorities, depending on the descriptors used.[19,20]

Despite the development of specialist palliative services, it is widely recognized that most patients who have progressive illness which is no longer curable (see page 187) receive much of their care from the primary care team and hospital staff. Specialist palliative care services have tended to concentrate on offering a service for cancer patients. They also receive those patients who have the most severe symptoms or for whom family distress is most severe.[2,1] However a recent joint report of the Standing Medical Advisory Committee and Standing Nursing Advisory Committee included among its recommendations that:

- all patients needing them should have access to palliative care services
- similar services should be developed for patients dying from diseases other than cancer.[4]

Health districts were encouraged to determine levels of need among all patients and to purchase an appropriate mix of services, including the specialist palliative care services. However this leaves health districts to determine what mix of services should be purchased to provide the most cost-effective and high quality care for their local population. Health commissioners also have to decide what constitutes a specialist palliative care service. These services vary in their levels of trained staff and there has been recent concern that some nursing homes or units without staff trained in palliative care will rename themselves as specialist services without being able to offer this type of specialized care. This chapter aims to provide assistance in the needs assessment for palliative and terminal care and follows the format proposed by Stevens and Raftery.[71]

3 Statement of the problem

Definitions of palliative care, terminal care and the specialist services

This section sets out the main definitions and terms relevant to this field.

Palliative care

There are various definitions of palliative care. The most straightforward is that of the National Council for Hospice and Specialist Palliative Care Services, which is based on an earlier definition from the World Health Organization:[22-24]

Palliative care is the active total care of patients whose disease is not responsive to curative treatment. Control of pain, of other symptoms and of psychological, social and spiritual problems is paramount. The goal of palliative care is achievement of the best possible quality of life for patients and their families. Many aspects of palliative care are also applicable earlier in the course of the illness, in conjunction with anticancer treatment. Palliative care:

- affirms life and regards dying as a normal process
- neither hastens nor postpones death
- provides relief from pain and other distressing symptoms
- integrates the psychological and spiritual aspects of patient care
- offers a support system to help patients live as actively as possible until death
- offers a support system to help the family cope during the patient's illness and in their own bereavement.

A similar definition is from the Standing Medical Advisory Committee and Standing Nursing and Midwifery Advisory Committee (1992):[4]

Palliative care is active total care offered to a patient with a progressive illness and their family when it is recognised that the illness is no longer curable, in order to concentrate on the quality of life and the alleviation of distressing symptoms within the framework of a co-ordinated service. Palliative care neither hastens nor postpones death; it provides a relief from pain and other distressing symptoms and integrates the psychological and spiritual aspects of care. In addition it offers a support system to help during the patient's illness and in bereavement. 'Family' is used as a general term to cover closely-attached individuals, whatever their legal status.

A key feature of this second definition is that the disease is described as 'progressive'. It distinguishes between chronic diseases which may not be curable but are unchanging – such as patients with unchanging diabetes – and those diseases that are progressive and likely to result in a patient dying – such as advanced lung cancer. For this reason and because of its comprehensiveness, it is the SMAC/SNMAC definition above which will be used in this chapter.

Other definitions include the above but tend to expand or elaborate on some of the aspects of care offered. Common other definitions include:

From the European Association for Palliative Care:[25]

Palliative care is care for the dying by providing active, total care at a time when disease is not responsive to curative treatment. Control of pain, of other symptoms and of psychological, social and spiritual problems is paramount. The goal of care for the dying is the highest possible quality of life for the patient and family.

Terminal illness and terminal care

Terminal illness refers to active and progressive disease for which curative treatment is neither possible nor appropriate and from which death is certain. This varies from a few days to many months.[4]

For the purpose of the DSS income support limits for people suffering from a terminal illness and within NHS executive letters a definition that 'terminally ill people are those with active and progressive disease for which curative treatment is not possible or not appropriate and from which death can reasonably be expected within 12 months' is adopted.[16,26]

Terminal care is an important part of palliative care and usually refers to the management of patients during their last few days or weeks or even months of life from a point at which it becomes clear that the patient is in a progressive state of decline.

Palliative medicine

Palliative medicine has been recognized as a specialty in its own right.[4] Postgraduate training is available for doctors intending to practise in this specialty in centres approved by the Joint Committee for Higher Medical Training and for general practitioners (GPs) during after-vocational training. Academic, medical and nursing posts have been created.[4]

When palliative medicine became a specialty the Association of Palliative Medicine provided the definition:

Palliative medicine is the appropriate medical care of patients with advanced and progressive disease for whom the focus of care is the quality of life and in whom the prognosis is limited (though sometimes may be several years). Palliative medicine includes consideration of the family's needs before and after the patient's death.[24]

Note that this definition refers to 'medicine' and thereby the activities of doctors. Clinical nurse specialists in palliative care must also complete post-registration training in palliative care.

Sub-categories of services: definitions of specialist care services

The principles and practices of palliative care are not the exclusive concern of the specialist services.[24] The relief of suffering is the general responsibility of doctors, nurses and other health care professionals over the whole continuum of diagnosis to death. General palliative care approaches and attitudes should be part of normal clinical practice.[24]

Specialist palliative care services are immediately concerned with only one segment of that spectrum of care. They are committed to controlling pain and other symptoms, easing suffering and sustaining the last phase of life in patients who have active, progressive and far advanced disease which is no longer amenable to curative treatment. Their work integrates the physical, psychological, social and spiritual aspects of care enabling dying patients to live with dignity and offering support to them, their families and carers during the patient's illness and their bereavement. All patients with progressive disease would benefit from a palliative approach and a smaller group need specialist care.

The following section outlines the main terms. Further information is given in Appendix II.

Hospice

The term hospice is used in two ways. The first refers to the philosophy of hospice care, which is in effect the same as the philosophy and principles of palliative care in the definitions above.[22] The second refers to a hospice unit. Usually this is a free standing unit with inpatient facilities, which practises palliative care emphasizing medical and psychosocial care. It will normally have medical and nursing staff specially trained in palliative care and the control of symptoms and has a high nurse to patient ratio. Hospices will usually offer symptom control and terminal, palliative and respite care. Many hospices also offer day care and home support teams. Some hospices do not offer inpatient care. To avoid confusion this chapter refers to the types of facilities offered by the hospice – e.g. inpatient care etc. Note also that there is a wide variety of types and grades of staff operating within different hospices. This is discussed in section 6.

Funding for hospices may be charitable, from the local community or national charities, or from the NHS, or a combination of these.[2] There is debate about what levels of staffing constitute an inpatient specialist service (Appendix II).[22]

Specialist palliative care teams

These teams are found in three main categories.

1 Hospital palliative care teams

These teams aim to bring the principles and benefits of palliative care into acute hospitals. The teams usually work in an advisory capacity providing symptom control and psychological support to patients and carers as well as playing an important role in education and advice within the hospital. Most teams are made up of two or more clinical nurse specialists and many are multi-disciplinary, including a doctor, social worker, chaplain and others.[2,4,22]

2 Domiciliary or home palliative care teams

These teams comprise specialist staff who offer advice and support to health workers in the community. It is usually centred on clinical nurse specialists (often Macmillan nurses) with medical and other professional support and the team may be attached to a general hospital with a cancer unit, inpatient hospice/palliative care unit or the community nursing service. The team does not take over responsibility from the community nurse or GP and does not usually deliver bedside nursing care.[2,4,22]

3 Palliative care teams

These teams combine elements of the hospital and domiciliary element, either with some team staff working in the community and others in the hospital or with staff working with individual patients and following them from setting to setting.[2,4,22,27]

Marie Curie nurses

These nurses offer a day and night nursing and sitting service, which complements the community nursing service.[4,5]

Multi-disciplinary care

This is the team approach to palliative care, which recognizes that many health care workers have roles to play. Each patient's key worker may vary according to the particular problem of the patient and local factors.

Day care

This is provided by a growing number of palliative care units and other facilities to enable patients to continue living at home. Day care is particularly valuable for patients who need more than outpatient and GP services and where carers need support. It also serves to introduce patients to a service without admission to inpatient care.[4,22]

Rehabilitation

In the context of palliative care, rehabilitation refers to assisting patients to achieve and maintain their maximum physical, emotional, spiritual, vocational and social potential, however limited this may be as a result of the progression of disease.[4]

If rehabilitation is effective and efficient, it may be of particular value to patients who are not terminal in enabling them to return home and obtain an improved quality of life.

Further descriptions of these services and terms are shown in Appendix II and in the definitions published by the National Council for Hospice and Specialist Palliative Care Services.[22] A national directory of services can be obtained from St Christopher's Hospice Information Service (see Appendix II).

Sub-categories of diseases and types of patient who need palliative care

This epidemiologically based needs assessment is very different from the previous disease based reviews and is more similar to the epidemiological reviews of a client group, such as the assessment for elderly people. As the earlier definitions suggest, palliative care encompasses patients who suffer from different diseases, with different rates of progression. Patients who need palliative care are not a homogenous group, although they are similar in having active, progressive disease where the emphasis needs to be on quality of life for the patient and their family.

Patients who have palliative needs can be grouped in several ways: by diagnosis, by symptoms or problems experienced or by type of care received. The first two of these would relate to the epidemiology of diseases and problems and thus are more useful in an assessment of need. The primary diagnosis can indicate whether a patient is likely to experience a palliative period, and whether they would develop problems and symptoms which would need a palliative approach or to be referred to a specialist palliative service. Data on the prevalence and incidence of diseases are available and can be obtained from mortality statistics. Some data on the likely incidence and prevalence of symptoms are available but much less is known about the incidence and prevalence of other problems – such as psychosocial, emotional or spiritual problems – experienced by patients, their families or carers.

The type of care received is affected by the availability of services across the country. This varies widely and so this indicator is less useful to assess need.

This chapter uses all of these three sub-categories but concentrates more on the first two.

The main primary diseases which can have a palliative period – i.e. a period when the disease is progressive, no longer curable and where the emphasis is the quality of life follow.

Types of illness

- Cancer, main categories are of:
  a) lung, trachea, bronchus
  b) ear, nose and throat
  c) female breast
  d) lymphatic
  e) digestive tract
  f) genitourinary
  g) leukaemia
  h) haemopoietic.
- Progressive non-malignant diseases, which can have a palliative period. These include:
  a) diseases of the circulatory system e.g. cardiovascular, cerebro-vascular diseases
  b) diseases of the respiratory system
  c) diseases of the nervous system and sense organs e.g. motor neurone disease, multiple sclerosis, dementia
  d) AIDS/HIV.
- Children's terminal illnesses and hereditary diseases, including:
  a) hereditary degenerative disorder e.g. muscular dystrophy
  b) cystic fibrosis.

To estimate the need among these populations we have estimated the numbers of patients who may experience the different symptoms encountered – e.g. pain, dyspnoea etc. Such symptoms and problems would require treatment, often involving a palliative approach. Alternative estimates have also been based on the current use of services.

4 Prevalence and incidence

Current situation

The incidence of patients needing palliative care (either the general approach and/or specialist input) can be estimated from death rates of common conditions[9,28] which may require palliative care (Table 1).

Table 1: Death rates per million population by age group for common conditions in England (1993)

Age (years)	Sex	Neoplasms	Diseases of the circulatory system	Diseases of the respiratory system	Diseases of the nervous system and sense organs
All ages	M	3017	4830	1174	222
	F	2648	5016	1175	228
1–4	M	41	14	27	40
	F	37	10	18	37
5–14	M	40	7	5	18
	F	29	6	4	16
15–24	M	63	29	15	42
	F	50	22	12	21
25–34	M	120	83	34	42
	F	142	46	13	27
35–44	M	388	443	70	66
	F	547	149	34	44
45–54	M	1402	1707	168	89
	F	1586	506	111	77
55–64	M	4864	6109	772	188
	F	3941	2356	518	153
65–74	M	12621	17517	3376	567
	F	7668	9034	1876	404
75–84	M	23532	43559	11575	1985
	F	12404	29517	5492	1187
85 and over	M	34529	88641	37272	4323
	F	16868	76305	22709	2752

Widening the definition of patients who may need palliative care beyond those with cancers could triple the number of people included. Only some people with these conditions would require specialist palliative care. Each disease would have roughly three groups of patients:

- those who have a palliative period of advancing, progressive disease
- those who have stable or no disease, relatively few symptoms but then deteriorate or die suddenly (e.g. from a myocardial infarct)
- those who suffer from chronic disease, where the disease is not clearly progressing, but who might have periods of progression and symptoms where they would benefit from palliative care and then periods of remission.

In cancer patients the period of progression is most clearly predicted and many would fall into the first category. However the other conditions, such as circulatory disease, may often fall into the other two categories. There is little research into the natural history of these diseases as death approaches and we do not know what proportion of patients experience a period of advancing disease suitable for specialist palliative treatment, although all would probably benefit from palliative approaches and principles. However symptoms experienced in the last year of life can provide us with some information about whether the patient was disease free or had symptoms which may be suited to palliative treatment. The likely symptoms in these groups for individual diseases are estimated below.

Calculating numbers of deaths in the population

This population needs assessment is based on a population of 1 000 000.

It is assumed that the population includes people from a range of different cultural and ethnic groups. It is also assumed that there is a range of health experiences across the different wards or localities within an area, with the most disadvantaged wards displaying higher rates of death and increased levels of illness, high levels of unemployment and poorer housing, with many single parent families and elderly people who live alone.

Mortality statistics provide details of the numbers of deaths occurring in the population, totally and for different causes. Within a population of 1 000 000 we would expect about 11 000 deaths per year.[28] Actual numbers for the population can be obtained from OPCS records. Anonymous records of the death registrations are made available to health authorities from OPCS via NHS executive regional health authorities, each year. Although a breakdown of the numbers and main causes of death are provided the raw data can be also obtained in a format suitable for local analysis in a spreadsheet or in a statistical package. For a small charge OPCS will also undertake specified analysis for individual populations if this is not possible locally. Some health authorities themselves collected and computerized data from the copies of death registrations which were automatically copied to them.

A breakdown of the likely data on deaths is shown in Table 2 and Figure 1. If the population follows the general pattern of England,[9,28] cancer would account for 25% of all deaths (27% for deaths in men and 23% for deaths in women). Cancers of the gastro–intestinal tract, trachea, bronchus and lung, and breast would be the most common (Table 2 and Figure 2). Circulatory disease would be the most common cause of death (45% men, 46% women). Respiratory disease would probably be the next most common after cancer (11% in men and in women).

Data from the public health common data set will provide the standardized mortality ratios (SMRs). These can be calculated for different causes of death and can be used to show whether cancers or other causes of mortality are more, less or equally common in the population compared with England and Wales. The SMR can also be calculated for different localities within the population, to show whether any of these vary in different ways. An example of the SMRs for one population is shown in Appendix III. Because the area shown appears to have an excess of cancer deaths, this may mean that higher than average palliative services are needed. However more accurate estimates of need for services are available by calculating the numbers of people who may have required palliative care locally and the prevalence of symptoms.

Cancer patients who may have required palliative care

The number of cancer patients with advanced disease and symptoms can be estimated from the number of cancer deaths. Some patients may have a short or not identified terminal period but the majority would have a clear period where they would require palliative care. The World Health Organization has recommended that for cancer patients the palliative approach should be a gradually increasing component of care from diagnosis onwards, rather than being confined to the last few weeks of life. This concept is shared by the

Table 2: Number of deaths in the population during one year for the most common causes (total population 1 million)

Cause of death	Men	Women	Total
Neoplasms[a]	1464	1341	2805
Circulatory system	2429	2624	5053
Respiratory system	595	626	1221
Chronic liver and cirrhosis	34	26	60
Nervous system and sense organs[b]	88	88	176
Senile and pre-senile organic conditions	22	22	44
Endocrine, nutritional, metabolic, immunity	187	123	310
Total of these diseases	4819	4850	9669
Total deaths from all causes[c]	5356	5644	11000
Cause of death			
Neoplasms include:			
Lip, oral, pharynx, larynx	41	34	75
Digestive and peritoneum	449	339	788
Trachea, bronchus, lung	394	291	685
Female breast	0	255	255
Genitourinary	243	178	421
Lymphatic and haemopoietic	154	54	208
Other, unspecified	7	7	14
Nervous system and sense organs include:			
Parkinson's disease	37	28	65
Multiple sclerosis	1	1	2
Meningitis	4	4	8

[a,b] For a breakdown of main groups see lower half of table.
[c] Deaths in those aged under 28 days excluded.

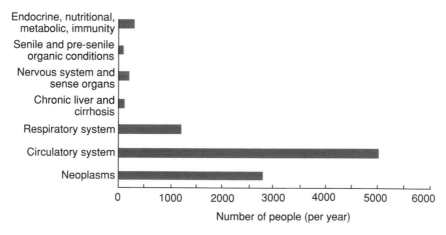

Figure 1: Main causes of death in the district: excluding those aged below 28 days.

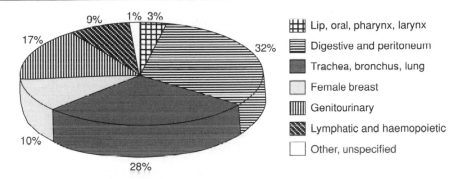

Figure 2: Main cancers in the district.

Expert Advisory Group on Cancer in their report on commissioning cancer services.[29] Implementation of this report's recommendations is underway.[30]

The data from Table 1 suggest that there may be 2800 people who die from cancer each year within a population of 1 000 000. Estimates of the proportions of these with symptoms should suggest the numbers who would benefit from palliative care advice, the palliative approach and, in some cases, specialist services such as hospice or home care.

Estimating the prevalence of symptoms and other problems in cancer and in patients with progressive non-malignant diseases

Studies which estimate the prevalence of symptoms among patients with cancer have been confined to selected populations, such as patients attending oncology clinics or patients admitted to a hospice service. Prospective data on the prevalence of symptoms and problems among patients with advancing non-malignant disease are rare and usually confined to those few patients referred to a palliative service. There is no prospective data on the prevalence of problems among patients not referred to these services, and such data are needed for an epidemiologically based needs assessment.

However one method of overcoming this sample bias is to identify patients after their death using the death registration. This approach has two drawbacks. First death registrations include inaccuracies – for example the recording of diagnosis is unreliable especially in elderly patients.[31] Second assessment of problems is made by the bereaved carers or spouse rather than the patient. Studies have suggested that spouses or carers may unreliably record some symptoms and anxieties when compared to patients' assessments.[32,33] On average carers or spouses tended to record slightly more severe problems than did the patients.[33] Psychological symptoms may be less accurately recorded.[34] Assessments made during bereavement appear to concord less than those made prospectively.[35] It may be that the carers' assessment is altered by their own grief and anxieties. Furthermore for some aspects of care, e.g. anxiety, the carers' and staff assessments agreed and recorded problems, whereas patients' ratings did not. Until prospective data on the prevalence of symptoms in complete populations of patients with advanced disease become available, these estimates based on the retrospective views of carers are needed. They at least provide the carers' views of whether patients need help for these symptoms. Given that the carer is part of the unit of palliative care, their view has some validity.

Prevalence of symptoms and other problems in cancer patients

The prevalence of symptoms in a random sample of national deaths in 1987 has been used to calculate the numbers of patients with symptoms, as viewed by bereaved carers, in the population.[8,36] A more recent study (1991) which examined the prevalence of symptoms in random samples of deaths within selected health districts showed similar findings.[37-40] These suggest that, among the population of 1 000 000 people, each year 2400 cancer patients have pain which requires treatment, 1300 have trouble with breathing and 1400 have symptoms of vomiting or nausea. The patients usually have several symptoms and the prevalence is shown in Table 3.

Table 3: Cancer patients: prevalence of problems (per 1 000 000 population)

Symptom	% with symptom in last year of life[a]	Estimated number in each year
Pain	84	2357
Trouble with breathing	47	1318
Vomiting or nausea	51	1431
Sleeplessness	51	1431
Mental confusion	33	926
Depression	38	1065
Loss of appetite	71	1992
Constipation	47	1318
Bedsores	28	785
Loss of bladder control	37	1038
Loss of bowel control	25	701
Unpleasant smell	19	533
Total deaths from cancer		**2805**

[a] As per Cartwright and Seale study,[8,36] based on a random sample of deaths and using the reports of bereaved carers.
Note: Patients usually have several symptoms.

Patients with cancer are known to have a higher prevalence of anxiety and depression when compared to the normal population. Anxiety and depression are often under-diagnosed.[31,41] High patient anxiety and family distress and anxiety are known to be associated with multiple symptoms, distressing or socially unacceptable symptoms (e.g. unpleasant smell) and poor symptom control.[3]

There are no population-based epidemiological studies which describe the levels of anxiety among patients and their families in the general cancer population. However studies based on referrals to palliative care teams have suggested that approximately one-third of families and one-quarter of patients describe severe anxiety, fears or worries.[34,42-44] This would translate into approximately 930 family members or family groups and 700 patients per 1 000 000 population. These people would need more intensive support and some would require specialist services.

Estimates based on use of specialist care services in cancer patients

Studies have suggested that in the UK between 15 and 25% of cancer deaths received inpatient hospice care and between 25 and 65% of cancer deaths received input from a support team or Macmillan nurse.[8,36-38,42,43,45,46] Applying these figures to the population would suggest that 700–1800 cancer patients require support team care and 400–700 should require inpatient hospice care (Table 4). Some patients will require both services and some patients would be admitted to hospice care two or more times.

Table 4: Cancer patients: need for specialist palliative services based on national and regional estimates of use (per 1 000 000 population)[a]

	Number of adults	%
Deaths from cancer in one year	2805	
Needing support team	701–1824	25–65
Needing inpatient hospice care	421–701	15–25

[a] Studies used include: Bennett and Corcoran (1994),[42] Cartwright (1991),[8] Seale (1991);[36] Higginson, Wade, McCarthy (1992);[43] Addington-Hall (1991);[37-40] Frankel (1990);[16] Eve and Jackson (1994).[45]

Given the fairly high prevalence of symptoms in cancer, it is likely that this figure is a conservative estimate. Furthermore national studies of the needs of cancer patients, given current provision, have demonstrated unmet needs for patients in terms of home support, symptom control and respite care.[8,36-38] As outlined on page 184 services have often developed in a piecemeal fashion; this limits the value of estimates based on current national use.

Patients with progressive non-malignant diseases who may have required palliative care

The numbers of patients with other causes of advanced disease and symptoms can be estimated from the numbers of non-cancer deaths within the health authority. Patients may have short or no identified terminal periods, some will die suddenly, but many who die from circulatory disorders, respiratory disorders, diseases of the nervous and sense organs and senile and pre-senile conditions will have a recognized period where they could require palliative care. This period is less clearly identified for patients with progressive non-malignant diseases than for patients who have cancer.

The data in Table 1 suggest that there may be 6900 people who die from other causes, mainly circulatory or respiratory disorders each year.[9,28]

Although the numbers of people with multiple sclerosis, motor neurone disease and similar disorders are small, these diseases have a much longer duration of symptoms than many of the cancers or other disorders. This factor should be taken into account when planning services.

As for cancer patients the prevalence of symptoms can be used to suggest the numbers who may benefit from palliative care advice, a palliative approach and in some cases specialist services such as hospice or home care.

Prevalence of symptoms and other problems in patients with progressive non-malignant diseases

As for cancer patients the prevalence of symptoms in a random sample of national deaths has been used to calculate the prevalence of symptoms in the population.[8,36-38] These suggest that, among the population of 1 000 000 people, each year 4600 patients with progressive non-malignant diseases have pain, 3400 have trouble with breathing, 1900 have symptoms of vomiting or nausea and 2600 have mental confusion. There are many other symptoms (Table 5).

Table 5: Patients with progressive non-malignant disease: prevalence of problems (per 1 000 000 population)

Symptom	% with symptom in last year of life[a]	Estimated number in each year
Pain	67	4599
Trouble with breathing	49	3363
Vomiting or nausea	27	1853
Sleeplessness	36	2471
Mental confusion	38	2608
Depression	36	2471
Loss of appetite	38	2608
Constipation	32	2196
Bedsores	14	961
Loss of bladder control	33	2265
Loss of bowel control	22	1510
Unpleasant smell	13	892
Total deaths from other causes, excluding accidents, injury and suicide and causes very unlikely to have a palliative period		6864

[a] As per Cartwright and Seale study,[8,36] based on a random sample of deaths and using the reports of bereaved carers.

Note: Patients usually have several symptoms.

High patient anxiety and family distress and anxiety are known to be associated with multiple symptoms, distressing or socially unacceptable symptoms (e.g. unpleasant smell) and poor symptom control. If the prevalences of severe patient anxiety and family anxiety is similar to those among cancer patients, this would suggest that within a population of 1 000 000 severe anxiety would be experienced by approximately 2200 families and 1600 patients.

Estimates based on use of specialist palliative care services by patients with progressive non-malignant diseases

Estimates of the use or need for specialist services among patients with progressive non-malignant diseases are rare. Many specialist palliative services have only recently begun to accept patients who do not have cancer. Services which accept or encourage referrals of patients needing palliative care, irrespective of diagnosis, have reported caseloads where up to one-third or a half have diseases other than cancer.[47,48] Similar figures are found from studies of patients receiving inpatient hospital care.[49] Applying these data to the population would suggest that 350–1400 patients with progressive non-malignant diseases may require a support team for their palliative care and up to 200–700 may require inpatient palliative care (Table 6).

Table 6: Patients with progressive non-malignant diseases: need for specialist palliative services based on local studies of use or need (per 1 000 000 population)[a]

	Number of adults	%
Deaths in one year	6864	
Needing support team	350–1824	0.5–1 times numbers of cancer patients needing care
Needing inpatient palliative care	210–701	0.5–1 times numbers of cancer patients needing care

[a] Studies used include: Hockley *et al.* (1988);[47] Severs and Wilkins (1991);[48] Noble (1993).[49]

People with HIV/AIDS who may need palliative care

Since reporting began in 1982 a total of 10 304 cases meeting the European AIDS case definition were reported in the UK up to the end of December 1994. Of these 7019 were known to have died.[50] The number of deaths has increased over the years; 1065 deaths occurred during 1994 (Table 7). In the same period there were 23 104 laboratory reports of first confirmed HIV-1 antibody positive tests.

Table 7: UK AIDS cases by year of diagnosis and date of known death

Year	Diagnosis	Date of known death
1982 or earlier	17	8
1983	33	15
1984	107	47
1985	240	119
1986	464	270
1987	671	345
1988	884	409
1989	1051	660
1990	1201	772
1991	1340	970
1992	1492	1067
1993	1546	1231
1994	1189	1065
Unknown	69	41
Total	10304	7019

Source: AIDS/HIV Quarterly Surveillance Tables[50]

Assessing the palliative care needs for people with HIV/AIDS will depend on the underlying prevalence within the population served, the symptoms and problems experienced and the extent to which there is a palliative period. Calculating these is complex. When estimating prevalence in central London, the OPCS death registrations did not prove useful: we found very few cases were identified. Instead data from the Public Heath Laboratory Surveillance appeared to be more accurate.[50] The number of AIDS related deaths varies greatly across the UK and in many populations the numbers are very small. For example, in 1994 it varied from two (Northern Ireland) or eight (Northern Region) to 141 (North West Thames) or 64 (NE Thames).[50] Even within the North East Thames area the number of deaths within health districts in 1993 varied from 0–33 deaths per year.[51] One other district in central London had higher rates than this, with

40–50 HIV/AIDS related deaths per year (personal communication – Kensington & Chelsea and Westminster Health Authority).

The prevalence of symptoms among total populations of people with advancing HIV/AIDS is not well researched. Studies to date have tended to include self-selected samples, such as those patients referred to particular services. However, studies have suggested that the prevalence of symptoms and psychosocial problems in people with HIV/AIDS is as high or higher than among cancer patients, although the nature of many of the symptoms differs. Among patients with advanced HIV/AIDS at least 60% experienced pain[52–54] and over a third needed opioid (e.g. morphine or diamorphine) treatment,[55] 90–100% experienced other symptoms and for 70% these were moderate or severe,[53,54,56] 90–100% experienced anxiety and for 70% this was moderate or severe and at least 50% needed practical support or practical aids.[56] Patients with HIV/AIDS may come from various different cultures and backgrounds which may need quite different support, e.g. for drug users.[57] The natural course of HIV/AIDS includes remissions, acute infections which may require intensive treatment and in some patients the long-term deteriorations associated with HIV/AIDS encephalopathy or cognitive impairment.[52,53,58] Although only a small proportion will develop encephalopathy, those who are affected and their carers need intensive support.[59,61] However the high prevalence of symptoms among people with HIV/AIDS suggests that most would need some palliative support towards the end of life.

Children who may need palliative care

A small proportion of the deaths described on page 192 were among children. Within a population of 1 000 000, if the population is similar to that of the UK,[9,28] there would be approximately 70 deaths in children aged 28 days to four years and 28 among those aged 5–14 years. The majority of these deaths would be due to illnesses or accidents which did not have a palliative period.[9–28] However within a population of this size, current data from England and Wales suggest that approximately three children aged 28 days to four years and five aged 5–14 years would die from cancers. The numbers of children who die from other diseases which may have a palliative period would also be small – two children aged 28 days to four years and one aged 5–14 years from endocrine, nutritional or immune disorders; five aged 28 days to four years and two aged 5–14 years from diseases of the nervous system and senses; and 11 aged 28 days to four years and two aged 5–14 years from congenital disorders.[9,28] Data from OPCS can be used to calculate the exact numbers locally.

Characteristics of patients needing palliative care and local trends

To consider the palliative care for patients within the population in more detail, the OPCS death registration data (page 193) can be analysed to examine:

- the characteristics of those people who will need palliative care in terms of age, sex, etc.
- the trends in place of death over five years
- place of death by electoral ward or locality (five or more years' data should be combined, to avoid very small numbers)
- effect of factors such as social deprivation, ethnicity or services available on place of death.

An example of the results of this for the district of Kensington, Chelsea and Westminster is shown in Appendix IV.

Likely findings would be that there are roughly equal numbers of men and women who died and the rate is constant over the years. The majority of patients who die will be elderly (over 75% will be aged over 65 years and over 50% over 75 years). The majority of deaths will have occurred in hospital (approximately 60–70%) and less at home (24–30%). The number of deaths in hospices will be difficult to calculate from OPCS records because hospices are not coded with a specific category. Free-standing hospices are likely to be coded as 'other communal establishment', hospices within an NHS hospital are likely to be coded as 'NHS hospital' and those hospices operating in private hospitals are likely to be coded as 'private hospital'.

Key issues for health commissioners

Key issues for health commissioners following the analysis of this incidence and prevalence data are as follows. Within a population of 1 000 000 the estimated need for palliative and terminal care is estimated by:

- approximately 2800 cancer deaths each year
- approximately 6900 deaths due to potentially progressive non-malignant disease. Within this there will be three main groups:
  a) those who had a palliative period of advancing, progressive disease
  b) those for whom death was sudden and followed a period where the disease was absent or stable and where they had relatively few symptoms
  c) those for whom there was a chronic disease, where the disease was not clearly progressing, but who might have periods of progression and symptoms where they would benefit from palliative care, and then periods of remission.

This estimates needs as follows:

- approximately 2400 cancer patients will experience pain, 1300 have trouble with breathing and 1400 have symptoms of vomiting or nausea
- approximately 4600 patients with progressive non-malignant diseases have pain, 3400 have trouble with breathing, 1900 have symptoms of vomiting or nausea and 2600 have mental confusion
- if patterns of average national use are followed, 700–1800 cancer patients would require hospital or home palliative care team care and 400–700 should require inpatient hospice or specialist unit care
- if patterns of use where such services exist are followed, up to 350–1800 patients with progressive non-malignant diseases may require a support team for their palliative care and up to 200–700 may require inpatient palliative care
- there may be up to 30 children aged up to 14 years who have a palliative period; most (20) would be under five years of age and half of these would be as a result of congenital disorders. The number of cancer deaths among children would be small – less than ten
- for people with HIV/AIDS the numbers needed in palliative care would depend on the local prevalence of AIDS. Numbers would be nil or small, except in high prevalence areas.

More accurate local estimates can be fairly easily calculated using the data from OPCS death registrations. This would ensure that the estimates take account of local variations within the population.

The commission should also consider the following.

- What proportion of deaths currently occur at home? How does this compare with the national average of 24% and does it vary across the population? How should this influence the way in which services are provided? Variation across the district may mean that some localities need to be targeted for an increase in support services, home nursing or specialist palliative care services.

- What trends have occurred in the place of death for patients – for example over the last ten years – and how might these trends be explained? The development of a hospice or home care service may have impact. Are the percentages of people who die at home increasing or decreasing?

5 Services available

This section outlines palliative care services available for different types of illnesses. The range of clinical and supportive services which should be considered in any district policy for palliative care is described in the following sections. As patterns of provision vary between districts the average national level of use has been included, where available, as indication of availability. These levels of use are not the recommended levels for optimum care.

This section is divided by the sub-categories described on page 191 – underlying type of illness. For each of these the palliative care services and their use is described.

Estimates of service use can be varied throughout the country and may have changed markedly in recent years as the numbers of specialist hospices, units and home care services have expanded. The most comprehensive and up-to-date information on service use is that collected by Addington-Hall and colleagues[37–40] in 1991. This study selected random samples of cancer and non-cancer deaths from death certificates in 20 health districts in the UK and interviewed the nearest carer or family member about the death. It is the largest sample of deaths in this country – and provides information on 2074 cancer deaths and 1622 non-cancer deaths. Many of the findings regarding the prevalence of symptoms and service use were similar to an earlier study in 1987 by Cartwright and Seale,[8,36] except for the use of hospices and specialist services which had increased since that time.

Funding arrangements for the services differ as outlined on page 186. About 75% of hospices and some other specialist palliative care services are organized by voluntary groups.[17] Much of their costs are met by charitable donations with health authorities meeting the remaining costs.

There are difficulties in linking numbers of patients requiring services and the services available. Service activity is often measured in contacts with a range of services some of which are non-NHS. The advent of the NHS number in 1996 onwards will help, although the non-NHS sector will still be omitted.

Cancer

The following list is of palliative care services which provide some degree of palliative care available to people with all types of cancer.

Primary health care

Primary care teams consisting of GP, practice nurse and district nurse provide care for all people in the community and are used by almost all people with cancer in the last year of life (Table 8).

The survey by Addington-Hall et al.[37–40] showed that 99% of cancer patients had contact with GPs in their last year of life, but for almost half (43%) this was fewer than ten contacts. Just over a quarter (29%) had over 20 contacts. Although fewer patients (59%) had district nurses when these were available, visits were more frequent – 34% had ten or under visits, 14% 11–20, 26% 21–50 and 27% 51 or more visits in the last year of life.

Some GPs and district nurses have postgraduate training or qualifications in palliative care, symptom control and psychosocial care. Those organizing courses report that high numbers wish to attend and this

Table 8: Use of services by patients in the last year of life. Uses data from Addington-Hall 1993[37-40]

Service	Cancer[b] $n = 2074$ (%)	Non-cancer[b] $n = 1622$ (%)
Primary health care		
GP	99	95
Home visit by GP	92	79
Nurses at home	67	36
District nurse	59	32
Health visitor	3	2
Night nursing	19	8
Other community services		
Home help	20	28
Home help if lived alone	40	48
Home help if lived with others	11	16
Meals on wheels if lived alone	22	27
Meals on wheels if lived with others	4	6
Specialist home or hospital palliative care services		
Support team or Macmillan nurses	29	nil
Marie Curie nurses[a]	2	nil
Inpatient care		
Admitted to hospital or hospice	91	72
Hospice		
Hospice inpatient admission	19	<1
Day hospice	3	not available
Spiritual and emotional support		
Chaplains (post-bereavement)	38	34
Support and information groups	11	13
Lived in a nursing or residential home at some point during their last 12 months of life	13	29

[a] Note: In the survey families may not have been able to clearly identify Marie Curie nurses. This finding is disputed by Marie Curie. Data from Marie Curie obtained separately suggest that Marie Curie nurses care for more than one-third of all those who die at home from cancer.
[b] National percentage of people who used the service in their last year of life.

suggests considerable interest and motivation (personal communications from course organizers in the UK). The number who undertake extra training is not known.

Other generic community services

This can include social services such as day care, meals on wheels, home help or home care workers, social workers, laundry and incontinence services, or occupational therapist and other health services such as a health visitor, chiropodist, physiotherapist or clinical nurse specialist from other areas of care, e.g. stoma care. There are also volunteer sitters and workers in many areas and bereavement visitors and support workers.

These services are available in many districts, although to varying extents. Their use by people in the last year of life is fairly limited (Table 8).

Home and hospital specialist palliative care teams and Marie Curie nurses

There are now various forms of services available (see page 189).

Specialist palliative care team (home and hospital)

This team includes doctors, nurses and social workers, although the number in a 'team' can range from 1–11 staff (strictly speaking, one person does not constitute a team). Their function is to provide specialist knowledge in symptom management, control and support, supplement the care of the dying, co-ordinate care, emotional and bereavement support and teaching of staff, carers and patients. They aim to work alongside the primary care team and hospital staff, providing advice and additional support.[1,2]

The teams can be referred to as home care teams and work primarily in the community, or as hospital teams working mainly in hospital. However the boundaries are blurred and many teams will work in both hospital and the community. Teams can be based within a hospice (most common), a hospital, community unit or be independent.

There are over 400 palliative care teams working in hospitals or in the community in the UK and Republic of Ireland[17,62] (Appendix V). Of these about 260 are free standing, community based teams and almost 150 are attached to hospice inpatient units (calculated from[17,62]). Most districts in the UK would have one or more such teams, usually working in a defined catchment area. Just over a quarter of cancer deaths would be cared for by such a service – 57% of patients having help for 1–12 weeks with 2–6 visits per week (Table 8).

Macmillan nurses

Macmillan nurses sometimes work in isolation and sometimes work as part of a palliative care team. Macmillan nurses provide symptom control and support, specialist advice, support, training and liaison with the patient, family and staff involved in caring but do not take over the patient's care. They are self-funding for three to five years after which the district health authority or trust takes over.

Marie Curie nurses

These nurses provide a night and day practical nursing service in patients' homes. There are about 5000 Marie Curie nurses in the UK and they care for about 20 000 patients at home.[5] They are jointly funded by Marie Curie and health authorities. These are not classified as specialist palliative care services.

A survey conducted by the Hospice Information Service showed that in the UK approximately 100 000 patients per year were seen by palliative care nurses. This is over half the number of cancer deaths (160 000) per year.[17,45]

Hospital services

Oncology and radiotherapy services

These offer expert technical facilities and treatment. Treatment may often be given in conjunction with the support care team. The Expert Advisory Group on Cancer to the Chief Medical Officer report on cancer treatment has recommended that cancer treatment centres should be clearly identified and that these should include palliative care.[29]

Hospital inpatient beds

Palliative or terminal care may occur in hospitals for patients who, during their illness have reached the terminal phase of their illness or have been admitted for acute episodes with the possibility of it being the terminal stage and are now comfortable with the hospital as their choice for place of care, and are familiar with the environment and staff. 50% of patients with cancer die in hospital (Table 9).

Table 9: Place of death in 1991 of patients who were identified has having a terminal or palliative period[37-40]

Place of death	Cancer deaths (n = 2074) (%)	Non-cancer deaths (n = 1622) (%)
Home	29	22
Hospital	50	57
Hospice	13	0
Nursing/residential home	7	16
Ambulance/street	0	5

Hospital palliative care teams

These are one form of special palliative care team (see page 204), although in some hospitals there may be only one nurse providing support. This nurse will usually liaise with a community team if patients are discharged. There are now over 250 hospitals in the UK with support teams or support nurses (Appendix V).[17,62]

Hospice

Hospices provide a variety of services including day support, home support teams, night nursing, inpatient units, pain clinics, counselling and training. They admit patients for symptom relief and control, respite and terminal care if the family or patient cannot manage at home.

The Hospice Information Service in 1995 identified 208 units with 3182 beds with various sources of funding,[17,62] (Table 10 and Appendix V). The number of beds in an inpatient hospice unit varied from 2–62.

Table 10: Number and type of inpatient hospice and specialist palliative care services, as of January 1995[17]

Type of inpatient unit	Number of units	Number of beds
Independent or voluntary	142	2196
NHS managed units	46	533
Marie Curie cancer care centres	11	290
Sue Ryder homes	9	163
Total	208	3182

Of cancer deaths Addington-Hall *et al.* showed that in 1991 19% were admitted to a hospice during some part of the last year of life; 13% died in a hospice.[37-40] A survey conducted by the Hospice Information Service in 1994 suggested that in the UK approximately 28 000 deaths occurred in a hospice.[45] The majority would be cancer patients, so this could represent up to 18% of the 160 000 annual cancer deaths.[45]

Nursing homes and residential homes

Nursing homes and residential homes provide intermittent or continuous respite and continuing care. The NHS tends to take responsibility for individuals who have high nursing needs, while social services combined with the individual take responsibility for others. Many patients already in nursing or residential homes will eventually die there. Nursing homes do not have the specialist facilities of hospices or palliative care teams. Support teams can work with nursing and residential homes (as they work with hospitals or in patients' own homes) to assist and advise in the care of patients who need palliative care.

Other professional services

Pain clinics

These offer pain control and support and are usually run by anaesthetists based in hospitals. The patients are seen in outpatient departments. In 1994 there were over 200 pain clinics operating in the UK.[63] Almost all clinics will accept referrals of malignant pain and chronic pain. A directory of pain clinics was published by the College of Health,[63] and an up-to-date list is available from the Pain Society, British and Irish Chapter of the International Association for the Study of Pain. Pain clinics vary, some being comprehensively staffed and others being very small. Not all clinics will accept GP referrals, some only accept hospital or consultant referrals. Some individuals suggest that the number of patients with cancer pain seen in pain clinics has been reducing in recent years while the number seen with non-malignant pain has increased. This change has sometimes been attributed to the growth of specialist palliative care services for cancer patients (personal communications).

Most districts have dieticians, physiotherapists and occupational therapists who will offer some support for patients dying from cancer although the liaison with the specialist services is varied.

Spiritual and other support

This can be provided by:

- chaplains or other religious leaders, who may work in hospitals, hospices and/or in the local community
- support and information groups and voluntary support organizations run in local hospitals, hospices or palliative care teams by local groups of charities such as Cancer Link. Palliative care teams and hospices have information on most groups being organized locally.

A most useful source of information on local services or contacts is available from the St Christopher's Hospice Information Service (including a directory of services in the UK and Republic of Ireland and information on hospices and services abroad) and the National Council for Hospices and Specialist Palliative Care Services. Leaflets and advice are also available from the BACUP (British Association of Cancer United Patients). Help the Hospices offers education and research support for palliative services or staff and can provide advice.

Other psychological support and alternative therapies are sometimes available such as: aromatherapists, manicurists, beauticians and hairdressers.

Family bereavement support

This is varied and can be provided by:

- social workers – via social services or specialist palliative services and hospices. Social workers are also found in some hospitals
- hospices, support teams who may offer individual support and counselling, organize groups for bereavement and post-bereavement support, or self-help groups
- CRUSE and BACUP are voluntary organizations that also offer support nationally.

Cancer diagnosis specific services

Other care is available from the list below, although this is not confined to palliative patients.

- Clinical nurse specialists e.g. pressure care, continence promotion, nebulizer, Hickman Line nurses for all cancers, chest nurse for cancer of lung, trachea or bronchus and stoma nurse for digestive tract cancer.
- Counsellors for specific groups of patients e.g. mastectomy/breast cancer counsellors for women with breast cancer.

Patients with progressive non-malignant diseases

Very similar services apply for cancer patients as for patients with progressive non-malignant disease although there is less information available. Therefore this section concentrates on the main differences in services.

- **Primary health care** This is used by almost all people with non-cancer in the last year of life (Table 8). Contact is often slightly less than that for cancer patients.
- **Other community services** Services are available in most districts and estimates of use suggested these are used by a higher percentage of non-cancer patients, compared to cancer patients (Table 8).
- **Home and hospital specialist services** Some palliative care teams will accept referrals of patients who do not have cancer. However only a very small proportion of patients are referred to such services (Table 8 shows use in the last year of life) A few teams have a stated policy of accepting all patients but even in these teams the majority of referrals continues to be of cancer patients, with up to 30% of referrals of non-cancer patients.[47,48]
- **Hospital services** Hospital acute ward beds and hospital inpatient beds are important, because about 60% of patients with non-cancer die as hospital inpatients nationally (Table 9).
- **Hospices** 62% of hospices will accept patients who do not have cancer but require palliative care.[62] Reports suggest that hospices are used by very few people who do not have cancer (Tables 8 and 9).
- **Nursing homes** These are increasingly common as a place of care and death in the last year of life, especially among elderly and frail patients (Table 9).
- **Pain clinics** These play an increasing role in the care of patients with advanced non-malignant diseases for pain control and support.
- **Other psychological support and alternative therapies** For example aromatherapists, manicurists, beauticians and hairdressers are available in many hospices and occasionally in hospitals or long-term care facilities.

Additional services for non-cancer patients

The following additional services are available to people with specific non-cancer terminal illnesses. Most are not confined to people who need palliative care.

Hereditary degenerative disorder

For example muscular dystrophy.

- genetic counselling support and information services
- family support groups and support and information groups – voluntary.

Dementia

- community care assistants
- sitting services for respite for carers
- domiciliary home services including mental health teams for elderly people, Admiral nurses (funded by the charity Dementia Relief and working to support the family), community psychiatric nurses
- home help daily personal care with: hygiene, eating, pensions, shopping, cleaning
- incontinence laundry service – social services
- special beds in nursing homes
- hospital wards for people with dementia. Many long stay wards seek to provide homely care in small units. There is at least one hospital which has converted a house and developed a 'hospice like' model of care for people with dementia. However this is the exception
- voluntary support and information groups and associations for carers and for people with dementia
- charities such as the Alzheimer's Disease Society and the Mental Health Foundation provide information, have support groups in some areas and support research
- co-ordinators to inform carers of services that are available and how to access them.

Circulatory disease

- support and information groups in some areas
- advice and leaflets, plus support groups in some areas via the British Heart Foundation or via stroke groups.

Cystic fibrosis

- specialist community nursing service enabling a family to care for their child at home in the terminal phase of their illness
- hospices for children accept this condition. There are few hospices for children (page 209)
- cystic fibrosis physiotherapists
- genetic advice for cystic fibrosis
- parental and family support, information and counselling, including bereavement counselling are available in some districts.

Motor neurone disease and multiple sclerosis

- hospices – almost all hospices will admit people with motor neurone disease and multiple sclerosis if they have far advanced disease or for respite care
- there are special support groups and associations for people with motor neurone disease and multiple sclerosis and their families available from the voluntary sector.

Services for people with HIV/AIDS

Existing social and health services are available together with some of the services described for patients with cancer. Services specializing in support for people with HIV/AIDS can be found, particularly in high prevalence areas. These include the following.

- **Other community services** Advocacy workers, voluntary services including Buddy schemes, Terrence Higgins Trust and volunteers organized from local groups or hospices.
- **Specialist services** These may be:
  a) special AIDS teams – multi-professional teams similar to the home support team for cancer patients which may care for people with AIDS are found in areas where AIDS is most common e.g. London districts
  b) home support teams for cancer patients which may care for people with AIDS/HIV
  c) clinical nurse specialists who are found in many districts, especially where AIDS/HIV is common. They offer advice for patients with HIV/AIDS at all stages of the illness.
- **Hospital services** Beds reserved for people with AIDS.
- **Hospices** Many hospices will accept people with HIV or AIDS, although in some instances only when the person has a cancer-like illness. Inpatient and day care services specifically for people with HIV/AIDS are found especially in places where HIV/AIDS is common, for example in the London area, London Lighthouse, Mildmay Mission Hospital and, offering residential care for people with HIV/AIDS related encephalopathy, Patrick House.

Terminal illnesses in children

Children with terminal illnesses and their families receive the following additional services in some areas.

Mobile specialist services

Specialist community nursing service can enable families to care for their child at home in the terminal phase of their illness. Many of the teams caring for adults will care for children, but there are a few specialist teams which deal only with children from children's hospitals, e.g. Gt Ormand Street, London.

Hospice/inpatient

Children's hospices are available in a few areas. The Association for Children with Life Threatening or Terminal Conditions and their Families (ACT) lists eight established and ten planned hospices for children in England. The established hospices are:

- Acorns, Birmingham (ten beds)
- Derian House, Rochester, Lancashire (nine beds)
- Francis House, Manchester (seven beds)
- Helen House, Oxford (eight beds)
- Martin House, Wetherby, West Yorkshire (nine beds)
- Quidenham Children's Hospice, Norfolk (six beds)
- Rainbows Children's Hospice, Loughborough, Leicestershire (eight beds)
- Children's Hospice, Milton, Cambridgeshire (12 beds).

Those planned are:

- Hope House, Oswestry, Shropshire
- Children's Hospice Association Scotland, Edinburgh
- Children's Hospice South West, Barnstaple, Devon
- Claire House, Liverpool, Merseyside
- Demelza House, Rochester, Kent
- Little Haven, Southend-on-Sea, Essex
- Rainbow House, Walsall
- Richard House Appeal, Canning Town, London
- Ty Hafan Appeal, Barry, Glamorgan
- Wessex Children's Hospice Trust.

In addition to inpatient care most of the hospices offer home care services, hospice at home, day care and/or respite care.

Other professional services

Other professional services may include psychosocial support from clinical psychologists and social workers, specialist paediatric oncology nurses to improve communication between patient and family and patient and health care workers.

Charities

Charities such as Dreams Come True and the Starlight Foundation provide special treats and holidays for terminally ill children.

6 Effectiveness and cost-effectiveness of therapies and services

This section reviews the effectiveness and cost-effectiveness of therapies and services used in palliative care. Following the guidelines for these needs assessments of Stevens and Raftery[21] the quality of the evidence and strength of recommendation for each procedure are graded (see Appendix VI for grades).

Effectiveness in palliative care is judged in terms of the quality of life before dying, quality of life at the time of dying, a 'good death' and the impact on the family or carers. These can include elements such as the control of pain and symptoms, relief of psychosocial or emotional problems for the patient or family, subsequent resolution of grief and in some cases the achievement of particular wishes, such as developing a new interest or activity.

Efficacy and cost-effectiveness of individual therapies and treatments

There is a large body of work which assesses the efficacy of drug therapies and interventions in these patients (for detailed reviews and summaries, see many of the available textbooks, including *The Management of Terminal Malignant Disease*[3] and the *Oxford Textbook of Palliative Medicine*[64]). It is not appropriate to describe this in detail, but some of the common recommendations follow.

Pain and symptom control

The management of pain requires a detailed assessment.[3,64] There are many different types of pain. Evidence has demonstrated that, in particular, cancer patients will have several different pains, each with a different cause.[65] The prevalence of and the ability to control the pain is related to its aetiology.[66] The World Health Organization (WHO) has recommended a regimen for the treatment of morphine-sensitive pain, which advocates that drugs should be given a) orally, b) regularly according to the half-life of the drug and c) following the WHO analgesic 'ladder', which moves from non-opioid (morphine-like) drugs to weak opioids to strong opioids.[67–68]

Quality of the evidence is (I) – large multicentre and randomized controlled trials have demonstrated that cancer pain can be controlled in the majority of patients,[3,64,67–71] strength of recommendation (A). Improvements in the use of the analgesic ladder and its use for different types of pain is being further researched.

There is good evidence that there are also types of pain that are only partially (or not at all) responsive to morphine.[67–72] These include pains due to the spread of the cancer to the bone, and pains due to destruction of nerve tissue. There are many other adjuvant therapies for these particular types of pain including non-steroid anti-inflammatory drugs, steroids, anticonvulsant, antispasmodic, anti-arrhythmic and anti-depressant drugs.[68–73] Radiotherapy, surgery, neural blockade and other physical measures (e.g. transcutaneous nerve stimulation, acupuncture) and psychosocial interventions also may have a role. Evaluations of these therapies are under way and reviews of effectiveness of treatments such as non-steroidal anti-inflammatory drugs are available.[73] Therefore the management of pain in terminal illness is complex and in a proportion of patients requires specialized assessment.[68,72] This area remains under investigation. However quality of the evidence for the use of adjuvants, if indicated, is (II-1) and given the need to control symptoms, if the WHO ladder is insufficient, the strength of recommendation is (A). Specialist advice may be needed to ensure that up-to-date treatments are given. The National Council for Hospice and Specialist Palliative Care Services has recently published straightforward clinical guidelines for pain control in palliative care.[68]

The control of other symptoms is similarly complex and often requires specialized knowledge. Evaluations of the drug therapies and interventions is fairly well established and comprehensive reviews of their efficacy are available.[74–77]

The delivery system of drugs has been revolutionized during the last decade and in particular studies it has been shown that the delivery of some analgesics and anti-emetics (anti-sickness) drugs subcutaneously using a battery-operated pump[66,78] has enabled people to be cared for at home when otherwise they might require hospital treatment. The most notable example of this is the management of patients with gastro-intestinal obstruction where it was demonstrated that this simple treatment was as effective and often better than the previous treatment, which involved inserting a naso-gastric tube and removing the contents of the stomach by suction, and inserting an intravenous line and providing fluids by that route.[79,80] Quality of the evidence is (II-2 and II-3), patients can be involved in the choice of delivery system and the evidence of the efficacy of the drugs is (I) as above. Therefore strength of recommendation is (A).

Few studies have compared the costs of these recommended treatments. There are two possible reasons for this. First the control of symptoms is often considered to be an essential requirement in care. Second many of the therapies, for example morphine, diamorphine or delivery systems with battery-operated syringe drivers, are relatively inexpensive, especially if compared with an extended inpatient stay due to uncontrolled symptoms. These therapies are also in line with moves towards 'appropriate technologies' as suggested by the WHO in their primary health care programme,[81] in that the treatments and technologies are relatively cheap, simple and can be used away from the hospital.

Emotional support and communication

Emotional support is a common desire by some patients and their families and communication is one of the most common concerns expressed by patients and families. There have been frequent complaints that doctors and nurses do not provide sufficient information about the diagnosis and are not well skilled at talking to patients and families.[44,82-85] There is some evidence (quality II-2 and II-3) that hospices and specialist palliative care services are successful in meeting emotional needs (page 213). In 1985 Lunt demonstrated that two hospices met emotional needs as well as those concerning anxiety, depression and physical symptoms better than a district general hospital.[86]

Co-ordination

Co-ordination is also a frequent concern; many patients and families complain of poor co-ordination of services. There are various ways of addressing this problem, and often Macmillan or support team nurses have a significant role in co-ordinating services. There is some evidence (quality = II-2 and II-3) that they are successful in this role.[43,86]

However the model of an extra independent co-ordinating service was not found helpful in one randomized controlled trial. Two co-ordinating nurses did not appear to have any benefits over and above existing conventional and specialized palliative care services.[87] Therefore there is fair evidence not to utilize this type of 'special' co-ordinating service (level D).

Bereavement

Bereavement and grief for carers is known to be a risk factor for increased mortality and ill health, particularly among elderly men.[88] Risk assessment tools to identify those patients at highest risk of prolonged grief are available[89] and there is some evidence that such support is welcomed by bereaved relatives, but this is patchy. (Quality of evidence = II-2, II-3 and III, strength of recommendation B.) However, the proportion of families requiring bereavement follow-up is currently disputed[89] and bereavement support is known to vary greatly.[90]

Effectiveness of conventional care

During the 1970s and 1980s many studies demonstrated deficiencies in conventional care for dying people both in hospitals and the community. Dying patients suffered severe unrelieved symptoms particularly pain, had unmet practical, social and emotional needs and suffered as the result of poor co-ordination of services and because health professionals appeared unwilling to share information.[91-94] In hospital staff were observed to withdraw from patients and to pay little attention to their symptoms, emotional needs or needs for care.[94]

Their families also suffered because of poor communication by health professionals and had unmet needs for emotional, practical and bereavement support.[84-86,93,95,96] Cancer patients were found to have depression and anxiety more commonly than in the 'normal' population, while their families also were at risk of developing social and psychiatric problems.[97]

Attention shifted to home care when further work emphasized the increased severity of many problems while the patient was at home, where the patient spent most of their time.[98,99] Also studies have estimated that 50-70% of cancer patients would prefer to be cared for or to die at home.[100,101] A longitudinal study of patients in the care of a domiciliary palliative care team suggested that as death approached patients changed their preferences: hospital and home became less preferred and hospice more preferred, although even one week before death 50% still wished to be cared for at home.[102] However far fewer achieve this and the number of people who die at home has fallen in recent years (from 42% in 1969 to 24% in 1987).[8] 29% of cancer deaths included in the Regional Study of Care for the Dying (RSCD) by Addington-Hall et al. died at home.[40] The RSCD, which examined care in the last year of life for random samples of cancer and non-cancer deaths, demonstrated continued problems of unrelieved pain and other symptoms and that relatives bore the brunt of caring.[40]

Therefore the quality of evidence that conventional care alone failed to meet the needs of many patients and families was strong (quality of evidence = II-1, II-2, II-3 and III) and there is poor evidence to support the use of conventional care alone (level D).

Effectiveness and cost-effectiveness of specialist palliative services compared with conventional care

Hospices and specialist palliative teams were developed to try and fill the deficiencies described in conventional services. However there are very few randomized controlled trials of these services. Evidence for the different services is summarized as follows.

Inpatient hospices

Controlled and comparative studies of inpatient hospices versus other forms of inpatient care have suggested that the hospice model is at least as effective as conventional models of care in terms of the management of pain and symptoms. In some instances it has shown benefits in terms of symptom control, anxiety, depression and bereavement outcome and it has nearly always shown benefits in terms of patient and family satisfaction with care. Quality of evidence ranges from I – but note that the randomized controlled and multi-centre trials were in North America and have not been repeated in the UK – to III. Most of the services evaluated accepted exclusively or mainly cancer patients. Therefore, the strength of recommendation is (B/A), for reviews of studies see.[2,94,103–114] Multi-centre studies of the effectiveness and costs of inpatient hospices, especially in the care of patients with progressive non-malignant diseases are needed.

There is also evidence that hospices use a higher number of nursing staff per patient than conventional care, but use fewer invasive therapeutic procedures and investigations.[101,105,115] The costs of inpatient hospice care versus conventional care suggest that hospice care is similar to or cheaper than conventional care.[94,106,116,117] However all but one of these studies are from North America, which has a very different health system compared with the UK. There is little information on comparison costs in the UK. Because when setting contracts with voluntary hospices the NHS does not have to cover the full costs, while this arrangement continues voluntary hospices can represent very good value for NHS commissioners. The costs of inpatient hospice care vary considerably from hospice to hospice. Hill and Oliver[118,119] demonstrated that very small hospices had higher costs, but also a higher throughput when compared with larger hospices. They recommended that the optimal size of a hospice, in general, was 15 beds or larger.

Hospices do vary considerably in their activity, types of staffing and procedures undertaken.[120–122] Organizational standards have been developed by various bodies including the Royal College of Physicians[123] by a Delphi exercise of participating experts,[124] NAHAT,[26] the Royal College of Nursing[125] and by the Cancer Relief Macmillan Fund, which later became an organizational audit programme.[126] These include guidelines on the nature and training of hospice doctors and nurses, and the environment and nature of services. They are based on the opinions of those experts on the panels and some aspects of all the standards agree – e.g. use of staff trained in specialist palliative care etc. However, they are rarely well referenced and their use has not been evaluated. Therefore the quality of evidence for these organizational standards is III. Research is needed to compare the effects of different hospices, before details of the most effective structure of care delivery is known.

Specialist palliative care teams and specialist advice

A wide range of different structures and processes of specialist palliative care teams has developed. Teams commonly work most closely with or within the NHS, offering shared care, advice and support by working alongside GPs and hospital staff. Teams were often originally planned by district health authorities either independently or in conjunction with the charity the Cancer Relief Macmillan Fund, which pump-primed posts, providing the trust and/or district health authority took over funding after three to five years.[7] However a 'team' can vary in size from one nurse to 11 nurses and may have doctors, social workers and in some cases a chaplain, occupational therapist, physiotherapist, psychologist, dietician, administrator or secretary.[7] Catchment populations have been found to range from 43 000 to 500 000 per 'team', with variations in the nurse caseload from 11 to 57 current patients per nurse.[7,127] One team may offer both home care and hospital support. Teams usually confine their remit to advice and emotional support and the nursing members do not provide 'hands on' nursing care: this is carried out by existing services.

Some of the larger, multi-professional home care teams have been evaluated in randomized controlled trials and various other comparative studies. The home care teams were able to demonstrate their ability to keep patients at home for longer than when such services did not exist. They also resulted in lower costs to the health service (between 18% to eight times lower costs than inpatient care) and in equivocal or improved pain control,[2,43,106–107,109–111,116,117,128–137] except for one comparative study which suggested that relatives reported more pain in patients kept at home compared with those in hospital.[99] Much of the cost data are from North America rather than the UK. All studies showed higher patient satisfaction in home care teams compared to conventional care.[2,85,99,129,131,135] A study comparing patient satisfaction with home care teams, GPs and hospital services demonstrated that patients were more satisfied with the home care team than with their GP and district nurses and least satisfied with the hospital service.[85]

Therefore there is strong evidence that adding a multi-professional support team can provide a higher quality care than conventional care alone: quality of evidence = I (note again the randomized controlled trials were in North America and not in the UK), II-1, II-2, II-3 and III. Some of the services did care for patients with progressive non-malignant diseases, and in one cost-effectiveness study for HIV/AIDS.[137] There is good evidence to support its use (level A).

Studies which compare the different types of teams, for example larger multi-professional teams with smaller teams comprising only nurses are not available. One study has reported better symptom control for a team approach comprising GP, district nurse and specialist palliative nurse, compared to GPs operating alone.[138] Otherwise, the nurse-only teams have not been rigorously evaluated.

Harper *et al.* showed that a consensus of palliative care doctors and nurses favoured multi-professional teams rather than nurse-only teams.[124] Other reports have also recommended a multi-professional approach.[68,123,126]

Hospital support services

The evaluation of hospital support teams is less well evolved than that of other services. However there have been a few studies that have demonstrated the effectiveness of the service in terms of its ability to assist in the control of symptoms and have reported that patients and families have benefited from the service.[36,43,47,139] Again the evaluations have mainly considered the larger multi-professional teams rather than single-handed nurses. (Quality of evidence = II-3 and III, strength of recommendation B, although further research is needed.)

Day care

Day care has been largely unevaluated and varies considerably throughout the country. It can be offered as part of an inpatient hospice service or associated with a home care team, or both. Research into the effectiveness, appropriateness and costs of day care is urgently needed before further growth occurs.

Practical support and respite care

There is also some evidence to demonstrate that practical and respite support is needed by patients and carers and the provision of this is patchy throughout the country. In 1991 Addington-Hall and colleagues advocated the transfer of funds from acute hospital services to community-based services.[44] The provision of practical and respite support for palliative carers remains largely unresolved.[140,141] Such support is not usually provided by mobile support teams. There is also anecdotal evidence that many 'respite' admissions to hospices are too late in the course of illness and carry a distinct mortality

In some instances, the provision of respite care is met by inpatient hospices but the provision of practical support at home is an issue for many patients and families. To assist this, in many areas hospices also run teams of volunteers to provide an additional sitting service, as does the Marie Curie Cancer Care Service. Evaluation of a relative support team, which was part funded by Marie Curie Cancer Care showed high satisfaction among relatives.[142]

Hospice at home

A new model of care has developed recently which seeks to combine the specialist advice of specialist palliative care services (which do not usually provide hands-on nursing care), existing district nursing services and practical support, in terms of nursing, sitting and basic care, at home.[143] The care offered is very like that of hospital at home,[144] but with specialist palliative support from the local hospice or home care team added. This service is usually called hospice at home, but note that two services which operate in a similar way to home care support teams and do not offer practical nursing care at home, have already called themselves hospice at home.

Hospital at home was shown to benefit terminally ill patients in a comparative trial.[144] Therefore this development of hospice at home appears promising. At least two pilot schemes are under way and are in the process of evaluation. One scheme was developed in an area where there was no existing night or day sitting/nursing service generally available. It was specifically geared towards patients with advanced HIV/AIDS where Marie Curie nurses could not be used. Early data from this scheme, which was led by a consultant in palliative medicine, suggested that the proportion of patients cared for at home was increased and that symptoms were controlled. A more detailed evaluation is planned.[143]

Social variations

Eight-fold differences in the proportions of cancer patients dying at home have been found between areas of high and low deprivation, suggesting that this has an impact on care.[145]

Services for patients with progressive non-malignant diseases and HIV/AIDS

Studies which demonstrated failings in conventional care included cancer and non-cancer patients. Patients also appear to have a poorer quality of care if they are of lower social class.[146] However there is little evaluation of new services for patients with progressive non-malignant diseases. This may be partly because specialist care for these patients is rare and partly because the teaching and textbooks which consider the care for patients with these diseases frequently omit the palliative aspects. A randomized controlled trial of a mobile palliative care team demonstrated benefits for elderly patients, whatever their condition.[128] The evaluation of the hospital teams has also assessed the care of non-cancer patients.[47] Severs and Wilkins described how they were able to convert part of a ward caring for elderly people into one which provided inpatient palliative care and successfully cared for elderly people, where 79% had cancers and 21% other diseases.[48] (Quality of evidence = I and III.) Expansion of home care teams to include more patients with non-cancer diagnoses has shown increased cost savings.[147]

Evaluations have also demonstrated that the model of hospice and home support can be successfully transferred to care for patients with HIV/AIDS, although some symptoms are more common or have different presentations.[136,137,148–150] General practitioners have also indicated that they would like extra support and advice for terminally ill patients with all diseases,[151–155] although studies have found that some GPs were unaware of the local services available or did not know how to refer to a palliative service.[154]

What proportion of patients and families experience a palliative period, with what characteristics and nature of problems that would benefit most from these types of service needs further study.

Services for children

Many of the specialist palliative care teams and hospital support teams described will care for children and their families.[17,62] However the numbers of children cared for are small and no evaluations are available. Descriptive studies of hospices are available but these do not include an evaluative component. Evaluation is made difficult by the small numbers of children cared for. Hospices for children are subject to much debate, and experts disagree on whether such services should be supported.[156,157] Research into the needs of children and their families and the effectiveness of models of care is needed.

Key issues

For a health authority considering the data on effectiveness key issues in relation to their services would be as follow.

- Strength of recommendations for multi-disciplinary palliative home care teams is A and for inpatient hospices is B/A. The recommendation for hospital teams is B. Conventional care alone within a district is inadequate.

     Do the methods of staffing, size and methods of working of the specialist palliative services concord with those types of services which have been demonstrated to be effective, cost-effective and efficient? Other specialist palliative care developments need to be evaluated as they are introduced.
- Are the services offering a multi-professional approach, as is generally recommended?
- Are there mechanisms for co-ordination of care between NHS, voluntary and social services – is this carried out by palliative care teams, do they work and can they be improved – given that this is often considered to be one of the major problems for patients and families nationally?
- Given that many patients will not be cared for in specialist palliative settings, what are the systems for educating and insuring staff are sufficiently trained in the palliative aspects of care such as the correct range of techniques for pain and symptom control, emotional support, staff with good communication skills and bereavement care?
- Given that many more patients wish to be cared for at home or to die at home than currently achieve this, what alteration in mix of services would be needed to increase the proportion of people who can be offered palliative care at home?

7 Models of care

This section sets out models of palliative provision which are indicated by the previous sections on prevalence, incidence, effectiveness and service provision. A range of levels of service provision is given – these levels will depend on the components included.

Cancer patients

A cost-effective programme for palliative care would include the following.

- Multi-professional home care and hospital support for 25–60% of cancer deaths.
- Inpatient hospice care for approximately 15–30% of cancer deaths. Very small units, i.e. less than 10–15 beds, should be avoided if possible because of their higher costs when compared with larger hospices. The nature of the service provided by the hospice should be multi-professional, with a high nurse–patient ratio and medical staff trained in palliative medicine, as suggested by the current standards. (This may need to be amended when better data of the most effective structure of care are available.)
- An education programme and quality standards for hospital and community staff who care for patients with advanced cancer – including symptom control, communication, patient and family referral and information on appropriate services.
- Quality standards which would probably include the development of clinical protocols for the management and referral, where appropriate, of patients and families with particular problems or symptoms. Protocols for symptoms and pathologies would be based on therapies which have known efficacy.
- Local systems which should be developed to provide hospital and community staff with information about the palliative services available locally. Each district may have knowledge about the systems which will work best, but in some areas GPs have complained about excessive distribution of paper. In these cases a small, short 'placemat' of services would be appropriate.[158] Other districts have found short directories were useful.[159]
- Developments in day care, hospice at home or additional home support may be needed locally, especially if districts wish to increase the proportion of patients cared for at home. However these should only occur as part of evaluative studies, preferably comparative studies, which include details of costs. Also the multi-professional home care and hospital support and inpatient hospice care might effectively be expanded, but if this occurs development should be evaluated to determine the costs, numbers of patients cared for and effects, including the impact on acute hospital care.
- Audit and monitoring of the outcomes of care in all settings.
- Quality standards agreed between purchasers and providers would be needed to ensure the integration of services and good co-ordination across all sectors.

Patients with other diseases

- Existing specialist palliative care services should be encouraged to take patients who have diseases other than cancer which require palliative care, up to one-third or one-half of their workload. Their involvement should be audited and evaluated.
- Education, training and quality standards should be developed for all settings where palliative care is needed and these should be monitored through audit. These might include the development of clinical protocols for the management and referral, where appropriate, of patients and families with particular problems or symptoms, as above. Protocols would need more testing than that for cancer patients, above,

because there are less data on the efficacy of palliative treatments. All settings where palliative care occurs should be included in this (section 5). Note that an increasing proportion of patients remain in nursing, residential and warden aided homes until their death and that these settings too may need specialist palliative advice, support and training.

These services should be encouraged to call for specialist advice when caring for more complex patients and families.

- Other service developments, mechanisms for providing information about local services, audit and outcomes, should as much as possible be integrated into the existing arrangements for cancer patients. These should also include those services already caring for many non-cancer patients with advancing disease, as described in section 5.

Services for children

- The small numbers within many health districts and the lack of evaluative information suggest that districts should ensure that existing palliative support services, especially the mobile community teams, will include care, advice and support for children and their families.
- Specialist teams from tertiary referral centres, e.g. the Great Ormond Street Team, may be used to support and advise the local palliative care teams, if appropriate.
- Hospices for children should be developed only if these are part of a rigorous evaluation. Alternatively, it may be argued that the existing hospices for children require evaluation, along with a better assessment of children's and families' wishes for care, before any further developments are supported.

Different models

Having carried out the needs assessment, the options for a population might be as follow.

- To move towards increasing community support in palliative care, perhaps by increasing the input of specialist home care support teams or developing hospice at home models. This might be particularly appropriate in areas where few patients are able to be cared for at home. Note that any hospice at home development would need evaluation.
- To increase the inpatient hospice care. This might be a very attractive choice, if there are few patients currently cared for within hospices, particularly if there are local voluntary hospices where the health authority does not have to fund the full costs. There may be hospices with unused capacity, or they may wish to develop more hospice beds. Note, however, that this relationship would depend on the continued availability of voluntary funding. NHS hospices are likely to have similar costs to NHS hospitals and are often considered preferable; therefore NHS hospices may also be an attractive option for a health authority.
- To move away from providing specialist palliative care and try to incorporate this with all generic services. There is no research evidence to support such a move, nor is there evidence that without specialist palliative care services generic services improve by themselves.
- To increase the emphasis of the specialist palliative care services on education programmes. This might be an option for health authorities which already have a provision of specialist palliative care but which they feel is rather isolated from existing services and is not providing any educational input. This would also be an option for districts wishing to improve the care for patients who do not have cancer, without significantly increasing the resources to specialist palliative care services.
- To increase the hospital support through hospital palliative care teams. This may be an option for populations where there is no current hospital support and many patients are dying within hospitals.

Examples from other districts

Assessments of need from other districts and countries have included analysis of incidence and prevalence, but usually of only cancer patients, and analysis of local opinions, activity or trends.[46,158,160 162,170] In some instances districts have undertaken special surveys.[46,163–169] The study by Addington-Hall included 20 health districts, each of whom have been given local data, to provide them with better information on the characteristics and needs of patients and their families.[37–40,171] An example of a service specification from one district, which includes details of some of the quality aspects and their monitoring, is shown in Appendix VII.

A health authority may wish to determine how the estimates of incidence, prevalence of symptoms and likely numbers of patients needing care relate to local provision in terms of completed episodes, new referrals or spending on different services.

In 1990 Frankel[46] undertook a needs assessment for the Bristol area and concluded that approximately 50 inpatient hospice beds were required for a population of one million. This was based on the estimates of GPs and hospital staff on the number of patients with cancer who would require palliative care. Kensington & Chelsea and Westminster Health Authority undertook a survey of GPs, to obtain their views about the appropriate direction of palliative care and found that they were particularly concerned about the availability of 24-hour support.[154] A survey of district health authorities in England identified 67 which had planned or completed reviews of palliative care services.[170]

Further examples from the National Council for Hospice and Specialist Palliative Care Services

The National Council for Hospice and Specialist Palliative Care Services has produced guidance on setting contracts, describing services and assessing need. Although much of the information in this document is rather general it does contain examples of needs assessments and contracting experiences.[172] They have published further information for purchasers, to provide a background for available specialist palliative care services.[24] This provides an up-to-date and detailed description of the type of staff, services and modes of operating which are found and are recommended for specialist palliative care services.[24] This report is accompanied by another providing details of outcome measures[173] and their uses in palliative care, which expands on the following section of this chapter. They have also published a statement of definitions of specialist palliative care services.[22]

8 Outcome measures

Palliative care cannot be measured with commonly used outcome measures such as mortality or disability, but requires measurement of aspects which are important to patients with progressive disease and their families. It therefore deals with the quality of life, quality of death and dying and the bereavement outcome. Examples of the aspects of care within these three areas which might be measured by outcomes are shown in Box 1. Clearly outcomes may reflect positive or adverse events within the area of care; although most of the available outcome measures tend to measure the presence, absence or degree of problems, such as pain, anxiety, symptoms, rather than positive events such as fulfilment in life.

Box 1: Examples of aspects for outcome measurement in palliative care

General areas

- quality of life – all aspects, physical, emotional, social, spiritual
- quality of dying – all aspects as for quality of life including resolving last issues, planning
- bereavement outcome

Specific examples

- control of pain and symptoms
- relief of anxieties and fears for patient and family
- meet wishes for place of care and death (e.g. at home)
- meet needs for practical care, financial help
- patient and family feel that the communication and information given have been given as they would wish
- last wishes before death are met – e.g. meeting with estranged family
- satisfaction with care
- relief of depression
- lessened mortality and morbidity during bereavement

Quality of life measures or adaptations of these measures are often used to assess outcomes in palliative care. Early definitions of quality of life concentrated on physical function. Then these were extended to include symptoms of the disease, emotional and psychological functioning. Most recently aspects of social functioning, sexual needs and spiritual needs have been added.[174,175] Although the definition of quality of life currently lacks a consensus, the commonly identified domains include:[173-176]

- physical concerns (e.g. symptoms, pain, etc.)
- functional ability (activity, self-care)
- emotional well-being, psychological function
- social functioning
- occupational functioning
- spirituality
- sexuality (including body image)
- treatment satisfaction
- financial concerns
- future plans/orientation (hope, planning)
- family well-being – emotional and physical.

Measuring palliative care outcomes within other national outcomes initiatives

Some measures of outcome are being set nationally. One relevant to palliative care is pressure sores. The NHS Executive 1994/95 Planning Guidance stated that health authorities should ensure that contracts specify that providers record the incidence and prevalence of pressure sores 'differing between those acquired in hospital and others', and are 'encouraged to set annual targets for an overall reduction of at least 5% working from a baseline 1993/94 figures'. A guide on pressure sore measurement, risk assessment and management has been published[177] and these measures are being monitored in hospices throughout the country.

The results of this measurement need to be adjusted for the characteristics of patients receiving palliative care. Patients who are weak and close to the end of life are often at a high risk of developing pressure sores. Also it is difficult in such debilitated patients to know if they have a 'true' pressure sore, or if it is tumour eroding the skin. The results from some settings have shown that patients arrive in the hospice unit having already acquired pressure sores (personal communications). The management of pressure sores must also be viewed within the context of a patient's complete care and the distress caused by the pressure sore, rather than simply its size.

Some difficulties in outcome measurement in palliative care

Case-mix and attributability

The patients and families who receive palliative care are not a homogenous group but have different diagnoses and aetiologies of symptoms and problems which have varying prognoses. For example in many instances a patient's pain(s) are relatively easy to control, but some are not, especially neuropathic pains. Therefore where possible the results of outcome measurement need to be adjusted for case-mix – especially if these are likely to be different, e.g. in an inpatient hospice versus a hospital ward. Similarly it is difficult to be certain that the intervention affected the change in outcome, outside the context of a randomized controlled trial.

Accounting for individual wishes

Patients vary in their individual wishes for care while they are dying and these wishes may change over time, depending upon a person's experiences. For example, although many patients wish to die at home, a substantial proportion do not.[100 102] Although some patients wish for close communication with their family or for spiritual support when they are close to death, others do not.[3,82,83] Therefore when measuring outcomes it is important to try to ensure that these reflect the wishes of individual patients and families.[178] This is often not easy, especially with standard instruments which are designed for use in populations and when patients and families have different wishes or expectations.

Accounting for differences between patient, family and professional assessments and wishes

Patients, their family, professionals and external assessors have all been used to assess outcomes in different ways. The main advantages and drawbacks of using the different assessors are considered in detail elsewhere.[179] There is probably no ideal choice of assessor and it is best to choose who is most appropriate for the setting being considered and the way in which the outcomes will be used.

Measures which can be used to assess outcome

Outcome measures are being tested among patients and families who need palliative care. These include the Support Team Assessment Schedule[32,178,179] and the Edmonton Symptom Assessment System,[180] both of which were designed for the quick assessment of outcomes in clinical practice. The first of these was developed in the UK in community settings, the second was developed in Canada in inpatient settings. Both are now used in many countries and in both inpatient and community settings. Measures developed for research are also being tested and adapted for use as outcome measures. These include the measures of quality of life developed for cancer patients, such as the Rotterdam Symptom Checklist[181] and the European Organisation for Research into Quality of Life Instrument,[182] and psychosocial measures such as the Hospital Anxiety and Depression Scale.[183] Details of these measures are shown in Table 11.

Other approaches to assessing the quality of care

Other approaches to the assessment of the quality of palliative care have developed. They include the Cancer Relief Macmillan Fund Organisational Audit, which provides a method to examine the organizational structure in which palliative care is offered. This is described in detail elsewhere.[125] It provides a framework and programme of inspection which purchasers and providers may wish to examine or adapt to their own circumstances.[125] More sophisticated assessments of the process of care than simply assessing the number of visits could also be used. This might involve assessing the way that staff work with patients and families, their communication skills or observing the interactions which take place.[94] Some health authorities have monitored the percentage of patients who die at home as a very crude indicator.

9 Targets

Health gain targets can be developed to improve the control of pain and symptoms and the relief of anxieties, and service targets to ensure service delivery in these areas. Examples are shown below.

Health gain targets

Targets suitable for national monitoring

- The percentage of cancer patients who are cared for or die at home, in a hospice or specialist palliative care unit.
- The percentage of patients receiving specialized palliative care – including all settings: home, hospital, residential, hospice.

Local targets

- Increase the proportion of patients and families who report their pain and symptoms are controlled, or that symptoms do not affect them. (Note: the prevalence of symptoms may not be affected but the success of control and the degree to which symptoms affect the patient may be reduced.)
- Increase the proportion of patients and families who feel that communication from health staff has met their requirements.
- Increase the proportion of patients and families who are cared for in the place of their choice.
- Reduce the mortality and morbidity following bereavement.
- Increase the satisfaction of patients and families with the palliative care provided.

Table 11: Some outcome measures which have been used, or are proposed for use, in palliative care

Name and source	Number of items and domains included	How developed and setting	Comments on use
Rotterdam symptom checklist[131]	34 symptoms covering: physical and psychosocial problems, for the patient	Items identified from three studies – cancer patients undergoing chemotherapy or follow-up with early disease; cancer patients undergoing chemotherapy for advanced ovarian cancer; cancer patients who were disease free	Used widely. Different formats available. Shown to be valid and reliable. Assessments are completed by patients – therefore evidence of missing data in one half or more in patients close to death
Hebrew Rehabilitation Centre for Ageing – Quality of Life index (HRCA-QL)[107,108]	Five items covering: health, support, outlook, daily living and mobility	Adapted from a quality of life index developed by Spitzer – the item mobility replaced one called activity. Items were identified by consensus of patients, the general public and professionals and aimed to apply to patients with all stages of disease	Used in the largest US evaluation of hospice care – the US National Hospice Study. Designed for completion by professionals, although has been completed by patients. The original Spitzer's index was validated, but the adapted index was not revalidated. Criticized for a lack of responsiveness in patients with advanced disease
The Support Team Assessment Schedule (STAS)[32,178,179]	17 items covering: pain and symptoms, psychosocial, insight, family needs, planning affairs, communication, home services and support of other professionals	Collaboration with five palliative support teams and revised in light of presentations at professional meetings, observation of palliative care, interviews with patients and families. Now used in different settings	Used widely. Time to complete or one patient averages two minutes. Validated to ensure professional ratings reflect patient views. Reliable. Reliance on professionals' assessments may be a problem but, where possible, has been tested with patients completing the assessments directly. Testing use of individual items, expanding symptom assessment and database under way
Edmonton Symptom Assessment System[180]	Nine visual analogue scales: pain, activity, nausea, depression, anxiety, drowsiness, appetite, well-being, shortness of breath	By members of hospice service	Inpatient hospice. In use and being validated

Continued

Table 11: *Continued*

Name and source	Number of items and domains included	How developed and setting	Comments on use
European Organisation for Research and Treatment of Cancer QLQ-C30[182]	30 items – multi-items and single scales	International collaboration of professionals – to devise items and scales. Measure tested in the different countries. Tested before and during chemotherapy in lung cancer patients	Being tested widely, in settings other than where originally developed. Patient completed – 11 minutes to complete. Shown to distinguish between patients at different stages of disease and valid, and reliable in those settings originally developed
Palliative Care Core Standards[184]	Six standard statements and 56 process and outcome items: collaboration with other agencies, symptom control, patient/carer information, emotional support, bereavement care and support, specialist education/training	Regional collaboration of hospice and home care units Inpatient hospice and community teams	Standards and measures developed and planning a pilot audit study to evaluate and review the core standards and to determine the criteria for the standards usage
Regional study of care of the dying[37–40,171]	Questionnaire administered to the person who knows most about the patient, approximately seven months after their death. It assesses services received, symptoms during the last year of life, communication, satisfaction with care and mental status of the carer	Adapted from studies by Cartwright in 1967 and Cartwright and Seale in 1987	It builds on information collected 20 years ago and five years ago, so that patterns of care and symptoms can be compared The new study has interviewed the carers of 3500 people who died in 20 districts in England
Short Form-36 (SF-36)[185,186]	36 items assessing bodily pain, self-reported general health, mental health, limitations, energy, social functioning, change in health in last year (this last item is not a core domain and the time period can vary)	Is one of several health status questionnaires developed in the US by the Medical Outcomes Study (MOS). This is a 36-item short form of a longer questionnaire. Developed to assess the outcomes of hospital care in the US. Designed for patients at all stages of disease – from completely well to those with symptoms	Becoming very widely used. English (not American) version now available. Very quick to complete – a few minutes. This is its main advantage over other general (generic) measures such as the Nottingham Health Profile. The validity, reliability and responsiveness are often well regarded but the measure is undergoing further testing. Not yet tested in patients with advanced disease but has been tested in elderly patients and seems to be of most use to assess populations. Caution urged when trying to assess therapies or services

Continued

Table 11: *Continued*

Name and source	Number of items and domains included	How developed and setting	Comments on use
Hospital Anxiety and Depression scale (HAD)[41,183]	14 items – divided into two subscales; seven items to assess anxiety and seven to assess depression	Developed for patient completion in sick populations, translated into several languages. Validated against other scales	Described as quick and easy to use. Used widely in cancer patients but its use in palliative care is still being tested
Karnofsky index[187]	Single item of mobility and functioning rated 0–100	Developed for completion by professional to assess chemotherapy	Limited because it only assesses functioning. Widely used in clinical records to give a quick indication of how sick a patient is. Shortened version – scored 0–5 – is available as European alternative
McGill pain questionnaire[188]	Pain is assessed by the patient ratings of the severity of a series of descriptors (e.g. throbbing)	Developed for completion by patients. At least five versions of the index are available – ranging from short form (15 descriptors) to longest version (128 descriptors)	Assesses only pain, not other aspects. Self-completion and verbal versions are available, although the originator recommended the verbal form. Good test–retest reliability
Standards of care for palliative nursing[25]	Seven topics – symptom control, spiritual support, family care, bereavement care, multi-professional team, ethical practice and staff support, each with structure, process and outcome criteria	Developed by a working group of the Royal College of Nursing which included five senior nurses for various settings. Standards follow the principles of the Dynamic Standard Setting System. Designed for a wide range of settings	This is the second revision of an earlier document. Standards can be adapted for local use. Like the Palliative Care Core Standards outcome criteria are given, but not ways to measure these. Such measures would need to be developed

Note: Other measures are available. See refs[173,189–190] for reviews of measures in palliative care and/or cancer care and refs[174,191–194] for reviews of measures in general.

Baseline data, to enable the monitoring of these targets, are usually lacking. The most important targets, e.g. controlling pain and symptoms or meeting communication needs, are the most difficult to monitor. However baselines could be established locally, through audit and outcomes projects and then monitored. Information on place of death is available routinely and this can be monitored. Note however that there is evidence that place of death is associated by social factors such as deprivation: in underprivileged areas fewer patients die at home compared with areas of higher privilege.[145] Therefore any targets which were monitored would need careful interpretation.

Service targets

More detailed examples of service targets can be found in the example service specification (Appendix VII). However targets for services could be as follow.

- To ensure that clinicians communicate effectively with patients, families and colleagues in relation to:
  a) pain and symptoms
  b) treatment regimens
  c) diagnosis
  d) follow-up and arrangements for care
  e) services available
  f) psychosocial problems and care available.
- To ensure that clinical protocols are developed, applied and audited in the management of patients with advanced progressive disease, including the use of therapies and mechanisms for referral for specialist advice.
- To ensure that health care professionals undertake and apply basic training in palliative care.
- That there is a multi-professional approach among specialist palliative care services.
- That services provide care suited to patients' individual cultural and ethnic needs. (Note there is evidence that the needs of patients from different ethnic groups may differ.[187,188,195,196]) Patients and families experience a range of emotional stages.[197]
- That non-cancer patients to be accepted by specialist palliative care services.

Process targets

- Full awareness among all GPs and relevant hospital staff of how to refer to palliative care services, and knowledge of the services available.
- Increase in the proportion of appropriately timed referrals for specialist palliative care.
- Increase in the proportion of patients being cared for at home and dying at home.

These targets may be monitored through the service specifications or clinical audit, providing that clinicians as well as managers are fully signed up to them.

10 Research and information priorities

Priorities for further research

Main priorities, where research information is lacking, are as follow.

- Comparison of models of care, including different models of specialist palliative care, to determine:
  a) the most effective and cost-effective structure and process of care
  b) at what stage and for which patients and families specialist care is most effective.
- Evaluation of hospice at home and day care in terms of impact and cost-effectiveness.
- Evaluation of models of palliative care and treatment for non-cancer patients in terms of impact and cost-effectiveness.
- Comparison of different potential outcome measures of palliative care, in terms of their validity, reliability, responsiveness to clinical change, appropriateness and cost implications of their use.
- Evaluation of palliative care services for children and their families.
- Assessment of the needs of people from different backgrounds, cultural situations and ethnic groups.

Evaluations should ensure that appropriate outcome measures are used to assess effectiveness. Cost-effectiveness studies are particularly needed. Past studies have been criticized for weaknesses in these areas.[2,198]

Information priorities

- Nationally, for OPCS – the recording of hospice as a place of death should be included as a separate category. Coders could be provided with details and listings, for example from the St Christopher's Hospice Directory. This would allow study of the trends of hospice as a place of death.
- Nationally, trends in place of death should be monitored.
- For purchasers – as much as possible, purchasers should agree the details and coding of information required from specialist palliative services, to ensure that data can be aggregated at regional or national levels. Ideally, a core minimum data set should be agreed. One is currently being piloted by the National Council for Hospice and Specialist Palliative Care Services.
- For providers – standardized data collection should be used which includes demographic details including ethnic group, place of care, diagnosis, problems or symptom profile, and outcomes. Examples of such systems are available.[199-201] Coding systems should be compatible with the NHS and include the NHS number.
- For providers – details of service costs are needed.

Appendix I Purchasing specialist palliative care services 1994/95

Allocations

The allocation of funds to each region for 1994/95 is based on the estimated distribution of population in the 65–84 age group as follows.

Region	Amount in £000s
Northern	2308
Yorkshire	2710
Trent	3498
East Anglian	1679
North West Thames	2358
North East Thames	2624
South East Thames	2906
South West Thames	2304
Wessex	2426
Oxford	1646
South Western	2805
West Midlands	3772
Mersey	1747
North Western	2917
Total	**35700**

Source: EL(94)14 Annex A[15]

Appendix II Specialist palliative care services (adapted from information for purchasers: background to available specialist palliative care services[24])

Community services in patients' own homes

Specialist service	Availability[a]	Nature/role
Home care team from local IP unit[b]	Widely available 100+ in UK	Generally work in conjunction with primary care team. Advise on symptom control and availability and relevance of other services. Often have direct access to other specialist palliative care services and round-the-clock nursing services
Macmillan community-based free-standing team	200+ in UK	
Hospice at home staff clinical nurse specialist – hospital or community-based	Not known	
Marie Curie nursing service	Over 5000 'bank' nurses available in almost all areas	Hands-on nursing around the clock. Accessed via district nurse or Macmillan nurse. Increasingly organized by Marie Curie Cancer Care regional nurse manager[b]
Rapid response teams home respite care hospice at home services (some)	Limited availability as yet but developing	These services are multi-disciplinary and are provided on a 24-hour basis to avoid admission where this would otherwise be necessary and/or to fill in gaps until other services come into play. Apart from hospice at home services, these are additional responsibilities being developed by inpatient units
Specialist medical service	Widely available	Telephone advisory service generally provided by all inpatient Specialist Palliative Care Units (SPCUs) and multi-disciplinary teams. Visits to patients made by arrangement with GP. Not limited to cancer
Social work physiotherapy occupational therapy	Limited service given by same SPCUs	May be available to work with patients direct or advise the primary care team on patients referred and accepted by the specialist palliative care unit
Bereavement services	Widely available but generally limited to families/friends of patients cared for by the SPCU	Increasingly part of services offered by SPCUs through trained staff (often volunteers)

[a] Figures in column 2 are drawn from the 1995 *Directory of Hospice and Palliative Care Services.*
[b] Historical focus on cancer (not Sue Ryder) but patients with other diagnoses are increasingly accepted.

Institution-based services for patients not requiring admission or after discharge

Service	Availability[a]	Nature/role
Day care free-standing or attached to a specialist palliative care unit	Widely available. 220 units providing day care	Accent on rehabilitation and independence. A variety of services offered, e.g. physio/ OT/aromatherapy, as well as nursing and medical care, if appropriate
Outpatient clinics	Often offered by specialist palliative care inpatient units	Medical or other specialist service, e.g. lymphoedema, available through referral from GP or hospital doctor

Inpatient facilities

Service	Availability[a]	Nature/role
NHS specialist palliative care units voluntary/hospice[b] (Marie Curie/Sue Ryder and many others)	2500+ beds (England and Wales)	Specialist inpatient care with accent on symptom control, support for families, etc.
Hospital palliative care/ support team or nurse	200+ (England and Wales)	Teams, increasingly multi-disciplinary, working in an advisory capacity in a hospital setting. Not limited to either cancer or patients with very late stage disease
Hospital clinical nurse specialists or physicians (some Macmillan)	Increasing	Individuals with palliative remit, usually based on oncology departments
Hospital physicians in palliative medicine	Increasing	Consultants in the specialty, not necessarily with associated teams and often based in a local SPCU, but with committed sessions for advising colleagues and treating patients by arrangement

[a] Figures in column 2 drawn from the 1995 *Directory of Hospice and Palliative Care Services*.
[b] Historical focus on cancer (not Sue Ryder) but patients with other diagnoses are increasingly accepted.

Appendix III Standardized mortality ratios for selected causes, all ages (1990–94); example

		1990/94 Standardized mortality ratio
All malignant neoplasms (ICD 140–208)	Men	100
	Women	140
	Total	102
Malignant neoplasm of trachea, bronchus and lung (ICD 162)	Men	103
	Women	142
	Total	115
Malignant neoplasm of:		
female breast (ICD 174)	Women	93
cervix uteri (ICD 410–414)	Women	105
Ischaemic heart disease (ICD 430–438)	Men	81
	Women	72
	Total	77
Cerebrovascular disease (ICD 430–414)	Men	79
	Women	62
	Total	68
Motor vehicle traffic accidents (ICD E810–819)	Men	68
	Women	87
	Total	74
Suicide and self-inflicted injury and injury undetermined (ICD E950–959, E980–989)	Men	190
	Women	248
	Total	208
Suicide and self-inflicted injury (ICD E950–959)	Men	142
	Women	273
	Total	179
All above causes (except all malignant neoplasms)	Men	87
	Women	78
	Total	83
All causes (all ages) (ICD 001–999)	Men	100
	Women	87
	Total	93

Note: ICD 9 coding used.

Appendix IV An example of the results of analysis of characteristics of patients who may need palliative care for the district of Kensington, Chelsea and Westminster (KCW)[a]

Analysis of place and cause of death in KCW (1988–92)

To consider the palliative care for patients within KCW in more detail, place of death has been analysed separately for people dying from cancer, circulatory diseases and other disease. The following have been examined:

- the trends in place of death over the five years
- place of death by ward (using all the five years data combined, to avoid very small numbers).

The sample (five years in KCW)

The sample consists of 15 805 deaths registered between 1988 and 1992 inclusive. This accounts for all the deaths of residents of KCW.

There were 6481 deaths within Kensington & Chelsea and 9324 deaths within Westminster (Table A1).

Table A1: Number of deaths in KCW: 1988–92

Borough	*n*	%
Kensington & Chelsea	6481	41.0
Westminster	9324	59.0
Total	15805	100.0

There were approximately equal numbers of men and women who died and the rate was constant over the years (Tables A2, A3). (Note: a few deaths in 1987 are included in this sample because of the delay in registering. Similarly a few deaths in 1992 will not be recorded until 1993.)

Table A2: Sex of deaths in KCW: 1988–92

Sex	*n*	%
Men	7945	50.3
Women	7860	49.7
Total	15805	100.0

---

[a]Source: Higginson *et al.*[158]

Table A3: Year of death in KCW sample

Year	n	%
1987	64	0.4
1988	3281	20.8
1989	3342	21.1
1990	3066	19.4
1991	3150	19.9
1992	2902	18.4
Total	15805	100.0

The majority of patients who died were elderly (Table A4).

Table A4: Number of deaths by age in KCW: 1988–92

Age (years)	n	%
<15	129	0.8
16–35	508	3.2
36–64	2942	18.6
65–74	3389	21.4
75+	8837	55.9
Total	15805	100.0

Cause of death (five years in KCW)

The most common causes of death were diseases of the circulatory system, neoplasms or diseases of the respiratory system. Table A5 shows the number of people who died from these diseases and other diseases, which may potentially have a terminal period, such as dementia, liver cirrhosis. etc. There were 2213 (14%) deaths which were unlikely to have had a terminal period.

Table A5: Cause of death in KCW: 1988–92

Disease recorded on death certificate	n	%
Neoplasms (cancers)	4171	26.4
Nutritional and metabolic	326	2.1
Dementia	122	0.8
Nervous system	296	1.9
Circulatory system	6316	40.0
Respiratory system	2015	12.7
Liver cirrhosis	225	1.4
Musculo-skeletal system	121	0.8
Other diseases, not at all likely to have a terminal/palliative period	2213	14.0
Total	15805	100.0

Place of death (five years in KCW)

The majority of deaths occurred in hospital (69%) and 24% occurred at home (Table A6).

Table A6: Place of death in KCW: 1988–92

Place	n	%
NHS non-psychiatric hospital	9524	60.3
Non-NHS psychiatric hospital	2	0.0
NHS psychiatric hospital	22	0.1
Private hospital	1316	8.3
Other communal establishment	679	4.3
At home	3735	23.6
Elsewhere	527	3.3
Total	15805	100.0

Analysis of place of death by cause, borough and ward: 1988–92

The percentage of patients who died at home and in hospital have been analysed for those who died from neoplasms, circulatory diseases and other potentially terminal conditions for the years from 1988 to 1992. The 2213 cases unlikely to have had a terminal period have been excluded from this analysis.

Deaths due to neoplasms

Examination of trends over the years suggests a slight increase in the percentage of patients dying at home from neoplasms within Kensington & Chelsea. There may be also a slight increase within the City of Westminster, although there appears to have been a fall between 1991 and 1992 (Figures A1–A3).

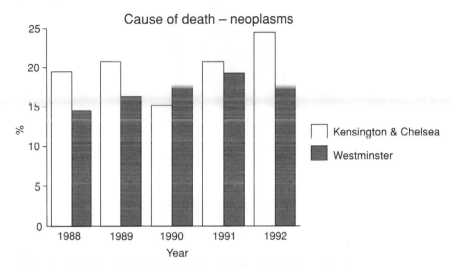

Figure A1: Percentage of people who die at home.

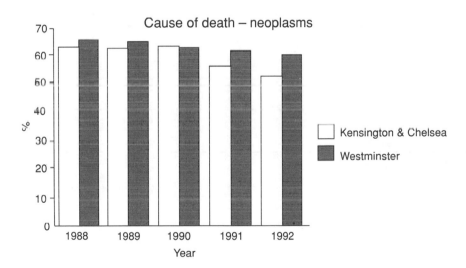

Figure A2: Percentage of people who die in NHS non-psychiatric hospitals.

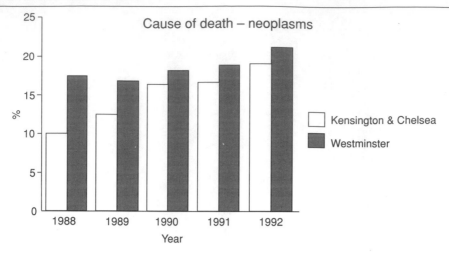

Figure A3: Percentage of people who die in private hospitals.

The proportion of people dying in NHS non-psychiatric hospitals has fallen in both boroughs between 1988 and 1992. The proportion of people who have died in institutions recorded by OPCS as private hospitals has increased during this period – especially in Kensington & Chelsea.

Circulatory diseases

The proportion of people who died in each setting from circulatory diseases is largely unchanged over these years – there appears to be a slight reduction in home deaths. However in general there is a higher proportion of deaths at home for circulatory diseases than from neoplasms (Figures A4–A6) especially in Westminster. In this borough in 1992, 17% of deaths from neoplasms died at home, compared to 29% of deaths from circulatory diseases.

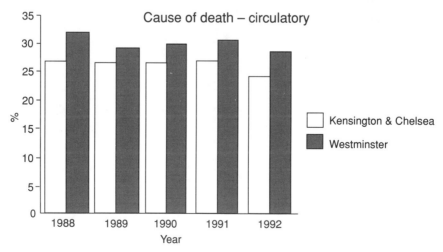

Figure A4: Percentage of people who die at home.

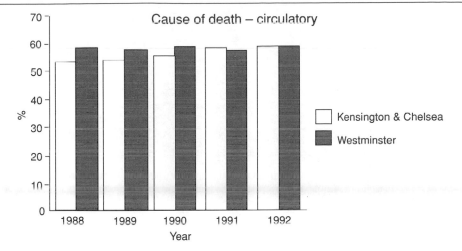

Figure A5: Percentage of people who die in non-psychiatric hospitals.

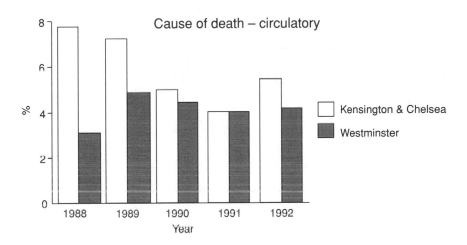

Figure A6: Percentage of people who die in private hospitals.

Other terminal diseases

There appears to be no trend over the years for people who have died of other terminal diseases, apart from a suggestion of an increased use of private hospitals (Figures A7–A9).

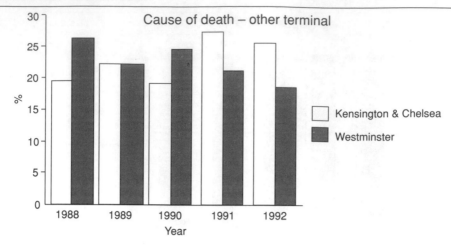

Figure A7: Percentage of people who die at home.

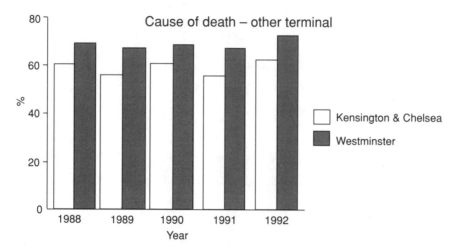

Figure A8: Percentage of people who die in non-psychiatric hospitals.

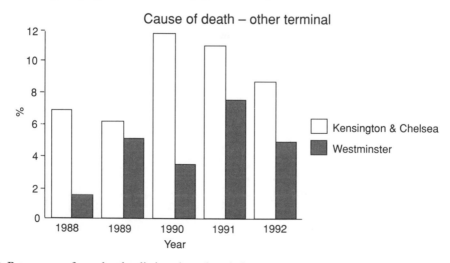

Figure A9: Percentage of people who die in private hospitals.

All data combined for neoplasms, circulatory and other terminal diseases

Figures A10 to A12 show the percentage of people who died from all the aforementioned diseases. The only apparent trend is an increase in the use of private hospitals, as was found separately for neoplasms.

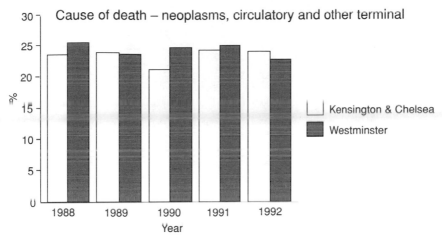

Figure A10: Percentage of people who die at home.

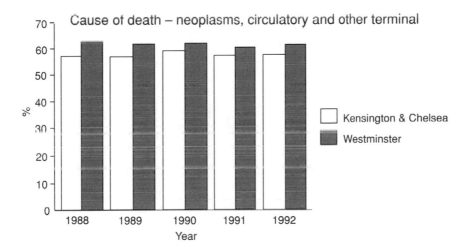

Figure A11: Percentage of people who die in non-psychiatric hospitals.

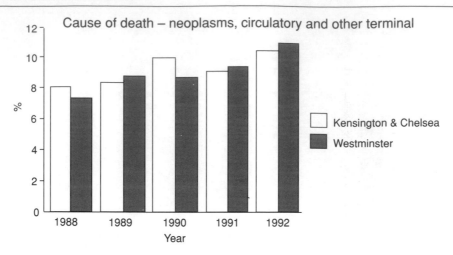

Figure A12: Percentage of people who die in private hospitals.

Analysis of data by ward

Figures A13 to A16 show the proportions of deaths occurring at home for the different wards during the five-year period for patients who died from neoplasms, circulatory diseases, other terminal diseases and these catagories combined. Certain wards appear consistently to have a higher percentage of deaths at home, notably Knightsbridge and the wards to the south and west of this area. This distribution is similar to that of the indicators of social deprivation within KCW.[202]

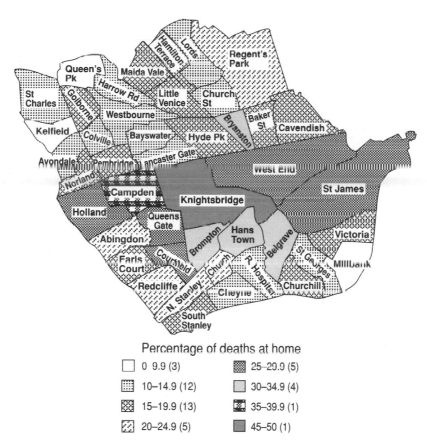

Percentage of deaths at home

☐	0 9.9 (3)	▨	25–29.9 (5)
▥	10–14.9 (12)	☐	30–34.9 (4)
▩	15–19.9 (13)	▨	35–39.9 (1)
▨	20–24.9 (5)	■	45–50 (1)

Figure A13: Percentage of deaths at home by electoral ward: neoplasms.

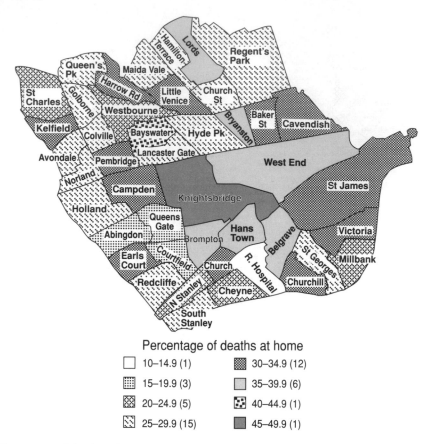

Figure A14: Percentage of deaths at home by electoral ward: circulatory disorders.

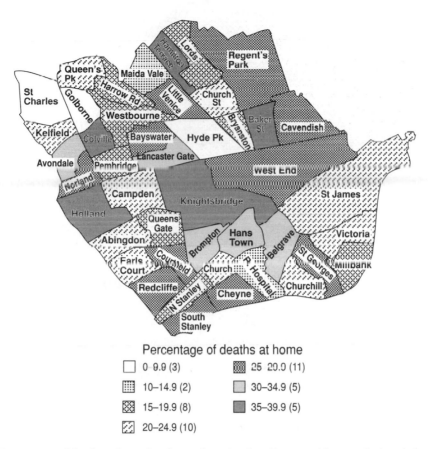

Percentage of deaths at home

☐ 0–9.9 (3)		▓ 25–29.9 (11)	
▦ 10–14.9 (2)		▢ 30–34.9 (5)	
▨ 15–19.9 (8)		▩ 35–39.9 (5)	
▧ 20–24.9 (10)			

Figure A15: Percentage of deaths at home by electoral ward: other diseases with a terminal period.

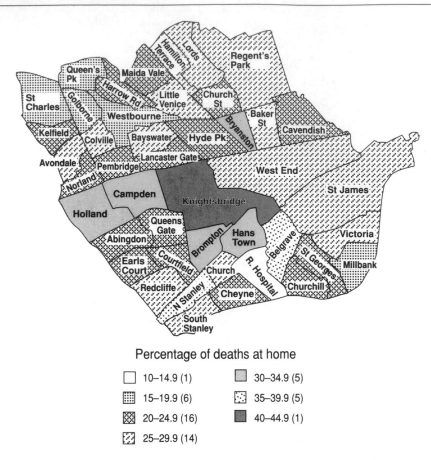

Percentage of deaths at home

☐	10–14.9 (1)	▨	30–34.9 (5)
▦	15–19.9 (6)	▦	35–39.9 (5)
▨	20–24.9 (16)	■	40–44.9 (1)
▨	25–29.9 (14)		

Figure A16: Percentage of deaths at home by electoral ward: neoplasms, circulatory and other terminal disorders combined.

Appendix V Growth in palliative care in UK and Ireland: 1965–95

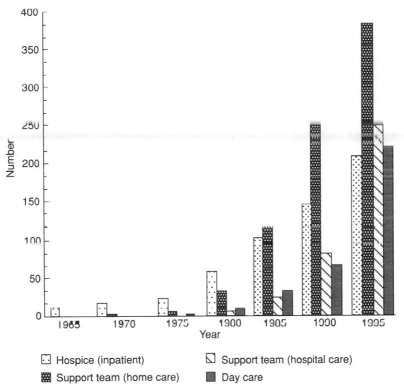

☐ Hospice (inpatient)   ▨ Support team (hospital care)
▨ Support team (home care)   ■ Day care

Appendix VI Grades for assessment of quality of scientific evidence

Analysis of service efficacy – strength of recommendation

A	There is good evidence to support the use of the procedure
B	There is fair evidence to support the use of the procedure
C	There is poor evidence to support the use of the procedure
D	There is fair evidence to reject the use of the procedure
E	There is good evidence to support the rejection of the use of the procedure

Source: Stevens and Raftery (1994)[21]

Quality of the evidence

(I)	Evidence obtained from at least one properly randomized controlled trial
(II-1)	Evidence obtained from well designed controlled trials without randomization
(II-2)	Evidence obtained from well designed cohort or case controlled analytic studies, preferably from more than one centre or research group
(II-3)	Evidence obtained from multiple timed series with or without the interventions, or from dramatic results in uncontrolled experiments
(III)	Opinions of respected authorities based on clinical experience, descriptive studies or reports of expert committees
(IV)	Evidence inadequate owing to problems of methodology, e.g. sample size, length or comprehensiveness of follow-up, or conflict in evidence

Table adapted from US Task Force on Preventive Health Care.
Source: Stevens and Raftery (1994)[21]

Appendix VII Kensington & Chelsea and Westminster Health Authority service specification: palliative care services

Introduction

Kensington & Chelsea and Westminster Health Authority (KCWHA) has recently undertaken a detailed and in-depth review of specialist palliative care services. Following the production of a report and a seminar with all major providers of palliative care services, this service specification outlines KCW's requirements for palliative care services.[a]

The specification relates to all services apart from paediatric and HIV palliative care services. (There is currently a separate specification for HIV services but we would aim to integrate both these specifications in the future.)

For the purposes of this specification the following UK definition of palliative care has been adopted.

Palliative care is active total care offered to a patient with a progressive illness and their family when it is recognised that the illness is no longer curable, in order to concentrate on the quality of life and the alleviation of distressing symptoms within the framework of a co-ordinated service. Palliative care neither hastens nor postpones death, it provides a relief from pain and other distressing symptoms, integrates the psychological and spiritual aspects of care. In addition it offers a support system to help during the patient's illness and in bereavement. 'Family' is used as a general term to cover closely attached individuals, whatever their legal status. (Standing Medical Advisory Committee and Standing Nursing and Midwifery Advisory Committee 1992.)

Strategic principles

KCWHA wishes to incorporate the following principles into the palliative care services it commissions.

- To ensure the authority commissions a comprehensive range of specialist palliative care services which are of high quality and cost-effective.
- To secure equity of access to these services for differing groups of diagnoses, by ensuring services are appropriate to the specific needs of KCW residents and that details of services available are widely known, particularly with regard to how to refer into the service.
- To commission services which will allow patients and their carers choice of care models, in particular ensuring that patients can remain within their own home settings for as long as they may wish.
- To ensure that service provision to patients and their carers is seamless even if the care is being shared between a range of different providers, including other social services, housing and voluntary providers.
- To ensure that all health staff involved in direct patient and family care are well versed in good practice principles of palliative care.
- To ensure that services commissioned are of the highest quality standards and that these standards are regularly monitored.
- To ensure that service providers are regularly involved in clinical audit and measurement of effectiveness of outcomes of interventions, which will be jointly agreed with purchasers.

---

[a] Copies of the report are available from the authority and contain a reference list.

Context

Considerable changes are currently taking place within specialist palliative care services, which have caused some uncertainty particularly to voluntary hospice providers; these are as follow.

- Monies previously ring-fenced specifically for voluntary hospices have now been devolved from regional health authorities to districts and can now be used for any specialist palliative care services.
- 1994 sees voluntary hospice providers for the first time having to come into the market and set contracts with health authorities. This has involved the setting of agreed levels of activity and finance and setting clearer criteria for admission. Service developments now must be agreed with purchasers in advance.
- There has been an increase in the number of hospice providers within greater London, which has caused current providers concerns as to their viability with increased competition.
- A growing awareness of an inequity in access to palliative care services for non-cancer patients.
- The Calman report on cancer services suggesting a reduction in the number of treatment centres providing specialist care within acute hospitals will influence the distribution of services locally.

Population/health needs

Kensington, Chelsea and Westminster covers an area of 13 square miles in North West London and is coterminous with its two constituent local authorities. According to the OPCS mid-1991 population estimates, the resident population of the district is 323 900 (141 400 in the Royal Borough of Kensington & Chelsea and 182 500 in the City of Westminster).

The population is an inner-city population and includes people from a range of different cultural and ethnic groups. There is a wide range of health experiences across the different wards within the area. The most disadvantaged wards display higher rates of death and increased levels of illness, high levels of unemployment and poorer housing, with many single parent families and elderly people who live alone.

Analysis of potential needs for palliative care showed that 830 KCW residents die from cancer each year. The majority of these are aged over 75 years. National statistics suggest that of these almost 700 would experience pain in the last year of life, almost 400 would have trouble with breathing and 400 would have symptoms of vomiting or nausea. Many would have other symptoms. KCW residents who die from other causes were also considered, such as circulatory diseases, which may have a palliative period. Each year approximately 1700 KCW residents die from these diseases, as for cancer the majority are elderly. National statistics would suggest that of these almost 1200 would experience pain in the last year of life, 850 would experience trouble with breathing and 450 would have symptoms of vomiting or nausea. Again many had other symptoms or a combination of symptoms.

Patients will also need emotional, spiritual and social support. Many of the families of these patients would require support during care and in bereavement.

Within KCW approximately 24% of deaths occur at home and 69% occur in hospital. For cancer patients an even smaller proportion – 18% – die at home. The percentage of patients who die at home varies greatly across KCW ranging from less than 10% in some of our electoral wards to greater than 40% in others. The distribution appears to mirror that of the Jarman indicators for social deprivation within KCW.

Examining trends over the years indicates that there has been a slight increase in the percentage of cancer patients who die at home in the Royal Borough of Kensington & Chelsea but probably not in the City of Westminster. There was also a fall in the proportion of people who died in NHS hospitals and an increase in the proportion who died in private hospitals.

Preferred model of service

In the review KCW identified current service provision and the report and the seminar highlighted areas where service changes were required. From specialist providers KCW will wish to commission a package of care which will range through symptom control, psychological support for the patient and the carers, respite care within the community, terminal care and bereavement care. Other providers will assist in the provision of a seamless, comprehensive service to the patient and their carers.

The main recommendations in response to the concerns raised in the KCW review report were as follow.

- Links between Macmillan and support nurses working in acute hospitals and the hospices and specialist palliative care teams needed to be more formalized.
- There was a need to cascade support from the specialist services through into generic services, perhaps in the form of in-reach teams into acute hospitals.
- There needed to be more accurate reporting of activity, particularly the activity of the Macmillan nurses in the Chelsea and Westminster Hospital should be clearly indentified for purchasers.
- For data collection there needed to be greater clarity in the requirements and reasons for process data. This would ensure that personnel could improve the quality of their data collection.
- Data collection was also needed on the outcomes and quality of care given, for example symptom control, safe discharge and appropriateness of interventions.
- Links between acute providers and hospices needed to be formalized.
- Similarly links between hospices and specialist palliative care services and primary care staff needed to be improved.
- GPs required better information on the services available, but rather than have this in the form of directories it was suggested that the KCW 'place mats' would be a useful approach. Advertising information was not felt to be helpful.
- There was a need to develop patient agreements or protocols between services to ensure that duplication did not occur but that good liaison did.
- A 24-hour service provision was thought to be essential for home care in collaboration with appropriate social services.
- GPs should be made aware of those services which provide 24-hour advice and support and where patients in the care of a service or already known to a hospice may be admitted out of hours as an emergency.
- Greater investigation of the access to services for people from black and ethnic minority groups was needed and in particular KCW needs to determine how many patients from this group are likely to need palliative care services and what their preferences may be.
- Work is also needed to determine the language needs of people from ethnic groups and the availability of translators for patients who are cared for at home.
- Training is needed for generic workers to ensure that all staff are aware of good practice in palliative care.
- There was a general need to be mature about interprofessional working relationships.

Attached to this service specification is a range of standards which outline the preferred model of services that KCW wishes to commission.

Although all standards are not appropriate to all providers it is essential to note that patients will move between the varying providers and their care must be a continuum so that all services are linked.

These standards cover general quality requirements, data requirements and clinical audit. It should be noted that it is not anticipated that all standards will be regularly monitored. An initial position statement from each provider will be prepared and agreement reached between the provider and KCW as to which specific standards will be monitored in any one year.

Monitoring

KCW places great emphasis on information and the monitoring of not only activity, but of the quality of the service commissioned and the agreed outcome. It is anticipated that reporting on achievement of specific quality standards as outlined in this specification will be incorporated into schedule 4 of KCW contracts and will therefore be monitored on a twice-yearly basis.

Audit and outcome

Arrangements for clinical audit and development of outcome measures

- An audit is requested of the treatment and management of symptoms of pain, anxiety and family problems using or adapting already established outcomes tools such as the Support Team Assessment Schedule (STAS). Providers are requested to present results of this to purchasers and to demonstrate what action they are intending to take as a result of any problems found with the services.
- Providers are requested to demonstrate and to audit joint initiatives with local practitioners and primary care teams or acute hospitals in enhancing the quality of care offered to terminally ill patients and in particular including those who do not have cancer and their families or carers.

To commission a comprehensive range of palliative care services

Standard	Ability to comply	Monitoring mechanism

Specialist palliative care providers will provide packages of care that will include:
 • Inpatient care
    a) symptom control
    b) psychological support
    c) respite care
    d) terminal care
 • Day care – at current levels only until evaluation has been undertaken
 • Care within the community
    a) symptom control
    b) psychological support
    c) maintenance
    d) terminal care
 • Bereavement and after-care services		

Pain control • Patients will have access to specialist pain control advice which complies with agreed clinical guidelines		
Emotional support • Emotional support will be available to the patient and their carer by staff with an understanding of/or training in general counselling techniques. Specialist counselling advice will be available from suitably trained personnel when appropriate		

Continued

To commission a comprehensive range of palliative care services: *continued*

Standard	Ability to comply	Monitoring mechanism
• Bereavement after-care services will be available to relatives and carers, linking with voluntary services where appropriate		
Co-ordination		
• Patients should have access to a range of professionals with specialist palliative care skills		
• Where the multi-disciplinary team is not centrally managed, formal interprofessional working arrangements should be in place, with a designated head of service, which includes medical care		
• Specialist palliative care nurses and multi-disciplinary teams should have formal working agreements with a hospice with whom KCW holds a contract		
• Recognized complementary therapies, which are known to be clinically effective should be available to patients where appropriate		
• Link nurses (in addition to specialist palliative care nurses) should be identified within the community and on hospital wards to act as a resource on palliative care services		
• Prior to discharge from inpatient care there will be a clear mechanism for co-ordination of care on discharge with named lead care provider		

To secure equity of access to services by ensuring they are appropriate to the specific needs of KCW residents

Standard	Ability to comply	Monitoring mechanism
Availability		
• Urgent referrals can be made to the service seven days a week		
• Specialist providers will offer a single contact number for GPs and hospitals to obtain advice about a patient		
Cultural beliefs		
• Provision should be made to allow patients to observe their own faith (or non-faith) and facilitate their spiritual leaders to enter the hospice		
• Providers will not impose their personal religious beliefs on patients unless the patient initiates/requests support		
• Cultural beliefs about death and dying will be properly observed		
• Meals should meet cultural and religious requirements		
• Patients and their carers should have access to interpreting advocacy services where necessary		

References

1 Working Group on Terminal Care (chairman: E Wilkes). National terminal care policy. *J Roy Coll Gen Practit* 1980; **30**: 466–71.

2 Higginson I. Palliative Care: a review of past challenges and future trends. *J Public Hlth* 1993; **15(1)**: 3–8.

3 Saunders C, Sykes N. *The management of terminal malignant disease*. 3rd edn. London: Edward Arnold, 1993.

4 Standing Medical Advisory Committee and Standing Nurse and Midwifery Advisory Committee. *The Principles and Provision of Palliative Care*. London: Joint Report of the Standing Medical Advisory Committee & Standing Nurse & Midwifery Advisory Committee, 1992.

5 Marie Curie Memorial Foundation. *The Marie Curie Memorial Foundation; a brief history 1948–1984*. London: Marie Curie Memorial Foundation, 28 Belgrave Square, 1985.

6 Lunt BJ, Hillier ER. Terminal care: present services and future priorities. *Br Med J* 1981; **283**: 595–8.

7 Lunt B. Terminal cancer care services: recent changes in regional inequalities in Great Britain. *Soc Sci Med* 1987; **20(7)**: 753–9.

8 Cartwright A. Changes in life and care in the year before death 1969–1987. *J Pub Hlth Med* 1991; **13(2)**: 81–7.

9 Office of Population Censuses and Surveys. Mortality statistics general. Series DH1 No. 26 Review of the Registrar General on deaths in England and Wales, 1992. London: HMSO, 1994.

10 Bowling A. The hospitalisation of death: should more people die at home? *J Med Ethics* 1983; **9**: 158–61.

11 Department of Health. London: DoH Circular HC(87)4(2).

12 Department of Health. Press release. *Extra £8 million Government money for hospices*. London: Department of Health Press Office, 1989: 89/556.

13 Department of Health. Press release. *Government gives £17 million more for hospices*. London: Department of Health Press Office, 1991: H91/6.

14 Department of Health. Press release. *£37 million more for hospices*. London, Department of Health Press Office, 1992: H92/96.

15 NHS Management Executive. Contracting for specialist palliative care services. NHS Management Executive 1994: EL(94)14.

16 NHS Executive. Specialist palliative care services including Drugs for Hospices scheme. NHS Executive 1995: EL(95)22.

17 1995 Director of Hospice Services in the UK and the Republic of Ireland. St Christopher's Hospice Information Service. London: St Christopher's Hospice, Sydenham, 1995.

18 Heginbotham C. Rationing. *Br Med J* 1992; **304**: 496–9.

19 Department of Public Health. *Health and Lifestyle Survey*. London: Department of Public Health, Kensington, Chelsea and Westminster Health Authority, 1994.

20 Caroll G. *Priorities for health care*. Essex: Department of Public Health, Essex Health Authority, 1992.

21 Stevens A, Raftery J. The epidemiological approach to needs assessment. In *Health Care Needs Assessment* (eds A Stevens, J Raftery). Oxford: Radcliffe Medical Press 1994; pp. 21–30 (volume 1).

22 National Council for Hospice and Specialist Palliative Care Services. *Specialist palliative care: a statement of definitions*. London: National Council for Hospice and Specialist Palliative Care Services, 1995.

23 WHO Expert Committee. *Cancer pain relief and palliative care*. No. 804. Geneva: World Health Organization Technical Report Series, 1990.

24 Working party on clinical guidelines in palliative care (drafted by G Ford). *Information for purchasers. Background to available specialist palliative care services*. London: National Council for Hospice and Specialist Palliative Care Services, 1995.

25 European Association for Palliative Care – European Association for Palliative Care Constitution, Milan 1988.

26 National Association of Health Authorities and Trusts. *Care of People with a Terminal Illness*. Birmingham Research Park, Vincent Drive, Birmingham B15 2SQ, 1991.

27 McCarthy M, Higginson IJ. Clinical audit by a palliative care team. *Palliative Medicine* 1991; 5(3): 215–21.

28 Office of Population Censuses and Surveys. *Population Trends 74*, Winter 1993. Tables 13 and 14. Deaths rates by age, sex and selected causes. London: HMSO, 1994.

29 Expert Advisory Group on Cancer to the Chief Medical Officers of England and Wales. A policy framework for commissioning cancer services. London: Department of Health, 1995.

30 NHS Executive. A policy framework for commissioning cancer services. NHS Executive 1995: EL(95)51.

31 Gau DW, Diehl AK. Disagreement among general practitioners regarding cause of death. *Br Med J* 1982; 284: 239–445.

32 Higginson I, McCarthy M. Validity of the support team assessment schedule: do staffs' ratings reflect those made by patients or their families? *Palliat Med* 1993; 7: 219–28.

33 Epstein AM, Hall JA, Tognetti J et al. Using proxies to evaluate quality of life. Can they provide valid information about patient's health status and satisfaction with medical care. *Medical Care* 1989; 27(3): S91–S98.

34 Field D, Douglas C, Jagger C et al. Terminal illness: views of patients and their lay carers. *Palliat Med* 1995; 9: 45–54.

35 Higginson I, Priest P, McCarthy M. Are bereaved family members a valid proxy for a patient's assessment of dying? *Soc Sci Med* 1994; 38(4): 553–7.

36 Seale C. A comparison of hospice and conventional care. *Soc Sci Med* 1991; 32(2): 147–52.

37 Addington-Hall JM. *Regional study of care for the dying*. Feedback for district health authorities. Cancer deaths only. London: Department of Epidemiology and Public Health, University College London, 1993.

38 Addington-Hall JM. *Regional study of care for the dying*. Feedback for district health authorities. Non-cancer deaths only. London: Department of Epidemiology and Public Health, University College London, 1993.

39 Addington-Hall JM, McCarthy M. Regional study of care of the dying: methods and sample characteristics. *Palliat Med* 1995; 9: 27–35.

40 Addington-Hall JM, McCarthy M. Dying from cancer: results of a national population-based investigation. *Palliat Med* 1995; 9: 295–305.

41 Hopwood P, Howell A, Maguire P. Psychiatric morbidity in patients with advanced cancer of the breast: prevalence measured by two self-rating questionnaires. *Br J Cancer* 1991; 62(2): 349–52.

42 Bennett M, Corcoran G. The impact on community palliative care services of a hospital palliative care team. *Palliat Med* 1994; 8: 237–44.

43 Higginson I, Wade A, McCarthy M. Effectiveness of two palliative support teams. *J Pub Hlth Med* 1992; 1: 50–6.

44 Addington-Hall JM, MacDonald L, Anderson H et al. Dying from cancer: the view of bereaved family and the friends about the experiences of terminally ill patients. *Palliat Med* 1991; 5: 207–14.

45 Eve A, Jackson A. Palliative care, where are we now? *Palliat Care Today* 1994; 1: 22–3.

46 Frankel S. Assessing the need for hospice beds. *Hth Trnd* 1990; 2: 83–6.

47 Hockley JM, Dunlop R, Davis RJ. Survey of distressing symptoms in dying patients and their families in hospital and the response to a symptom control team. *Br Med J* 1988; 296: 1715–7.

48 Severs MP, Wilkins PS. A hospital palliative care ward for elderly people. *Age and Ageing* 1991; 20(5): 361–4.

49 Noble B. A snapshot survey of hospital and hospice patients. In: *Older peoples: palliative care strategy.* Sheffield: Family and Community Services, Health Authority and Family Health Services Authority, 1993, Appendix B.

50 PHLS AIDS Centre – Communicable Disease Surveillance Centre and Scottish Centre for Infection and Environmental Health. Unpublished Quarterly Surveillance Tables No.25, December 1994 Tables 2 and 3a.

51 Butters E, Higginson I, Hearn J *et al. Prospective audit of community care for people with HIV/AIDS provided by health, social and voluntary sector teams.* Report to North Thames Region. London: London School of Hygiene and Tropical Medicine, 1995.

52 Moss V. Care for patients with advanced HIV and AIDS disease. *Palliat Care in Terminal Illness* 1994; **2**: 84–93.

53 Cole RM. Medical aspects of care for the person with advanced acquired immunodeficiency syndrome (AIDS): a palliative care perspective. *Palliat Med* 1991; **5**: 96–111.

54 Welch JM. Symptoms of HIV disease. *Palliat Med* 1991; **5**: 46–51.

55 Dixon P, Higginson I. AIDS and cancer pain treated with slow release morphine. *Postgrad Med J* 1991; **67** (Suppl. 2): S92–S94.

56 Butters E, Higginson I, George R *et al.* Assessing the symptoms, anxiety and practical needs of HIV/AIDS patients reviewing palliative care. *Quality of Life Research* 1992; **1**: 47–51.

57 Bulkin W, Brown L, Fraioli D *et al.* Hospice Care of the Intravenous Drug User AIDS Patient in a Skilled Nurse Facility. *J Acq Imm Def Synd* 1988; **1**: 375–80.

58 Rosci MA, Pigorini F, Bernabei A *et al.* Methods for detecting early signs of AIDS dementia complex in asymptomatic HIV-1-infected subjects. *AIDS* 1992; **6(11)**: 1309–16.

59 Bornstein RA, Nasrallah HA, Para MF *et al.* Neuropsychological performance in symptomatic and asymptomatic HIV infection. *AIDS* 1993; **7**: 519–24.

60 McKeogh M. Dementia in HIV disease: a challenge for palliative care. *J Palliat Care* 1995; **11(2)**: 30–3.

61 Higginson I, Mallandain I, Butters E *et al.* What services are needed to care for people with HIV/AIDS encephalopathy in North Thames. London: London School of Hygiene and Tropical Medicine, 1995.

62 *1994 Directory of Hospice Services in the UK and the Republic of Ireland.* St Christopher's Hospice Information Service. London: St Christopher's Hospice, Sydenham, 1994.

63 Crone S, Rigge M, Whalley P. *The Pain Clinic Directory 1994.* London: College of Health, 1994.

64 Doyle D, Hanks GWC, MacDonald N (eds). *Oxford Textbook of Palliative Medicine.* Oxford: Oxford University Press, 1993.

65 Twycross RG. Cancer pain a global perspective. The Edinburgh Symposium on Pain and Medical Education. In *Royal Society of Medicine International Symposium Series (149)* (RG Twycross ed.), London, 1989, pp. 3–16.

66 Larve F, Colleau SM, Brasseur L *et al.* Multicentre study of cancer pain and its treatment in France. *Br Med J* 1995; **310**: 1034–9.

67 Ventafridda V, Tamburini M, Caraceni C *et al.* A validation study of the WHO method for cancer pain relief. *Cancer* 1987; **59**: 850–6.

68 Working Party on Clinical Guidelines of the National Council for Hospice and Specialist Palliative Care Services (drafted by R Dunlop). *Clinical Guidelines for Pain Control.* London: National Council for Hospice and Specialist Palliative Care Services, 1994.

69 Walker VA, Hoskin PJ, Hanks GW *et al.* Evaluation of WHO analgesic guidelines for cancer pain in a hospital-based palliative care unit. *J Pain Symp Management* 1988; **3(3)**: 145–9.

70 Takeda F. Results of field-testing in Japan of the WHO draft interim guidelines of relief of cancer pain. *Pain Clin* 1986; **1**: 83–9.

71 Schug SA, Zech D, Dorr U. Cancer pain management according to WHO analgesic guidelines. *J Pain Symp Management* 1990; **5(1)**: 27–32.

72 Portenoy RK. Adjuvant analgesics in pain management. In *Oxford Textbook of Palliative Medicine* (eds D Doyle, GWC Hanks, N MacDonald). Oxford: Oxford Univeristy Press, 1993, pp. 229–44.

73 Pace V. The use of non-steroidal anti-inflammatory drugs in cancer. *Palliat Med* 1995; **9**: 273–86.

74 Twycross RG, Lack SA. *Control of alimentary symptoms in far advanced cancer*. Edinburgh: Churchill Livingstone, 1986.

75 Ventafridda V, Ripamonti C, Sbanotto A *et al*. Mouth care. In *Oxford Textbook of Palliative Medicine* (eds D Doyle, GWC Hanks, N MacDonald). Oxford: Oxford University Press, 1993, pp. 434–7.

76 Hanratty J, Higginson I (eds). *Palliative Care in Terminal Illness*. Oxford: Radcliffe Medical Press, 1994.

77 Regnard C, Ahmedzai S. Dyspnoea in advanced nonmalignant disease – a flow diagram. *Palliat Med* 1991; **5**: 56–60.

78 Johnson I, Patterson S. Drugs used in combination in the syringe driver – a survey of hospice practice. *Palliat Med* 1992; **6**: 125–30.

79 Baines M, Sykes N. Gastrointestinal symptoms. In *The management of terminal malignant disease* (eds C Saunders, N Sykes). 3rd edn. London: Edward Arnold, 1993, pp. 63–76.

80 Regnard C, Comiskey M. Nausea and vomiting in advanced cancer – a flow diagram. *Pall Med* 1992; **6(2)**: 146–51.

81 World Health Organization. *Targets for health for all – targets in support of a European strategy for health promotion*. Copenhagen: WHO, 1985.

82 Maguire P, Faulkner A. Communicating with cancer patients: 1 Handling bad news and difficult questions. *Br Med J* 1988; **297**: 907–9.

83 Maguire P, Faulkner A. Communicating with cancer patients: 2 Handling uncertainty, collusion, and denial. *Br Med J* 1988; **297**: 972–4.

84 Parkes CM. Home or hospital? Terminal care as seen by surviving spouses. *J Roy Coll Gen Practit* 1978; **28**: 19–30.

85 Higginson I, Wade A, McCarthy M. Palliative care: views of patients and their families. *Br Med J* 1990; **301**: 277–81.

86 Lunt B. A comparison of hospice care for terminally ill cancer patients and their families. Final report. Research funded under grant DHSS JR/121/692, 1986.

87 Addington-Hall JM, MacDonald L, Anderson H *et al*. Randomised controlled trial of effects of coordinating care for terminally ill cancer patients. *Br Med J* 1992; **305**: 1317–22.

88 Bowling A. Mortality after bereavement: a review of the literature on survival periods and factors affecting survival. *Soc Sci Med* 1987; **24(2)**: 117–24.

89 Bereavement. In *Oxford Textbook of Palliative Medicine* (eds D Doyle, GWC Hanks, N MacDonald). Oxford: Oxford University Press, 1993.

90 Bromberg M, Higginson I. Bereavement follow-up: what do support teams actually do? *J Palliat Care* 1996; **12(1)**: 12–17.

91 Wilkes E. Terminal cancer at home. *Lancet* 1965; **i**: 799–801.

92 Wilkes E. Dying now. *Lancet* 1984; **i**: 950–2.

93 Cartwright A, Hockey L, Anderson JL. *Life before death*. London: Routledge & Kegan Paul, 1973.

94 Parkes CM. Terminal care: evaluation of in-patient service at St Christopher's Hospice. Part I. Views of surviving spouse on effects of the service on the patient. *Postgrad Med J*, 1979; **55**: 517–22.

95 Mills M, Davis HTO, Macrae W. Care of dying patients in hospital. *Br Med J* 1994; **309**: 583–6.

96 Bowling A, Cartwright A. *Life after a death. A study of the elderly widowed*. London: Tavistock, 1982.

97 Maguire P. Monitoring the quality of life in cancer patients and their relatives. In *Cancer: assessment and monitoring*. London: Churchill Livingstone, 1980, pp. 40–52.

98 Ward AWM. Terminal care in malignant disease. *Soc Sci Med* 1974; **8**: 413–20.

99 Parkes CM. Terminal care: home, hospital, or hospice? *Lancet* 1985; **i**: 155–7.

100 Townsend J, Frank A, Fermont D *et al*. Terminal cancer care and patients' preference for place of death: a prospective study. *Br Med J* 1990; **301**: 415–17.

101 Dunlop R *et al*. Preferred versus actual place of death: a hospital palliative care support team study. *Palliat Med* 1989; **3**: 197–201.

102 Hinton J. Which patients with terminal cancer admitted from home care? *Palliat Med* 1994; **8**: 197–210.

103 Seale CF. What happens in hospices: a review of research evidence. *Soc Sci Med* 1989; **28(6)**: 551–9.

104 Kane RL, Klein SJ, Bernstein L *et al*. Hospice role in alleviating the emotional stress of terminal patients and their families. *Medical Care* 1985; **23(3)**: 189–97.

105 Kane RL, Wales J, Bernstein L *et al*. A randomised trial of hospice care. *Lancet* 1984; **i**: 890–4.

106 Higginson I, McCarthy M. Evaluation of palliative care: steps to quality assurance? *Palliat Med* 1989; **3**: 267–74.

107 Greer DS, Mor V, Morris JN *et al*. An alternative in terminal care: results of the National Hospice Study. *J Chron Dis* 1986; **39**: 9–26.

108 Greer DS, Mor V, Sherwood S *et al*. National Hospice Study analysis plan. *J Chron Dis* 1983; **36(11)**: 737–80.

109 Mor V, Greer DS, Kastenbaum R (eds). *The Hospice Experiment*. Baltimore: John Hopkins University Press, 1988, pp. 88–108.

110 Mor V, Morris JN, Hiris J *et al*. The effect of hospice care on where patients die. In *The Hospice Experiment* (eds V Mor, DS Greer, R Kastenbaum). Baltimore: John Hopkins University Press, 1988, pp. 133–46.

111 Morris JN, Sherwood S, Wright SM *et al*. The last weeks of life: does hospice make a difference? In *The Hospice Experiment* (eds V Mor, DS Greer, R Kastenbaum). Baltimore: John Hopkins University Press, 1988, pp.109–32.

112 Parkes CM. Terminal care: evaluation of in-patient service at St Christopher's Hospice. Part II. Self-assessments of effects of the service on surviving spouses. *Postgrad Med J* 1979; **55**: 523–7.

113 Parkes CM, Parkes J. Hospice versus hospital care – re-evaluation after 10 years as seen by surviving spouses. *Postgrad Med J* 1984; **60**: 120–4.

114 Field D, Ahmedzai S, Biswas B. Care and information received by lay carers of terminally ill patients at the Leicestershire Hospice. *Palliat Med* 1992; **July 6(3)**: 237–45.

115 Mor V, Greer DS, Goldberg R. The medical and social service interventions of hospice and non-hospice patients. In *The Hospice Experiment* (eds V Mor, DS Greer, R Kastenbaum). Baltimore: John Hopkins University Press, 1988.

116 Kidder D. The impact of hospice on the health-care costs of terminal cancer patients. In *The Hospice Experiment* (eds V Mor, DS Greer, R Kastenbaum). Baltimore: John Hopkins University Press, 1988, pp. 48–68.

117 Kidder D. Hospice services and cost savings in the last weeks of life. In *The Hospice Experiment* (eds V Mor, DS Greer, R Kastenbaum). Baltimore: John Hopkins University Press, 1988, pp. 69–87.

118 Hill F, Oliver C. Hospice – the cost of in-patient care. *Hlth Trnd* 1984; **16**: 9–11.

119 Hill F, Oliver C. Hospice – an update on the cost of patient care. *Hlth Trnd* 1988; **20**: 83–7.

120 Smith AM, Eve A, Sykes NP. Palliative care services in Britain and Ireland 1990 – an overview. *Palliat Med* 1992; **6**: 277–91.

121 Johnson I, Rogers C, Biswas B *et al*. What do hospices do? A survey of hospices in the United Kingdom and Republic of Ireland. *Br Med J* 1990; **300**: 791–3.

122 Kirkham S, Davis M. Bed occupancy, patient throughput and size of independent hospice units in the UK. *Palliat Med* 1992; **6**: 47–53.

123 Working Group of the Research Unit, Royal College of Physicians. Palliative care: guidelines for good practice and audit measures. *J R Coll Phys London* 1991; **25(4)**: 325–8.

124 Harper R, Ward A, Westlake L *et al*. *Good Practice in Terminal Care. Some standards and guidelines for hospice inpatient units and day hospices.* Sheffield: Department of Community Medicine, University of Sheffield Medical School, Beech Hill Road, 1988.

125 RCN Dynamic Quality Improvement Programme. *Standards of care for palliative nursing.* London: Royal College of Nursing, 1993.

126 Cancer Relief Macmillan Fund. *Organisational standards for palliative care.* London: Cancer Relief Macmillan Fund, 1994.

127 Ward AWM. Home care services – an alternative to hospices? *Comm Med* 1987; **9(1)**: 47 54.

128 Zimmer JG, Groth-Juncker A, McCusker J. Effects of a physician-led home care team on terminal care. *J Am Ger Soc* 1984; **32(4)**: 288–93.

129 Hughes SL, Cummings J, Weaver F *et al.* A randomized trial of the cost effectiveness of VA hospital-based home care for terminally ill. *Hlth Serv Res* 1992; **26(6)**: 801–17.

130 Cox K, Bergen A, Norman I. Exploring consumer views of care provided by the Macmillan nurse using the critical incident technique. *J Adv Nurs* 1993; **18**: 408–15.

131 Parkes CM. Terminal care: evaluation of an advisory domiciliary service at St Christopher's Hospice. *Postgrad Med J* 1980; **56**: 685–9.

132 Ventafridda V, De Conno F, Vigano A *et al.* Comparison of home and hospital care of advanced cancer patients. *Tumori* 1989; **75**: 619–25.

133 Creek LV. A homecare hospice profile: description, evaluation, and cost analysis. *J Family Practice* 1982; **14(1)**: 53–8.

134 Higginson I, McCarthy M. Measuring symptoms in terminal cancer: are pain and dyspnoea controlled? *J Roy Soc Med* 1989; **82**: 1761–4.

135 Seale C. Death from cancer and death from other causes: the relevance of the hospice approach. *Palliat Med* 1991; **5**: 12–19.

136 Hughes SL, Cummings J, Weaver F *et al.* A randomised controlled trial of VA hospital-based home care for the terminally ill. *Hlth Serv Res* 1992; **26(6)**: 801–17.

137 Tramarin A, Milocchi F, Tolley K *et al.* An economic evaluation of home-care assistance for AIDS patients: a pilot study in a town in northern Italy. *AIDS* 1992; **6(11)**: 1377–83.

138 Jones RVH. Teams and terminal cancer at home: do patients and carers benefit? *J Interprofess Care* 1993; **7(3)**: 239–44.

139 Irvine B. Development in palliative nursing in and out of the hospital setting. *Br J Nurs* 1993; **2(4)**: 218–24.

140 Griffin J. *Dying with dignity.* London: Office of Health Economics, 1991, pp. 4–45.

141 Theis S, Deitrick E. Respite Care: A community needs survey. *J Comm Hlth Nurs* 1987; **4(2)**: 85–92.

142 Johnson IS. The Marie Curie/St Luke's Relative Support Scheme: a home care services for relatives of the terminally ill. *J Adv Nurs* 1988; **13**: 565–70.

143 Koffman J, Higginson I. *Evaluation of a new hospice at home scheme.* London: Department of Public Health, Kensington, Chelsea and Westminster Health Authority, 1994.

144 Anand JK, Pryor GA. Hospital at home. *Hlth Trends* 1989; **21**: 46–8.

145 Higginson I, Webb D, Lessof L. Reducing beds for patients with advanced cancer. *Lancet* 1994; **344(8919)**: 409.

146 Cartwright A. Social class differences in health and care in the year before death. *J Epidem Comm Hlth* 1992; **46**: 54–7.

147 McCusker J, Stoddard AM. Effects of expanding home care program for the terminally ill. *Med Care* 1987; **B25(5)**: 373–84.

148 Butters E, Higginson I, George R *et al.* Palliative care for people with HIV/AIDS: views of patients, carers and providers. *AIDS Care* 1993; **5(1)**: 105–16.

149 Butters E, Higginson I, George R *et al.* Assessing the symptoms, anxiety and practical needs of HIV/AIDS patients receiving palliative care. *Qual Life Res* 1992; **1(1)**: 47–51.

150 Moss V. Patient characteristics, presentation and problems encountered in advanced AIDS in a hospice setting – review. *Palliat Med* 1991; **5**: 112–16.

151 East Anglian Regional Health Authority. *A Quality Framework for the Dying and Bereaved*. East Anglian Regional Health Authority. October 1992.

152 Finlay I, Wilkinson C, Gibbs C. Planning palliative care services. *Hlth Trnd* 1992; **24(4)** 139–41.

153 Haines A, Booroff A. Terminal care at home: perspective from general practice. *Br Med J* 1986; **292(6527)**: 1051–3.

154 Winget C, Higginson I. Palliative care – questionnaire survey of local general practitioners' views. In *Commissioning Specialist Palliative Care Services* (eds I Higginson, R Bush, P Jenkins, M Collins). London: Kensington & Chelsea and Westminster Health Commissioning Agency, 1994.

155 Copperman H. Domiciliary hospice care: a survey of general practitioners. *J R Coll Gen Practit* 1988; **38(314)**: 411–13.

156 Chambers E, Oakhill A, Cornish J *et al.* Terminal care at home for children with cancer. *Br Med J* 1989; **298**: 937–40.

157 Chambers T. Hospices for children? *Br Med J* 1987; **294**: 1309–10.

158 Higginson I, Bush R, Jenkins P *et al.* Commissioning specialist palliative care services. London: Kensington & Chelsea and Westminster Health Commissioning Agency, 1994.

159 Barnet Local Medical Committee. *Palliative care in Barnet – a guide for general practitioners and practice staff*. London: Department of Public Health, Barnet Health Commissioning Agency, 1993.

160 Ford GR, Pincherle G. Arrangements for terminal care in the NHS (especially those for cancer patients). *Hlth Trnd* 1978; **10**: 73–6.

161 Nicholas A, Frankenberg R. *Towards a strategy for palliative care - a needs assessment for Nottingham Health*. Nottingham: Department of Public Health, Nottingham Health, 1992.

162 Welsh Health Planning Forum. *Pain, discomfort and palliative care*. Cardiff: The Welsh Office NHS Directorate, 1992.

163 Robbins M, Jackson P. *Somerset study of patients and carers*. Bristol: Health Care Evaluation Unit, Department of Epidemiology and Public Health Medicine, University of Bristol, 1993.

164 Rutman D, Parke B. Palliative care needs of residents families and staff in long term care facilities. *J Palliat Care* 1992; **8(2)**: 23–9.

165 Murphy D, Bahr R, Kelly J *et al.* A needs assessment survey of HIV-infected patients. *West Indian Med J* 1992; **Jun**: 291–5.

166 Kincade J, Powers R. An assessment of palliative care needs in a tertiary care hospital. *QRB* 1984; **August**, 230–37.

167 Barnett M, McCarthy M. Identification of terminally-ill patients in the community. In *1986 International Symposium on Pain Control* (ed. D Doyle). London: Royal Society of Medicine: 78–80. (123 in International Symposium Series), 1987.

168 Neale B, Clark D, Heather P. *Purchasing palliative care: a review of the policy and research literature*. Sheffield: Trent Palliative Care Centre, 1993.

169 Zalot GN. Planning a regional palliative care services network. *J Palliat Care* 1989; **5(1)**: 42–6.

170 Robbins MA, Frankel SJ. Palliative care: what needs assessment. *Palliat Med* 1995; **9**: 287–93.

171 Addington-Hall JM, McCarthy M. Audit methods: views of the family after the death. In *Clinical audit in palliative care* (ed. I Higginson). Oxford: Radcliffe Medical Press, 1993, pp. 88–100.

172 National Council for Hospice and Specialist Palliative Care Services. Needs Assessment for Hospice and Specialist Palliative Care Services: from philosophy to contracts. *Occasional paper 4*. London: National Council for Hospice and Specialist Palliative Care Services, 1993.

173 Working party on clinical guidelines in palliative care (drafted by I Higginson). Outcome measures in palliative care. London: National Council for Hospice and Specialist Palliative Care Services, 1995.

174 Bowling A. *Measuring health. A review of quality of life measurement scales*. Milton Keynes: Open University, 1991.

175 Katz S. The science of quality of life. *J Chron Dis* 1987; **40(6)**: 449–63.

176 Quality of life. In *Oxford Textbook of Palliative Medicine* (eds D Doyle, GWC Hanks, N MacDonald). Oxford: Oxford University Press, 1993.

177 Department of Health. *Pressure sores and key quality indicator.* Heywood: Health Publication Unit, 1993.

178 Higginson I, McCarthy M. Validity of a measure of palliative care – comparison with a quality of life index. *Palliat Med* 1994; **8(4)**: 282–90.

179 Higginson I. A community schedule. In *Clinical Audit in Palliative Care* (ed. I Higginson). Oxford: Radcliffe Medical Press, 1993 pp. 34–47.

180 Bruera E, Macdonald S. The Edmonton Symptom Assessment System. In *Clinical Audit in Palliative Care* (ed. I Higginson). Oxford: Radcliffe Medical Press, 1993, pp. 61–77.

181 de Haes JCJM, van Knippenberg FCE, Neijt. Measuring psychological and physical distress in cancer patients: structure and application of the Rotterdam Symptom Checklist. *Br J Cancer* 1990; **62**: 1034–8.

182 Aaronson NK, Ahmedzai S, Bergman B *et al.* The European Organisation for Research and Treatment of Cancer QLQ-C30: a quality of life instrument for use in international clinical trials in oncology. *J Nat Cancer Inst* 1993; **85(5)**: 365–75.

183 Zigmond AS, Snaith RP. The Hospital Anxiety and Depression Scale. *Acta Psychiatrica Scandinavica* 1983; **67**: 361–70.

184 Trent Hospice Audit Group. *Palliative Care Core Standards: a multidisciplinary approach.* Nightingale Macmillan Continuing Care Unit, Trinity Street, Derby, 1992.

185 Dixon P, Heaton J, Long A *et al.* Reviewing and applying the SF-36. *Outcomes briefing* (UK Clearing House on Health Outcomes) 1994; **4**: 3–25.

186 Hill S, Harris U. Assessing the outcome of health care for the older person in community settings: should we use the SF-36? *Outcomes briefing* (UK Clearing House on Health Outcomes) 1994; **4**: 26–7.

187 Karnofsky DA, Abelmann WH, Craver LF *et al.* The use of nitrogen mustards in the palliative treatment of carcinoma. *Cancer* 1948; **I**: 634–56.

188 Melzack R. The McGill pain questionnaire: major properties and scoring methods. *Pain* 1975; **I**: 277–99.

189 Maguire P, Selby P. Assessing quality of life in cancer patients. *Br J Cancer* 1989; **60(3)**: 437–40.

190 Fallowfield L. *The quality of life. The missing measurement in health care.* London: Souvenir Press, 1990.

191 Wilkin D, Hallam L, Doggett MA. *Measures of need and outcome for primary health care.* Oxford: Oxford University Press, 1992.

192 Bowling A. *Measuring disease.* Milton Keynes: Open University Press, 1995.

193 Slevin ML. Quality of life: philosophical question or clinical reality? *Br Med J* 1992; **305**: 466–9.

194 Spitzer WO. State of science 1986: Quality of life and functional status as target variables for research. *J Chron Dis* 1987; **40(6)**: 465–71.

195 Thomas VJ, Rose FD. Ethnic differences in the experience of pain. *Soc Sci Med* 1991; **32(9)**: 1063–6.

196 Clarke M, Finlay I, Campbell I. Cultural boundaries in care. *Palliat Med* 1991; **5**: 63–5.

197 Cassidy S. Emotional distress in terminal cancer. *J Royal Society Med* 1986; **79**: 717–20.

198 Goddard M. The role of economics in the evaluation of hospice care. *Hlth Policy* 1989; **13**: 19–34.

199 Higginson I, Butters E, Murphy F *et al.* Computer database for palliative care. *Lancet* 1992; **340**: 243.

200 Higginson I, Butters E, Murphy F *et al.* Audit experience: using a data base to audit care. In *Clinical Audit in Palliative Care* (ed. I Higginson). Oxford: Radcliffe Medical Press, 1993, pp. 156–67.

201 National Council for Hospice and Palliative Care Services and The Hospice Information Service. *Data manual. Minimum data sets project.* London: National Council for Hospice and Palliative Care Services, 1995.

202 Department of Public Health. *1993 Annual Public Health Report.* London: Kensington, Chelsea and Westminster Health Commissioning Agency, 1993.

Acknowledgements

I am very grateful to a number of individuals who have provided me with help and useful suggestions in the preparation of this document. In particular I would like to thank Dr Derek Doyle, Dr Gill Ford, Dr Julia Addington-Hall, Dr Andrew Stevens, Dr James Raftery and the external referees for their helpful comments on earlier drafts of this document; my colleagues in Kensington & Chelsea and Westminster Health Authority (KCWHA) with whom I developed a palliative needs assessment, which formed the pilot for much of the work outlined here, and in particular Robina Bush, Paul Jenkins, Mary Collins and Catherine Winget and colleagues in the local hospices and specialist palliative care services, who provided helpful advice and comments on the KCWHA needs assessment – Dr Anne Naysmith, Dr Philip Jones, Dr Joe Chamberlain and Dr Rob George. I would like to thank Professor Michael Clarke and colleagues in Leicester for sharing information on the epidemiologically based needs assessment for the elderly, which they were preparing and which helped me formulate some of my ideas. Finally I am indebted to Franky Eynon and Sarah Scutt for their help in preparing the manuscript.

5   Dermatology

HC Williams

1 Summary

Introduction

This chapter sets out the major issues which health service purchasers need to consider in specifying services for people with skin problems. Skin disease is very common, affecting around one-quarter to one-third of the population. Apart from being the largest organ in the body, the skin has a vital social function and relatively minor skin complaints often cause more anguish to people than other more serious medical disorders. With the exception of melanoma skin cancer, the majority of skin diseases are not life threatening. However it is the product of this morbidity multiplied by the high prevalence of skin disease which results in a large burden of disease in absolute terms. Small changes in health policy could have large health and financial implications simply because they affect so many people.

Increase in future demand

Demand for dermatological services is likely to increase over the next decade for the following reasons.

1   **There is a large iceberg of unmet dermatological need** Previous surveys have suggested that approximately one-quarter of the population has a skin problem which could benefit from medical care, yet about 80% do not seek medical help. With increased public and professional awareness of effective treatment this submerged sector of the population is likely to surface and place heavy demands on the current system.
2   **The prevalence of some of the commonest skin diseases is increasing** Three of the commonest and most costly skin diseases, viz skin cancer (a Health of the Nation target), atopic eczema and venous ulcers are becoming more common and are set to consume a higher proportion of scarce resources within future health services budgets.
3   **The distinction between skin disease and 'cosmetic' skin problems is unclear** Even a small reduction in the threshold of what the public and health professionals regard as a skin complaint worthy of medical attention could lead to a large increase in future dermatology service requirements. The division between what constitutes reasonable need (e.g. somebody worried that a mole may be cancerous) and demand (e.g. somebody requesting removal of an 'ugly' mole) is especially blurred in dermatology.

Over 1000 skin diseases

Making generalizations about the need for dermatology services is difficult with such a vast range of disorders. Fortunately around 70% of the dermatological workload in primary and secondary care in the UK is currently taken up by just nine categories of skin disorders and effective treatments are available at low cost for the majority of these. The disorders covered include:

- skin cancer
- acne
- atopic eczema
- psoriasis
- viral warts
- other infective skin disorders
- benign tumours and vascular lesions
- leg ulceration
- contact dermatitis and other eczemas.

Priorities in ensuring a quality future service

Most people with skin diseases can be treated in the community but some will always require specialist services because of diagnostic difficulties or disease severity. Many skin diseases, especially skin cancer, are theoretically preventable but prevention programmes have not yet been evaluated adequately. There is reasonably good evidence to support the effectiveness of most treatments used for the common skin disease sub-categories. Less is known about the differential health gain of specialists versus generalists in the diagnosis and treatment of common skin diseases. The diagnosis and surgical removal of skin cancer is best carried out by, or with the involvement, of dermatologists. Retention of a central core of hospital-based dermatological medical and nursing expertise is essential and there is considerable scope for improving and expanding links between specialist and community services to provide seamless care for patients and for developing strategies aimed at disease prevention. Three models of health care are considered in this chapter in relation to dermatology services.

1 The current system which offers the least flexibility to predicted future trends in need and demand.
2 A model where dermatologists conduct community 'outreach' clinics; an approach of unproven benefit to patients which would require a costly four-fold increase in dermatologists.
3 A hybrid model consisting of hospital-based dermatology assessment centres, community-based treatment centres run by dermatology nurses accountable to district dermatology liaison teams and shared care clinics for common chronic skin diseases seen in primary care. This model offers the most flexibility and potential health gain building on local skills for a modest investment.

Despite the magnitude of skin disease morbidity in the general population, health services research for dermatological disorders has been minimal. Urgent research into the prevalence, incidence and cost of skin diseases is required in order to formulate public health strategies to respond to the impending crisis of increased demand for services. Public involvement in distinguishing between need and demand is crucial and this may vary considerably throughout the UK according to the demographic mix of the population.

2 Introduction and statement of the problem

General approach

The main purpose of this chapter is to help health care purchasers to develop purchasing plans for dermatology based on epidemiological data. Attempting to cover the entire range of a thousand or so dermatological diseases is akin to trying to cover the whole of general medicine in a single chapter. Each of the sub-categories of skin disease mentioned here merits a chapter in its own right because of the high prevalence and economic importance of each of these disease groups. However dermatology services have traditionally been considered as a single group and an attempt will be made to provide an overview of skin diseases in general at the expense of some of loss of detail for individual skin diseases. Despite the high prevalence of skin disease no NHS reports have ever been commissioned for skin disease and the inclusion of skin disease in this volume is to be welcomed as a promising start.

What is dermatology?

Dermatology is the study of the skin and associated structures such as hair and nails. The skin is not a simple inert covering but a sensitive dynamic boundary between ourselves and the outside world. Its functions include defence against infections and infestations, protection against irritants, ultraviolet radiation and trauma. The skin is essential for controlling water and heat loss and it is an important sensory organ which distinguishes pain, touch, itching and heat and cold. Vitamin D is synthesized in the skin. The skin is also an important organ of social and sexual contact. Perhaps the greatest disability of all is to be unwelcome and to have no confidence in one's appearance. In addition to the epidermis and dermis, the skin contains other structures including hair, blood vessels, nerves, sweat and sebaceous glands, all of which can become involved separately or in combination to produce a wide range of skin diseases such as alopecia, vasculitis, generalized pruritus, hyperhidrosis and acne. Skin failure is as worthy of medical attention as cardiac or renal failure and encompasses all of the functions described above.[1]

Why is dermatology important?

Skin disease which might benefit from medical care is very common, affecting around 22.5–33% of the population at any one time.[2,3] Historically there has been a tendency to trivialize skin disease within the medical profession and accord it a low priority in research programmes. However the public and those involved in primary care have a very different view. The psychological effects of relatively minor skin complaints can often cause more distress to the public than other more serious medical disorders.[1]

Whilst it is true that most skin diseases are not life threatening the product of high disease prevalence and low morbidity still results in a large burden of disease in absolute terms. Minor changes in health policy such as campaigns to increase public awareness of the potential dangers of pigmented lesions, have large health and financial implications simply because they affect so many people. In addition several important skin diseases such as skin cancer,[4] venous ulcers[5] and atopic eczema[6] are becoming more common and these are set to consume a higher proportion of scarce resources in future health services budgets.

Although skin disease is very common, only a fraction of people with skin conditions currently seek medical help. Even so skin conditions were the fourth most common reason for people consulting with general practitioners (GPs) in England and Wales in 1991/92,[7] accounting for at least 1500 consultations per 10 000 person–years at risk. Skin conditions comprise 4.4% of all medical outpatient activity[8] and around

1.6% of all hospital bed occupancy.[9] Skin disease accounts for 0.46% of all deaths at all ages from all causes.[10] Melanoma skin cancer alone accounted for 1142 deaths in England and Wales in 1992;[10] one-half of whom were in younger economically active age groups. Skin disease is one of the commonest reasons for injury and disablement benefit and spells of certified incapacity to work in the UK.[11,12] Total direct NHS expenditure for diseases of the skin and subcutaneous tissues in 1994 (excluding outpatient consultations) was estimated to be around £617 million, approximately 2% of total NHS health expenditure.

Where does skin disease begin and general medicine end?

Because the skin is a large and visible organ which is in direct contact with the outside environment, it has been possible to observe and describe a vast range of disease reaction patterns affecting the skin, hair and nails. Unlike most other medical specialties which usually cite around 50 diseases, dermatology has a complement of between 1000 to 2000 conditions.[13] Most of the major systemic diseases (e.g. infectious, vascular and connective tissue diseases) have manifestations which frequently affect the skin and, conversely, skin failure (e.g. caused by a severe drug reaction) has many systemic effects ranging from dehydration to heart failure, septicaemia and death. The division into what should be considered purely as a 'skin disease' is necessarily arbitrary.

The problem of defining need

The accepted definition of need as 'the population's ability to benefit from health care' [14] is not helpful in distinguishing between genuine medical need and demand that is not needed within dermatology. People who do not like the cosmetic appearance of a facial mole or a large seborrhoeic wart certainly 'benefit from health care' and express a high degree of satisfaction when such lesions are removed within the NHS. Although some might feel that such procedures should not be performed within the NHS, the concept of what constitutes a 'dis-ease' is largely couched in social terms and it is essential that both purchasers and providers are aware of the public's perception of what constitutes dermatological need and demand. Twenty years ago many cases of acne were ignored despite effective treatment being available as acne was considered to be relatively minor by physicians. The key issue is for physicians, purchasers and members of the public to work together closely in order to develop clearer guidelines as to what should constitute reasonable need for NHS dermatology services so that a system can be developed which is both fair and explicit. Because of the subtle ways in which skin diseases affect individuals and society, definition of dermatological need is best viewed as a corporate process[14,15] which should be reviewed periodically to incorporate developments in treatment and social attitudes towards the skin.

Why should further research concern purchasers?

Some of the recommendations in this chapter refer to the urgent need for research in estimating the need, supply and demand of dermatology health requirements in the UK. Although this may not at first appear to fall within the remit of purchasers covering limited geographical areas, without such vital and up-to-date information it is impossible to formulate an appropriate purchasing strategy. Simple epidemiological studies of skin disease conducted at a regional level are basic requirements of health care which could be built into purchasing contracts. Without such evidence-based health technology the potential for wastage of health care services is large.

Classification of skin diseases

The rationale for classification of skin disease[16] is currently a mixture of symptom-based terms such as 'general pruritus', purely descriptive terms such as 'papuloerythroderma' (literally meaning protruding spots on a red background), terms of anatomical distribution (e.g. leg ulcer), terms which refer to the pathology as seen on histological examination (e.g. histiocytoma), immunological staining pattern (e.g. linear IgA disease), genetic terms (e.g. X-linked ichthyosis), terms which utilize elements of disability (e.g. hand dermatitis) and uppermost on the nosological hierarchy, terms which imply a cause (e.g. vinyl chloride disease or herpes simplex).

Methods of skin disease classification

International Classification for Diseases version 9

The important ICD 9 codes for skin diseases[17] are listed in Appendix I. A very detailed alphabetical list of over 3000 dermatological categories found in ICD 9 has been published by Alexander and Shrank.[10] Cutaneous manifestations have been described in almost all diseases which affect human populations. Appendix I should therefore be viewed as a minimum list which identifies the most important and common skin diseases.

The usefulness of the ICD 9 chapter on diseases of the skin and subcutaneous tissues is discussed in more detail in Appendix I. It is at best only a very crude indicator of skin disease. The problems encountered with nebulous disease codes and exclusion of important skin complaints such as skin cancer and localized infections and the inappropriate inclusion of some 'surgical' disorders such as finger abscess make regional comparisons of common skin diseases difficult.

The system does not distinguish the serious from the trivial and it does not permit separation of conditions which may or may not benefit from available health care.

International Classification for Diseases version 10

Relevant codes are outlined in Appendix I. The ICD 10 chapter for diseases of the skin and subcutaneous tissues [19–20] contains a more comprehensive listing of relevant skin diseases than ICD 9 (L00 to L99), and exclusions to this section are clearly listed in the handbook.[20] Many rare skin diseases are listed in great detail, whereas the listings for the commonest disease groupings may be less useful in operative terms. Anomalies exist, such as the classification of atopic dermatitis (one of the commonest reasons for consultation) into many categories of obscure clinical significance (L20.0 Besnier's prurigo – a term used in some European countries which is synonymous with atopic dermatitis; L20.8 Other atopic dermatitis: flexural, infantile and intrinsic and L20.9 Atopic dermatitis unspecified). In contradistinction basal and squamous cell carcinoma of the skin, the commonest forms of cancer to affect the UK population, are not differentiated (both C44) but are separated by site codes.

Diagnosis-related classifications

The British Association of Dermatology (BAD) has formed a diagnostic coding group[21] in conjunction with the clinical terms project of the NHS centre for coding and classification (Read Codes).[22] The result of this endeavour is a very detailed, comprehensive hierarchical classification structure for skin diseases designed by dermatologists for use by UK dermatologists. The disease classifications are logically ordered and sub-categories are based on aetiology and anatomical site. This coding index also offers the opportunity for revision and updating at frequent intervals and it should be possible in the future to cross-map the BAD diagnostic codes to ICD 10 via Read Codes. The BAD diagnostic coding index is primarily intended for use by dermatologists and it is perhaps too detailed for use in primary care e.g. acne alone has 35 different categories.

In addition to the BAD coding index a detailed lexicon of dermatological terms has been allocated to ICD 10 codes, in conjunction with the International League for Dermatological Societies (of which the BAD is a member). This is yet to be published partly because the authors are awaiting confirmation of appropriateness of ICD 10 codes from the statistical division of the WHO (A Shrank, personal written communication, December 1994). The new lexicon of dermatological terms should represent a considerable improvement over ICD 9 for those seeking more comprehensive dermatology data from international data sources which use ICD classifications.

Other diagnostic coding systems

The four national morbidity surveys from general practice have utilized the Royal College of General Practitioner's diagnostic codes for skin disease.[5] These are broadly similar to ICD 9 codes with an added advantage of including disease severity status.

Summary

- Dermatology covers a wide range of over 1000 disorders affecting the skin, hair and nails.
- Skin disease is common and consumes a significant amount of NHS resources.
- Since the causes of many skin diseases are unknown, current methods of classifying skin disease are a hybrid of systems based on symptoms, signs, pathology, anatomical site, mode of inheritance and aetiology.
- The ICD 9 codes for 'diseases of the skin and subcutaneous tissues' are of limited use but those categories highlighted in Appendix I are likely to cover the nine most common disease sub-categories.
- ICD 10 codes for 'diseases of the skin and subcutaneous tissues' are more comprehensive than ICD 9 but they still do not include some common skin infections, infestations and benign and malignant skin tumours, which form a large portion of dermatological workload.
- The BAD diagnostic coding index is likely to be a useful tool for recording diagnosis of skin conditions seen by specialists.

3 Sub-categories

The following skin diseases are dealt with in full because:

- they are common
- collectively they account for around 70% of consultations in primary and secondary care [23–27]
- some data on the prevalence and effectiveness of services for these sub-categories are available
- the categories may correspond to purchasers' targets such as skin cancer.[4]

The diseases discussed are:

- skin cancer (including melanoma)
- acne
- atopic eczema
- psoriasis
- viral warts
- other infective skin conditions
- benign tumours and vascular lesions
- leg ulceration
- contact dermatitis and other eczemas.

Two potential problems exist with the proposed sub-categories:

1   Oversimplification is a danger to purchasers and consideration needs to be given to further diagnostic groups and severity gradings within these sub-categories. For example the sub-category 'skin cancer' includes several types of neoplasm ranging from very benign slow-growing lesions such as carcinoma *in situ*, to metastatic melanoma which is invariably fatal. Similarly acne can range from a physiological disorder of excessive greasiness of the skin with a few comedones (blackheads), to a severe nodulocystic process resulting in extensive permanent scarring and severe psychological disability. The corollary is that a patient with severe acne might be seen more quickly than someone with carcinoma *in situ* under the appropriate circumstances.[28]

2   In considering the sub-categories it is important to be aware that services for some skin diseases included in the remaining 30% of 'other disorders' seen by health practitioners are also important. Some common skin disorders such as urticaria and vitiligo fall into this group. Also within this group are rare but extremely disabling or fatal conditions such as epidermolysis bullosa (an inherited blistering disorder), life-threatening drug reactions and other immunobullous disorders such as pemphigus which virtually always require some form of specialist intervention.

4 Prevalence and incidence

Prevalence

Special surveys

Self-reported skin disease

In 1986 the Proprietary Association of Great Britain commissioned a detailed nationwide survey of 1217 adults and the parents of 342 children to determine how people in the UK manage minor ailments and some chronic recurring illness.[29]

Skin complaints were the most common ailment reported in the last two weeks, affecting 25% of 6009 adult 'ailments' and 36% of 806 child 'ailments'.

In addition to estimating the age and sex-specific incidence of skin complaints over a two-week period (Table II.1), the study provides a useful estimate of the proportion of skin complaints that are not considered by the public to be sufficiently severe to seek medical care and the potential service implication should that threshold change. For example of the 291 people complaining of acne/spots/greasy skin; 47% took no action, 34% used or bought an over the counter (OTC) preparation and 12% used medicines prescribed by a doctor, the remaining 7% using home remedies.

Similar proportions of self-reported skin disease in the last two weeks have been recorded in two earlier studies.[30,31] A survey in Gothenburg, Sweden of 20 000 randomly chosen residents aged 20–65 years found that 27% of females and 25% of males reported symptoms of skin disease in the last 12 months.[32]

Examined skin disease

Only one study in the UK has ever estimated the prevalence of skin diseases in the general population according to some form of physical examination. In 1975 Rea *et al.* sent a questionnaire on skin symptoms to a stratified sample of 2180 adults in Lambeth, London.[2] All positive respondents and one-fifth of those responding negatively were then interviewed and examined at home by a team of seven doctors and 11 nurses trained in the recognition of common skin disorders. Only exposed skin (face, scalp, neck, forearms, hands, knees and lower legs) was examined and the overall response rate was 90.5%. Because of difficulties in agreeing on objective criteria for skin disease severity, skin disease was classified into trivial (not justifying medical attention), moderate (justifying medical attention) and severe (needing early medical attention because of severe symptoms or risk of progression) based upon the judgement of the examiner. Medical need in this study was therefore defined as those people, who, in the opinion of a team of four dermatologists, three GPs and 11 nurses, had a skin condition 'justifying medical attention'. Such a normative definition is probably an unstable one, depending upon prevailing medical opinion, accuracy of diagnosis and knowledge of effective treatment. There is some evidence in this study that the dermatologists were more likely to categorize conditions as moderate/severe when compared with the other observers. The key findings of this study were as follows.

- The overall proportion of the population found to have any form of skin disease was 55% (95% confidence intervals 49.6 to 61.3%).
- The overall proportion considered to have skin disease worthy of medical care (i.e. moderate or severe) was 22.5% (95% confidence intervals 17.8 to 27.2%).

The breakdown according to broad diagnostic group by sex is summarized in Table 1.

The group containing tumours and naevi has the highest overall prevalence (20.5%) but 90% were considered as trivial by the examiners. In the eczema group on the other hand, with an overall prevalence of 9%, more than two-thirds were graded as moderate/severe so that the highest prevalence of conditions justifying medical care fell into this group (6.1%). The prevalence of skin disease according to severity and age group (children were not included in this study) is shown in Table II.2. Clear age trends emerge for specific disease groupings e.g. acne and warts in younger age groups, although age, sex and social class trends were not found when all forms of skin disease were considered together since several conditions had trends in opposite directions.

Usage of medical care was also recorded in this study (Table II.3). The key findings were that:

- of those with moderate/severe skin disease, only 24% made use of any medical service in the past six months
- a further 30% used self-medication
- around 20% of those with moderate/severe conditions had consulted their GP and 7% had been referred for specialist help
- medical usage was still considerable for those with trivial skin disease with 10% using medical services and 33% self-medicating.

Table 1: Prevalence of examined skin disease expressed as rates for 1000 in a survey of 2180 adults in Lambeth[2]

Skin condition	Both sexes		Male		Female	
	All grades	Moderate and severe	All grades	Moderate and severe	All grades	Moderate and severe
Tumours and vascular lesions	204.7	14.1	141.9	0.6	264.1	26.8
Eczema	90.1	61.2	99.5	80.2	81.1	43.4
Acne	85.0	31.6	109.0	31.5	61.1	31.7
Scaly dermatoses	84.7	28.7	118.3	39.2	53.0	18.9
Scalp and hair disorders	82.1	13.6	79.0	7.9	95.0	18.9
Prurigo and allied conditions	82.1	38.9	60.8	16.9	95.0	59.6
Erythematous and other dermatoses	75.0	21.4	30.9	20.8	116.8	22.0
Infective and parasitic conditions	46.0	6.7	48.2	10.9	43.9	2.8
Warts	34.3	1.5	35.9	–	32.8	2.8
Nail disorders	33.0	18.8	23.9	12.5	41.8	24.8
Psoriasis	15.8	5.8	24.4	3.7	7.7	7.7
Mouth and tongue disorders	8.9	0.7	15.4	–	2.7	1.3
Chronic ulcer	1.7	–	3.5	–	–	–
Any skin condition	554.7 (495.9–613.5)	225.0 (178.2–271.8)	479.1 (399.7–558.5)	213.0 (164.4–279.6)	606.7 (520.0–693.3)	236.0 (170.1–301.9)

Despite the large number of observers, limited nature of the skin examinations and ambiguous definition of medical need, this important study suggests that:

- skin conditions that may benefit from medical care are extremely common in the community
- most sufferers do not seek medical help.

Given the scarcity of epidemiological data on skin disease within the UK, mention should also be made of another detailed cross-sectional study of skin diseases contained within the first US Health and Nutrition Examination Survey (NHANES).[3]

This study was conducted on a representative population sample of 20 749 persons aged one to 74 years from 65 primary sampling units throughout the US during 1971–74 and included a detailed structured skin examination by 101 dermatologists. Clinical findings were backed by laboratory investigations such as mycology culture and skin biopsy where possible. The following indicate that significant skin pathology is common.

- Nearly one-third (312.4 per 1000 population) had one or more significant skin conditions which was considered by the dermatologist to be worthy of evaluation by a physician at least once (Table III.1).
- The prevalence of significant skin pathology increased rapidly with age (Figure III.1) from 142.3 per 1000 children aged 1–5 years to 362.0 per 1000 youths age 1–17 years and to 365.2 per 1000 young adults aged 18–24 years, due primarily to the increase in acne at puberty.

- After a slight decline at age 25–34 years the prevalence of skin pathology again increases steadily reflecting the increase in chronic diseases such as psoriasis, vitiligo, malignant and benign tumours, actinic and seborrhoeic keratoses.
- In this study significant skin pathology was slightly commoner in males (Table III.2).
- An additional 12.5% of the population were deemed to have a skin condition that was clinically inactive at the time of examination.

Minor degrees of skin disease or abnormalities were also recorded by the dermatologists for each disease group and these are shown in Table III.3. There was a considerable mismatch between what the dermatologists considered to represent medical need and the population's concerns.

- Nearly one-third (31%) of persons with significant skin pathology diagnosed by the dermatologists expressed concern about these specific skin conditions, whereas nearly 18% of those who complained about their skin conditions were not considered as serious by the dermatologists.

The following findings were found in relation to disability and handicap.

- Skin conditions were reported to limit activity in 10.5 per 1000 of the population aged 1–74 years, or 9% of those persons with such skin conditions.
- About 10% of those persons with skin complaints considered the condition to be a handicap to their employment or housework and 1% considered themselves severely handicapped.
- About one-third (33%) of those persons with skin conditions indicated that the condition(s) was a handicap in their social relations.
- The dermatological examiner rated more than two-thirds of those persons with skin complaints as disfigured to some extent from the condition and about one-fifth of those were rated moderately or severely disfigured.
- More than half of those persons with skin complaints reported some overall discomfort from the condition such as itching or burning.
- An estimated 62.8 per 1000 US population (or 56% of those with skin complaints) indicated that the conditions were recurrent, with 49% active in the preceding seven to 12 months.

The following outlines findings for sub–optimal care.

- Only one-fifth of those with significant skin pathology were considered by the dermatologist to be receiving optimal care.
- Of the remaining 81% who were not receiving optimal care nearly all (94%) could, in the judgement of the survey dermatologists, be improved with more expert care (84% in pre-school children to 96% among the elderly).
- Nearly one-fourth (23.9%) of adults aged 18–74 years of age with significant skin pathology indicated that their condition might have been caused or worsened by occupational exposures.

The following information was found on medical advice.

- About one-half of the US population aged 1–74 years of age with skin complaints had not sought medical advice for the problem.
- Males were more likely than females to not seek medical advice (56 compared with 44% respectively).
- Nearly 15% were given inadequate medical advice in the view of the dermatologist in those who received medical advice.
- About 6% did not co-operate with the doctors they had consulted.

To minimize examiner variability in this study the 101 dermatologist examiners underwent a training period and findings were recorded on a structured form. Even so there was considerable variation between these dermatologists in the degree to which they recorded banal lesions such as freckles and normal variations. Age-adjusted prevalence rates of significant skin pathology ranged from zero to 90.4% according to the examiner, the average being 31.2%. The range in the proportion expressing complaints about skin conditions to the examiner was from 0 to 70.8%, the average being 11.4%. The study is therefore limited by the wide variation in what the 101 dermatologist examiners considered as need and physicians' views might have changed since the early 1970s. Given the predominantly private care system in the US, it is also possible that US dermatologists had a lower threshold than UK dermatologists for what skin conditions might benefit from medical intervention. Nevertheless the study provides us with the most detailed account of skin pathology and its relation to disability and health-seeking behaviour to date. Population surveys in other European countries have indicated a similar high prevalence of skin disease in the community.[33–35]

Summary of prevalence studies of skin diseases in general

- There are no recent population studies on the need, supply and demand for skin care in the UK.
- Studies conducted in the UK and US 20 years ago suggest that skin disease is very common, affecting around one-quarter to one-third of the population at any one time.
- Around 10% of those with skin disease report that the condition seriously interferes with their activities.
- Only 20% of those with a skin condition which might benefit from medical care sought medical help in the UK.
- Around 10% of those with trivial skin conditions also seek medical help.
- Region of residence, sex, age, social class, ethnic group, skin type, occupation and leisure activities are all important determinants of skin disease prevalence in the UK.
- Generalizations about the determinants of the entire range of skin diseases are limited because subgroups may exhibit trends in opposite directions.

Routinely collected data

Morbidity statistics

Most morbidity data refer to those who seek medical help in the primary care setting. With the exception of a few conditions such as cellulitis where incidence and demand are closely related, the extent to which routine morbidity data reflect demand or genuine dermatological need is unclear. Despite these limitations routine statistics such as the four morbidity surveys from general practice[5,7,36,37] are useful in that they provide us with an estimate of the magnitude and determinants of those who seek medical care. Data validity is discussed in Appendix IV. Patient consulting rates in general practice for diseases of the skin and subcutaneous tissues have steadily increased over the last 40 years as shown in Figure 1, although some of these changes could be due to differences in the age structure of the populations studied.[5,7]

In the second general practice morbidity survey of 1970–72[37] diseases of the skin and subcutaneous tissues were among the top eight reasons for people seeking help, accounting for 6.5% of patient contact. The referral rate for specialist opinion for those who contacted their GP because of a skin problem was 4.5 per 100. A more detailed social class analysis revealed very little difference in consultation rates between social classes defined by occupation and marital status. Benign skin neoplasms had a higher standardized patient

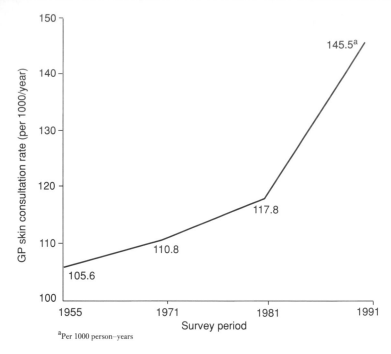

Figure 1: Increase in consulting rates in general practice for diseases of the skin and subcutaneous tissue over the last 40 years.
Source: Data obtained from the four general practitioner morbidity surveys.[5,7,36,37]

consultation ratio in the non-manual classes (especially men) and in manual classes for women. There was little evidence to support differences in urban and rural consultation rates.

In the third 1981/82 morbidity survey[5] diseases of the skin and subcutaneous tissues were one of the ten most common diagnoses made in general practice. Around 6% of all GP diagnoses made in the RCGP study involved the skin and 5% of these were referred for specialist opinion, a similar proportion to other specialties.

Data from the fourth national morbidity study[7] by GPs in England and Wales (1991/92) show that about 15% of the population per year seek advice regarding conditions relating to the skin or subcutaneous tissues (the fourth commonest reason for seeking GP advice). These estimates are to be viewed as a minimum since they exclude those consulting for skin neoplasms and some skin infections such as herpes simplex. The average number of consultations per person–year for each skin condition was 1.26. Approximately 3.5%, 7.6% and 4.9% of people consulted their GP each year because of skin infections, inflammatory skin conditions and 'other diseases of the skin and subcutaneous tissues' respectively. Around 2% of the population consulted about eczema/dermatitis and 0.75% for psoriasis.

Although none of the skin conditions seen in this survey were considered life threatening, only one-quarter of the skin conditions were considered by GPs to be minor in severity (defined as commonly treated without recourse to medical advice or requiring no specific treatment). This survey covered around half a million people in 60 practices in England and Wales and had a bias towards larger, computerized practices with younger principals. Around 4.2% of those with a skin complaint were referred for specialist opinion from the survey practices. When compared with the 1981/82 survey there was a 24% increase in consultation rates for those aged five to 14/15 years of age and a 16% increase for those aged 15/16 to 24 years of age, compared with a 8% and 7% increase for all diseases within each age group.[38] Table 2 shows age-specific consultation rates for diseases of the skin and subcutaneous tissues (excluding skin tumours and some infections) for 1991/92.[7] Highest consultation rates are found in the very young, followed by a decline and subsequent smaller peak in the 16–24 year age group. Consultation rates remain lower throughout adulthood except for a more progressive increase with increasing age above 65.

Table 2: Patients consulting GPs for diseases of the skin and subcutaneous tissues of minor and intermediate severity in 1991/92 expressed as rates per 10000 person–years at risk[7]

Chapter XII	Total	Age							
		0–4	5–15	16–24	25–44	45–64	65–74	75–84	85+
Total	1455	2715	1418	1697	1288	1177	1387	1472	1613
Intermediate	1100	2295	1014	1339	950	852	1044	1110	1235
Minor	455	602	498	477	421	407	451	473	506

Mortality and skin disease

Overall mortality is relatively low for skin diseases, accounting for at least 2578 deaths in 1992 (or 0.46% of deaths from all causes and all ages).[10] Melanoma skin cancer alone accounted for a total of 1142 deaths in England and Wales in 1992 (565 male and 577 female), with 48% occurring in economically active adults.[10] Other malignant neoplasms of the skin (basal cell carcinoma, squamous cell carcinoma and cutaneous lymphoma) accounted for 298 male deaths and 222 female deaths in 1992. Six deaths were recorded for 'benign' neoplasms of the skin in 1992.[10]

Mortality from skin diseases other than skin cancer has increased slightly over the last ten years. In 1991 there were 240 male deaths due to diseases of the skin and subcutaneous tissues and 688 female deaths; a 20% relative increase when compared with 1988.[39] Chronic ulcer of the skin accounted for two-thirds of the female deaths (an increase of 19% from 386 deaths in 1990 mainly due to women aged 80 and over).[39]

Pharmaceutical services

In the 1992 Health Survey for England[40] skin disease was the sixth commonest reason for issuing a prescription, yet it represented one of the lowest cost per items when compared with other prescribed medicines, with an average gross ingredient cost of £4.49 compared with £8.15 for respiratory disorders and £13.47 for gastrointestinal disorders.

In 1993 total prescription costs for dermatology (all items included in *BNF* Chapter 13) amounted to £143.6 million (Prescription Pricing Authority, written communication, 1994). This compares with OTC sales of skin and acne preparations of £138.8 million in 1993.[29] Over-the-counter sales of skin and acne preparations represented an 18.2% increase compared with 1992, due mainly to OTC treatments for vaginal thrush and topical acyclovir for cold sores (K Fitzsimons, Proprietary Association of Great Britain, written communication, 1994).

Summary of routinely available data on prevalence and costs of skin disease

- About 15% of the population consult their GP each year because of a skin complaint.
- General practice consultation rates for diseases of the skin increase with age and are slightly higher for females.
- GP consultation rates also probably vary with other factors such as ethnic group, skin type and social class. Summary statistics for skin diseases as a whole may obscure these trends.

- Consultation rates for skin disease in general practice have probably increased over the last 20 years both in absolute and relative terms.
- About 5% of those who seek help from their GP are referred for further specialist advice.
- Mortality from skin diseases is low, accounting for 2578 deaths in 1992, or 0.46% of deaths from all causes at all ages.
- Over-the-counter sales for skin preparations accounted for £138.8 million in 1993, or 11.8% of total OTC sales.

Incidence data

Unfortunately no population-based studies on the incidence of examined skin disease considered as a whole have been conducted. Incidence data are available for some skin disease sub-categories such as new diagnoses of melanoma and these are discussed below. Many skin diseases such as psoriasis are chronic and persistent and their impact may be estimated reasonably well from cross-sectional prevalence studies such as those outlined on pages 267–271.

Many infectious skin diseases such as impetigo, on the other hand, are transient and incident data are required to assess their importance. In the absence of appropriate population studies, GP morbidity statistics provide us with some information on demand incidence for these transient disorders.[7] Although it is likely that all cases of impetigo presenting to doctors represent medical need, it is not known how many resort to self-treatment in the community. Some skin diseases are both chronic and intermittent (e.g. atopic eczema) and other measures such as the one-year period prevalence are the most appropriate measure of disease burden.

Common skin disease groupings

Skin cancer

Skin cancer has become a Health of the Nation target 'to halt the year-on-year increase in the incidence of skin cancer by 2005'.[4] The term skin cancer usually refers to three main diseases:

1   malignant melanoma
2   basal cell carcinoma
3   squamous cell carcinoma.

The last two are often considered jointly as non-melanoma skin cancer. Other forms of cancer such as cutaneous T-cell lymphoma also affect the skin and, although they are comparatively rare, can be miserable conditions which require specialist care. Melanoma, basal cell and squamous cell carcinoma are discussed in more detail in Appendices V and VI.

Key points for skin cancer in general are:

- halting the year-on-year increase in the incidence of skin by 2005 is a Health of the Nation target
- because of the long latent period between exposure and disease, the overall incidence of both melanoma and non-melanoma skin cancer will probably continue to increase for the next 30 years
- skin cancer is largely preventable.

Melanoma skin cancer

- Melanoma is a comparatively rare but potentially lethal tumour, accounting for 1265 deaths in the UK in 1992.[41]
- The incidence and mortality of melanoma has increased substantially over the last 30 years.
- Melanoma incidence increases with age but it also affects proportionately more economically active people than other cancers.
- Risk factors for melanoma include increased number of moles, atypical moles, episodes of severe sunburn, fair skin type, red or blonde hair, tendency to freckle and a positive family history.
- Melanoma is almost twice as common in females than in males in the UK, with 2722 and 1716 newly registered cases in 1988 for females and males respectively.
- Early diagnosis and surgical removal of a thin (<1.5 mm) melanoma is usually curative.

Non-melanoma skin cancer

- Non-melanoma skin cancer is the commonest cancer in the UK, affecting around 2% of people over the age of 60.
- The incidence of non-melanoma skin cancer has increased substantially over the last 20 years but it is difficult to say how much of this change is due to increased registration.
- Non-melanoma skin cancer registrations show considerable regional variation throughout the UK.
- The incidence of non-melanoma skin cancer rises sharply with age, with most tumours occurring above the age of 60.
- The incidence of non-melanoma skin cancer is likely to increase with an increasingly ageing population.
- Subjects with one non-melanoma cancer are at high risk of developing further new lesions.
- Deaths from non-melanoma skin cancer are uncommon, amounting to 486 deaths in 1992 in the UK.

Acne

Acne refers to a group of disorders characterized by abnormalities of the sebaceous glands. Although over 40 types of acne have been described,[21] acne vulgaris, which commonly affects teenagers and acne rosacea which typically affects adults form the bulk of this disease subgroup. Because of the lack of data for acne variants such as acne rosacea, only acne vulgaris is discussed in more detail in Appendix VII.

The key points on the prevalence of acne are:

- prevalence surveys must take acne severity into account because minor degrees of acne are almost universal in teenage years
- acne which is deemed as clinically significant by physicians affects around 1% to 14% of teenagers
- although considered to be a 'teenage' disease acne continues to affect around 3.5% of those aged 25 to 34 years
- severe acne with cysts and scarring affects around 0.6% to 1.4% of young adults
- acne forms a considerable burden of psychological misery in the population (Figure 2)
- recent surveys suggest that there might have been a shift in the distribution of acne severity towards the milder end over the last 20 years, perhaps due to better treatment.

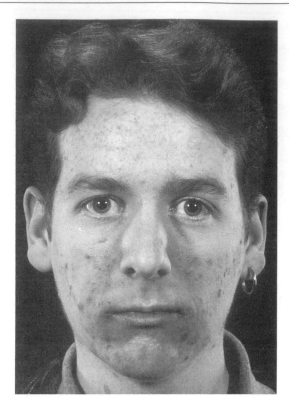

Figure 2: Despite trivialization of skin disease, it can have a devastating effect on peoples' lives. Acne is just one example where social stigmatization is still common. Would this man's appearance influence your decision to employ him?
(Photograph reproduced with written permission from the subject.)

Atopic eczema

Atopic eczema (or 'childhood eczema') is an inflammatory skin disorder characterized by itching, involvement of the skin creases and onset in early life and is discussed in Appendix VIII. Key points on the prevalence of atopic eczema are:

- atopic eczema currently affects between 5% to 20% of children by the age of seven in the UK
- the intractable itch of atopic eczema causes sleep loss and misery to children and disruption to family life
- although eczema prevalence is higher in childhood, adults may form the bulk of cases when entire populations are considered
- atopic eczema is commoner in wealthier families and in Afro-Caribbean children for reasons which are not clear at present
- past studies suggest that there may be considerable regional variation in eczema prevalence throughout the UK
- there is reasonable evidence to suggest that the prevalence of atopic eczema has increased substantially over the last 30 years for reasons which are unclear.

Psoriasis

Psoriasis is a chronic inflammatory skin disorder characterized by red scaly areas which commonly affect the knees, elbows, lower back and scalp and is discussed in more detail in Appendix IX.

The key points of prevalence studies suggest:

- the prevalence of psoriasis in the general population is around 1% to 3%
- between one- and two-thirds of psoriasis sufferers have clinically significant disease according to physicians
- psoriasis exhibits a bimodal age distribution with a first peak in early adulthood and a smaller peak in later life
- psoriasis tends to be a chronic condition.

Viral warts

Viral warts are discussed further in Appendix X.

The key points of prevalence studies are:

- viral warts affect between 4% to 5% of children in the UK aged 11 to 16
- the Lambeth study found that 3.5% of adults aged 25–34 years also had viral warts
- around 60% to 90% of warts clear spontaneously within two years
- there is considerable regional variation in wart prevalence in the UK with highest rates in Northern districts
- wart prevalence is also less in children born to parents with non-manual occupations and in smaller families
- warts may be less common in children from ethnic groups other than white European.

Other infective disorders

This category refers to a miscellaneous range of other bacterial, viral and fungal infections which are discussed further in Appendix XI.

The key points of prevalence studies are:

- taken as a whole, prevalence rates for this category range from 4.6% to 9.3%
- these point prevalence rates probably underestimate the true burden of skin infections by a considerable degree, since most are transient
- at least 4% of the population consulted their GP for a skin infection other than warts in 1993/94
- the age distribution of skin infections differs according to the infectious agent and clinical pattern
- impetigo and scalp ringworm usually affect children, boils peak in young adulthood and chronic fungal infections are common in older adults
- fungal infection of the toe webs (athletes' foot) may affect 3.9% of the population
- certain occupational groups working in wet conditions are more prone to fungal infections of the feet and toenails.

Benign tumours and vascular lesions

This sub-category refers to a range of cutaneous lesions which either cause discomfort or concern because of the need to exclude malignant or premalignant disease and they are discussed further in Appendix XII.

The key points of prevalence studies are:

- white adults usually have between 40 to 60 moles on their body
- small changes in public anxiety about moles can have large service implications
- prevalence surveys conducted by physicians suggest that around 1.4% to 5.1% of the population have a benign skin tumour which may warrant medical attention
- the prevalence of benign tumours and precancerous lesions shows a striking increase with age from 2% in children to 13% in those aged 65–74 years
- solar keratoses are premalignant skin lesions which affect around 23% of those aged over 65
- the risk of malignant transformation of solar keratoses is probably less than 1% per year and 10% to 27% remit spontaneously
- port wine stains are permanent vascular malformations which are usually found on the face. They occur in around two to four of every 1000 live births
- the psychological consequences of port wine lesions can be devastating for the sufferer.

Leg ulcers

Leg ulceration may be due to a range of disorders from squamous cell carcinoma through to sickle cell disease, diabetes and rheumatoid arthritis. In the UK the commonest causes are venous disease, arterial disease or a mixture of both. These are discussed more fully in Appendix XIII.

The key points of prevalence studies are:

- leg ulcers may occur for a number of reasons but venous (70%) or arterial disease (10%) or both (20%) are the commonest causes in the UK
- venous leg ulcers affect around 0.1% to 2% of the population
- the prevalence of leg ulcers increases with increasing age
- leg ulcers are an important cause of pain and morbidity in the elderly and consume a large proportion of nursing time
- approximately one-half to two-thirds of venous ulcers recur within a year
- the proportion of people with leg ulcers is likely to rise considerably in the future because of an increasingly ageing population.

Contact dermatitis and other eczemas

These are discussed in Appendix XIV.

The key points of prevalence studies are:

- in the UK the term eczema usually refers to an endogenous process whereas dermatitis usually denotes a contact factor such as exposure to irritants or specific allergens
- the prevalence of contact dermatitis and endogenous eczemas (other than atopic eczema) is around 9% in the UK
- one large US survey has suggested that about one-quarter of cases in this subgroup are clinically significant
- hand dermatitis can be crippling and lead to permanent disability and loss of earnings (Figure 3)
- certain occupations pose high risks for individuals to develop contact dermatitis
- eczema and contact dermatitis account for 84% to 90% of occupational skin disease.

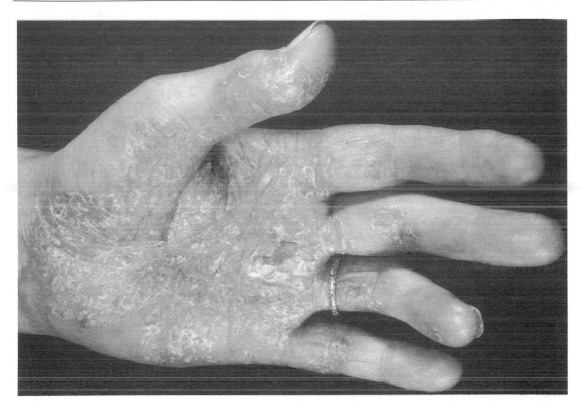

Figure 3: The hand that cannot work. Hand eczema can be crippling and lead to permanent disability and loss of earnings.

Other important skin diseases

These are discussed in Appendix XV

The key points from prevalence studies are:

- because of the heterogenous nature of this remaining group of skin diseases there will be a temptation to allocate it with a low priority, yet skin conditions in this group still affect around 3.9 million people in the UK
- included in this group are rare but potentially fatal skin disorders such as blistering diseases, lymphoma and severe cutaneous drug reactions
- other common skin disorders such as vitiligo and urticaria are included in this group
- because skin disease is so common, around 7% of the population will have more than one skin disease (or around one-quarter of those with significant skin disease).

5 Services available

Introduction

People with skin problems require a range of health services from simple advice to specialist investigation and management. The most usual routes of help currently in use are summarized in the flow chart (Figure 4). The estimated number of people using current dermatology health services at various entry points for a population of 100 000 over a one-year period is summarized in Box 1.

Box 1: A guide to the number of persons per 100 000 per year using dermatology services

• Number with a skin complaint	=	25000 (at least 25% of total population)[29]
• Number who will self-treat	=	7500 (30% of those with skin complaint)[2]
• Number who will seek advice from GP	=	14550[a] (15% of total population or 19% of all GP consultations)[7]
• Number referred on to dermatologist	=	1162 (8% of those attending their GP for skin problems, or 1.2% of the total population)[42]
• Number admitted to hospital	=	24 to 31 (2% to 3% of all new dermatology referrals)[43]
• Number of deaths due to skin disease	=	5[b] (0.4% of all new dermatology referrals)[10]

[a] Excludes skin neoplasms, viral warts, herpes simplex and scabies.
[b] Includes people dying from cellulitis, chronic ulcer of the skin and severe drug reactions who might not have been admitted under a dermatologist's care.

Self-help

Although self-help and self-medication are not traditionally regarded as a health service, the range and availability of OTC skin products is an important element in the equation of balancing need, supply and demand. Around 30% of those with a skin complaint decide to self-medicate and this proportion is similar for trivial and moderate to severe disease.[2] Many effective skin treatments are available OTC such as 1% hydrocortisone for mild eczema, topical acyclovir cream for cold sores, topical benzoyl peroxide for acne and numerous anti-fungal preparations and wart removers.

Pharmacists occupy a key role in advising the public on the use of these products but whether this advice is beneficial or whether it simply delays appropriate medical consultation has not been studied adequately in the UK.[44] Self-help groups such as the National Eczema Society, Psoriasis Association and Acne Support Group are well organized and are a useful source of advice to those with mainly chronic skin diseases. They have recently joined forces to form a Skin Care Campaign to increase public and government awareness regarding skin disease.[45]

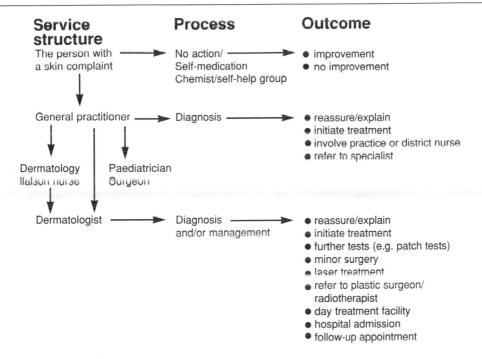

Figure 4: Routes of help currently available for a person with a skin complaint. Other routes of help such as referral to occupational health doctors, other specialists, attendances at the A and E department and contact with practice or hospital nurses are also used occasionally.

Primary care

The majority of those with a skin complaint who seek medical help are treated by their GP. In addition to making a diagnosis and prescribing medication, treatment may well include simple reassurance or explanation and advice. The GP contract in April 1990 introduced payment for minor surgical procedures and many GPs now conduct their own minor surgery for benign and sometimes malignant skin lesions.

Around 6–8% of all GP diagnoses involve the skin [26,46] The most recent GP morbidity statistics[7] suggest that 1455 people per 10 000 person–years at risk (approximately 15% per year) consult their GP because of a skin condition (excluding benign and malignant skin neoplasms and some skin infections). Despite this only one in ten GPs has received special training in dermatology and most of those who had no training wished they had.[47] A more recent study of 456 GPs in Avon found that most were willing to shoulder more of the dermatological burden, yet 57% said they had little interest in the subject and had not attended any dermatology teaching since qualifying.[48] The average 'block' allocated to dermatology undergraduate training is less than 40 hours and in some centres dermatology is entirely optional. In a recent survey of 165 UK GPs 97% felt that undergraduate training in dermatology was essential and that more time should be allocated to the subject.[49] Some GPs gain further experience working as clinical assistants in dermatology and some have undergone further training leading to a diploma in dermatology qualification. General practitioners interested in skin care have recently formed a primary care dermatology society.[50]

Practice nurses and district nurses are involved to a variable extent in the treatment of skin diseases, with up to 50% of their time employed in administering dressings for leg ulcers. In a recent survey 33% of 800 practice nurses reported that they saw five to ten patients with skin disease each week but less than 7% felt that they had the knowledge to deal with them.[47]

The range of skin disorders seen in general practice is similar to that in the general population, with the nine sub-categories mentioned in this report accounting for the majority of consultations.[5,26] A greater proportion of incident diseases such as skin infections (e.g. impetigo, herpes simplex and viral exanthems) are commoner in general practice settings than in secondary care.[5,7]

Use of specialist services

Outpatients

Most specialist dermatology activity is concentrated in the outpatient department. Persistent waiting list problems occur[51] and overbooking of clinics to expedite long waits by patients distressed by their skin condition and to accommodate emergency referrals such as acute drug eruptions and skin infections is common. Currently there are only 312 dermatologists throughout the UK, providing a ratio of 1 per 217 000 members of the population;[7] the lowest specialist ratio throughout the EU by a factor of around three (Table 3). The ratio of specialists to the population is generally much lower throughout all specialties within the UK than elsewhere in the EU, although the ratio of dermatologists to population in the UK in 1992 (1 : 217 000) is still quite low compared with other comparable specialties such as ENT (1 : 128 000), ophthalmology (1 : 115 000) and general medicine (1 : 41 000).[52] In 1990 there were 537 worked outpatient sessions per dermatology consultant in the UK compared with 149 sessions per general medicine consultant.[8] Diagnosing skin disease takes time to learn and constant practice to refine and dermatologists spend a period of around ten years training, although this period will be reduced when the Calman proposals for training are introduced.

Table 3: Ratio of dermatologists to population in Europe[47]

Country	Total	Ratio/population
France	2800	1 : 20 400
Italy	2900	1 : 20 000
Belgium	450	1 : 22 000
Greece	400	1 : 25 000
West Germany	1600	1 : 39 000
Spain	900	1 : 43 000
Portugal	300	1 : 44 700
Denmark	100	1 : 50 000
The Netherlands	300	1 : 80 000
UK	312	1 : 200 000

What does the specialist do?

In addition to diagnosis, explanation and treatment in routine clinics which can be accomplished without recourse to further investigations in most patients,[51] the dermatologist offers a range of services. Most teaching centres run clinics which specialize in contact dermatitis and industrial skin diseases and a patch-testing service, paediatric dermatology, pigmented lesions, supervision of ultraviolet light treatment and combined plastic surgery/radiotherapy clinics for skin tumours.

Other clinics which reflect the special interest of local dermatologists may also exist in some areas, such as those which deal with vulval conditions, somatic disorders, eczema, blistering disorders and laser clinics. Dermatological surgery is performed by all dermatologists and services may range from diagnostic biopsy to more complicated surgical techniques for skin tumours. Some forms of immediate surgical procedure (excision, biopsy, cryotherapy, curettage and cautery) are conducted in around a third of new patients.[51] Some centres also offer laser treatment for vascular lesions.

Assessment and removal of tumours is a major part (40%) of the specialist's workload and dermatological surgery is recognized by the Royal College of Surgeons of London as an important part of the practice of dermatology. All dermatologists are trained in removal of tumours with repair by a variety of closure techniques involving simple closure, skin grafts and skin flaps. Some dermatologists have been trained in advanced surgical techniques such as Mohs micrographic surgery, which is not practised by plastic surgeons and has the lowest recurrence rates of all procedures for removal of skin cancers.[53] Dermatologists work closely with a range of other specialists such as plastic surgeons and radiotherapists for skin tumours and also with paediatricians in genetic disorders and chronic skin diseases in childhood such as atopic eczema. The dermatologist also undertakes an important role in educational activities which includes teaching medical students, pharmacy students, nurses, postgraduates and GPs. Some dermatologists have conducted 'outreach' clinics in the community but a recent survey by BAD has indicated that dermatologists see, on average, only ten patients per session against the BAD recommended figure of 12 to 24.

Despite the vast range of dermatological disorders that a dermatologist may encounter the majority of disorders encountered in the outpatient department are covered within the subgroups mentioned in this chapter.[13,51,54] Around 12% of referrals were considered inappropriate by dermatologists in a West Midlands study.[51] Another study in Leicester showed that even a senior house officer with three months training in dermatology considered that 26% of 490 consecutive referrals were probably unnecessary[55] and that 75% of these unnecessary referrals belonged to just seven disease categories (warts, eczema, naevi, basal cell carcinoma, acne, psoriasis and seborrhoeic warts).

Age-specific attendance rates are more common in female patients and also increase with increasing age (Table 4). Other studies such as the Oxford Regional study have recorded a similar excess of female and older patients.[24] Of 3678 referrals to dermatology (8.1% of all outpatient referrals), 42.7% of these were males and 57.3% female. Age- and sex-specific referral rates for Oxford are shown in Figure 5. In nearly two-thirds of referrals the GP expected the patient to be treated or taken over by the specialist (Table 5).

Table 4: Age-specific attendance rates per 1000 population for new patients attending dermatology clinics in West Midlands in November 1988[51]

Age (years)	0–4	5–14	15–29	30–44	45–64	65–74	75+	Total
Male	6.7	6.6	7.6	6.6	7.6	12.1	13.9	7.8
Female	5.2	9.9	12.7	10.7	11.5	10.4	10.9	10.9
Total	6.0	8.2	10.1	8.6	9.5	11.1	11.9	9.3

Table 5: Main reasons for a GP to refer a patient for specialist dermatology advice in the Oxford Region[24]

Diagnosis/ investigation (%)	Advice only (%)	Treatment/ management (%)	Second opinion/ reassure (%)	Other (%)
26.4	13.5	63	2.2	0.2

Private referrals accounted for 21.2% of referrals to dermatology in this region and these were spread fairly evenly across age groups. Another retrospective national survey of a clinical caseload of 217 private hospitals in England and Wales recorded 28 706 consultations for the 1992/93 financial year for diseases of the skin and subcutaneous tissues (excluding plastic surgery), or 4.2% of all procedures carried put in private hospitals.[56] This represents a three-fold rise in private dermatology episodes when compared with 1981 data,

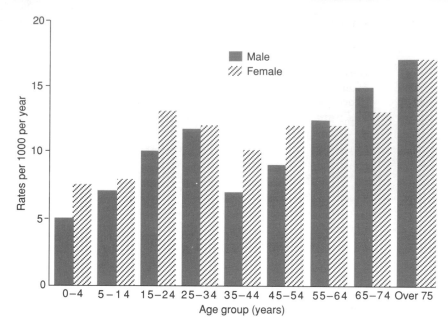

Figure 5: Age- and sex-specific outpatient referrals for dermatology in the Oxford Region in 1992[24]

whereas all medical and surgical procedures taken as a whole rose approximately two-fold. It is difficult to state whether this increase in private dermatology truly reflects individual's desire to pay for skin care treatment since most of these private episodes were paid by insurance schemes but the figures provide us with some idea of the magnitude of dermatology services in the private sector.

How much does the specialist do?

In the year ending 31 March 1994 the attendance rate for dermatology referrals in the whole of the UK was 11.62 per 1000 population (Statistical Information Unit, Trent Regional Health Authority, 1995). The number of dermatology referrals per year in the UK has increased by 150 282 (33%) over the past three years, representing a change in referral rate from 9.4 to 12.5 per 1000 over the same period.[42] Referral rates in different regions varied slightly in the year ending March 1994 from 10.55 in North West Region to 12.95 in South Thames (Table 6). A further 22.48 per 1000 population were given follow-up appointments, giving an overall new/follow-up ratio of approximately 1 : 2. Around 6% of newly referred patients did not keep their appointments.

These numbers probably underestimate a dermatologist's workload by around 10% as they do not include ward referrals and consultations with staff members.[54] Private outpatient consultations accounted for an overall 0.5% of all new and follow-up dermatology patients seen in the UK in 1990,[8] compared to 0.3% of total general surgery and general medicine activity. This proportion of private activity shows considerable regional variation from 0.2% in Yorkshire to 2.6% in North West Thames.[57]

These figures probably underestimate the current private dermatology activity carried out by recently opened laser clinics and GPs with some training in dermatology.

Although 30% to 40% of new dermatology outpatients undergo some form of minor surgical procedure, these have only recently been recorded by hospitals.[52] Similarly other activities such as dressings and attendance for PUVA are not recorded in routinely published hospital statistics.

Table 6: Consultant outpatient activity for dermatology in the UK in the year ending March 31 1994 by new NHS regions.

Region (new NHS regional offices)	Population (000)[a]	Referral attendances	Rate per 1000 population	Consultant initiated attendances[b]	Rate per 1000 population	Total GP written referral requests	Rate per 1000 population
North West	6935	73194	10.55	126809	18.29	86283	12.44
North East and Yorkshire	6314	74039	11.73	187026	29.62	77508	12.28
Trent	4777	57062	11.95	129946	27.20	51715	10.83
Anglia and Oxford	5325	54812	10.29	97076	18.23	60788	11.42
North Thames	6892	87635	12.72	151459	21.98	92803	13.47
South Thames	6809	88196	12.95	144877	21.28	100509	14.76
South West	6397	72432	11.32	156511	24.47	76254	11.92
West Midlands	5294	56723	10.71	95881	18.11	56397	10.65
Special HAs	–	2361		6042	–	2295	–
UK	48743	566454	11.62	1095627	22.48	604552	12.40

[a] 1994 Mid-year population (1991 projection).

[b] Consultant initiated attendances means follow-up visits initiated by a consultant.

Variations in referral rates

In the third GP morbidity survey, regional referral rates for dermatology varied from 3.1 to 12.2% of all those seen.[5] The overall rates in this survey are lower than for the rest of the UK probably because of the unrepresentative nature of the GPs selected for this survey. The study does however suggest a considerable variation in referral rates by GPs. Severity of skin disease does not appear to be a major determinant of referrals, since 8.1% of serious and 6.5% of trivial ones were sent to hospital in the 1981/82 study.[5] Referral rates for individual districts within the Trent Region also vary considerably from 4.92 to 17.7 per 1000 in 1994 (Statistical Information Unit, Trent Regional Health Authority 1995), although less variation is seen within each district with time (Table 7). Small area referral rates for new patients in the Bristol District for 1991 to 1994 also show a wider variation in referral rates, ranging from 9.5 to 49.1 outpatient attendances per 1000 population (C Kennedy, personal written communication,1994). There was a strong relationship between referral rates and accessibility to hospital services in this small area study.

There is some evidence to suggest that much of the regional variation in referral rates may be governed by established patterns of care such as number of available consultants rather than reflecting any special dermatological need related to the demographic constitution of the local population. A study by Roland and Morris failed to show any relationship between referral rates for dermatology services and medical need as suggested by standardized mortality ratios or mean number of prescriptions issued by GPs (standardized regression coefficient of 0.1).[58] It is possible that mortality ratios are not a suitable surrogate measure for dermatological need. A strong relationship between dermatology referral rates and the number of dermatology consultants per 100 000 population was present however (standardized regression coefficient of 0.82, $p < 0.001$). Given that skin diseases are undertreated and that treatments for many skin diseases are

Table 7: General practitioner written referral requests for dermatology per 1000 population for the districts within Trent Region over the last seven years. (Data kindly supplied by the Statistical Information Unit, Trent Regional Health Authority)

District	1988	1989	1990	1991	1992	1993	1994
North Derbyshire	10.07	11.01	11.70	9.88	10.62	9.14	10.09
South Derbyshire	10.21	11.07	11.07	9.17	8.96	8.42	10.39
Leicestershire	8.98	9.33	9.33	8.80	8.34	8.26	4.92
North Lincolnshire	7.91	7.44	7.44	6.86	9.11	10.06	9.99
South Lincolnshire	7.42	7.65	7.65	7.55	7.98	8.39	9.05
Bassetlaw	6.58	6.25	6.25	5.80	–	–	12.71
Central Nottinghamshire	9.38	11.80	11.80	11.72	–	–	11.52
North Nottinghamshire					11.17	12.02	
Nottingham	14.25	11.55	11.55	8.94	12.48	10.83	10.07
Barnsley	10.99	9.42	9.42	9.54	11.37	13.72	17.71
Doncaster	12.20	13.53	13.53	11.49	13.20	14.85	17.20
Rotherdam	10.90	11.94	11.94	10.54	9.45	11.09	12.65
Sheffield	12.66	19.61	19.61	17.12	10.81	8.13	14.93
Trent	10.52	11.37	11.37	10.23	11.11	10.91	10.67

effective, another interpretation of between-practice variations in referral rates is that of simple rationing according to individual practice priorities.

Secular trends in dermatology specialist workload

Data from the first three GP morbidity surveys suggest that dermatology referral rates have increased substantially over the last 40 years.[5,7] More recent data suggest that this trend has been accentuated with a 33% rise in the dermatology referral rate for the UK in 1993/94 (12.5 per 1000) when compared with 1990/91 (9.4 per 1000).[42] Reasons for this increasing secular trend in dermatology referrals have not been studied adequately but probably include an increase in public demand for specialist referral and an increased willingness to refer by GPs. New outpatient attendances for Amersham and High Wycombe[13] rose by 62% in the 20 years from 1958 to 1988, thought mainly to be due to an increasing proportion of moles, keratoses and skin tumours. In another study of new dermatology outpatients in South East Scotland increases of 29% and 28% were noted between 1981 and 1988 for new and follow-up patients respectively.[59] This was accounted for largely by rises of 173% and 106% in benign and malignant tumours respectively, with a concomitant 98% increase in surgical procedures. This increase in pigmented lesions coincided with national campaigns which encouraged the early diagnosis of malignant melanoma. The population increase in the same period was 1.5%. Others have noted similar changes in workload because of pigmented lesions.[60–62]

Role of the dermatology nurse

The dermatology specialist nurse is a vital person in the provision of dermatology services.[63,64] Dermatology specialist nurses provide a range of services including leg ulcer assessment, assistance with patch testing, counselling for chronic skin diseases, practical instruction in using skin treatments, support groups (e.g. healed ulcer group) and day treatment facilities for ultraviolet light therapy or topical applications (e.g. dithranol therapy for psoriasis) as well as the traditional role of providing a secure and accepted environment for the care of dermatology inpatients. Some centres employ dermatology liaison nurses to provide a link between the hospital based specialist and the community in an attempt to foster continuing care.[65] Since 1988 in addition to a 20% decrease in dermatological beds, 35% of dermatology consultants have lost the services of trained dermatological nurses.[47]

Inpatient services

Hospital inpatient statistics show that 82 950 hospital discharges/deaths in the UK in 1985, or 1.6% of all admissions, were due to diseases of the skin and subcutaneous tissue (ICD 9 codes 680–709 which exclude skin cancer and lymphoma).[9] This number of admissions has shown a steady increase from 68 980 in 1979, despite a 20% reduction in dermatology beds.[9,47] In the financial year 1993/94 there were 109 806 ordinary admissions for diseases of the skin and subcutaneous tissue (excluding infections and tumours of the skin), or 1.4% of all ordinary admissions for the UK.[66] Many such patients were cared for by non-dermatologists since only about one-quarter of these inpatient episodes were for inflammatory dermatoses, the rest being made up from disorders such as cellulitis, pilonidal sinus, leg ulceration etc. Diseases of the skin accounted for 1.4% of all inpatient bed days in 1993/94 and the mean and median duration of stay was 10.6 and three days respectively.[66] In 1994 there were 2900 patients awaiting admission for a dermatological disorder in the UK, with 14.4% waiting between six to 11 months and 5.2% waiting 12 months or longer (Statistical Information Unit, Trent Regional Health Authority). Day cases (e.g. those attending for a skin operation) have only recently been recorded fully, but even in 1993/94 diseases of the skin and subcutaneous tissues accounted for 84 597 day case episodes (or 4.0% of all day case episodes).[66]

A detailed study of inpatient workload in the Oxford region using linked data for 1976 to 1985 showed that age-specific admission rates were considerably higher in people aged over 50 years.[13] Age-specific admission rates declined over time in those aged below 70 years but increased above this age. Unlike most other medical specialties, length of patient's stay did not decrease substantially over the ten years and most inpatient work consisted of treatment of people with psoriasis, eczema and leg ulcers. Although overall inpatient admission rates were roughly the same over the ten years, new dermatology outpatients rose by 41% in that same period suggesting that innovations in dermatology practice had been greater for those in an ambulatory setting than those requiring prolonged inpatient care.

Costs of services

Direct costs to the NHS

The only study that has attempted to estimate the direct costs of skin disease to the NHS was conducted by the Office of Health Economics in 1970.[67] They estimated that at least £50 million (or 2.9% of total NHS expenditure) was spent in direct costs on skin disease (£12.8 million on hospital inpatient costs, £6 million on dermatology outpatients, £12.2 million on general practice and £18.3 million by the pharmaceutical service). Skin conditions took up just over 1% of hospital inpatient expenditure but accounted for 7% and 9% respectively of the costs of general practice and prescribed medicines. There is no clear evidence that advances in medical technology have altered the amount or the nature of direct expenditure on dermatological services. In 1994 the direct costs of treating diseases of the skin and subcutaneous tissue were estimated as £617 million (Office of Health Economics, personal communication) still only 2% of total NHS direct costs (Table 8) despite many more expensive drugs being available. Costs for outpatient consultations (the bulk of a dermatologist's work) are excluded from these estimates because of the variation in methods of costing. Benton's study of dermatology services estimated the cost of a single outpatient visit as £4.30 in 1983, compared to £106 for one day as an inpatient.[54] Current methods for costing dermatology outpatient consultations vary between regions and are often based on simple formulae such as total staff and overhead costs divided by the number of new and follow-up patients based on the previous year's contracted figures. At University Hospital Nottingham, the charge to fundholding practices for first and subsequent visits to the dermatology department was £53 and £27 respectively (T Foan, personal communication, December 1994).

Table 8: Breakdown of direct NHS costs for diseases of the skin and subcutaneous tissues for 1994. Overall costs for dermatology outpatient activity are not available

Nature of direct costs to NHS	Cost (£ million)
GP consultations[a]	155
Hospital inpatients	245
Drug costs[b]	175
Drug dispensing costs	42
Total	617

[a] Derived from the fourth national GP morbidity study.[7]

[b] Refers to all prescriptions included in the *BNF* chapter on skin diseases. Although dermatology accounts for a large amount of NHS activity, it accounted for only 2% of NHS expenditure in 1994.

Source: R Chew, Office of Health Economics, personal communication, 1994

As a specialty dermatology incurs a relatively low average drug bill when compared with other hospital disciplines.[68]

Indirect costs

Perhaps the most useful sources of estimating the magnitude of indirect costs of loss of productivity due to skin disease are sickness absence and Industrial Injuries Fund statistics. In 1970 0.3 million spells of work absence were attributed to skin disease, or over 7 million working days lost in 1970/71.[12] Despite this more recent data suggest that the spells of absence attributed to skin disease have declined through the last 20 years possibly due to improved working practices and the introduction of topical corticosteroids and antibiotics.[11,12]

Diseases of the skin were still amongst the top 14 reasons for spells of certified incapacity due to sickness in 1992/93 accounting for 10 000 out of a total of 606 000 claims for men in those years.[11] Extrapolation of these figures to 1996 may not be appropriate due to recent changes in classifications of incapacity to work. Skin diseases were also cited as one of the most common reasons for injury and disablement benefit in the period 1977 to 1983.[12]

Personal disability/handicap of skin disease and additional costs

The 1989 General Household Survey estimated that 16 per 1000 persons were affected by a longstanding skin disorder (i.e. those covered by ICD 9 Chapter XII) sufficiently to limit their activities.[69] Another survey of disability amongst 14 000 adults conducted in the mid 1980s found that 1% of complaints causing disability in private households and 2% in communal establishments were due to skin disease.[70] In the US HANES-1 study skin conditions were reported to limit activity in 10.5 per 1000 of the population aged 1–74 years, or 9% of those persons with such skin conditions.[3] About 10% of those with skin complaints considered the condition to be a handicap to their employment or housework and one-third (33%) indicated a handicap in their social relations as a result of skin disease. Quantification of such disability in monetary terms has not been evaluated. In addition to disability and handicap some chronic skin diseases such as atopic eczema also incur considerable additional direct costs to families, such as purchasing of moisturizers and special soaps, extra laundry expenses and extra cotton clothing and bedding. The Lothian atopic dermatitis study estimated these costs to patients to range from £0 to £70 per two months (median £3.00) compared with health service costs ranging from £0 to £61 (median £7.50) per two months.[71]

Relationship between need, supply and demand

This is summarized in the form of Venn diagrams[14] for skin disease as a whole and for disease sub-categories (Figures 6 and 7).

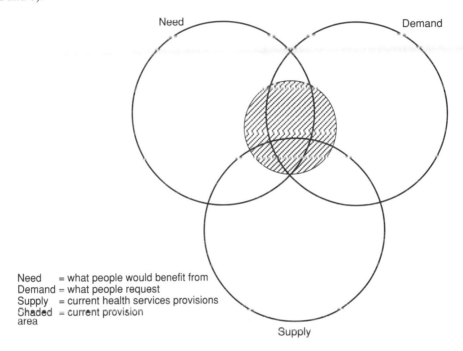

Need = what people would benefit from
Demand = what people request
Supply = current health services provisions
Shaded = current provision
area

Figure 6: A schematic representation of the relationship between the need, supply and demand for dermatological health care for skin disease as a whole.

These representations are intended only as a visual guide given the limitations in current data on the relationship between the three categories of need, supply and demand for skin disease and the limited nature of defining need in such a normative way. Different patterns are seen for different subgroups. For skin cancer much disease amenable to treatment (need) is not asked for (demand), and would probably outstrip current supply if it were identified. Many benign tumours on the other hand, may not represent medical need in the eyes of physicians but are demanded by people and only dealt with to some degree, possibly at the expense of more urgent priorities such as a patient distressed with an inflammatory rash. If one defines medical need as the ability to benefit from medical care, then even people with benign tumours such as seborrhoeic warts, which may be unsightly or catch in clothing, will certainly benefit from medical care such as cryotherapy or curettage, again illustrating the need for providing explicit corporate definitions of dermatological need.

Generalizations for the whole of skin disease are difficult since different sub-categories for skin disease may have different service requirements. The summary in Table 9 provides a rough guide. It is reasonable to summarize the whole of skin disease as a service where the core pattern of services is good for most major disease groupings, but allowances need to be made for lack of recent data. In particular, demand for treatment of benign skin tumours has increased and is likely to continue increasing with a better informed population empowered by the patient's charter. Overall, there is considerable unmet need, and some services are demanded which probably do not require supply.

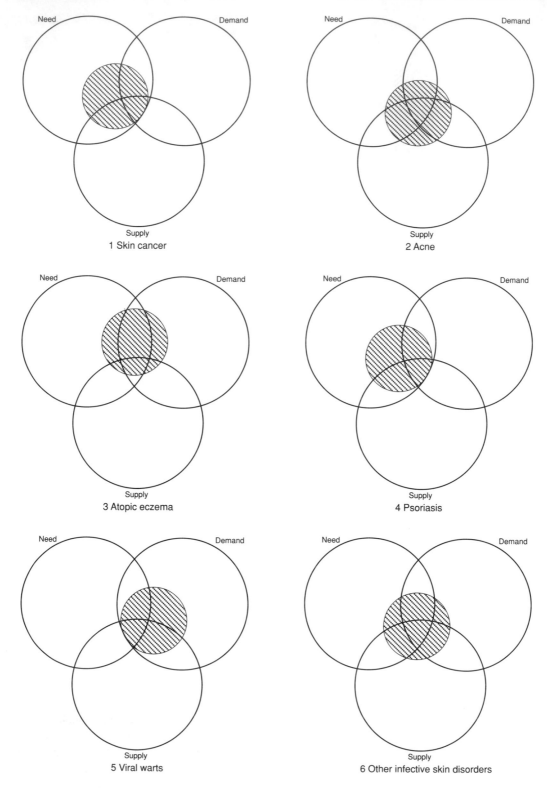

Figure 7: The relationship between the need, supply and demand of health care services for the main sub-categories of skin disease.

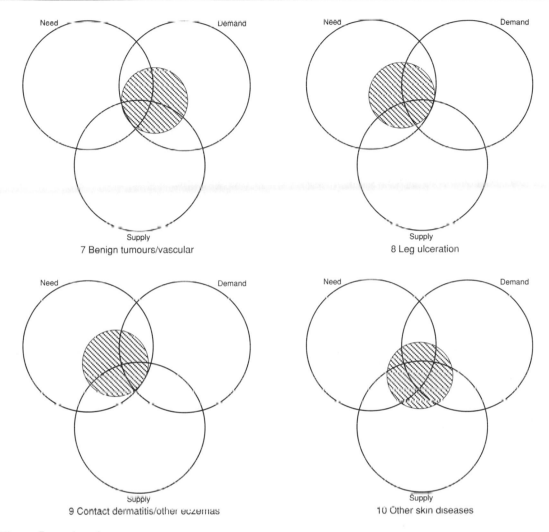

7 Benign tumours/vascular

8 Leg ulceration

9 Contact dermatitis/other eczemas

10 Other skin diseases

Figure 7: continued.

Table 9: The relationship between dermatology services and population need and demand

Need, supply and demand pattern	Skin disease sub-category
1 Large need, large demand, modest supply	Atopic eczema, contact dermatitis and other eczemas
2 Large need, modest demand, modest supply	Skin cancer
3 Moderate need, demand and supply	Psoriasis, acne, other infective skin conditions, leg ulceration, other skin conditions
4 Large demand, small need, moderate to large supply	Viral warts, benign skin tumours

Summary

- People with skin conditions require a range of services from self-help groups to specialist inpatient care.
- Around 15% of the population consults the GP each year because of a skin complaint.
- The UK has the lowest ratio of dermatologists to population in Europe (around 1 : 200 000).
- At least 12.5 per 1000 people are referred to a dermatologist each year in the UK.
- Considerable variation in specialist referral rates exist for dermatology.
- There is some evidence to suggest that these variations in referral rates may be related partly to established patterns of care.
- In addition to diagnosis and management, dermatologists offer a range of services such as surgery for skin cancer, laser treatment, patch testing, ultraviolet light therapy and other special clinics such as pigmented lesion and paediatric dermatology clinics.
- Around 30% of a dermatologist's work involves a minor surgical procedure.
- The dermatology nurse is a vital person in the dermatology team.
- Dermatology inpatients account for 1.4% of all admissions.
- Dermatology accounted for £617 million in direct costs to the NHS in 1994 (2% of the total NHS budget for direct costs).
- Skin diseases are still one of the commonest occupational disease, and accounts for a considerable amount of absence from work and sickness benefit.
- Generalizing the relationship between the need, supply and demand of skin disease over all disease sub-categories is difficult.
- Apart from a large iceberg of unmet need, the current core pattern of services for dermatology generally fits the evidence except for uncertainties regarding the relative merits of care settings.

6 Effectiveness of services

This section summarizes what is known about the effectiveness of current dermatological services in different care locations, focusing on diagnostic accuracy and appropriateness of treatment where this information is available. Strength of recommendation will be based on the quality of evidence[72] (Appendix XVI). Discussion will also include primary and secondary prevention of skin disease where this is relevant. Effectiveness of currently available treatments by dermatological disease sub-categories is also discussed, together with examples of cost-effectiveness and cost utility data where these are available.

Dermatology services as a whole

Over-the-counter preparations and pharmacists' advice (BIV)

Although some OTC preparations such as 1% hydrocortisone, anti-fungal creams, topical acyclovir for herpes simplex and topical benzoyl peroxide have been rigorously tested (AI to BI), many others are less well tested or have not been tested at all (CII to CIV). It is likely that the availability of OTC acne preparations has resulted in less patients consulting with their doctors but whether this is appropriate in terms of correct diagnosis or choice of treatment and satisfactory outcome has yet to be examined. Wastage of family income on ineffective skin treatments has been shown to be a problem in other countries[73] but this has yet to be studied in the UK. Little is known about the way in which availability of OTC substances affects the total burden of skin disease, as is the quality and appropriateness of advice given by pharmacists on skin matters.[44,74]

Primary care (CIII)

Apart from specific diseases such as viral warts and pigmented lesions, very little work has examined the outcome of consultation and treatment of skin diseases in general practice.[5] Some GPs trained in dermatology have reported high rates of positive diagnosis (85%).[46] The low ratio of benign lesions to melanoma in UK hospitals (40 : 1 compared to 253 : 1 in US skin cancer fairs) has been cited as an illustration of the usefulness of GPs in screening such lesions[75] but such an assessment does not take into account those lesions dismissed or incorrectly diagnosed by GPs. Despite considerable personal experience in dermatology, Horn pointed out that with an expected frequency of one malignant skin condition once every two to three years GPs cannot be expected to diagnose skin malignancy reliably.[26] General practitioners with some specialist training probably have higher but more appropriate overall referral rates to hospital specialists.[76]

Although minor skin surgery conducted by GPs may offer a more personal and convenient service to patients[77] a recent UK study of pathology requests submitted by GPs for minor surgical procedures found that the overall correct diagnosis rate for skin malignancy and seborrhoeic warts was below 30%.[78] Most of the three-fold increase in workload in the local pathology department generated by GPs was due to benign lesions such as moles, cysts and seborrhoeic warts. None of the four melanomas in this study was correctly identified. Only nine out of 21 squamous cell carcinomas were adequately excised. Similar rates of correct diagnoses for seborrhoeic warts by non-specialists (35%) have been found elsewhere.[79]

The study by Stevenson *et al.* of 2940 dermatology patients in the West Midlands found that 12% of referrals were considered inappropriate by the dermatologist (mainly viral and seborrhoeic warts).[51] Around one-quarter to one-third of referrals for atopic eczema, acne and psoriasis were also considered inappropriate in that adequate primary treatment had not been given prior to referral. In another study of 686 consecutive new referrals to a dermatology unit in London[80] 32% were judged to have been inappropriate on the grounds of not requiring specialist diagnosis or management. Some of these inappropriate referrals might have been due to increased patient demand for specialist referral. It is also not clear whether these problems are likely to be resolved simply by intensive training programmes. A study by Sladden *et al.* showed that over 75% of their inappropriate referrals belonged to just six diagnostic categories,[55] suggesting that focused educational programmes might be beneficial. One recent study which set out to train GPs in distinguishing malignant from benign lesions found that although the proportion of melanomas diagnosed correctly rose from 65% to 81% after training the proportion of seborrhoeic warts diagnosed correctly remained unchanged at 54%.[81]

Specialist services (BIII)

Except for sub-categories of skin disease and meeting reports[28,82,83] (BIII) no systematic research into the differential health gain of referral to dermatologists has been undertaken (CIV). In a comprehensive study of hospital outpatients in 1970[84] Forsyth and Logan commented that 'Of all out-patient departments dermatology had the clearest function and is the least suspect of impinging on territory which might safely be left to a retrained and revitalised corps of general practitioners'. It seems obvious that the consequences of non-referral of a patient with a diagnostic or management problem to a dermatologist could be serious (e.g. missing a melanoma or death due to generalized pustular psoriasis) but little is known about the threshold and reasons for referral for common skin disorders. One study by Roland and colleagues in Cambridge has suggested that many more patients with skin disease might benefit from specialist help.[85] This study identified 22 patients with skin problems whose GPs were satisfied with their management and had no intention of sending them to hospital. These patients were reviewed by a dermatologist who made treatment recommendations in 14 cases, six of whom reported a definite improvement in their skin condition six weeks later and the GPs themselves found the consultation helpful in 17 cases.

Although these patients might have improved anyway, the authors have drawn attention to a large and understudied group of patients who might benefit from brief assessments by specialists. The views of consumers with regards to satisfaction of dermatological health care services have not been examined, except in a small study of satisfaction with hospital versus outreach clinic appointments.[86]

In addition to outpatient referrals generated by GPs, dermatologists also see referrals for inpatients from other specialties who have skin disease. In a recent study Falanga et al. found that dermatologic consultation changed dermatologic diagnosis and treatment in more than 60% of patients, usually common conditions with established treatment.[87] In a study of 500 non-dermatological inpatients referred for a dermatological opinion, 37% were considered to have a skin condition which contributed substantially to the diagnosis of the systemic disease.[23]

Another study of melanoma cases seen in a London hospital over an 18-year period showed that dermatologists were more likely to enter the correct clinical diagnosis on pathology forms when compared with general surgeons (85% compared with 61% respectively).[88]

Although there are compelling arguments for ensuring that dermatologically trained nurses should be key members of the specialist team[63–65,89] no studies have examined the cost-effectiveness of this professional group in dermatology (CIV). Similarly the cost-effectiveness of liaison dermatology nursing has not been assessed.

The effect of outreach dermatology clinics (DIII) has been monitored in terms of activity.[28] Preliminary results suggest that around half as many patients are seen than in a dedicated dermatology outpatient set up, at the possible expense of patients who do not have the benefit of outreach clinic services. Shorter waiting times and ease of access have been reported with such clinics but they have not increased interaction between specialists and GPs.[90]

Specific services for skin disease sub-categories (AI to BII-2)

Although many excellent clinical trials have been conducted in dermatology, the vast number of skin disorders and small number of dermatologists has meant that many treatments for less common skin conditions have not been fully tested by means of randomized placebo-controlled studies. In assessing the quality of evidence it is important to distinguish procedures which lack adequate evaluation (where currently there may be no alternative treatments) from those where there is some evidence to reject the use of the procedure.

Other problems exist such as a lack of agreement on suitable end-points[91,92] and a profusion of studies that are too small to answer the questions posed.[93] Recent work on the development of patient-derived measures of skin disability such as the Dermatology Life Quality Index are a welcome development in patient-centred assessment of effectiveness of skin treatments but requires further evaluation.[94] Little work has been conducted in implementing research findings in dermatology and a few studies point to a considerable gap between intended and actual practice.[95]

In considering effectiveness of newer and more expensive dermatological treatments it is important not to consider initial purchase costs in isolation. Several cost-effectiveness and cost utility analyses have shown that treatments with high initial costs such as isotretinoin (a potent oral treatment for acne),[96–98] terbinafine (an anti-fungal agent),[99] cyclosporin A (for treatment of resistant psoriasis)[100] and calcipotriol ointment (a new topical vitamin D preparation for treatment of psoriasis)[101] may be offset by reduced frequency of follow-up visits, better compliance and higher clearance rates.

Skin cancer

Primary prevention of melanoma (BII-3)

Concerns that excessive exposure and burning in the first ten years of life may be critical in the development of melanoma have led the Health of the Nation to encourage efforts directed at informing school children of the dangers of excessive sun exposure.[4]

Preliminary studies in school children indicate that knowledge of skin cancer can be enhanced by such schemes[102] but studies in the UK have been unable to show that people's sun exposure behaviour actually changes as a result of such knowledge.[103] No studies have yet showed that sunscreens reduce numbers of melanoma cancers.[4]

Since 1993 issues pertaining to skin cancer have been co-ordinated by a national UK Skin Cancer Working Party composed of representatives from dermatology, cancer charities and the Health Education Council.[a] This working party is further divided into four sections which deal with the following:

1 cancer registration problems
2 helping the primary care team
3 helping hospital skin cancer services
4 public education.[104]

Secondary prevention of melanoma (BII-3)

Since thin melanomas have a relatively good prognosis, rapid access to specialists has been a priority for health professionals. Many dermatologists run specially designated pigmented lesion clinics. The establishment of a pigmented lesion clinic does not in itself influence melanoma prognosis in a population. The main source of delay in seeking medical help has been shown to be because of patients' lack of knowledge of the significance of the lesion. Pigmented lesion clinics may provide an administrative focus for skin cancer services and they may also play a part in public education and generation of important research data.

Publicity campaigns to alert the public to the early signs of malignant melanoma have been evaluated on a before and after basis in the UK with mixed results and the effects on melanoma mortality are awaited. Population screening for melanoma has not been adequately assessed, although the disease fulfils most of the requirements for screening, especially in high risk groups such as those with fair skin.

Evidence that skin cancer screening is effective for melanoma skin cancer is incomplete.[105] Secondary prevention does not seek to reduce the incidence rates of these diseases.

Treatment of melanoma

Management is mainly by surgical excision. Narrow excision margins for thin lesions have been associated with an excellent prognosis (AI). Thicker lesions may require wider excision and further surgery or other treatment modalities (BII-2). The treatment of disseminated disease is disappointing (CII-2).

Non-melanoma skin cancer

Although non-melanoma skin cancer is a potentially preventable disease, the cost-effectiveness of primary and secondary prevention of non-melanoma skin cancer in the UK is unknown (BIII). Surgical excision produces excellent results in basal cell and squamous cell carcinomas of the skin (AII-1) and other treatment modalities such as radiotherapy and cryotherapy may also be effective (BII-3). Some invasive tumours in

---

[a] c/o British Association of Dermatologists, 19 Fitzroy Square, London W1P 5HQ.

certain anatomical locations may require more advanced techniques such as Mohs micrographic surgery, an intensive time-consuming procedure which requires special training (usually in the US). Recurrence rates however are the lowest for all procedures for removal of skin cancer (AII-2). Although people with one non-melanoma skin cancer are at a high risk of developing further lesions, the optimum frequency and level of review is unknown.

Acne (AI)

Treatments for acne vulgaris have been well evaluated.[106] Consideration of disease severity[107] and whether lesions are inflammatory or non-inflammatory and compliance are the main determinants of therapy. Mild disease is usually treated with topical agents such as benzoyl peroxide, tretinoin and isotretinoin, antibiotics and azelaic acid. Long-term systemic antibiotics (minimum six months) and anti-androgens are used in more extensive disease. Oral isotretinoin is used under specialist supervision for severe and unresponsive disease, with excellent long-term results. Around 40% will be cured, 21% will require topical therapy only and the remaining 39% relapsing usually with milder disease within three years of treatment.[98]

Cost-effectiveness (AII-2)

Although a four-month course of oral isotretinoin for severe acne may appear to carry high initial costs (£650 including outpatient costs, 1991 prices), this was considerably less than the cumulative costs of conventional treatment with rotational antibiotics and return visits to GPs (£2108).[97] Simpson in 1993 calculated that the cost per subsequent disease-free year was £192 for oral isotretinoin and a median cost per QUALY of £899.[96]

The severity threshold where oral isotretinoin is no longer cost-effective in acne vulgaris is unknown. Small changes in this threshold brought about by more demanding and articulate groups of patients with high expectations of treatment, could have serious financial implications and alteration in the cost : benefit ratio as illustrated in Figure 8.

Atopic eczema (BI to BII-2)

One randomized study has suggested that prevention of atopic eczema in children born to parents with atopic disease may be possible by restricting maternal allergens and reducing household house dust mite levels.[108] Further studies are needed to assess the impact in unselected populations. Observational studies on the effect of exclusive breastfeeding on the development of atopic eczema is conflicting and beneficial effects are likely to be small (CIV).

The mainstay of treatment of mild to moderate atopic eczema is with emollients to moisturize the skin (BIII) and mild to moderate potency topical corticosteroids (BI). Other treatments such as bandaging limbs (BIII), topical tar (BIII), antibiotics for secondary infection (BIII) and evening primrose oil are also used, although the additional benefits may be small. The roles of allergy testing and environmental manipulation have not been adequately assessed. No treatments have been conclusively shown to alter the natural history of established atopic eczema. Given such limitations in treatment patients value adequate time to have the nature and prognosis of the disease explained to them, as well as easy access to a specialist during exacerbations.[109] Severe atopic eczema is usually treated with potent topical corticosteroids (BII-2) and other measures such as short courses of oral corticosteroids (BII-3), ultraviolet light (BII-3), traditional Chinese herbs (BII-1) and other immunosuppressive agents such as azathioprine or cyclosporin A (BII-1), or hospital admission (BIII). Cost-effectiveness studies are absent but one study has suggested that costs to patients incurred by prescription charges for topical treatments are considerable even for milder cases in the community (mean two month expenditure by patients of £22.50 compared with £16.20 direct NHS costs in 1993).[110]

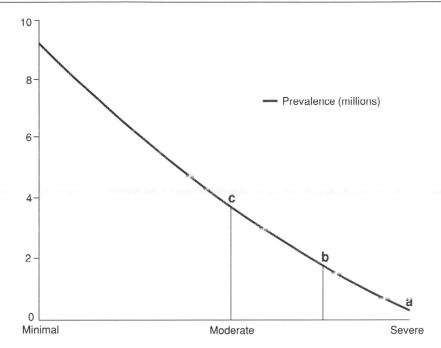

Figure 8: Acne severity in females and the possible implications of changes in the threshold for treatment with powerful agents such as isotretinoin. Even a small change in treatment threshold from **a** (severe disease) to **b** (moderately severe) would result in a seven-fold increase in prescriptions. A change in treatment threshold from a (severe) to c (moderate) would result in a fifteen-fold increase in prescriptions in absolute terms
(Source: Based on actual data on acne severity in US females.[107])

Psoriasis (AI to BII-2)

Smoking and alcohol are both risk factors for psoriasis which are amenable to public health manipulation (BII-2) but their avoidance as a means of prevention or treatment of established psoriasis has yet to be studied. Mild cases of psoriasis may be treated with a variety of effective topical treatments such as coal tar (AI), dithranol (AI), topical corticosteroids (AI) and calcipotriol (AI). Ultraviolet light both in the form of long-wave ultraviolet light (UVB) and oral PUVA is well established and is an effective method of treating more extensive psoriasis (AI), although there is a small risk of long-term skin cancer in those receiving high cumulative doses (BII-2). Severe disease may also be treated by immunomodulators such as oral acitretin (AI), cyclosporin A (AI) and low dose oral methotrexate (AI). Day case topical treatment (AII-3) or hospital admission is occasionally required for assistance in treating widespread or life-threatening disease. Cost of methotrexate per year has been estimated at £875 (1993), £586 of which is due to the initial liver biopsy required to monitor possible liver damage. Phytochemotherapy treatment for one year has been estimated to cost around £560 and a six-week course of UVB ultraviolet light and tar baths at £222 (1993).[101]

Cost-effectiveness

Although the unit cost of new drug developments such as calcipotriol (a topical vitamin D analogue) may be high (£23.49 per 100 g tube compared with £2.06 for diluted betamethasone valerate ointment in 1993) this may bare little relationship to its overall cost-effectiveness as savings may be made in terms of fewer follow-up visits, less recourse to second-line therapy and possibly less inpatient admission which may be costly.[101] Similarly although second-line treatments such as cyclosporin A are expensive, preliminary cost-comparison analyses suggest that such drugs may be up to four times less costly than conventional treatments such as short-contact dithranol plus UVB therapy in a supervised outpatient setting.[100]

Viral warts (AI to DIII)

Treatment of simple viral warts on the hands or feet is usually either by topical salicylic acid paints or liquid nitrogen cryotherapy. There is little evidence to suggest that cryotherapy at three-weekly intervals is any more effective than topical application of salicylic acid for simple hand and foot warts, each having a three-month cure rate of around 60% to 70% after three months treatment (CII-2).[111] Double freezing is probably no more effective than a single freeze except for warts on the feet (AI).[112] There is reasonable evidence to suggest that considerable savings could be made by the provision of liquid nitrogen to GPs or by health authorities employing nurses to treat warts (BIII).[113] The cost-effectiveness of medical practitioners in treating simple warts with liquid nitrogen has not been assessed (CIV). Although liquid nitrogen is cheap, treatment is time consuming and this needs to be weighed against the fact that around 65% of viral warts on the hands and feet clear spontaneously within two years.[111]

It is probably wasteful of resources for dermatologists to be concerned with the routine treatment of warts (DIII) but they may need to see patients with resistant warts, where a number of treatments such as intralesional bleomycin, interferon, retinoids, topical sensitization and more prolonged or aggressive cryotherapy have been tried (BII-1 to CIII).

Other infective skin disorders (AI to AII-3)

Controlled trials have shown that both oral and topical antibiotics are effective in treating bacterial skin infections such as impetigo (AI). The pain and duration of herpes simplex infections may be reduced by specific anti-viral agents such as acyclovir, either given topically or orally (AI). Short- and long-term pain due to Herpes zoster infection (shingles) may also be reduced by high dose acyclovir administration (BI). Many effective topical and systemic anti-fungal agents have been evaluated for the treatment of fungal infections of the skin, hair and nails (AI). Systemic anti-fungals are required to treat fungal nail and scalp infections and although the unit cost of newer treatments such as terbinafine and itraconazole may be high, the cost-effectiveness of these drugs may be higher than cheaper alternatives because of shorter duration of treatment,[99] better cure rates and fewer follow-up visits (BII-3).

Benign tumours and vascular lesions (AII-3 to C4)

Benign tumours such as naevi, dermatofibromas and sebaceous cysts which cause discomfort or concern for other reasons can all be treated by surgical removal with good cosmetic results and high patient satisfaction (BII-3). No studies have examined the cost-effectiveness of treatment and its relation to the threshold of intervention; although treatment by dermatologists is considerably cheaper than treatment by general surgeons because of lower theatre and overhead costs. In Watford General Hospital for example, excision of a skin lesion by a dermatologist was charged at a rate of £28, whereas an identical procedure performed in the main theatre by surgeons cost £250 (JK Schofield, personal written communication, 1994). Treatment of unsightly seborrhoeic warts with topical liquid nitrogen is highly effective with high degrees of patient satisfaction (AII-3). The Candela flash lamp pumped pulsed tunable dye laser is considered as the gold standard for treating facial port wine stains in children because of its high efficacy and low incidence of side-effects such as scarring or pigmentary changes (AII-3), although techniques are continually being refined. Treatment is likely to produce 50% lightening of the stain in 70% to 80% of patients and around 20% may clear completely. Best results are seen in small children where the mean number of treatments may be reduced. Treatment costs are related to the number of treatments which are required but an estimate of costs would be between £150–£300 per treatment episode with an expected number of treatments ranging from 6–15 (S Lanigan, personal written communication, 1995).

Although cost-effectiveness of such laser treatment has not been evaluated, the social stigma and psychological morbidity for patients with these disfiguring marks can be very serious.

Treatment of solar keratoses with topical liquid nitrogen or 5-fluorouracil cream is effective (AIII) but the extent to which treatment of visible lesions prevents the development of subsequent squamous cell carcinomas is unknown. Large long-term trials will be needed to address this important question because of the very low rate of malignant transformation of these common lesions and substantial rates of spontaneous regression. Although the presence of solar keratoses is a marker of solar damage indicating a possible increased risk of skin malignancy, the evidence that all such patients need to be followed-up is poor (CIV).

Leg ulceration AII 1

Primary and secondary prevention of leg ulcers in high risk populations such as the elderly has not been assessed in the UK (CIII). Treatment of leg ulcers is tailored to the cause. Most venous ulcers respond readily to adequate external graduated compression, wound cleansing, leg elevation and exercises. Healing rates for venous ulcers with adequate external compression therapy vary from 33% to 60% at 12 weeks[114,115] (AII-1). Basic treatment is simple and is designed to counteract the effects of raised venous pressure in the affected limb. Although many new topical ulcer preparations and dressings are available their advantage in terms of cost-effectiveness over simple hydrocolloid alternatives for most venous ulcers is doubtful (BII-1) Other treatments such as skin grafting may accelerate the healing of large ulcers and reduce costly inpatient care (AII-1). Support groups such as healed ulcer clinics may play an important role in encouraging self-care and prevention of ulcer recurrences (AIII).

Ischaemic ulcers require a different treatment approach as external compression may lead to irreversible ischaemia and amputation. Vascular surgeons offer a range of treatments including arterial bypass surgery, angioplasty or sympathectomy for ischaemic leg ulcers (AIII).

Costs associated with the treatment of leg ulcers may be high (£400 to £600 million in 1992) mainly due to nursing time. One study has examined the cost-effectiveness of establishing community leg ulcer clinics versus existing hospital-based services and found that community clinics were associated with higher healing rates (80% and 22% healed at three months respectively) and less cost (£169 000 compared with £433 600 per year, 1993 prices for 500 ulcer patients in a district with a population of 270 000).[116] This study referred to a well-motivated research group in the community and caution should be exercised in generalizing costs and healing rates to other settings. The study does however show that good healing at lower costs can be achieved in well-run community clinics (AIII).

Contact dermatitis and other forms of eczema (AIII-3)

Contact dermatitis is a preventable disease and skin protection in high risk occupations such as cleaning work is encouraged to a variable degree (AIII). Although most eczematous skin reactions respond to treatment with topical corticosteroids and emollients to hydrate and protect the skin, treatment without investigation is not cost-effective as the avoidance of external causes such as irritants or allergens identified through patch testing may offer a permanent cure. Not all patients require referral for specialist assessment if features elicited in the history and examination suggest an obvious cause. Treatment (including avoidance of provoking factors) results in clearing or improvement of around 40% to 70% of those with hand eczema, regardless of the cause. A range of effective treatments is available for 'other eczemas' such as seborrhoeic, discoid, stasis, photosensitive and asteatotic eczema depending on the underlying cause (AII-3).

Other skin diseases (AI to CIII)

Too many skin diseases are included within this category to make any generalizations of effectiveness of services. Treatment of some of the more common diseases such as symptomatic relief of urticaria by antihistamines has been well evaluated (A1), whereas the treatment of many rare skin disorders is based on case reports or uncontrolled series (CIII) because of practical difficulties in organizing randomized controlled studies. It is important that purchasers appreciate that 'treatment' does not necessarily imply drug treatment. Effective drug treatment may not yet be available in some serious skin diseases such as epidermolysis bullosa but explanation, practical advice and special footwear to avoid skin trauma, surgical procedures to release fingers trapped by scar tissue and access to specialist nursing care may be very valuable for sufferers and their families (AIII).

Key points on service effectiveness

- The effectiveness of OTC preparations and pharmaceutical advice on the burden of skin disease in the community is unknown.
- Little is known about the differential health gain of specialists versus generalists in the diagnosis and treatment of common skin diseases.
- Some evidence suggests that the diagnosis and surgical removal of skin cancer is best carried out by dermatologists.
- General practitioners are in the best position to manage mild to moderate common recurrent skin diseases such as acne, psoriasis and atopic eczema.
- Better management of these conditions could reduce unnecessary referrals to specialists.
- Most viral warts do not require referral to a specialist.
- Outreach specialist clinics are probably not an efficient use of the limited specialist care currently available in the UK.
- The cost-effectiveness of liaison dermatology nurses is unknown.
- There is reasonably good evidence to support the effectiveness of most treatments used for the common skin disease sub-categories.
- Many skin diseases, especially skin cancer, are theoretically preventable but prevention programmes have not been evaluated adequately.

7 Models of care

This section deals with a variety of alternative scenarios for delivering dermatological care and examines the possible consequences of these models. By considering both ill-deployed services and opportunities for investment in health care gain, an agenda is set for some potential changes in dermatological health care provision. With such scanty and out-of-date information on the prevalence of skin disease and even weaker data on economic costs of skin disease, the emphasis on direct costing estimates has been reduced in favour of suggestions as to where shifts in the provision of skin care need to be explored, based upon available evidence. The models of care topic requires further discussion and piloting before any decisions are made.

Public health approach

Prevention of skin disease is more desirable than investment in expensive treatments and technologies for sick individuals who present themselves at the end of a long chain of pathological events. The high prevalence of many skin conditions combined with knowledge of their causes makes some of them an ideal target for future public health intervention programmes. Infectious skin diseases such as scabies,[117] head lice and scalp ringworm outbreaks are obvious examples of appropriate management utilizing a public health approach in order to facilitate disease control at a population level.

Skin cancer, a Health of the Nation target,[4] is the most common form of cancer in the UK yet it is largely a preventable disease. Already there is sufficient information on the link between ultraviolet light and skin cancer and predisposing factors such as skin type to suggest primary and secondary prevention strategies are worthy of further evaluation.

There is a chasm however between what might at first appear to be a sensible approach and what has been shown to be effective in terms of skin disease prevention. For example although skin cancer fulfils most of the requirements for a successful screening programme, randomized population studies examining the cost-effectiveness of such approaches in various risk groups have not yet been performed. Urgent research is required if costly programmes with low diagnostic yields and unnecessary public anxiety are to be avoided.[105]

Early intervention of incident cases of leg ulcers when they are at a small stage in elderly groups is another area where secondary prevention may be cost-effective. More research is required into the effects of manipulating environmental risk factors for atopic eczema (e.g. reducing house dust mite and cow's milk exposure during pregnancy in high risk groups), psoriasis (reducing smoking and alcohol consumption) and contact dermatitis (protection, education and use of substitutes for potent sensitizers) in order to formulate the most efficient preventative strategies.

However lack of adequate research data should not be a reason for inaction over primary prevention of skin cancer by attempts at altering public attitudes and behaviour (especially children) because the results of such endeavours may not be known for several decades and the cost of forgoing such programmes are potentially high in terms of mortality, morbidity and future treatment costs. Greater emphasis on prevention of skin cancer by reducing excessive sun exposure in early and adult life can be justified, as well as the continued emphasis on early diagnosis of melanoma skin cancer. Widespread screening for skin cancer cannot be currently recommended until further research is conducted.[105]

Service approach

This approach considers possible changes in existing services in the light of the prevalence and incidence of skin disease and available effective treatments so that people are treated in the appropriate health care setting by appropriate personnel. Generalizations for skin disease as a whole may be difficult since different skin disease sub-categories may have different health care requirements. For example the shift in services for viral warts should be from secondary towards primary care because hospital treatment is expensive and no more effective than in the community;[113] whereas there is a strong argument that dermatologists should see all patients with skin malignancy because the cost of missing a case or inadequate excision of a lesion could be high.[78]

Current evidence would suggest that demand for dermatological services is likely to increase over the next 30 to 40 years because:

1 prevalence surveys have indicated a large iceberg of people with unmet dermatological needs, most of whom would like treatment if they knew effective treatment was available [2,3,118]

2 the public exposed to a US-style culture which encourages use of specialist services and empowered by the Patient's Charter are more likely to request specialist referral for milder common chronic skin diseases, thereby exerting greater pressure on GPs to reduce their threshold for specialist referral

3 the prevalence of three of the most common and most costly skin diseases – skin cancer,[119,120] atopic eczema[6] and leg ulcers[121] is increasing and will continue to increase with an ageing population[5]

4 there may be increased demand for attention to skin lesions which were formally considered as cosmetic problems by physicians.

The drug industry has been quick to recognize the large burden of untreated disease in the community and some companies are actively distributing posters in sports centres and advertisements in newspapers in order to increase the public's awareness of the particular condition that their product is used to treat.[122] Any health care strategy which focuses solely on the relationship between primary and secondary care is doomed to failure unless it considers the enormous and unstable burden of people with unmet dermatological needs. Small changes in awareness within this population are likely to have a far greater effect on dermatological services than minor changes in referral patterns.

Three scenarios for dermatology health service provision are now discussed in the light of these projected increased service demands.

Maintaining the current passive response model

Although the status quo model involves the least organizational disruption, such a passive response to demand is likely to perpetuate and possibly exacerbate the mismatch between need and supply at all levels of health care delivery and be the least cost-effective in the long term. Specialist services are already saturated and long waiting lists are the norm. Hospitals in the London area have been particularly hard hit, with waiting lists varying from four to 46 weeks whilst at the same time losing 68% of dedicated dermatology beds and 60% of trained dermatology nurses.[28] Such a stressed system lacks the flexibility to respond to even small further increases in demand without compromising the quality of patient care. The direct costs per 100 000 population of the current system at 1994 costs for one year are estimated at £1.26 million (GP consultations £0.29 million, inpatient costs £0.45 million, prescription costs £0.32 million, dispensing costs £0.08 million, dermatology outpatient costs £0.12 million).

The outreach clinic model

Dermatology is a unique specialty in that a considerable proportion of diagnoses can be made on the basis of history and examination alone. This makes it an appropriate specialty for developing in a community setting and the idea of employing dermatologists solely as community specialists serving a series of 'outreach' clinics might appear attractive at first. Whilst the provision of medical services at a location convenient to the patient is a desirable aim, such a scheme would result in giving undue attention to a few at the expense of others, given the current number of dermatologists in the UK. With around 223 dermatologists and 28 460 GPs (with an average of three per practice) currently in the UK,[52] one dermatologist would have to cover 42 health centres. Even if clinics were held once a fortnight at each centre, then with five clinics per week, each dermatologist could only manage to cover ten health centres.

If equity of coverage is to be maintained this strategy would require a four-fold increase in dermatology specialists. With only two extra dermatology unified training grade posts being announced by SWAG for the whole of England and Wales in 1996, it is hard to envisage how this approach could work. Such a top heavy service is probably least efficient in terms of costs and use of expertise. Some surveys have suggested that around half as many patients are seen in outreach clinics when compared with their hospital equivalents[28] and around one-third of such patients require further procedures for which referral to hospital might have been more appropriate.

Another problem is that funds (e.g. to employ retired dermatologists to run outreach clinics) may be directed into the private sector rather than into developing and training local dermatology services. Other studies have suggested that outreach clinics have not increased the interaction between GPs and specialists,[90] a finding echoed by the BAD survey which found that a GP or GP trainee sat in with the dermatologist in only 6% of outreach clinics.[123] Another study in Aylesbury found that GPs did not attend outreach clinics run by a consultant dermatologist,[124] despite initial agreement, although this study found that these clinics were an excellent setting for teaching dermatology to local nurses.

Although many GPs quite reasonably hold the view that outreach clinics can improve their access to and involvement with a dermatologist, a recent consumer survey in Stoke-on-Trent suggests that the provision of outreach clinics is not the wish of the majority of patients,[86] with most wishing to be followed-up by a specialist in a hospital centre.

The removal of dermatologists from a hospital base also holds potentially serious implications for the development of future services. Given the low ratio of specialists per population, specialists are best retained in hospital sites because of access to diagnostic facilities such as patch testing, specialist nursing support, specialist treatment facilities such as PUVA, access to counselling services for patients with chronic or disfiguring conditions and contact with other members of the professional team such as plastic surgeons, radiotherapists and paediatricians.

With a complement of over 1000 skin diseases support from other consultant colleagues over diagnostic or therapeutic difficulties is also important for patients. Dermatologists are also needed in hospitals to see patients with serious systemic diseases who also have dermatological manifestations as their input frequently helps in diagnosing or managing that condition.[87] Since skin cancer is the most common form of cancer in human populations dermatologists must be retained in cancer treatment centres because of their diagnostic skills and experience at surgically treating large numbers of people at low cost.

The removal of dermatology as a hospital based specialty would pose difficulties for training and research by losing a critical mass of patients and staff. Dermatologists also need access to hospital beds where patients can be cared for in an appropriate environment by appropriately trained dermatology nurses.

Whilst a shift in emphasis from hospital to community care for dermatology is desirable for most common skin disorders the *ad hoc* adoption of outreach dermatology clinics in the absence of a large expansion of dermatologists and financial investment is likely to result in unequal coverage of the whole population and possibly an erosion of the specialty in general. With an estimated four-fold expansion of dermatologists and reduced numbers of patients seen in outreach clinics (many of whom are likely to have milder skin disease and who might not have otherwise been referred) this model would also be the most costly option in the long run, representing an additional estimated £0.36 million per 100 000 population. This would increase the estimated service costs from £1.26 million for the status quo model in 1994 (page 302) to £1.63 million. This estimate does not take into account extra prescribing and dispensing costs and increased GP's time.

The other extreme of this model i.e. routine open access to specialist clinics could lead to fragmentation of patients' care and undermine the unique role of the GP as a generalist with higher rates of intervention and higher costs.[125] It would also lead to the overmedicalization of patients and propagate the 'collusion of anonymity' where many specialists see a patient but no one accepts overall responsibility.[126]

Such outreach clinics need to be distinguished from 'outpost' clinics conducted in remote areas by dermatologists on a firm basis of geographical need which have been in place long before the recent health service reforms.[123]

Other modifications of the outreach clinic approach exist such as moving a regular hospital clinic to a community location strategically located close to purchasing district boundaries (as opposed to a dermatologist visiting several individual general practices).[127] Offering more convenient locations to patients and direct training to GPs (providing attendance by GPs is mandatory) are advantages of this system but given that the same number of dermatologists will have to staff such clinics in the same number of sessions it is not clear how this approach offers any advantage over the status quo model in terms of waiting lists. Such a system may help to attract more business away from neighbouring services where there is an abundance of competition[128] but shortage of patients is unheard of in most dermatology departments. Given the shape and size of the dermatological iceberg there is clearly an enormous amount of dermatological demand that can be passed as 'business' in today's purchaser/provider culture but in over-stretched areas, such increases in business will need an equivalent service investment.

The hybrid model

This model proposes an integrated district approach to serving the dermatological needs of its community by building on the strengths of existing services. Within the next 20 years several factors will combine to reshape the pattern of the NHS into smaller more specialized acute centres with a focus on short day cases and complex treatments. The corollary is an extended role for primary and community health services which is capable of delivering some of what currently takes place in hospitals.[125] Purchasing, as a new strategic tool, could extend the scope of these boundary changes.[82]

A hybrid model is proposed of:

1 developing community services by the formation of district dermatology liaison teams
2 establishing dermatology treatment centres in the community set up at sites convenient to the public
3 maintaining a critical mass of expertise within hospitals
4 involvement of community pharmacists.

Research into such shifts of emphasis should start with the user's experience.

Developing community dermatology services by establishing a liaison team

This could be accomplished in a number of ways but the formation of a district liaison team of dermatologists, GPs, dermatology nurses, community pharmacists and public representatives could provide a framework for further development. The function of such a team would be to identify areas for releasing ill-deployed services (e.g. dermatologists treating simple warts or straightforward acne) which could be harnessed for areas of potential health gain such as improving services for the early assessment and treatment of skin cancer.

Issues such as current variations in referral patterns and unnecessary specialist referrals could also be addressed by such teams so that dermatologists are deployed for what they are best at doing i.e. diagnosing skin disease and suggesting management for severe/difficult cases. The dermatology liaison team would formulate targets for referral and management policies for common skin diseases based on guidelines developed by BAD and the Royal College of General Practitioners. Such an approach would present a more consistent and explicit approach to consumers of health care. Corporate needs assessments which are sensitive to issues such as age and ethnic group composition of the local population could be performed so that decisions regarding what should be considered cosmetic and what constitutes reasonable need could be made more explicit, enabling dialogue between consumers and health care providers.

Other ways of improving the practice of dermatology within the community could be through shared care schemes, such as those used for people with asthma and diabetes. These could serve as models for other common and occasionally severe skin diseases such as atopic eczema and psoriasis in order to use the resources of the primary care team already in place more effectively. Such a scheme would release dermatologists from following-up large cohorts of patients with chronic skin disease thereby reducing waiting lists so that his/her skills could be used more appropriately for new patient assessments.

Chronic skin disease management clinics in primary care could provide a useful educational setting for both patients and members of the primary care team and the establishment of registers could enable more appropriate services and audit to be carried out.[50] This requires the ability to distinguish those individuals with simple maintenance needs from those who need specialist care for stabilization or special treatment as well as a professional commitment and adequate funding to producing and developing guidelines.[82]

The use of technologies such as high resolution video cameras, high quality photographs, or digital images transmitted down telephone lines as a means of obtaining a rapid opinion from specialists, especially for straightforward disorders, needs further evaluation.[129,130] The concept of teledermatology as a means of increasing contact between GPs and dermatologists sounds promising and such an approach may be particularly useful for specialists covering remote communities in a large geographical area. It is unclear whether such a system will help dermatology waiting lists given the current number of available dermatologists, as, given the enormous size of the dermatological 'iceberg' it is possible that such a convenient system will simply encourage a large increase in teleconsultations for transient skin problems which GPs would have otherwise managed themselves. Whether the quality of images will be sufficiently high for dermatologists to make difficult diagnoses (e.g. over-pigmented lesions where the cost of false reassurance may mean the difference between life and death) is questionable but some preliminary work has suggested a role for teledermatology in triage of pigmented lesions.[129] Patients may value the convenience that teledermatology may offer them, although simple image transmission will deny them the opportunity of benefiting from a personal consultation with dermatologists to discuss treatment options and prognosis. High resolution audio-visual contact could offer a direct two-way consultation between a GP, patient and dermatologist but with the large demand for consultants' opinions, such a system might become quickly choked leading to on-line queues with patients waiting hours in order to get through. There is a danger that as this technology spreads it will become increasingly difficult for clinicians to invite patients to participate in randomized trials – a situation that implies that the position of clinical equipoise has been missed.[131] Further evaluation of teledermatology from the user's perspective, with consideration of diagnostic accuracy and cost-effectiveness from the provider's and purchaser's perspective along the lines of the US National Library of Medicine Teledermatology project[132] is urgently required.

Establishing dermatology treatment centres within the community

Many of the nursing activities of hospital dermatology outpatients such as day treatment for psoriasis, ultraviolet light therapy, leg ulcer treatment, wart treatment and counselling and treatment of common skin conditions such as atopic eczema could easily be carried out in the community providing adequate facilities and close supervision is made available (K Dalziel, personal communication, December 1994). Under this scheme hospitals will remain as assessment centres for new patients (or rapid access for those with unstable conditions) with the treatment being carried out in the community closer to patients' homes at flexible times to fit in with patients' work and school commitments. Senior dermatology nurses could run such centres with accountability to a named dermatologist and a group of GPs. Such a system would need further development of training nurses in dermatology and rigorous monitoring for compliance to guidelines such as those developed by the British Photodermatology Group for ultraviolet light therapy.[133] The extended role for GPs would require more incentives for educational development in dermatology and those with special interest in dermatology could play a key role in ensuring continuity of care in the treatment centres. The number of treatment centres required would be calculated from estimated numbers of patients currently attending hospitals for such treatment at present (approximatley one-third to half of follow-up visits, equating to around one centre per 100 000 population).

Maintain hospital-based specialists and use their skills more effectively

Dermatologists need their hospital facilities and colleagues in order to function effectively. Dermatologists would be responsible for rapid assessment of those who need help and for supervising treatment centres. Skin cancer is one area where there is strong argument for dermatologists to take the main responsibility for initial assessment. Establishing the 'correct' number of specialists will be difficult without further information about the differential gain of specialists over GPs for each skin disease sub-category. The British Association of Dermatology has recommended that in order to ensure a continuing quality service one dermatologist per 100 000 will be needed (still the lowest ratio in the EU). This ratio can only serve as a guide as it depends on other factors such as urban/rural mix, the availability of specialist dermatology clinics such as paediatric or tumour clinics and junior staff support. Lower follow-up ratios usually mean that those who are recalled for follow-up visits are often more complex than the traditional dermatology follow-up patients, and this along with an increasing tendency to practise defensive medicine will mean that dermatology consultation times will increase in the future. A maximum of 12 new patients or 24 return patients or a pro rata mix per single consultant session has been recommended by BAD. Some highly specialist services such as phototesting for light sensitivity or diagnosis of epidermolysis bullosa are probably best dealt with at a regional or supraregional level.

Involvement of community pharmacists

Better public information about effective OTC skin preparations and involvement of community pharmacists in providing better information regarding the treatment of common mild skin diseases such as acne could lead to substantial savings in consultation and prescribing costs,[44] given that around 50% of people with skin complaints self-medicate.[30,31] This may not appear at first to be the remit of purchasers but they could ensure that local pharmacists are linked with the district dermatology liaison team so that locally approved information leaflets concerning common skin diseases are made available to those who seek help at community pharmacists.

In summary the hybrid model emphasizes strengthening existing services by improving communication and co-operation between various health care providers, encouraging greater public participation in deciding appropriate levels of care and a shift of care towards developing treatment facilities in the community. It is a model which recommends improved co-ordination of available skills. The model offers a quality service which would:

- ensure many entry points into a system which provided consistent advice or support
- develop a real ownership between professionals and patients
- promote informed expectations and outcome measures
- develop an appropriate cascade of expertise with access to a named person/case manager.

Such a scheme would need adequate financial support for implementation of educational programmes and collaborative initiatives between local teams. The total running costs of such a hybrid model would depend on the needs and priorities of the local population but a for a mixed urban/semi-urban population of 100 000 in the Nottingham area, around £1.47 million would be required at 1994 prices (excluding initial building costs of community treatment centres). This estimate assumes a consultant/population ratio of 1 : 100 000 but with a 16% reduction in dermatology outpatient running costs due to the availability of community day treatment facilities (£0.2 million), a 11% reduction in inpatient costs due to day treatment facilities (£0.4 million), running costs for one community skin treatment centre treating 1000 patients per annum (£0.05 million), the appointment of three additional 'F' grade community specialist liaison dermatology nurses (£0.08 million), an implementation fund of £0.05 million and costs for GP consultations and prescription and dispensing remaining the same as current expenditure (£0.29, £0.32 and £0.08 million respectively).

Summary

- Care models that focus solely on the relationship between general primary and secondary dermatological care are likely to fail unless they consider the large and unstable burden of unmet dermatological needs.
- Most common skin diseases can and should be managed in the community.
- Some shift from secondary to primary care for dermatological services is desirable but it will need considerable investment in terms of GP education and/or specialist expansion.
- Initial assessment of all skin cancers should be performed by dermatologists.
- Retaining the current system of dermatology services without specialist expansion is likely to fail patients by not responding to unmet needs and responding inappropriately to increased demands.
- A shift of dermatologists away from hospitals into community-run outreach clinics would require a costly four-fold expansion of dermatology consultants in order to ensure equitable care, with serious implications for the future of dermatology development as a scientific discipline.
- A hybrid model consisting of hospital-based dermatology assessment centres, shared care clinics in primary care for chronic skin diseases and community-based treatment centres run by dermatology nurses accountable to district dermatology liaison teams is described.
- Individual skills are used more appropriately in such a scheme in that assessment is carried out in hospitals where appropriate facilities are available and treatment is carried out nearer patients' homes.
- The formation of a local dermatology liaison team of dermatologists, dermatology nurses, GPs, local pharmacists and public representatives could form the basis for corporate needs assessments which are sensitive to local issues.
- Cost estimates for the hybrid model (£1.47 million per 100 000, 1994 prices) are slightly higher than the status quo model (£1.26 million) but less costly than the outreach clinic model £1.63 million and offers additional flexibility for adjustment to future demands in skin health services.
- New technologies such as teledermatology which enhance communication between GPs and dermatologists require further evaluation before they become adopted in practice.

8 Outcome measures

The development of generic outcome measures in dermatology is still in its infancy and most practical measures which could be used to monitor effectiveness of current services are indirect. Given the vast differences in needs of patients with different skin diseases simplification of outcome measures for dermatology as a whole may be misleading. For example an elderly person who has had an incidental, symptomless basal cell carcinoma removed by his or her doctor may not record any change in a life quality index measurement, as it was not perceived as a problem by themselves in the first place. In contrast a family whose child has a severe atopic eczema which is unresponsive to most medical therapies may still find that the support and information given to them by their doctor are extremely useful but such a beneficial outcome would not be evident with a measure such as 'percentage reduction in surface area of affected skin'.

Direct outcome measures

- Simple surveys that assess patient satisfaction regarding adequacy of information provided by GP/dermatologist/nurse regarding their skin condition.
- Disease-specific outcomes such as improvement in acne disability index, improvement in sleep loss for atopic eczema sufferers, duration of remission following psoriasis treatment, percentage satisfied or symptom free after reassurance or removal of benign skin tumour, percentage warts clear at three months, venous ulcer healing rates of over 33% at three months and 45% at six months for uncomplicated ulcers treated in the community[114] and proportion of people with hand dermatitis who are able to return to work within six weeks.
- Further development of the use of generic skin disease disability scores such as the Dermatology Life Quality Index.

Indirect outcome measures

- Use of computerized pathology records to determine the thickness distribution of melanomas as an indicator of possible patient delay in presentation.
- Use of pathology records to determine diagnostic accuracy of skin cancer request forms and adequacy of excision margins.
- Use of pathology records to determine proportion of moles and seborrhoeic warts that have been excised for 'cosmetic' reasons.
- Melanoma mortality in relation to tumour thickness compared with national rates.
- Recurrence rates of non-melanoma skin cancer.
- Re-referral rates for patients seen in specialist settings with different new or follow-up ratios as an indicator of cost-effective use of specialist services.
- Appropriateness of referral for specialist advice as measured by proportion of warts referred and by variations in referral rates between practices.

9 Targets

Dermatology fulfils all of the Health of the Nation target requirements, i.e. it is a major cause of avoidable ill health, effective interventions are available and it is possible to set objective targets and monitor progress. Requesting evidence for efficacy of new technologies such as photophoresis for systemic sclerosis, teledermatology, laser treatment for strawberry haemangiomas etc. is a positive action. However insisting on high quality evidence for all dermatological interventions currently carried out on the 1000 or so skin diseases is unrealistic given the low priority accorded by central and local funding agencies in evaluating dermatological interventions.

Care must be taken in distinguishing between those procedures which urgently require further evaluation because of lack of evidence and those where there is reasonable evidence against the use of the procedure.

Purchasers are in a good position to specify service priorities and targets – for example in the diagnosis and treatment of skin cancer – but require close professional advice to ensure that, for example, carcinoma *in situ* is not given priority over scarring acne or a flare-up of pustular psoriasis. Purchasers should not be misled into believing that encouraging GPs to perform more minor surgery will cut the demand for dermatology surgery;[134,135] though it may well reduce standards.[78] Improved training of GPs in dermatology, while important for patients,[25] does not reduce referrals to dermatology departments, though it may change their nature.[76]

The following targets are suggestions for dermatology which could be realistically accomplished within the next ten years.

Prevention

- To educate every child on the dangers of excessive sun exposure through educational programmes co-ordinated by the UK Skin Cancer Working Party.[104]
- To inform outdoor workers on simple measures to reduce sunburn and cumulative ultraviolet light exposure.
- To reduce the incidence of skin cancer in younger people and the prevalence of skin cancer in the elderly.

Information

- For each district to commission simple population-based needs assessment exercises for skin disorders and to formulate service strategies based on the results.
- Each district to complete an assessment exercise on the direct and indirect costs of the dermatology service.
- Computerized patient records of diagnosis and severity of skin disease in both primary and secondary care.
- To achieve a 100% registration for melanoma and non-melanoma skin cancer for each district with regular review of the completeness and accuracy of data.

Service

- One dermatologist per 100 000 of the population.
- Retention of a core of hospital based diagnostic facilities with access to inpatient beds.
- Dermatology outpatient waiting lists of under six weeks for a routine appointment, under three weeks for a 'soon' appointment, within one week for an urgent referral and within 48 hours for a telephoned emergency request.
- Demonstrable benefits to patients based on a range of outcome measures (including improved coping with skin disability) in skin disease sub-categories in both primary and secondary care.
- Clear links between primary and secondary care with patient centred record keeping, combined audit exercises and a clear description of what patients can expect from each level of service.
- Shared care schemes for common chronic skin diseases linked with national guidelines.
- The establishment of local district dermatology liaison teams to improve unexplained variations in referral patterns and the establishment of community treatment centres.
- Inclusion of the commissioning of services located outside of normal working districts (such as laser treatment for port wine stains) into current purchasing arrangements.
- Development of a good skin care guide that covers both primary and secondary care which makes it clear to patients what they can expect from each service and who has responsibility for their care.
- An increase in dermatology training for GPs so that at least one in three have received additional training by the year 1998.

10 Further information and research priorities

Care has to be taken in distinguishing between health care requirements and distress caused by skin disease for which available treatment is not beneficial. Some degree of prioritization is inevitable with such a large burden of unmet dermatological needs but these priorities should be more open so that they can be debated, criticized and changed. Even with such explicit rationing some degree of implicit rationing will be necessary at the point of service as this is likely to be more sensitive to the complexity of medical decisions and the needs of personal and cultural preferences of patients,[136] especially in a field where perception of disease is intimately linked with personal and cultural factors. As Frankel has pointed out even if demand generally exceeds supply this does not mean that particular health care requirements cannot be satisfied.[137] Limited data from the NHANES study suggest that only a certain amount of those with skin disease feel the need to request help,[3] adding some support to the concept that infinite demand may be a myth. Providing future epidemiological surveys incorporate other factors which may influence health care requirements such as the relationship between symptoms, examination findings, handicap and effectiveness of treatment, there may be a realistic prospect of demand and supply achieving a balance for skin disease.

Because dermatology is such a vast and complex subject with health care requirements ranging from simple reassurance for benign moles to life-saving interventions for skin cancer or drug eruptions, dermatologists must be involved in future needs assessments if useful information is to be collected.

With the exception of protocols for better management of some common skin diseases in the population and the provision of liquid nitrogen to all GPs for treatment of warts, there seem to be no glaring examples of inappropriate distribution of existing services for dermatology. Rather the major omissions in NHS provision for skin diseases are those which can only be filled by adequate research and development of services.

Because of the vast nature of unmet dermatological needs, research should focus on skin disease in the community, rather than on minor differences in existing primary care and secondary care. Research into the determinants of health seeking behaviour is needed as well as research into how some of the population's dermatological needs might be met by other approaches, such as better OTC treatment and information.

The boundary between disease and cosmesis is especially blurred in dermatology and one which is likely to shift according to availability of effective treatments and social attitudes. Normative care is likely to vary according to local resources and interests. Just as patients are encouraged to participate in choices and decision making, so populations should participate in the process of deciding with doctors and purchasers about what constitutes reasonable demand,[138] so that boundaries are explicit and open to further debate if circumstances change. This is compatible with the NHS' and dermatologists' long-term strategic aim to promote a healthy skin for all.[139,140]

Ensuring a quality future service

- Urgent research to determine the prevalence and incidence of skin disease in different regions and age groups throughout the UK and to investigate factors which influence people to seek medical care.
- An explicit policy based on public consultation to determine guidelines which will distinguish between reasonable need and demand for dermatology services.
- Examination of the differential health gain and costs of specialist versus generalist or nursing care for skin disease.
- Investigation of the cost-effectiveness of liaison dermatology community nurses.
- The development of achievable outcome measures for the nine common skin disease sub-categories which could be built into contracts.

- Research into the use of information technology which could increase the flexibility of the primary/secondary care interface such as high resolution photography and shared computerized coding systems for diagnosis, severity and costing.
- The development of a more co-ordinated approach to health services research in dermatology such as the establishment of centres for systematic review and evaluation of outcome measures.
- Research into the effectiveness of OTC skin preparations and pharmacy advice for skin complaints.
- Cost-effectiveness of community skin treatment centres.
- Research into factors which enhance implementation of good practice guidelines.
- Randomized studies which examine the cost-effectiveness of screening for skin cancer in high risk groups.

Appendix I ICD codes relating to skin diseases

ICD 9

Only diseases that commonly have cutaneous manifestations have been included. Readers are referred to Alexander and Shrank for a more detailed alphabetical list of all possible dermatological entries in ICD 9.[18]
Conditions belonging to sub-categories discussed in more detail in the text are in **bold**.

Chapter I: Infectious and parasitic disease

017	Tuberculosis of other organs
022	Anthrax
030	Leprosy
031	Diseases due to other mycobacteria
034	Streptococcal sore throat and scarlatina
035	**Erysipelas**
053	**Herpes zoster**
054	**Herpes simplex**
078.1	**Viral warts**
057	Other viral exanthemata
091	Erysipeloid
102	Yaws
103	Pinta
104	Other spirochaetal infection
110	**Dermatophytosis**
111	**Dermatomycosis, other and unspecified**
112	Candidiasis
114	Coccidioidomycosis
115	Histoplasmosis
117	Other mycoses
118	Opportunistic mycosis
128	Other and unspecified helminthiasis
132	**Pediculosis (lice) and phthirius infestation**
133	**Acariasis (scabies)**
134	Other infestation
135	Sarcoidosis
137	Late effects of tuberculosis

Chapter II: Neoplasms

172	**Malignant melanoma of skin**
173	**Other malignant neoplasms of the skin**
174.0	Paget's disease of the breast
202.1	**Mycosis fungoides**
202.2	Sezary's disease
216	**Benign neoplasm of skin**
232	**Carcinoma *in situ* of skin**

Chapter III: Endocrine, nutritional and metabolic diseases and immunity disorders

277.8	Hystiocytosis X

706	Diseases of sebaceous glands (Acne vulgaris 706.1)
707	**Chronic ulcer of the skin**
708	Urticaria
709	Other disorders of skin and subcutaneous tissue

Chapter XIV: Congenital anomalies
757   Congenital anomalies of the integument

Chapter XV: Certain conditions originating in the perinatal period
778   Conditions involving the integument and temperature regulation of foetus and newborn

Chapter XVI: Symptoms, common signs and ill-defined conditions
782   Symptoms involving skin and other integumentary tissue

Chapter XVII: Injury and poisoning
995.1   Angioneurotic oedema
995.2   Unspecified adverse affect of drug, medicament and biological

Comment on usefulness of ICD 9 Chapter XII on skin disease

The ICD 9 chapter code for disorders of the skin and subcutaneous tissues (Chapter XII) is of limited operational use because of problems with completeness, accuracy, diagnostic transfer and appropriateness of diagnostic categories. Important exclusions from the ICD 9 chapter for disorders of the skin and subcutaneous tissues include neoplasms of the skin, localized cutaneous infections such as fungal infections and herpes simplex, perinatal skin disorders such as erythema toxicum, systemic diseases which commonly affect the skin such as sarcoidosis and a range of other miscellaneous conditions such as hirsutism and hyperhidrosis. Inappropriate inclusions within the ICD 9 coding for disorders of the skin and subcutaneous tissues include some categories which are perhaps best regarded as 'surgical' such as acute lymphangitis, and abscess of finger or toe.[17]

The rationale for some of the diagnostic codes used in ICD 9 is not especially helpful for the purchaser interested in common disease groupings. Some important categories are not mutually exclusive e.g. a child with atopic dermatitis could be classified under atopic eczema, flexural eczema, neurodermatitis, infantile eczema or intrinsic allergic eczema, permitting diagnostic transfer according to which is the predominant fashionable term. Thus in the first national morbidity survey,[36] there was apparently twice as much eczema as dermatitis in the South West, whereas in Wales the position was reversed with three times as much dermatitis recorded as eczema. The total incidence of the two however was almost identical in the two areas. Unfortunately ICD 9 173, which codes for non-melanoma skin cancer, does not distinguish between the two commonest forms of skin cancers, namely basal cell carcinoma (rodent ulcer) and squamous cell carcinoma.

ICD 10

Diseases of the skin and subcutaneous tissues are coded as L00 to L99.[19,20] The codes are grouped as follows:

L00–L08	Infections of the skin and subcutaneous tissues
L10–L14	Bullous disorders
L20–L30	Dermatitis and eczema
L40–L45	Papulosquamous disorders
L50–L51	Urticaria and erythema
L55–L59	Radiation–related disorders
L60–L70	Disorders of skin appendages
L80–L99	Other disorders of skin and subcutaneous tissues.

Important exclusions from L00 to L99 include:

- malignant skin neoplasms (malignant melanoma of the skin C43, other malignant neoplasms of the skin C44)
- carcinoma *in situ* D04 (excluding melanoma *in situ*)
- benign neoplasms of the skin (melanocytic naevi D22, other benign skin neoplasms D23)
- certain skin infections such as erysipelas A46, herpes simplex B00 (non-genital), molluscum B08.1, mycoses B35-B49, infestations such as scabies B85-89 and viral warts B07.

A detailed list of exclusions which include congenital, perinatal and connective tissue diseases are given in the opening section dealing with skin diseases of the ICD 10 handbook.[20]

Appendix II UK prevalence studies of skin diseases

The table shows the PAGB study of self-reported skin disease.[29]

Table II.1: Two-week incidence of ailments of the skin according to diagnostic group and age in a stratified sample of 1217 UK adults and 342 children (the PAGB study[29])

Base = all adults	All adults (%)	Men (%)	Women (%)	15–19 years (%)	20–34 years (%)	35–64 years (%)	65 years or over (%)	All children[a] (%)	Boys (%)	Girls (%)
Unweighted base	1217	589	628	140	334	526	215	342	185	157
Weighted base[b]	1217	595	622	126	347	531	212	354	194	160
	100	100	100	100	100	100	100	100	100	100
Minor cuts and grazes	16	23	10	35	23	13	4	21	25	17
Acne/piles/spots	14	13	15	41	25	5	1	3	2	4
Bruises	12	12	12	30	16	8	5	22	25	18
Oily/greasy skin	10	9	11	27	17	5	1	1	1	1
Bunions/corns/callouses	6	4	8	5	3	7	12	1 c	1	d
Discoloured skin/blotches/age spots	6	4	8	7	4	4	15	d	c	d
Thinning/losing hair/baldness	6	10	2	d	3	6	10	c	c	d
Irritated skin	5	3	6	3	5	5	5	2	2	1
Varicose veins	5	2	7	1	2	7	7	d	d	d
Rashes/skin allergies	4	3	5	4	5	5	3	5	7	3
Chapped skin	4	2	6	4	6	4	3 c	3	4	1
Minor burns/scalds (not sunburn)	4	3	3	5	6	4	d	3 c	1	c
Insect bites/stings	4	5	3	3	4	4	3	2	1	3
Piles/haemorrhoidal problems/itching	4	3	4	4	2	4	7	2	2	d
Athletes' foot	3	5	2	2	5	3	3	2	2	1
Ingrown toenail	3	2	4	4	2	4	4	1	1	1
Warts	2	2	3	6	3	2	1	1	1	d
Animal bites and scratches	2	2	3	7	4	1	d	1	2	d
Psoriasis	2	2	2	2	1	3	2 c	2 c	c	c
Sunburn	2	2	2	5	4	1	1	1	2	d
Severe dandruff	2	2	2	2	3	1	1	1	1	1
Eczema	1	1	2	2	2	1	d	2	3	1
Septic/infected cuts	1	1	1	1	2	2	1	1	1	d
Verruca	1	1	2	2	1	1	d	2	2	3
Boils	1	1	1 c	1	2	1	1	2	2	3
Headstroke/sunstroke	c	d	c	c	1	d	d	d	d	d
Head lice	d	d	d	d	d	d	d	d	1	1
Ringworm	d	d	d	d	d	d	d	d	1	d
Nappy rash	d	d	d	d	d	d	d	5	5	6
Cradle cap	d	d	d	d	d	d	d	4	3	4

[a] Data collected by proxy from mothers.
[b] Weighted to population structure of the UK.
[c] Less than 0.5% but not zero.

Table II.2: Estimated prevalence of skin diseases (per 1000) by age group and grade of severity in 2180 adults in Lambeth[2]

| Grade of severity | Age group (years) | | | | | | | |
| | 15–24 | | 25–34 | | 35–54 | | 55–74 | |
	All grades	Moderate and severe	All grades	Moderate and severe	All grades	Moderate and severe	All grades	Moderate and severe
Eczema	122.7	72.6	35.4	34.2	126.5	89.4	64.4	38.0
Acne	273.3	137.8	78.7	34.5	57.2	8.9	20.3	8.6
Scaly dermatoses	60.5	9.8	35.3	14.0	56.4	40.1	173.0	35.8
Prurigo and allied conditions	66.8	38.4	42.4	34.4	122.6	32.6	54.0	50.8
Erythematous and other dermatoses	14.2	–	99.4	4.1	89.4	15.2	73.0	55.1
Warts	61.5	–	35.3	7.1	3.1	–	59.1	–
Psoriasis	4.2	–	51.6	23.2	–	–	16.4	3.6
Any skin condition	614.1	308.0	543.3	246.0	514.0	186.0	545.9	211.0

Table II.3: Use of medical care for major sub-categories of skin disease by grade of severity in 2180 adults in Lambeth.

| Group | Grade of severity | No. of persons (= 100%) | Self medication | General Practitioner | Hospital | | Use of any medical service | No treatment |
					Outpatient	Inpatient		
Eczema and prurigo	Trivial	57	27	7 (12)	3 (5)	–	8 (14)	26 (45)
	Moderate/ severe	100	(47) 35 (35)	27 (27)	6 (6)	–	30 (30)	41 (41)
Acne	Trivial	40	17	9 (22)	1 (3)	–	9 (22)	18 (45)
	Moderate/ severe	43	(42) 14 (31)	5 (12)	1 (2)	–	6 (14)	25 (58)
Psoriasis	Trivial	6	–		1 (17)	–	1 (17)	5 (83)
	Moderate/ severe	11	2 (18)	3 (27)	1 (9)	–	4 (4)	6 (55)
All other conditions	Trivial	215	70 (33)	18 (8)	6 (3)	1	22 (10)	130 (60)
	Moderate/ severe	94	28 (30)	19 (20)	7 (7)	(0.5)	23 (24)	48 (51)

Percentages are shown in parenthesis

Appendix III Prevalence of examined skin disease in the US NHANES study

Table III.1: Prevalence of significant skin pathology among 20 749 US persons aged 1–74 years[3]

Condition	Male	Female	Both sexes
	Rate per 1000 population		
Persons with one or more significant skin conditions	339.8	286.6	312.4
Significant skin conditions, all types	499.4	383.4	439.7
Acne vulgaris	70.5	65.9	68.1
Cystic acne	3.3	0.6	1.9
Acne scars	2.0	1.3	1.7
Xerosis	5.3	7.7	6.5
Dermatophytoses	131.4	33.7	81.1
Tumours	59.6	53.7	56.5
Malignant	6.4	5.3	5.9
Basal cell epithelioma	4.7	3.5	4.1
Benign	35.8	40.5	38.2
Pre-cancerous and not specified	17.4	7.9	12.4
Actinic keratosis	13.9	5.5	9.6
Seborrhoeic dermatitis	26.7	30.1	28.5
Atopic dermatitis, eczema	19.5	17.4	18.4
Atopic dermatitis	8.2	5.6	6.9
Lichen simplex chronicus	4.7	4.4	4.5
Hand eczema	1.1	2.1	1.6
Nummular eczema	1.0	2.4	1.7
Dyshidrotic eczema	3.1	1.2	2.1
Contact dermatitis	13.4	13.8	13.6
Ichthyosis, keratosis	9.3	9.6	9.5
Verruca vulgaris	10.3	7.2	8.5
Folliculitis	12.3	4.0	8.0
Psoriasis	5.9	5.1	5.5
Seborrheic keratosis	4.6	5.8	5.2
Vitiligo	3.6	6.2	4.9
Urticaria (hives etc.)	3.8	5.6	4.8
Herpes simplex	4.0	4.5	4.2
All other skin conditions	106.7	105.0	106.2

See also Figure III.1 on page 321.

Table III.2: Significant skin pathology and its relationship to subject's concern according to sex category[3]

Age	Both sexes				Male				Female			
	Skin condition of concern	Significant skin pathology of		Non-significant skin pathology of concern	Skin condition of concern	Significant skin pathology of:		Non-significant skin pathology of concern	Skin condition of concern	Significant skin pathology of:		Non-significant skin pathology of concern
		Concern	No concern			Concern	No concern			Concern	No concern	
Rate per 1000 population												
Total 1–74 years	118.2	97.1	215.3	21.1	128.2	108.0	231.8	20.2	108.8	86.9	199.7	21.9
Standard error of rate												
Total 1–74 years	7.58	6.23	13.82	1.35	7.94	6.69	14.36	1.55	7.64	6.10	14.02	1.61

'Concern' implies that the subject expressed concern or complained about their skin condition

Table III.3: Proportion of skin conditions classified as significant by a dermatologist examiner in the NHANES study[3]

Condition	Total	Skin condition Significant	Non-significant	Proportion classed as significant
		Rate per 1000 population		%
Other skin disorders (vitiligo, traumatic scars, ephelides etc.)	516.2	27.5	488.7	5.3
Ichthyosis, keratosis	432.7	21.8	410.9	5.0
Tumours, malignant and benign and leukemias	357.1	56.7	300.4	15.9
Malignant tumours	11.6	5.9	5.7	50.9
Diseases of sweat and sebaceous glands	209.5	87.0	122.5	41.5
Other diseases of circulatory system (Osler's disease, telangiectasis etc.)	182.7	1.0	181.7	0.5
Corns, callosities	156.9	3.2	153.7	2.0
Lichen planus	140.6	0.8	139.8	0.6
Seborrhoeic keratosis	124.1	5.2	118.9	4.2
Seborrhoeic dermatitis	116.7	28.5	88.2	24.4
Dermatophytoses	81.1	81.1	–	7.8
Infections of skin (boils, impetigo, infectious warts etc.)	60.0	15.9	44.1	26.5
Contact dermatitides	53.9	13.6	40.3	25.2
Diseases of hair and hair follicles	50.5	15.8	34.7	31.3
Pruritus	25.8	13.7	12.1	53.1
Psoriasis	14.3	8.8	5.5	61.5
Injuries, adverse effects of chemical and other external conditions	3.8	3.7	0.1	97.4

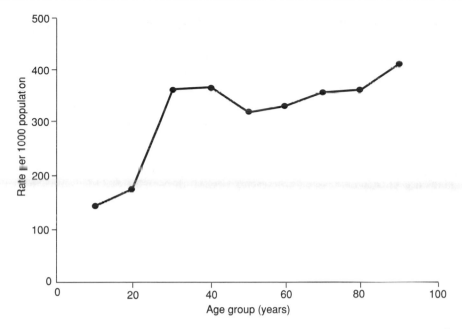

Figure III.1: Age-specific prevalence of one or more significant skin conditions in a US population.[3]

Appendix IV The general practitioner morbidity surveys

Every ten years, the Royal College of General Practitioners conducts a survey of 25 to 60 practices in England and Wales on every face-to-face consultation with patients over a one-year period.[5,7,36,37]

The sample is not fully representative of England and Wales in that practices from the North, Midland and Wales are over-represented whilst practices from the South are under-represented.

The studies also include too many practices with four or above principals and too many with larger list sizes. The surveys are also limited by employing similar classification systems to ICD 9 and no direct validation of diagnosis is available.

Despite these limitations the studies remain the most useful routinely available data on people who seek help through the first entry point in the health service. Each study covers a total of around a third of a million patients and slightly less patient–years. There have been no direct studies on validity of the diagnoses entered by GPs into these statistics but indirect validation is available in the from of the confidence expressed by the GP in the diagnosis given.[5] These are summarized in Table IV.1.

Table IV.1: Confidence expressed by GPs in diagnosis of skin disorders

Symptom	Diagnosis not advanced beyond presenting (%)	Provisional diagnosis (%)	Confident diagnosis (%)
Cough	4	20	76
Rashes	7	28	65
Sore throat	2	9	89
Abdominal pain	18	60	21
Back pain	8	52	40

Degree of confidence (%)

Appendix V Prevalence of melanoma skin cancer

Malignant melanoma is a comparatively rare but potentially lethal form of skin cancer which develops in the pigment-producing cells of the skin. There are three reasons why health professionals have expressed concern over what may be a largely preventable cancer.[41,119] First incidence rates in England and Wales have doubled over the last ten years[4,41](Figure V.1). Second the disease affects young adults and third survival rates could improve if more patients were treated at an early stage when excision may be curative.

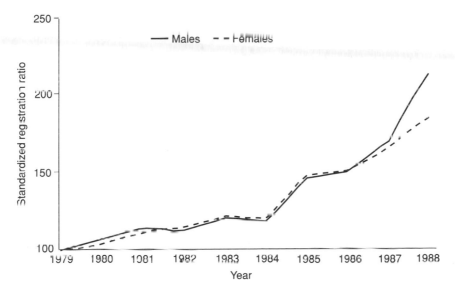

Figure V.1: Standardized registration ratios (SRRs) for melanoma skin cancer in England and Wales 1979 to 1988.[141]

Melanoma accounted for 1142 deaths in England and Wales in 1992.[10] In both men and women death rates at ages over 40 years rose three-fold between 1959 and 1989.[120] Mortality rates have also increased at younger ages, though not so dramatically. New cases of melanomas were recorded in 1354 males and 2249 females in England and Wales in 1989.[141] Estimates for the whole of UK are shown in Table V.1.[41] In Scotland it is the most rapidly rising cancer.[41] In a special survey in South Wales the crude cancer registration rates for melanoma were 7.4 and 13.7 per 100 000 per year for males and females respectively.[142]

Table V.1: Numbers of new cases and deaths from melanoma in 1988 for the UK[41]

| | Number of new cases UK 1988 | | | |
	England/ Wales	Scotland	Northern Ireland	UK
Males	1497	203	16	1716
Females	2394	300	28	2722
Persons	3891	503	44	4438
	Numbers of deaths UK 1992			
Males	565	46	12	623
Females	577	56	9	642
Persons	1142	102	21	1265

The most common type of melanoma is the superficial spreading melanoma – a lesion which can remain in a horizontal growth phase for a period of several years during which removal may be curative. Prognosis of melanoma which has not metastasized to lymph nodes is directly related to its depth of invasion into the skin. Lesions removed at a thin early stage have a very good prognosis (over 92% five-year survival for lesions less than 1.5 mm thick in females) whereas lesions presenting at a later thick stage fare poorly (five-year survival of around 37% for lesions thicker than 3 mm).[143,144] Melanomas are characterized by irregularity of shape, colour and border – features which are usually easily recognizable by health professionals.

In an attempt to alert people to the importance of early diagnosis of melanoma several public education campaigns were initiated by the Cancer Research Campaign in the late 1980s and early 1990s. These well-intentioned campaigns generated a considerable increase in workload of benign pigmented lesions in both GP and dermatology departments.[60–62,75] Since the campaigns, the proportion of thinner, better prognosis melanomas has increased, although these trends had been in place long before the campaigns were started.[62] Melanoma mortality has continued to increase in England and Wales although a flattening of melanoma incidence has been reported over the last ten years for females in Scotland.[145] Due to the long latency of melanoma (incidence to mortality ratio of 3.9 for females and 3.2 for men) it is too early to assess the effects of the public education campaigns for early diagnosis on melanoma mortality. Purchasers need to be aware that whilst the Health of the Nation Target 'to halt the year-on-year increase in incidence of skin cancer by the year 2005' is a noble one, it is most unlikely to be realized within the allotted time span because of the lag between exposure and the development of skin cancer and the fact that a cohort of older patients who have already received excessive ultraviolet light exposure through leisure activities will continue to develop skin cancers such as melanoma for the next 40 to 50 years.

Melanoma is more common in fair skinned populations living in sunny climates such as Australia and Southern USA.[144] The increased incidence of melanoma has affected both sexes and all ages and there is progressive risk for successive birth cohorts. These changes appear to be real as opposed to changes in diagnostic criteria or increased reporting.[144] Risk factors for melanoma include fair skin, red or blonde hair, blue eyes, tendency to burn easily on sun exposure, tendency to freckle, excessive number of benign moles and family history of melanoma. The importance of sunlight is illustrated by the association of melanoma incidence in white skinned people with latitude, although melanomas may occur on non-exposed sites. In addition to different susceptibility of melanoma, intermittent (recreational) exposure to sunlight is important.[146,147]

Unlike Australia and USA melanoma is more common in females in the UK, with a female to male ratio of 1.7 : 1, the reasons of which are unclear.[75] Melanoma exhibits a social class gradient with higher rates among professional and non-manual workers thought to be due to intermittent intense UV exposure. The age-specific incidence rates increase with increasing age (Figure V.2). Melanoma is very rare in childhood but around 20% of melanomas occur in young adults (20–39 years), whereas less than 4% of all neoplasms occur in this age group. Standardized registration rates (SRRs) show some variation with region, with highest rates in the Wessex and South Western regions (female SRRs 160 and 152 respectively) and lowest rates in Northern and Merseyside (female SRRs 68 and 70 respectively).[141]

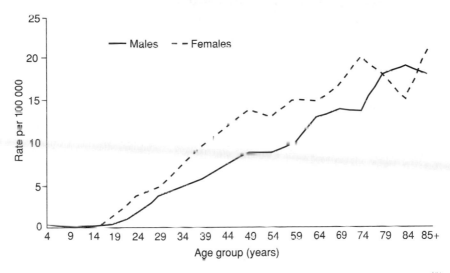

Figure V.2: Age and melanoma incidence per 100 000 population for England and Wales in 1988.[141]

Appendix VI Prevalence of non-melanoma skin cancer (NMSC)

Of the NMSCs around 80% are basal cell carcinomas (BCC) and most of the remainder are squamous cell carcinomas (SCC). In most countries NMSC is more common than melanoma skin cancer by a factor of ten and BCC is much more common than SCC by a factor of four. Melanoma skin cancer on the other hand causes more deaths than NMSC (1142 and 486 deaths respectively in 1992).[10]

Official cancer registration statistics probably underestimate the incidence of NMSC by a factor of at least two.[141,148] Despite under-registration it is by far the most common form of cancer in the UK. There was a total of 32 000 registrations for NMSC in England and Wales in 1988,[141] with the majority of tumours occurring in the over 60s age group. The incidence of both these tumours increases sharply with increasing age (Figure VI.1). Considerable regional variation in NMSC registration rates are seen within the UK but in the absence of complete data from special surveys it is difficult to comment on whether these differences are due to differences in registration/awareness or whether they are due to the age and skin type structure of the populations or whether they are due to total UVR exposure.[141] Coastal areas with a large proportion of retired people such as the South Western area have the highest rates (Figure VI.2). In a random sample of 560 subjects aged over 60 years in South Wales[142] the prevalence of non-melanoma skin cancer was 2.1% (95% confidence interval 1.1% to 3.7%) with a basal to squamous cell ratio of 5 : 1. The incidence of non-melanoma skin cancers was 5.4 per 1000 person–years (1.2 to 15.6 per 1000 person–years). Malignant melanoma was found in 0.2% of subjects (0.01% to 1%). Accurate and up-to-date statistics on the prevalence of NMSC in different regions of the UK according to age or other high risk groups is absent. This information is essential for the planning of appropriate services.

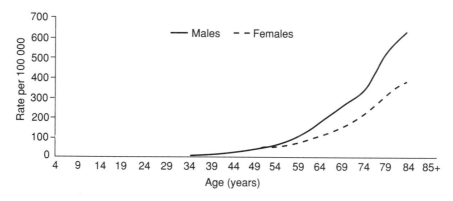

Figure VI.1: Incidence of non-melanoma skin cancer with age for England and Wales in 1988.[141]

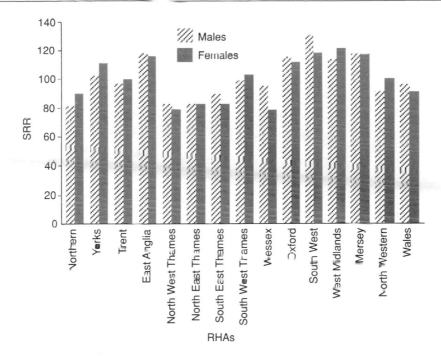

Figure VI.2: Standardized registration ratios (SRR) for non-melanoma skin cancer for different regions of England and Wales in 1988.[141]

Very few people die from NMSC. The five-year relative survival rates for men and women were about 97% for 1981 registrations[10] and the ratio of incidence to mortality is probably around 160:1 if known under-registrations are allowed for.

Susceptibility to both NMSCs is inversely proportional to degree of melanin pigmentation and most tumours occur on areas of the body which have received large amounts of ultraviolet radiation over many years, i.e. an effect of cumulative rather than intermittent exposure.[149] There has been a striking rise in the incidence of NMSC over the last 20 years in the UK (Figure VI.3). Some of this rise may be a pseudoepidemic caused by increased reporting[148] but increased recreational and occupational exposure to sunlight is also important and this will continue to affect successive population cohorts well into the next 30 years because of the long latent period (decades) between exposure and disease. The amount of ultraviolet radiation (especially UV-B) that will reach the earth's surface will also increase as a result of depletion of stratospheric ozone. It has been estimated that a 1% ozone depletion could give rise to a 1% to 3% increase in both melanoma and non-melanoma skin cancers.[149] It seems likely that the cohort effects of excessive recreational and occupational exposure to ultraviolet radiation, combined with an increasingly elderly population and diminished ozone will ensure that prevalent cases of NMSC will continue to rise for at least the next 30 years.

Although BCC and SCC are frequently grouped together in cancer statistics, there are some important differences in the behaviour of these tumours. Basal cell carcinomas are slow growing tumours (years) of the skin usually occurring on sun-exposed areas such as the face. If left untreated they eventually ulcerate and cause local problems. Secondary spread is extremely unusual and surgical removal is highly effective. People with a basal cell carcinoma are at a very high risk of developing further new lesions.[150]

Squamous cell carcinoma of the skin has been related to cumulative sun exposure, and also typically occurs on sun-exposed areas of the skin such as the head or backs of the hands in the elderly. These tumours grow

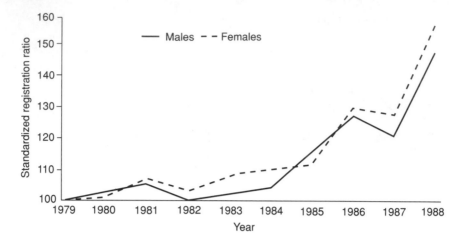

Figure VI.3: Standardized registration ratios for non-melanoma skin cancer for England and Wales 1979 to 1988.[141]

more rapidly (months) and can eventually metastasize if left untreated. As most NMSCs in white populations are probably due to UV-B exposure, a change in sun exposure habits could greatly reduce their incidence in future cohorts.

Appendix VII Prevalence of acne

Acne vulgaris is a very common condition characterized by papules, pustules, comedones (blackheads) and scars. It is caused by a combination of factors such as excessive and abnormal grease production, a bacterium (*Propionibacterium acnes*) and other abnormalities of the skin which lead to plugging of pilosebaceous openings. Mild degrees of acne are extremely common amongst teenagers and some have even considered it as a physiological disorder.[16] In discussing disease prevalence it is essential that some form of further breakdown according to disease severity is considered. It is also important to realize that whilst these severity gradings are reasonably objective they do not usually take into account the views of the sufferer. With increasing awareness of effective medical treatment and a decrease in the threshold of what both patients and doctor consider as a disease worthy of medical treatment, the distribution between the various severity categories could change substantially in the future. This would have major cost implications, as shown in Figure 8, page 297; as many more people exist with minor to moderate degrees of disease.

In a recent survey of Glasgow school children 83% of girls and 95% of boys had acne.[151] Most of these pupils had minimal disease and only 1.8% of boys and 0.3% of girls had moderate to severe disease in this study. 9% of boys and 14% of girls had visited their GP because of their acne and 0.3% were referred to a dermatologist.

Detailed analysis of 8328 people aged 15 to 44 years who were examined by dermatologists in the US in the early 1970s suggested that 20.7% of females had minimal disease (comedones and small pustular inflammatory lesions), 8.6% had moderate disease (comedones, pustules and deeper inflammatory lesions, considered by the examiner as a true disease as opposed to a passing cosmetic change), with a further 0.6% with severe disease (infected extensive cystic acne).[107] Corresponding prevalence rates for males were: 19% minimal, 11.3% moderate and 1.4% severe. Scarring secondary to acne was noted in 5.8% of females and 9.1% of males. Another US survey found that clinically significant inflammatory acne was present in 17.7% out of 435 boys aged nine to 15.[152]

The prevalence of moderate to severe acne in the Lambeth study was 13.8% in those aged 15–24 years.[2] Although much emphasis has been placed on teenage acne, moderate to severe disease may still affect a large number of older individuals affecting about 3.5% of those aged 25 to 34 years and 0.89% of those aged 35–54 years. Of all those with acne recorded in the NHANES study 17% were younger than 15 years old, 81% were aged 15 to 44 years and 2% were more than 44 years.[3] There is no evidence that ethnic group is an important determinant of acne prevalence when pubertal development has been adjusted for.[152]

No data are available on the incidence of acne in the population apart from GP morbidity statistics which reflects the incidence of those who choose to seek help.[5,7] With over £11 million spent on OTC acne preparations in the UK it is likely that the majority of sufferers do not seek a physician's assistance. In 1993 the cost of prescriptions for treatment of acne by GPs and dermatologists was £44.8 million.[153] An estimated 3.6 million consultations took place in GPs' surgeries, with 57 000 specialist referrals. Apart from the financial cost of acne, the human costs may also be high, since acne predominantly affects the face (Figure 2, page 276). Around 70% of acne patients experience shame or embarrassment because of their acne and 27% were depressed.[154] A specially designed acne disability index has been devised to assess the psychological effect of acne on the sufferer and disability correlates well with severity as measured by an objective grading system in most people.[155] There is however a small group of people whose disability appears to be out of proportion with severity. Little research has been conducted into the handicap caused by acne but a recent case-control study suggests that acne sufferers are more likely to be unemployed.[156]

It is possible that there has been a decrease in the proportion of people with moderate to severe acne over the last 50 years.[151] Although some of this shift could have been due to changes in defining disease severity, increased availability of effective treatment from chemists and GPs seems a more likely explanation.

Appendix VIII Prevalence of atopic eczema

Atopic eczema (or childhood eczema, infantile eczema, atopic dermatitis) is an inflammatory skin disorder characterized by itching, involvement of the skin creases and onset in early life.

Genetic factors are important[157] and hypersensitivity to a range of allergens and non-specific irritants may be implicated.[158] Although a tendency to dry irritable skin may be lifelong with atopic eczema, around 60% to 70% of children are clear of significant disease by their mid-teens.[158,159]

Recent prevalence studies of children in temperate developed countries suggest an overall cumulative prevalence of between 5% to 20% by the age of 11.[160-162] Point prevalences of visible dermatitis in populations of similar ages yield values approximately half of those for a history of ever having had atopic eczema,[163] compatible with the fluctuating nature of the disease. Data on the prevalence of severe disease is scanty but it is likely that most cases are mild and can be managed with simple treatments. In a recent study of 695 school children in London where 8.5% were noted to have visible atopic eczema 60% of eczema cases were considered to be very mild by the examining physician (i.e. required a moisturizer alone), 24% were mild (warranting a moisturizer and weak topical corticosteroid) and 16% were moderate or severe (requiring stronger topical preparations and a physician's supervision).[164] Prevalence estimates for adults suggest an overall frequency of atopic eczema of between 1.2% to 10%.[2,3,71]

Comparisons between different studies are limited, as diagnostic criteria which are suitable for epidemiological studies of atopic eczema have only recently been developed.[165] Even allowing for changes in diagnostic fashion, there is reasonable direct and indirect evidence to suggest that the prevalence of atopic eczema has increased two- to three-fold over the last 30 years.[6,166] The precise reasons for this increase in disease is not known but it is likely that environmental factors associated with urbanization are important.[158]

Atopic eczema in childhood shows a striking social class gradient for both reported and examined disease,[163] with higher rates in socio-economically advantaged groups and smaller families. Ethnic group may be an important factor for expression of atopic eczema. A recent study has found that the prevalence of atopic eczema (measured in three different ways) was twice as common in London born Afro-Caribbean children when compared with their white counterparts.[164] Generalizations to other ethnic groups may be unwise. For instance studies of Asian children in Leicester show that although they are three times as likely to be present in specialist clinics than white children, no differences in prevalence rates were seen in a community survey.[167]

Although there are no recent national prevalence studies of atopic eczema in the UK data for examined eczema from a national birth cohort study (the National Child Development Study or NCDS) points to considerable variation in disease prevalence and region, with highest rates in the South East and industrialized Midlands and lowest rates in Wales and Scotland.

Incidence figures are harder to obtain but unpublished data from the NCDS suggest around 50 cases per 1000 in the first year of life, falling to around five new cases per 1000 per year for the remainder of childhood.

Little is known about the direct and indirect costs of atopic eczema but it is clear that atopic eczema may be a source of considerable distress to both the children and their parents.[168] Atopic eczema consistently exhibits some of the highest scores on the Dermatology Life Quality Index[94] (a patient-derived tool for estimating the misery caused by skin diseases). A recent study of adult and childhood atopic eczema in Scotland has estimated that at least £288 million is spent annually on atopic eczema in the UK, with around one-third of costs being met by patients.[71] Although prevalence rates of atopic eczema were around five times higher in children than in adults, those aged over 16 accounted for 38% of all atopic eczema patients in absolute terms in this study.

Appendix IX Prevalence of psoriasis

Psoriasis is a chronic inflammatory skin disorder characterized by red scaly areas and tends to affect areas such as the knees, elbows, lower back and scalp. Onset of psoriasis is usually either in early adulthood or in later life and this bimodal onset may indicate different causative mechanisms.[169] Genetic factors are important in psoriasis and environmental factors such as skin trauma, streptococcal infection, certain medications, smoking, alcohol consumption and psychological stress may also play a role in disease expression.[170]

Epidemiological studies conducted in Northern Europe suggest an overall prevalence of between 1% to 3%.[33,34,171,172] Adult males and females are affected equally but age of onset may be earlier in females. The point prevalence of examined psoriasis was 0.5% (45/9263) and 0.8% (77/9263) at the ages of 11 and 16 respectively in the National Child Development Survey.[173] Psoriasis may be less common in blacks and oriental populations.[174] Longitudinal studies to examine the natural history of psoriasis have not been carried out but a retrospective questionnaire study suggested that between 36% and 55% of subjects experience some form of remission of their psoriasis for one to 54 years.[174] In this study 29% of patients considered that their psoriasis went into remission without physician-directed therapy.

The Lambeth study found that 1.6% (95% confidence intervals 0% to 3.3%) of the population had some psoriasis, a third of which was moderate to severe. Peak psoriasis prevalence was noted in the 25–34 years age group, with a second smaller peak 1.6% in the 55–74 years age group. Around two-thirds of the 1.4% of those noted to have psoriasis in the NHANES study were considered by the examining dermatologist to have clinically significant disease.[3]

A recent Gallup pole survey of 2019 people found that 5.5% of the public (or 8% of those aware of the disease) claimed to suffer from psoriasis.[175] This is considerably higher than examined psoriasis estimates from prevalence surveys but may reflect incorrect diagnoses by the public, differences between point and period prevalences and mild degrees of disease which might be ignored by physicians.

Although experience with hospital cases suggests that psoriasis is a chronic persistent condition,[174] care has to be shown in extrapolating this observation to milder community cases in the absence of appropriate studies of disease periodicity.

It is not known whether psoriasis prevalence rates vary throughout the UK but GP morbidity data suggest that a similar proportion of people seek advice about the condition throughout the UK.[5]

Appendix X Prevalence of viral warts

Warts are caused by human papilloma virus, of which over 50 subtypes have been described. Genital warts are usually treated in genitourinary departments and will not be discussed further here. Viral warts usually occur on exposed areas such as the fingers, hands and feet. Warts occurring on the soles of the feet are often referred to as verrucae.

The prevalence of examined warts according to medical officers in a representative sample of 9263 school children in the UK (NCDS) was 3.9% (95% confidence interval 3.5 to 4.3) and 4.9% (95% confidence interval 4.5 to 5.4) at the ages of 11 and 16 respectively.[176] Other surveys in the Northern Hemisphere quote prevalence rates of between 3% to 20% in children and teenagers,[177] the wide range possibly reflecting the conscientiousness with which warts were looked for. Further analysis of those ages with visible warts in the NCDS showed marked regional differences in wart prevalence with an increasing gradient of wart prevalence from the Southern to the northern regions at both 11 and 16 years of age.[178] In this study wart prevalence was also less in children born to parents with non-manual occupations, a finding echoed in the Lambeth study.[2] No sex differences in wart prevalence were noted in this study but children coming from smaller families had a lower prevalence of warts perhaps reflecting decreased opportunity for cross-infection. Visible warts were also twice as common in white Europeans when compared with other ethnic groups in the NCDS study. This study also suggested that over 90% of those children with warts at the age of 11 had cleared up by the age of 16.[176] Other studies have suggested two-year clearance rates of around 65%.[177,178] Although viral warts are often considered as a condition of childhood and adolescence the Lambeth study found that 3.5% of adults aged 25–34 years also had warts of which one-quarter were 'moderate to severe'.[2]

Appendix XI Prevalence of other infective skin disorders

The most common cutaneous bacterial infections in the UK include furunculosis (boils), impetigo, and folliculitis. Common viral infections other than warts include molluscum contagiosum, herpes simplex (cold sores) and herpes zoster (shingles). Fungal infections are usually described according to the site which they affect. The main forms include tinea corporis (affecting body skin), tinea capitis (affecting hair and sometimes referred to as ringworm) and onychomycosis (fungal infections of nails).

Prevalence rates for this category range from 4.6% to 9.3%.[2,3] These figures are to be viewed as a minimum, since most infective disorders are transient and might be missed in point prevalence surveys. As with any 'rag bag' category the prevalence rate will vary considerably with what is thrown into that bag and comparisons between surveys is difficult as different diseases have been included in the category. Cutaneous infections are also especially common in immunosuppressed individuals, such as those with AIDS[179] or transplant patients on immunosuppressive drugs and older surveys will underestimate the contribution of skin infections by such groups. Incidence data for cutaneous infective disorders are required in order to plan appropriate services but none are available for the UK. Morbidity statistics from general practice show that at least 4% of the population per year consult their GP for a skin infection other than warts.[7]

Bacterial impetigo and mollusca usually affect children, whereas boils and folliculitis peak in the 18 to 34 year age group. Herpes simplex shows a steady prevalence rate throughout the first four decades of life whilst new cases of herpes zoster peaks increase strikingly in later life.[5] In 1981/82 around 2.9 new episodes of herpes simplex infection (cold sore) and 3.7 new episodes of Herpes zoster (shingles) per 1000 people were recorded in general practice.[5] Fungal skin infections of the scalp typically occur in childhood and may form outbreaks in schools. Chronic fungal infection of the toe spaces (athletes' foot) is commonest in young adult life and this condition alone may affect as much as 3.9% of the population at any one time.[3] A recent survey of a representative sample of 9332 adults in the UK found that 2.8% of men and 2.6% of women suffered from fungal nail infections and this increased to 4.7% in those aged 55 and over.[118] Only 12% of those with nail infections had sought specialist medical advice and of those who had not sought help, 80% would have liked further treatment if they knew that effective treatment was available. This study estimated the incidence of fungal nail infection at 4.8 per 1000 per year. Fungal infection of the feet and toenails is more common in occupational groups such as miners and members of the armed forces, where it may affect 6.5% to 27% of the workforce.[180]

Appendix XII Benign tumours and vascular lesions

This category represents a heterogenous group of lesions such as moles, seborrhoeic warts, sebaceous cysts and pre-malignant lesions such as solar keratoses. From an operational point of view the common end-point of a consultation for a person with such a lesion is usually either to reassure and discharge, or perform minor surgery to remove/biopsy the lesion for discomfort or diagnostic reasons. Many benign vascular lesions occur on the skin but perhaps the most important lesions which purchasers need to be aware of are port wine stains because of their persistent nature and effective but expensive treatment.

The elasticity of this sub-category is considerable, since every person has some form of benign cutaneous lesion which may or may not cause them concern. Benign melanocytic lesions (moles) exemplify the difficulties in deciding what to include within this sub-category. Most white adults have between 40 and 60 moles on their body. Some moles can look very worrying to patients and many will seek medical advice to exclude malignancy. Some people may be very unhappy with the cosmetic appearance of their moles, whereas the majority of people are probably not bothered by their presence. Thus even for one common lesion there may be a range of concerns from none at all to cosmetic concerns or a wish to exclude malignancy. Purchasers are probably only concerned with the last category but the relative proportions of these categories are unstable. Small changes in the public's anxiety about moles, as has occurred in conjunction with media publicity directed at early diagnosis of skin cancer, or a small decrease in the threshold of what people regard as cosmetically unacceptable (as has occurred with the unrealistic media image of a blemishless skin), will have large implications for health services. Similar arguments apply to other benign tumours such as seborrhoeic warts, which are almost universal in later life.

Both the Lambeth and the NHANES study evaluated the prevalence of benign tumours which the examining physicians considered were worthy of medical attention.[2,3] Although 20.5% of the Lambeth study population were noted to have a tumour or vascular lesion of some sort, in only 7% of these was it considered 'moderate to severe'.[2] This corresponds to prevalence of 1.4% (95% confidence intervals 0.3% to 2.5%) in this adult population. In the NHANES study clinically significant benign tumours and precancerous lesions (excluding seborrhoeic keratoses) were noted in 5.1% of people.[3] The prevalence of benign tumours and precancerous lesions showed a striking increase with age from 2% in children to 13% in those aged 65–74 years.

It is possible that the threshold of what physicians might consider as worthy of medical attention might have changed considerably over the 20 years since these important surveys were conducted. During this time interest in the differential diagnosis of malignant melanoma has flourished and new concepts such as dysplastic naevus syndrome have emerged.

Solar keratoses deserve further mention in their own right because of their high prevalence and uncertainty regarding malignant potential. Solar keratoses are dysplastic epidermal lesions which occur in pale-skinned individuals who are chronically exposed to bright sunlight. Prevalence rates in the Northern hemisphere range from 11% to 25% with a striking increase in prevalence over the age of 65.[181] A recent study of 560 subjects aged 60 and over in South Wales reported a 23% prevalence (95% confidence interval 19.5% to 26.5%) of solar keratoses.[142] The incidence of new lesions after one year in this population was 88 newly affected persons per 100 person–years (95% confidence intervals 66–114 per 100 person–years). Very little is known about their natural history and role in carcinogenesis. Reported rates of malignant transformation have varied from fewer than 1 : 1000 to 20% but recent prospective studies suggest that this risk is likely to be less than 1% per year.[181] Around 10% to 27% of solar keratoses probably remit spontaneously.[142,182]

Port wine stains are rare vascular malformations composed of mature capillaries which are present at birth. Their presence can lead to considerable psychological disability if untreated. Unlike the more common strawberry haemangioma, spontaneous resolution does not occur and the affected area can become more prominent as the person becomes older. One previous study suggests an incidence rate of three per 1000 live births in the UK.[183] Similar rates have been shown in a Finnish study of 4346 consecutive live births who were examined by a dermatologist, where 0.23% (95% confidence intervals 0.09% to 0.37%) were born with a port wine stain.[184] Another study of 3345 Chinese infants born in Taiwan suggested 0.4% had a port wine stain, most of which occurred on visible areas of the head and neck.[185]

Appendix XIII Leg ulcers

The most common causes of leg ulceration in the UK are venous disease, arterial disease or a mixture of both. The distribution of different types of leg ulcer in earlier studies is venous ulcers 70–90%, arterial ulcers 5–15%, mixed venous/arterial 5–10% and other causes 1 to 15%.[186] In addition to a careful history and full examination various non-invasive techniques such as Doppler ultrasound testing which can be performed by trained nurses are used in assessing the relative contribution of venous versus arterial disease. The proportion of people with significant arterial ischaemia rises with age from 5% in patients under the age of 70 years to 31% over this age.[187]

Apart from pain,[188] discomfort and inconvenience, leg ulcers may become infected or develop superimposed contact dermatitis which requires further investigation with patch testing.[189] Recurrences of venous ulcers are high, with up to two-thirds of ulcers recurring within one year of discharge following intensive hospital inpatient admissions.[190]

Recurrence rates in the community have been studied less well but many ulcers remain unhealed for years. A recent study in Watford suggests that referral for specialist assessment of leg ulcers is a relatively late event (36% of 107 patients had their ulcer for over two years).[191] This delay was important as arterial disease was found to be the sole cause in 7% of cases and in four patients malignancies were found to be the cause of ulceration. Surveys suggest that district nurses spend between 25% and 65% of their time treating ulcers.[121] The UK cost of treating venous ulcers alone has been estimated as £400 to £600 million in 1992,[192,193] most of which is due to nursing costs.

Surveys have suggested that the prevalence of venous ulcers in the general population is around 0.1% to 2% of the population with a marked increase in rates with increasing age from 0.5% over 40 years to 2% in the over 80s.[121,187,194] Venous leg ulcers affect between 1% to 2% of people in their life time.[187,195]

The point prevalence of venous leg ulcers was 0.16% (95% confidence intervals 0.15 to 0.18) in a study of 270 800 Swedish people in a defined geographical area.[196] Prevalence rose markedly with age and over 85% of patients were older than 64 years. The median age was 78 years for women and 76 for men. Half of those with venous disease had onset before the age of 65 years and half had suffered from the ulcer for over one year. Venous ulcers were recurrent in 72% of cases. Duration of ulcer was more than one year in 54% of patients with venous ulcers and 44% with non-venous lesions. Dressing changes were painful in 31% of patients with venous ulcers and rest pain was reported by 28% of venous ulcer sufferers and by 29% of the others. The number of dressings per week for venous ulcers alone was 1100 per 100 000 population.

Another Swedish study of 5140 people in Gothenburg aged 65 years and above found that 2.15% (95% confidence intervals 1.73% to 2.57%) had a current leg ulcer.[197] Of these around one-third were found to have arterial disease/diabetes.

Morbidity data from general practice suggest leg ulcers are becoming more common, or at least that more people are seeking treatment. Some of these changes could be due to an increasingly ageing population but comparison of age-specific rates over the last 40 years shows increases in consultation rates within each age band (Table XIII.1).[5] In the decade 1981 to 1991 there was a 17.6% increase in those aged 75–84 and a 49.2% increase in people aged 85 and above[38] and with a 43% increase in the number of people over the age of 85 years projected by the year 2000 the prevalence of leg ulceration from venous and arterial disease is likely to increase.

Table XIII.1: Age-specific patient consulting rates for chronic ulcer of the skin 1955/56, 1971/72 and 1981/82[5]

Year	0–4	5–14	15–24	25–44	45–64	65–74	75+
1955/56		0.4		0.6		1.8	5.0
1971/72	0.1	0.1	0.5	0.4	2.0	4.8	9.1
1981/82	0.4	0.3	0.6	0.6	2.7	6.7	15.4

Rates per 1000 persons at risk

Appendix XIV Contact dermatitis and other eczemas

The terms dermatitis and eczema are synonymous and refer to a characteristic reaction pattern of the skin to a range of external and internal factors. In the UK the term dermatitis is usually used by the public and GPs to denote an exogenous process, such as contact dermatitis which may or may not be related to occupational exposure, whereas the term eczema refers to an endogenous disease such as atopic or seborrhoeic eczema.

This distinction is an important one for this sub-category as service requirements may differ. Contact dermatitis refers to either:

- irritant contact dermatitis (e.g. frequent exposure to mild irritant soaps seen in trained nurses or hairdressers)
- allergic contact dermatitis, where subjects develop a delayed type of allergic response to certain potentially sensitizing substances such as metals, perfumes, preservatives, or rubber compounds.

Although both mechanisms may occur simultaneously, distinction between the two requires further investigation by means of patch testing, a process whereby a standard battery of known allergens is applied in non-irritant concentrations on the subject's back and read 48 to 96 hours later. If the subject is found to be positive to a particular substance which is clinically relevant to that person's dermatitis, then complete avoidance of that substance offers the opportunity of a permanent cure.

Other eczemas in this section refer to any eczema that is not contact eczema or atopic eczema (Appendix VIII). Examples are seborrhoeic eczema, discoid eczema, asteatotic eczema, pompholyx eczema, varicose eczema, photosensitive eczema and lichen simplex. Detailed prevalence rates for the various endogenous eczemas are not available but the NHANES study suggested that around 1% of the population had clinically significant eczema that was not atopic eczema or contact dermatitis.[3] Seborrhoeic dermatitis was recorded separately in that study and clinically significant disease was found to affect 2.8% of the population, mainly adults. Asteatotic eczema may be especially common in old age, affecting around 29% of those in residential old people's homes.[197]

Contact dermatitis

Overall estimates of the prevalence and incidence of contact dermatitis in the general population are scarce, whereas a number of studies have looked at special groups such as occupations at high risk of disease. The Lambeth study found a bimodal distribution of eczema prevalence thought to warrant medical care with 7.3%, 3.4% 8.9% and 3.8% in age groups 15–24, 25–34, 35–54 and 55–74 years respectively.[2] This study did not distinguish between endogenous and contact eczema. Younger ages may also suffer from contact dermatitis and a recent study in Sweden found that 9% of school girls had nickel allergy, with highest rates in those with pierced ears.[198]

Significant contact dermatitis was noted in 1.4% of the population in the NHANES study and a further 4% was noted to have insignificant disease, with no overall sex differences.[2] Age-specific prevalence showed a similar bimodal distribution to the Lambeth study[3] probably corresponding to a peak of irritant dermatitis occurring in housewives in their 20s and occupational hand eczema in men and women in the 40 to 60 year age group. Coenraads has pointed out that age and sex are not risk factors for contact factors in themselves but that these characteristics are associated with exposure in occupational and household activities.[199] A recent study of an unselected population of Danish adults found that 15.2% were allergic to one or more substances when patch tested but the proportion with clinically relevant dermatitis was not clear.[200] Around half of those with irritant contact dermatitis and around one-third of those with allergic contact dermatitis were cured 4–7 years after attending a dermatology clinic.[201]

Occupational groups

Contact dermatitis is especially common in certain occupational groups such as the car, leather, metal, food, chemical and rubber industries and those frequently exposed to irritants such as hairdressers, nurses and nursing mothers. It has been estimated that eczema or contact dermatitis accounts for 85% to 98% of occupational skin disease.[202,203] Skin diseases are among the top three reasons for occupational diseases in Northern Europe and constitute 9% to 34% of all occupational disease. Despite differences in entry criteria for occupational skin disease in different European countries the incidence of occupational skin disease is of the same order of magnitude, with 0.5 to 0.7 cases per 1000 workers per year.

Hand eczema

A number of prevalence studies has specifically looked at hand eczema in adults and reported point prevalence rates of between 1.7% to 6.3% and 12-month period prevalences of 8.9% to 10.6%.[199,204] Although most of these studies have not distinguished between endogenous hand eczema and contact eczema the study of hand eczema *per se* is a useful concept since it is the form of eczema most frequently associated with work disability. In a study of 1992 adults in The Netherlands examined by a dermatologist, where hand/forearm eczema was seen in 6.2% of individuals, irritant factors were found to play a role in 73% of cases and contact allergy was detected in 30%.[205] A past history of atopic eczema is a strong risk factor for the development of subsequent irritant contact hand dermatitis.[204]

As with atopic eczema, consideration needs to be given to clinically significant disease. In the NHANES study for instance, only about one-quarter of all cases of contact dermatitis or seborrhoeic dermatitis were considered as significant by the examining dermatologist.[3]

Appendix XV Prevalence of skin diseases excluded from the main disease sub-categories

Although there are rational arguments for considering nine dermatological sub-categories on the basis that they constitute the bulk of skin disorders in the population and in primary care, the remaining 30% or so of disorders which do not fit neatly into the above system still represent a large sector of the UK population (around 3.9 million people). Because of the difficulties in making generalizations about this heterogenous group, there will be a temptation to ignore it or accord it a low status in purchasing plans. Whilst it is beyond the scope of this review to mention the 1000 or so remaining disorders contained in this group, some deserve special mention because of their service implications.

Included within this group are genetic disorders such as epidermolysis bullosa, a condition characterised by increased skin fragility. Although rare (one in every 50 000 live births) the consequences of more severe forms of this disease are devastating and diagnosis requires special expertise usually at specialized centres.

Urticaria (hives) is one of the 20 most common skin diseases affecting 1% to 5% of the general population. Vitiligo (loss of pigment) is another progressive and potentially disfiguring disorder affecting 0.5% of the US population.[3] Infestations with pediculosis capitis (nits) is also common in modern schools, although no recent incidence/prevalence estimates are available. Scabies outbreaks may also occur in old people's homes, nurseries and other institutions but incidence figures are lacking. Disorders of the hair and nails that could have benefited from medical help were found to affect 1.4% and 1.8% of adults respectively in the Lambeth study.[2] Also included in this group are blistering disorders such as pemphigus, which can be fatal if untreated. Cutaneous T-cell lymphoma and other skin lymphomas, whilst rare when compared to other skin diseases may require proportionately more services because of the unique treatments involved. Drug reactions which manifest themselves in the skin are also very common and most mild reactions are probably not reported. It has been estimated that around 1% to 8% of people taking antibiotics develop a skin reaction.[206] Of more concern are the rare but potentially fatal skin reactions characterized by skin necrosis (Stevens-Johnson syndrome). A recent West German register has estimated that at least 1.7 per million inhabitants per year develop such a reaction, with higher rates in the Asian population.[207]

There is also a temptation to consider the main nine sub-categories as mutually exclusive categories, whereas in reality many individuals have more than one skin disease, simply because skin disorders are so common and some skin diseases such as skin cancer and solar keratoses are related. The NHANES study found that 6% of the population had more than one significant skin pathology and 3% had more than two significant skin pathologies.[3] This implies that surveys and routine data which measure disease frequency according to persons consulting without regard to the total number of new skin problems will considerably underestimate the service requirements for dermatology.

Appendix XVI Strength of recommendations

Evidence

A   There is good evidence to support the use of the procedure
B   There is fair evidence to support the use of the procedure
C   There is poor evidence to support the use of the procedure
D   There is fair evidence to support the rejection of the use of the procedure
E   There is good evidence to support the rejection of the use of the procedure.

Quality of evidence

I   Evidence obtained from at least one properly designed, randomized control trial
II-i   Evidence obtained from well designed controlled trials without randomization
II-ii   Evidence obtained from well designed cohort or case control analytic studies, preferably from more than one centre or research group
II-iii   Evidence obtained from multiple time series with or without the intervention. Dramatic results in uncontrolled experiments (such as the results of the introduction of penicillin treatment in the 1940s) could also be regarded as this type of evidence
III   Opinions of respected authorities based on clinical experience, descriptive studies, or reports of expert committees
IV   Evidence inadequate owing to problems of methodology (e.g. sample size, or length or comprehensiveness of follow-up or conflicts in evidence).

References

1 Ryan TJ. Disability in Dermatology. *Br J Hosp Med* 1991; **46**: 33–6.
2 Rea JN, Newhouse ML, Halil T. Skin disease in Lambeth: a community study of prevalence and use of medical care. *Brit J Prev Soc Med* 1976; **30**: 107–14.
3 Johnson M-LT. *Skin conditions and related need for medical care among persons 1–74 years, United States, 1971–1974.* Vital and Health Statistics: Series 11, No. 212. DHEW publication No. (PHS) 79–1660. US Department of Health, Education and Welfare, National Center for Health Statistics 1978: 1–72.
4 *The Health of the Nation Key Area Handbook; Cancers.* London: Department of Health, 1993.
5 Royal College of General Practitioners. *Morbidity Statistics from General Practice.* Third National Study 1981–82. London: HMSO, 1986.
6 Williams HC. Is the prevalence of atopic dermatitis increasing? *Clin Exp Dermatol* 1992; **17**: 385–91.
7 Royal College of General Practitioners. *Morbidity Statistics from General Practice.* Fourth National Study 1991–92. London: HMSO, 1995.
8 Government Statistical Service. *Outpatients and ward attenders England – Financial Year 1989/1990.* London: HMSO, 1993.
9 Office of Population Census and Surveys. *Hospital Inpatient Enquiry 1979–85.* London: HMSO, 1989.
10 Office of Population Censuses and Surveys. *1992 Mortality Statistics.* London: HMSO, 1994.
11 Department of Social Security. *Social Security Statistics 1994.* London: HMSO, 1994.
12 Health and Safety Commission. *Annual Report 1991/1992.* London: HMSO, 1992.
13 Champion RH, Burton JL, Ebling FJG *Textbook of Dermatology.* 5th edn. Oxford: Blackwell Scientific Publications, 1992.
14 Stevens A, Raftery J. Introduction. In *Health Care Needs Assessment* (eds A Stevens, J Raftery) Oxford: Radcliffe Medical Press, 1994.
15 National Health Service Management Executive. *Local Voices.* London: Department of Health, 1992.
16 Burton JL. The logic of dermatological diagnosis. *Clin Exp Dermatol* 1981; **6**: 1–21.
17 *1975 International Classification of Diseases,* 9th Revision. Geneva: WHO, 1977.
18 Alexander S, Shrank AB. International Coding Index for Dermatology. Oxford: Blackwell Scientific Publications, 1978.
19 *International Statistical Classification of Diseases and Related Health Problems,* 10th Revision. Geneva: WHO, 1992.
20 *International Statistical Classification of Diseases and Health Related Problems,* 10th Revision. Volume 2. Geneva: WHO, 1993.
21 *The BAD diagnostic index issue 1.* London: British Association of Dermatology, 1994.
22 Department of Health. *Read Codes and the terms projects: a brief guide.* Loughborough: NHS Centre for Coding and Classification, 1994.
23 Hardwick N, Saxe N. Patterns of dermatology referrals in a general hospital. *Br J Dermatol* 1986; **115**: 167–76.
24 Bradlow J *et al.* Patterns of referral: a study of out patient clinic referrals from general practice in the Oxford Region. HSRU: Oxford University, May 1992.
25 Kelly DR, Murray TS. Twenty years of vocational training in the West of Scotland. *Br Med J* 1991; **302**: 28–30.
26 Horn R. The pattern of skin disease in general practice. *Dermatology in Practice* 1986; December Issue: 14–19.
27 Morrell DC. Symptom interpretation in General Practice. *J Roy Coll Gen Pract* 1972; **22**: 297.
28 Simpson NB, Allen BR, Douglas WS *et al.* Quality in the dermatological contract. *J Roy Coll Phys* 1995; **29**: 25–30.

29 *Everyday Health Care: a consumer study of self-medication in Great Britain.* London: The British Market Research Bureau Ltd, 1987.

30 Wadsworth MEJ, Butterfield WJH, Blaney R. *Without Prescription.* London: Office of Health Economics, 1968.

31 Dunnell K, Cartwright A. *Medicine takers, prescribers and hoarders.* Report of the Institute of Social Studies in Medical Care. London: Routledge and Kegan Paul, 1972.

32 Meding B. Normal standards for dermatological health screening at places at work. *Contact Dermatitis* 1992; **27**: 269–70.

33 Lomholt, G. Prevalence of skin diseases in a population. *Danish Medical Bulletin*, 1964; **11**: 1–8.

34 Hellgren L. *An epidemiological survey of skin diseases, tattooing and rheumatic diseases.* Stockholm: Almqvist and Wiksell, 1967.

35 Weismann K, Krakauer R, Wanscher B. Prevalence of skin diseases in old age. *Acta Derm Venereol (Stockh.)* 1980; **60**: 352–3.

36 Logan WPD, Cushion WW. *Morbidity Statistics from General Practice* Vol.1 London: HMSO, 1958.

37 Royal College of General Practitioners. *Morbidity Statistics from General Practice. Second National Study 1971–72.* Studies on Medical and Population Subjects No. 26. London: HMSO, 1974.

38 *On the State of the Public Health 1993.* London: HMSO, 1994.

39 Office of Population Censuses and Surveys. *1991 Mortality Statistics.* London: HMSO, 1993.

40 Breeze E, Maidment A, Bennett N *et al. Health Survey for England 1992.* OPCS. London: HMSO, 1994.

41 Cancer Research Campaign. *Malignant Melanoma Factsheet 1994.* London: CRC Promotions Ltd, 1994.

42 Carmichael AJ. Achieving an accessible dermatology service. *Dermatology in Practice* 1995; **Sept/Oct**: 13–16.

43 Ferguson JA, Goldacre MJ, Newton JN *et al.* An epidemiological profile of in-patient workload in dermatology. *Clin Exp Dermatol* 1992; **17**: 407–12.

44 Williams HC. Extended role of pharmacists in dermatology (editorial). *J Clin Pharm Ther* 1996; **20**:307–12.

45 Funnell C. Importance of patient self-help groups – a British Perspective. *Retinoids Today and Tomorrow* 1995; **41**: 6–8.

46 Steele K. Primary dermatological care in general practice. *J Roy Coll Gen Prac* 1984; **34**: 22–4.

47 Ryan T. *Dermatology – a service under threat.* London: British Association of Dermatology, 1993.

48 Harlow ED, Burton JL. What do general practitioners want from a dermatology department? *Br J Dermatol* 1996; **134**: 313–18.

49 Hay R J. Undergraduate teaching in dermatology and general practice. *Br J Dermatol* 1993; **129**: 356.

50 Mitchell T. A chronic skin disease management clinic in primary care? *Newsletter of the Primary Care Dermatology Society* 1994; **2**: 3.

51 Stevenson C, Horne G, Charles-Holmes S *et al.* Dermatology outpatients in the West Midlands: their nature and management. *Health Trends* 1991; **23**: 162–5.

52 Department of Health. *Personnel and social services statistics for England.* 1994 edn. London: HMSO, 1994.

53 Lawrence CM. Mohs surgery of basal cell carcinoma – a critical review. *Brit J Plastic Surgery* 1993; **46**: 599–606.

54 Benton EC, Hunter JAA. The dermatology out-patient service: a study of out-patient referrals in a Scottish population. *Br J Dermatol* 1984; **110**: 195–201.

55 Sladden MJ, Graham-Brown RAC. How many referrals to dermatology outpatients are really necessary? *J Roy Soc Med* 1989; **82**: 437–8.

56 Williams BT, Nicholl JP. Patient characteristics and clinical caseload of short stay independent hospitals in England and Wales, 1992–3. *Br Med J* 1994; **308**: 1699–701.

57 Griffin T, Rose P. *Regional Trends*. 1992 edn. London: HMSO, 1992.

58 Roland M, Morris R. Are referrals by general practitioners influenced by the availability of consultants? *Br Med J* 1988; **297**: 599–600.

59 Harris DWS, Benton EC, Hunter JAA. Dermatological audit: fact or friction? *Br J Dermatol* 1990; **123** (Suppl. 37): 20–1.

60 Whitehead SM, Wroughton MA. Education campaign on early detection of malignant melanoma. *Br Med J* 1988; **297**: 620–1.

61 Graham-Brown RAC, Osborne JE, London SM *et al*. The effect of a public education campaign for early diagnosis of malignant melanoma on workload and outcome – the Leicester experience. *Br J Dermatol* 1988; **119** (Suppl. 33): 23–4.

62 Williams HC, Smith D, du Vivier AWP. Evaluation of public education campaigns in cutaneous melanoma: the King's College Hospital experience. *Br J Dermatol* 1990; **123**: 85–92.

63 Jobling R. With and without professional nurses – the case for dermatology. In *Readings in the Society of Nursing* (eds R Dingwall, J McIntosh). Edinburgh: Churchill Livingstone, 1978, 181–95.

64 Ruane-Morris, Lawton S, Thompson G. *Nursing the Dermatology Patient*. Oxford: Blackwell Scientific Publications, 1996. (In Press.)

65 Venables J. Management of children with atopic eczema in the community. *Dermatology in Practice* 1995; **3**: S1–4.

66 Department of Health. *Hospital Episode Statistics. Volume 1*. Finished consultant episodes by diagnosis, operation and speciality. England: Financial Year 1993–4. London: HMSO, 1995.

67 Office of Health Economics. *Skin Disorders*. London: Office of Health Economics Publication No. 46, 1973, 1–32.

68 Editorial. Dermatologists incur lower drug costs. *Dermatology in Practice* 1993; **1**: 5.

69 Breeze E, Trevor G, Wilmot A. *The 1989 General Household Survey*. London: HMSO, 1991.

70 Martin J, Meltzer H, Elliot D. *The prevalence of disability among adults*. London: HMSO, 1988.

71 Herd RM, Tidman MJ, Hunter JAA *et al*. The economic burden of atopic eczema: a community and hospital-based assessment. *Br J Dermatol* 1994; **131** (Suppl. 44): 34.

72 Chalmers I, Enkin M, Kierse M (eds). *Effective care in pregnancy and childbirth*. Oxford: Oxford University Press, 1989.

73 Hay RJ, Castanon RE, Hernandez *et al*. Wastage of family income on skin disease in Mexico. *Br Med J* 1994; **309**: 848.

74 Rawlins MD. Extending the role of the community pharmacist. *Br Med J* 1991; **302**: 427–8.

75 Doherty V, MacKie RM. Experience of a public education programme on early detection of cutaneous malignant melanoma. *Br Med J* 1988; **297**: 388–94.

76 Reynolds GA, Chitnis JG, Roland MO. General practitioners outpatient referrals: do good doctors refer more patients to hospital? *Br Med J* 1991; **302**: 1250–2.

77 O'Cathain A, Brazier JE, Milner PC *et al*. Cost effectiveness of minor surgery in general practice: a prospective comparison with hospital practice. *Br J Gen Practice* 1992; **42**: 13–17.

78 Cox N, Wagstaff R, Popple A. Using clinicopathological analysis of general practitioner skin surgery to determine educational requirements and guidelines. *Br Med J* 1992; **304**: 93–6.

79 Stern RS, Boudreux C, Arndt KA. Diagnostic accuracy and appropriateness of care for seborrhoeic keratoses. A pilot study of an approach to quality assurance for cutaneous surgery. *JAMA* 1991; **265**: 74–7.

80 Basarab T, Munn SE, Russell Jones R. Diagnostic accuracy and appropriateness of general practitioner referrals to a dermatology outpatient clinic. *Br J Dermatol* 1996; **135**: 70–3.

81 Bedlow AJ, Melia J, Moss SM *et al.* Impact of skin cancer education on general practitioner's diagnostic skills. *Br J Dermatol* 1995; **133 (Suppl. 45)**: 29.

82 Plamping D, Gordon P. *Commissioning good skin care for a community.* Workshop Report, December 1992, London: King's Fund Centre.

83 Schofield J. Dermatological workload. Abstract in: *Medicine for Managers Seminar on Dermatology.* London: Institute of Health Services Management, May 1994.

84 Forsyth G, Logan R. *Gateway or dividing line?* Oxford: Oxford University Press, 1970.

85 Roland MO, Green CA, Roberts SOB. Should general practitioners refer more patients to hospital? *J Roy Soc Med* 1991; **848**: 403–4.

86 Heagerty AHM, Smith AG, English J. Dermatology outreach clinics – are they really what patients want? *Br J Dermatol* 1995; **133 (Suppl. 45)**: 28.

87 Falanga V, Schachner LA, Rae V *et al.* Dermatologic consultations in the hospital setting. *Arch Dermatol* 1994; **130**: 1022–5.

88 Williams HC, Smith D, du Vivier A. Melanoma: differences observed by general surgeons and dermatologists. *Int J Dermatol* 1991; **30**: 257–61.

89 Glover MT, Taylor C, Leigh IM. The contribution of the paediatric home care team to the management of atopic eczema in childhood. *Br J Dermatol* 1994; **131 (Suppl. 44)**: 25.

90 Bailey JJ, Black ME, Wilkin D. Specialist outreach clinics in general practice. *Br Med J* 1994; **308**: 1083–6.

91 Petersen LJ, Kristensen JK. Selection of patients for psoriasis clinical trials: a survey of the recent dermatological literature. *J Dermatol Treat* 1992; **3**: 171–6.

92 Eady EA. Topical antibiotics for the treatment of acne. *J Dermatol Treat* 1990; **1**: 215–26.

93 Williams HC, Seed P. Inadequate size of 'negative' clinical trials in dermatology. *Br J Dermatol* 1993; **128**: 317–26.

94 Finlay AY, Khan GK. Dermatology Life Quality Index (DLQI): a simple practical measure for routine clinical use. *Clin Exp Dermatol* 1994; **19**: 210–16.

95 Bilsland DJ, Rhodes LE, Zaki I *et al.* PUVA and methotrexate therapy of psoriasis: how closely do dermatology departments follow treatment guidelines? *Br J Dermatol* 1994; **131**: 220–5.

96 Simpson NB. Social and economic aspects of acne and the cost-effectiveness of isotretinoin. *J Dermatol Treat* 1993; **4 (Suppl. 2)**: S6–S9.

97 Cunliffe WJ, Gray JA, MacDonald Hull *et al.* Cost effectiveness of isotretinoin. *J Dermatol Treat* 1991; **1**: 285–8.

98 Layton AM, Knaggs H, Taylor J *et al.* Isotretinoin for acne vulgaris – 10 years later: a safe and successful treatment. *Br J Dermatol* 1993; **129**: 292–6.

99 Goodfield MJD, Andrew L, Evans EGV. Short term treatment of dermatophyte onychomycosis with terbinafine. *Br Med J* 1992; **304**: 1151–4.

100 Levell NJ, Shuster S, Munro CS *et al.* Remission of ordinary psoriasis following a short clearance course of cyclosporin. *Acta Dermato Venereol* 1995; **65**: 65–9.

101 Cork M. Economic considerations in the treatment of psoriasis. *Dermatology in Practice* 1993; **1**: 16–20.

102 Hughes BR, Wetton NM, Martin M *et al.* Health education about skin cancer: starting where children are at. *Br J Dermatol* 1993; **129 (Suppl. 42)**: 17.

103 Jarrett P, McLelland J. Do mothers 'slip, slap' in response to the sun in Sunderland? *Br J Dermatol* 1992; **127 (Suppl. 40)**: 22.

104 Mackie R. *Skin cancer co-ordinators newsletter.* UK Skin Cancer Working Party. London: British Association of Dermatology, November 1994. Issue 1.

105 Harvey I. *Prevention of skin cancer: a review of available strategies.* Bristol: Health Care Evaluation Unit, April 1995.

106 Healy E, Simpson N. Acne vulgaris. *Br Med J* 1994; **308**: 831–3.

107 Stern R S. The prevalence of acne on the basis of physical examination. *J Am Acad Dermatol* 1992; **26**: 931–5.

108 Arshad SH, Matthews S, Gant C *et al.* Effect of allergen avoidance on development of allergic disorders in infancy. *Lancet* 1992; **339**: 1493–97.

109 Long CC, Funnell CM, Collard R *et al.* What do members of the National Eczema Society really want? *Clin Exp Dermatol* 1993; **18**: 516–22.

110 Herd RM. Atopic eczema in the community: morbidity and cost: Proceedings of the fourth meeting of the British Epidermo-Epidemiology Society. *Br J Dermatol* 1994; **131**: 909.

111 Bunney MH, Nolan WN Williams DA. An assessment of methods of treating viral warts by comparative treatment trials based on a standard design. *Br J Dermatol* 1976; **94**: 667–79.

112 Berth-Jones J, Bourke J, Eglitis II *et al.* Value of a second freeze-thaw cycle in cryotherapy of common warts. *Br J Dermatol* 1994; **131**: 883–6.

113 Keefe M, Dick DC. Dermatologists should not be concerned in routine treatment of warts. *Br Med J* 1988; **296**: 177–9.

114 Thomson D, Powell R, Warin AP. Healing rates of venous leg ulcers in the community using the 'Charing Cross' four-layered system. *Br J Dermatol* 1995; **133 (Suppl. 45)**: 32

115 Moffatt CJ, Franks PJ, Oldroyd M *et al.* Community clinics for leg ulcers and impact on healing. *Br Med J* 1992; **305**: 1389–92.

116 Bosanquet N. Community leg ulcer clinics: cost-effectiveness. *Health Trends* 1993; **25**: 146–8.

117 Taplin D, Porcelain SL, Meinking TL *et al.* Community control of scabies: a model based on use of permethrin cream. *Lancet* 1991; **337**: 1016–18.

118 Roberts DT. Prevalence of dermatophyte onychomycosis in the United Kingdom: results of an omnibus survey. *Br J Dermatol* 1992; **126 (Suppl. 39)**: 23–7.

119 Acheson ED. Mortality form cutaneous malignant melanoma. *Health Trends* 1986; **18**: 73.

120 Coggan D, Inskip H. Is there an epidemic of cancer? *Br Med J* 1994; **308**: 705–8.

121 Bosanquet N. *Gravitational ulcers: the problem, what we know and what we need to know.* Department of Health. London: HMSO, November 1989.

122 Moss G. *STEPWISE.* Frimley: Sandoz Pharmaceuticals Ltd, 1994.

123 Monk B. Outreach clinics in dermatology – less heat, more light. *Dermatology in Practice* 1995; **3**: 9–13.

124 Burge SM. Dermatology clinics in the community. *Br J Dermatol* 1995; **133 (Suppl. 45)**: 29.

125 Coulter A. Shifting the balance from secondary to primary care. *Br Med J* 1995; **311**: 1447–8.

126 Sweeney B. The referral system. *Br Med J* 1994; **309**: 1180–1.

127 Editorial. Way forward for outreach clinics. *Medical Interface*, October 1995; 45–6.

128 McGill J. Outreach services can boost revenue and quality. *Medical Interface*, October 1995; 47.

129 Harris DWS, Parker A, Wills A *et al.* Teledermatology – The modern alternative to the GP referral letter for dermatological conditions: a six month appraisal. *Br J Dermatol* 1995; **133 (Suppl. 45)**: 28.

130 A picture of hope. *Hospital Doctor.* November 1994; 2.

131 MRC. *Developing high quality proposals in health services research.* London: Medical Research Council, 1994.

132 Perednia DA. Teledermatology in Oregon – report of the ongoing NLM/HPCC Teledermatology Project. *Skin Research and Technology* 1995; **1**: 156.

133 British Photodermatology Group Guidelines for PUVA. *Br J Dermatol* 194; **130**: 246–55.

134 Pitcher R, Gould DJ, Bowers DW. An analysis of the effect of general practice minor surgery clinics on the workload of a district general hospital pathology and dermatology department. *Br J Dermatol* 1991; **125 (Suppl. 38)**: 93.

135 Lowy A, Brazier J, Fall M *et al.* Minor surgery by general practitioners under the 1990 contract: effect on the hospital workload. *Br Med J* 1993; **307**: 413–7.

136 Mechanic D. Dilemmas in rationing health care services: the case for implicit rationing. *Br Med J* 1995; **310**: 1655–9.

137 Frankel S. Health needs, health-care requirements, and the myth of infinite demand *Lancet* 1991; **337**: 1588–90.

138 Dicker A, Armstrong D. Patient's views of priority setting in health care: an interview survey in one practice. *Br Med J* 1995; **311**: 1137–8.

139 Calnan K. On the state of the public health. *Health Trends* 1994; **26**: 35.

140 Ryan TJ. Healthy skin for all. *Int J Dermatol* 1994; **33**: 829–35.

141 Office of Population Censuses and Surveys. *1989 Cancer Statistics: registrations.* London: HMSO, 1994.

142 Harvey I. *Skin cancer in South Wales.* Proceedings of the 15th Commonwealth Universities Congress, Swansea, 1993. London: Association of Commonwealth Universities, 1994.

143 Malignant melanoma of the skin. *Drugs and Therapeutic Bulletin* 1998; **26**: 73–5.

144 Sober AJ, Lew RA, Koh HK *et al.* Epidemiology of cutaneous melanoma. *Dermatologic Clinics* 1991; **9**: 617–29.

145 Sharp L, Black RJ, Harkness EF. *Cancer registration statistics Scotland, 1981–1990.* Edinburgh: Common Services Agency, 1993.

146 Elwood JM, Gallagher RP, Hill GB *et al.* Cutaneous melanoma in relation to intermittent and constant sun exposure: the Western Canada Melanoma Study. *Int J Cancer* 1985; **35**: 427–33.

147 Marks R, Whiteman D. Sunburn and melanoma: how strong is the evidence? *Br Med J* 1994; **308**: 75–6.

148 Beadle PC, Bullock D, Bedford G *et al.* Accuracy of skin cancer incidence data in the United Kingdom. *Clin Exp Dermatol* 1983; **7**: 255–60.

149 Moan J, Dahlback A, Henriksen T *et al.* Biological amplification factor for sunlight induced non-melanoma skin cancer at high latitudes. *Cancer Research* 1989; **49**: 5207–12.

150 Schreiber MM, Moon TE, Fox SH *et al.* The risk of developing subsequent non-melanoma skin cancer. *J Am Acad Dermatol* 1990; **23**: 1114–8.

151 Rademaker M, Garioch JJ, Simpson NB. Acne in schoolchildren: no longer a concern for dermatologists. *Br Med J* 1989; **298**: 1217–20.

152 Lucky AW, Biro FM, Huster GA *et al.* Acne vulgaris in early adolescent boys. *Arch Dermatol* 1991; **127**: 210–16.

153 Hughes BR. Counting the real cost of acne. *Dermatology in Practice* 1994; **2**: 3–5

154 Jowett S, Ryan T. Skin diseases and handicap: an analysis of the impact of skin conditions. *Soc Sci Med* 1985; **20**: 425–9.

155 Motley RJ, Finlay AY. Practical use of disability index in the routine management of acne. *Clin Exp Dermatol* 1992; **17**: 1–3.

156 Cunliffe WJ. Unemployment and acne. *Br J Dermatol* 1986; **115**: 86.

157 Schultz-Larsen F, Holm NV, Henningsen K. Atopic dermatitis. A genetic-epidemiological study in a population-based twin sample. *J Am Acad Dermatol* 1986; **15**: 487–94.

158 Williams HC. On the definition and epidemiology of atopic dermatitis. *Dermatologic Clinics* 1995; **13**: 649–57.

159 Rystedt I. Hand eczema and long-term prognosis in atopic dermatitis. *Acta Derm Venereol* (Stockholm) 1985; **17 (Suppl. 1)**: 9–59.

160 Kay J, Gawkrodger DJ, Mortimer MJ *et al.* The prevalence of childhood atopic eczema in a general population. *J Am Acad Dermatol* 1994; **30**: 35–9.

161 Golding J, Peters TJ. The epidemiology of childhood eczema. *Paed Perinatal Epidemiol* 1987; **1**: 67–9.

162 Schmied C, Saurat J-H. Epidemiology of atopic eczema. In *Handbook of atopic eczema* (eds T Ruzicka, J Ring, B Pryzbilla). London: Springer-Verlag, 1991, 9.

163 Williams HC, Strachan DP, Hay RJ. Childhood eczema: disease of the advantaged? *Br Med J* 1994; **308**: 1132–5.

164 Williams HC, Pembroke AC, Forsdyke H *et al.* London-born black Caribbean children arc at increased risk of atopic dermatitis. *J Am Acad Dermatol* 1995; **32**: 212–17.

165 Williams HC, Burney PGJ, Hay RJ *et al.* The UK Working Party's Diagnostic Criteria for Atopic Dermatitis I: Derivation of a minimum set of discriminators for atopic dermatitis. *Br J Dermatol* 1994; **131**: 383–96.

166 Taylor B, Wadsworth J, Wadsworth M *et al.* Changes in the reported prevalence of childhood eczema since the 1939–45 war. *Lancet* 1984; **ii**: 1255–7.

167 Neame RL, Berth-Jones J, Kurinczuk JJ *et al.* Prevalence of atopic dermatitis in Leicester: a study of methodology and examination of possible ethnic variation. *Br J Dermatol* 1995; **132**: 772–7.

168 David LR, Garralda ME, David TJ. Psychosocial adjustment in preschool children with atopic eczema. *Arch Dis Child* 1993; **69**: 670–6.

169 Henseler T, Christophers E. Psoriasis of early and late onset: characterisation of two types of psoriasis vulgaris. *J Am Acad Dermatol* 1985; **14**: 450–6.

170 Williams HC. Smoking and psoriasis. *Br Med J* 1994; **308**: 428–9.

171 Kidd CB, Meenan JC. A dermatological survey of long stay mental patients. *Br J Dermatol* 1961; **73**: 129–33.

172 Brandrup F, Green A. The prevalence of psoriasis in Denmark. *Acta Derm Venereol* 1981; **61**: 344–6.

173 Williams HC, Strachan DP. Psoriasis and eczema are not mutually exclusive diseases. *Dermatology* 1994; **189**: 238–40.

174 Farber EM. Epidemiology: Natural history and genetics. In *Psoriasis*. 2nd edn. (eds HH Roenigk, HI Maibach). New York: Marcel Dekker Inc., 1991, 209–58.

175 Lipscombe S. Galloping psoriasis. *Dermatology in Practice*. November 1993; 8–9.

176 Williams HC, Pottier A, Strachan D. The descriptive epidemiology of warts in British schoolchildren. *Br J Dermatol* 1993; **128**: 504–11.

177 Van der Werf E, Lent T. Een onderzoek naar het vóókomen en het verloop van wratten bij schoolkindren. *Ned Tijdschr Geneeskd* 1959; **103**: 1204–8.

178 Massing AM, Epstein WL. Natural history of warts. *Arch Dermatol* 1963; **87**: 306–10.

179 Stern RS. Epidemiology of skin disease in HIV infection. *J Invest Dermatol* 1994; **102**: 34S–37S.

180 Williams HC. The epidemiology of onychomycosis in Britain. *Br J Dermatol* 1993; **129**: 101–9.

181 Frost CA, Green AC. Epidemiology of solar keratoses. *Br J Dermatol* 1994; **131**: 455–64.

182 Marks R, Foley P, Goodman G *et al.* Spontaneous remission of solar keratoses: the case for conservative management. *Br J Dermatol* 1986; **115**: 649–55.

183 Jacobs AH, Walton RG. The incidence of birthmarks in the neonate. *Pediatrics* 1976; **58**: 218–22.

184 Karvonen S-L, Vaajalahti P, Marenk M *et al.* Birthmarks in 4346 Finnish Newborns. *Acta Derm Venereol* 1992; **72**: 55–7.

185 Tsai F-J, Tsai C-H. Birthmarks and congenital skin lesions in Chinese newborns. *J Formos Med Assoc* 1993; **92**: 838–41.

186 Andersson E, Hansson C, Swanbeck G. Leg and foot ulcer prevalence and investigation of the peripheral arterial and venous circulation in a randomised elderly population. *Acta Derm Venereol* 1993; **73**: 57–61.

187 Baker SR, Stacey MC, Jopp McKay AG *et al.* Epidemiology of chronic venous ulcers. *Br J Surgery* 1991; **78**: 864–7.

188 Taylor G, Goodfield MJD, O'Neill S. Pain associated with venous leg ulceration. *Br J Dermatol* 1995; **133 (Suppl. 45)**: 33.

189 Baldursson B, Sigurgeisson B, Lindelöf B. Leg ulcers and squamous cell carcinoma. *Acta Derm Venereol* 1993; **73**: 171–4.

190 Monk BE, Sarkany I. Outcome of treatment of venous stasis ulcers. *Clin Exp Dermatol* 1982; **7**: 397–400.

191 Schofield JK, Tatnall FM. Leg ulcers in a district general hospital: duration, diagnosis and outcome. *Br J Dermatol* 1995; **133 (Suppl. 45)**: 33.

192 Freak L, McCollum CN. The effective management of venous ulceration. *Vasc Med Rev* 1992; **3**: 53–62.

193 Local applications to wounds – II dressings for wounds and ulcers. *Drugs Ther Bull* 1991; **29**: 98.

194 Cornwall JV, Dore CJ, Lewis JD. Leg ulcers; epidemiology and aetiology. *Br J Dermatol* 1986; **73**: 693–6.

195 Gilliland EL, Wolfe JHN. Leg Ulcers. *Br Med J* 1991; **303**: 776–9.

196 Nelzen O. Venous and non-venous leg ulcers: clinical history and appearance in a population study. *Br J Surg* 1994; **8**: 182–7.

197 Weismann K, Krakauer R, Wanscher B. Prevalence of skin diseases in old age. *Acta Dermato Venereol* 1980; **60**: 352–3.

198 Larsson-Stymne B, Widström L. Ear piercing – a cause of nickel allergy in schoolgirls. *Contact Dermatitis* 1985; **13**: 289–93.

199 Smit J, Coenraads PJ. Epidemiology of contact dermatitis. In *Epidemiology of clinical allergy* (ed. ML Burr). Monogr. Allergy. Basel: Karger, 1993, **31**: 29–48.

200 Nielsen NH, Menné T. Allergic contact sensitisation in an unselected Danish Population. *Acta Derm Venereol* 1992; **72**: 456–60.

201 Driessen LHHM, Coenraads PJ, Groothoff JW *et al.* A group of eczema patients: five years later. *Tijdschr Soc Geneesk* 1982; **60**: 41–5.

202 Mathias CGT. The cost of occupational disease. *Arch Dermatol* 1985; **121**: 332–4.

203 Emmet EA. The skin and occupational disease. *Arch Environ Health* 1984; **39**: 144–9.

204 Meding BE, Swanbeck G. Prevalence of hand eczema in an industrial city. *Br J Dermatol* 1987; **116**: 627–34.

205 Lantinga H, Nater, Coenraads PJ. Prevalence, incidence and course of eczema on the hands and forearms in a sample of the general population. *Contact Derm* 1984; **10**: 135–139.

206 Hoigné R, Schlumberger HP, Vervloet D *et al.* Epidemiology of allergic drug reactions. In *Epidemiology of clinical allergy* (ed. ML Burr). Monogr. Allergy. Basel: Karger, 1993, **31**: 147–70.

207 Rzany B, Mockenhaupt M, Holländer N *et al.* Incidence of Stevens-Johnson syndrome (SJS) and toxic epidermal necrolysis (TEN) in West Germany among different ethnic groups. *J Invest Dermatol* 1994; **102(4)**: 619.

6 Breast Cancer

P Dey, E Twelves, CBJ Woodman

1 Summary

Breast cancer is the most common cause of death from cancer in women in the UK.
Effective interventions exist:

- population-based breast cancer screening using mammography has been shown to reduce mortality in women aged 50–69 by 25–30%
- breast conservation therapy with post-operative radiotherapy is as effective as mastectomy in prolonging disease-free and overall survival in women with early breast cancer
- adjuvant therapies improve overall survival in women with early breast cancer. After ten years of follow-up adjuvant therapy will have:
  a) prevented ten deaths for every 100 women under the age of 50 treated with chemotherapy
  b) prevented 11 deaths for every 100 women under the age of 50 treated with ovarian ablation
  c) prevented eight deaths for every 100 women over the age of 50 treated with tamoxifen.

Ineffective interventions exist:

- there is no evidence to support the use of routine investigations to detect asymptomatic metastases in the follow-up of women with breast cancer.

The National Health Service Breast Screening Programme (NHSBSP) provides a co-ordinated mammographic breast cancer screening service for women aged between 50–64 years. Issues of relevance to purchasers include:

- the age limits for screening
- the interval between screens.

The diagnosis and treatment of women with breast cancer is often variable. Issues of relevance to purchasers include:

- paucity of information on hospital activity and costing information
- variations in provision leading to sub-optimum care or resulting in inefficient services
- the recommendations of the Report of the Expert Advisory Group on the Commissioning of Cancer Services.

Areas of current research which could have major resource implications for purchasers include:

- primary prevention with tamoxifen
- predictive genetic testing
- annual screening of women aged 40–49
- changes in the indications for chemotherapy in women with early breast cancer
- high-dose chemotherapy with autologous bone marrow treatment.

2 Statement of the problem

Breast cancer is a major public health problem. It is a significant cause of mortality and morbidity and is a national target area in the Government's Health Strategy The Health of the Nation.[1] The Expert Advisory Group on the Commissioning of Cancer Services has recommended the establishment of breast cancer units situated in local trusts for the diagnosis and treatment of breast cancer.[2] Therefore the optimum configuration of services for women with breast cancer must be a prime concern for NHS purchasers.

Scale of the problem

One in 12 women in England and Wales will develop breast cancer during their lifetime. England and Wales have the highest mortality rates for breast cancer in the world.[3] The number of years of life lost in women below the age of 65 is higher for breast cancer than for coronary heart disease.[4]

Strategies to reduce breast cancer mortality and morbidity

There are no proven primary preventive strategies.

Small localized breast cancers have a favourable prognosis.[5] Mammography can be used as a screening test in population settings to detect asymptomatic breast cancers.[6] The NHSBSP aims to reduce mortality from breast cancer by regularly screening women aged 50–64 in order to identify such lesions.[7]

Effective interventions exist for the treatment of women with early breast cancer.[8,9]

Resource consequences

Breast cancer services consume substantial resources. The NHSBSP costs £29 million per annum.[10] Women with breast cancer account for almost 1% of inpatient admissions.[11]

Health care professionals and organizations involved in breast cancer services include family health services authorities (FHSAs), primary health care teams, public health physicians, health promotion officers, surgeons, radiologists, radiographers, breast care nurses, pathologists, medical and clinical oncologists, psychiatrists and palliative care teams. Voluntary agencies and social services provide information, psychosocial care and practical support.

Male breast cancer

Male breast cancer is rare accounting for less than 1% of new diagnoses of breast cancer.[12] Treatment strategies reflect those recommended for women.[13] It is not considered further.

Classification

Appendix I lists the relevant coding classifications related to breast cancer.

Summary

The key issues for purchasers are:

- breast cancer is a significant public health problem
- health gain can be maximized through early detection and appropriate clinical management
- there are major resource implications relating to screening, diagnosis and treatment.

3 Sub-categories

There are four main sub-categories of women accessing breast cancer services:

1 women attending the NHSBSP
2 women with a family history of breast cancer
3 women presenting for assessment of symptoms suggestive of breast cancer
4 women requiring treatment for breast cancer.

Women attending the NHSBSP

The NHSBSP invites all women aged between 50–64 years for breast screening at intervals of three years and is responsible for the assessment and diagnosis of mammographically detected abnormalities.

Family history of breast cancer

Women with a first degree relative with breast cancer have a two- or three-fold increased risk of developing the disease. If two or more relatives are affected the risk of breast cancer may be more than ten-fold that of the general population.[14]

Women presenting with symptoms of breast cancer

The most common presenting symptom is a painless lump. Other symptoms include skin dimpling, bloody discharge from or retraction of the nipple.

A third of all women attending surgical outpatients with a breast-related problem will have a painless breast lump of whom one in eight or nine will have a breast cancer.[15,16,17]

Women with breast cancer

Women with breast cancer can be allocated to one of five clinical staging groups according to the extent the disease has spread at time of presentation (Appendix II). When discussing treatment strategies it is more useful to collapse these into three subgroups:

1   women with ductal carcinoma *in situ* (DCIS), Stage 0
2   women with early breast cancer, Stages I and II
3   women with advanced breast cancer, Stages III and IV.

The distribution of these subgroups in two population-based series of women with breast cancer is outlined in Table 1.

Table 1: Distribution of subgroups of women with breast cancer

	Number of women (%)	
	Wessex[18]	East Anglia[19]
1 DCIS	7.3	5.6
2 Early breast cancer	77.0	75.2
3 Advanced breast cancer	15.8	19.2

Ductal carcinoma *in situ*[20,21]

Ductal carcinoma *in situ* may present as a palpable mass or an asymptomatic mammographic abnormality. It is distinguished from invasive disease by the absence of stromal invasion on histological examination.

The natural history of DCIS has not been adequately clarified. The risk of invasion is not precisely known but there is some evidence that it varies with subtype of DCIS.

Early breast cancer

The majority of women with breast cancer present with early stage disease. Early breast cancer is confined to the breast tissue with or without local spread to axillary lymph nodes on the same side as the tumour. These breast cancers are amenable to local surgical intervention.

The most common invasive breast cancers are infiltrating ductal carcinoma (75% of all invasive tumours) and lobular carcinoma (10–15%). These tumours commonly metastasize to axillary lymph nodes.[22]

Other less common histological types include tubular, mucinous and medullary carcinomas. These are generally associated with a better prognosis.

Advanced disease

Advanced disease includes locally advanced disease and distant metastases.

Locally advanced disease may invade the chest wall and/or overlying skin and involved lymph nodes may be fixed to or invade other structures.

Distant metastases occur most frequently in bone, skin, liver and lung.[23]

4 Prevalence and incidence

Incidence, mortality and survival are used to describe the impact of cancer in a population.

Regional cancer registries collect information on all new cancers occurring in their population and these data are used to estimate incidence rates (the number of new cases per 100 000 population per year). Mortality rates are derived from information contained within death certificates but these have often been shown to be both incomplete and inaccurate.

The incidence of cancer increases with age. In order to compare different populations it is necessary to allow for differences in the age structure. This process is called age standardization and the measure derived the age standardized incidence rate. Directly standardized incidence rates are calculated by applying local rates to a notional (standard) population, e.g. World Standard Population or European Standard Population.

Population based survival rates are derived from matching death registrations with cancer registrations and are expressed as a proportion of patients alive at some defined point subsequent to the date of diagnosis. The 'relative' survival rate allows for deaths from other causes among the population under study and is calculated as the ratio of crude survival to that which would be expected given the general mortality experience of England and Wales.

It is conventional to quote five-year relative survival rates as it is frequently assumed that a person surviving five years from the time of diagnosis is cured. However women with breast cancer may develop local recurrence or distant metastases many years after initial diagnosis and conversely, some women with metastases may survive longer than five years.[24] Therefore it may be more appropriate to report ten-year survival rates.

International and temporal comparisons of population based data sets should be interpreted with some caution due to possible variations in the definition of disease status and the completeness of ascertainment of cases and deaths.

Incidence and mortality

Breast cancer is the most common cause of cancer in women in England and Wales. In 1989 there were 27 768 new registrations of breast cancer[12] and the age standardized incidence rate for England and Wales was 68.2 per 100 000. In 1992 13 663 deaths were attributed to breast cancer.[25]

Breast cancer incidence increases with age (Appendix III). Three-quarters of all registrations occur in women aged over 50 and a third in the age group eligible for screening.

Although nearly 90% of breast cancer deaths occur in women aged over 50 years, it is the most common cause of death in women under 50.

Regional health authorities (RHAs) in Southern England have the highest incidence and mortality rates in the UK.

Temporal trends in incidence and mortality

There has been a steady increase in the incidence of breast cancer over the last two decades (Figure 1). The largest increase has occurred in women aged 50–64 and although recent changes in this age group can be attributed to the NHSBSP the incidence was increasing even before the introduction of screening.[26] It has been suggested that secular changes in the incidence of breast cancer may be due, in part, to changes in the distribution of known risk factors for breast cancer e.g. late age at first pregnancy, early menarche and prolonged use of oral contraceptives.[27]

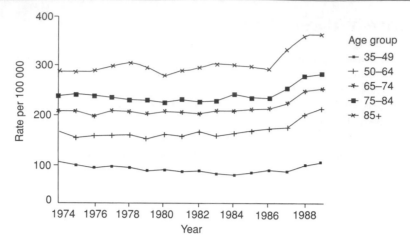

Figure 1: Temporal trends in age-specific incidence rates of breast cancer in England and Wales 1974–89.
(Source: OPCS Series MB1.)

There has also been an increase in registrations of DCIS following the introduction of screening (Figure 2).[25] DCIS accounts for 20% of screen-detected tumours.

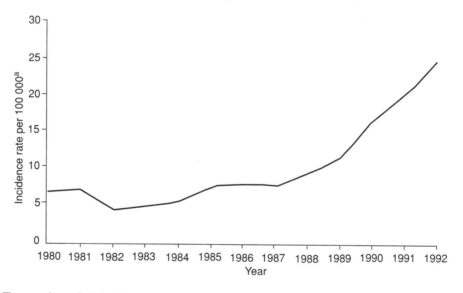

Figure 2: Temporal trends in incidence of *in situ* breast cancer in women aged 50–64 in the UK 1980–92.
[a] Standardized to the 1980 population.
(Source: Regional Cancer Registries.)

All ages mortality rates which rose during the 70s and early 80s have begun to decline in the late 80s and 90s[28] (Figure 3). This decrease predates any impact on mortality that might be expected following the introduction of the NHSBSP.[29]

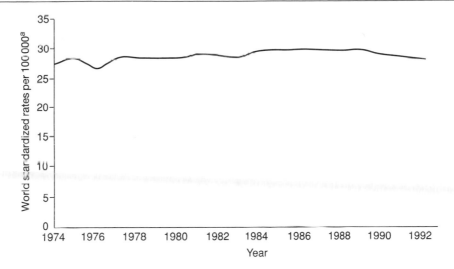

Figure 3: Temporal trends in mortality from breast cancer in England and Wales 1974–92.
ᵃ Standardized to world population (3 point moving averages).
(Source: OPCS Statistics Series DH2.)

Survival

The relative survival rate for breast cancer has been reported as 63% and 53% at five and ten years respectively.[30] It decreases with age in women over 40 (Figure 4).[31]

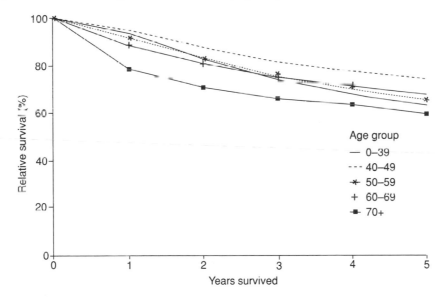

Figure 4: Relative survival rates for breast cancer by age group.
(Source: North Western Regional Cancer Registry.)

International and inter-regional variations in five year relative survival rates are shown in Figure 5 (see page 371).[31–38]

The extent of disease at presentation is an important prognostic indicator. Ten-year relative survival rates for women with no metastases, women with axillary node metastases but no distant metastases and women with distant metastases at presentation have been reported as 65%, 40% and 8% respectively.[30]

In early breast cancer the number of diseased axillary nodes is the most important predictor of recurrence. Large or high grade tumours (WHO pathological grade 3) have a poorer prognosis even in the absence of axillary node metastases.[5,39,40]

5 Service provision

This section describes the current level of provision of breast cancer services. Evidence of the effectiveness and efficiency of specific interventions is discussed in section 6. Palliative care services are not discussed.

The National Health Service Breast Screening Programme

The NHSBSP commenced in 1987. The programme aims to reduce mortality from breast cancer by screening women between the ages of 50 and 64 every three years.[6] The programme has benefited from clear central policy guidance, 'earmarked' funding and a strong quality assurance (QA) structure.[7]

National structure

A national co-ordinating body, with a national co-ordinator, was established at the inception of the NHSBSP. Its role includes training, QA and information systems. Policy and professional advice is supplied by a Department of Health Advisory Committee. Networking and advisory bodies, 'the Big 18s', have been established for the major disciplines within the programme including radiologists, surgeons, pathologists, radiographers, nurses, administrators, regional co-ordinators and QA managers. Each has representation from all RHAs in the UK; the health boards of Wales, Scotland and Northern Ireland and the private sector. There is a National Project Board for information systems.

Regional and district structure

Regional health authorities were responsible for the revenue costs of screening centres. Subsequent to changes in the structure of RHAs, the purchase of screening services became the responsibility of purchasing authorities in 1995.

Regional health authorities were required to nominate a QA manager and establish a QA reference centre to co-ordinate all aspects of the QA programme. The QA team includes a professional co-ordinator from each of the main groups contributing to screening i.e. radiology, radiography, pathology, surgery, nursing, administration and medical physics. Quality assurance was devolved to lead purchasing authorities in 1996.

Local purchasers and providers are required to offer a three-yearly mammographic screening programme and to attain national QA standards.

Quality assurance includes the following functions:

- standard setting (Appendix IV)
- monitoring progress towards meeting these standards
- providing professional advice e.g. QA guidelines for pathologists[41] and medical physics[42]
- co-ordinating professional QA schemes and ensuring they are in place
- local initiatives.

Setting

Breast screening and assessment of screen-detected abnormalities should be undertaken in specifically dedicated centres.

Breast cancer screening involves a core team of radiologists, radiographers, surgeons, pathologists/cytologists and administrative and technical support staff. Primary health care teams, the FHSA, breast care nurses and health promotion officers contribute to the acceptability and uptake of breast screening.

A screening centre is responsible for providing primary mammographic screening and assessment facilities to a defined population. A screening centre consists of the following.

- **Screening office** This is the administrative unit responsible for liaising with FHSAs, inviting eligible women for primary screening, informing women and general practitioners (GPs) of results and recalling women with abnormal mammograms for assessment.
- **Primary mammographic screening unit(s)** There may be one or more units per centre located on permanent sites or on mobile vans. Over 80% of screening centres have a mobile van.[43]
- **Assessment unit(s)** Women with abnormal mammograms are requested to attend for further assessment. This may involve clinical examination, further mammograms and/or ultrasound. Fine-needle aspiration cytology (FNAC) and/or excision biopsy may be undertaken to provide pathological confirmation prior to definitive surgery. Assessment should be by a multi-disciplinary specialist breast team including a radiologist, surgeon and pathologist/cytologist.

Screen-detected lesions may be palpable or impalpable. Impalpable lesions present specific assessment problems and may require the use of stereotactic equipment or ultrasound to guide FNAC. Mammography or ultrasound is required to aid localization of the tumour for excision. The excised area should be imaged to identify completeness of excision of the tumour prior to pathological assessment.

Utilization

There are nearly 4 000 000 women eligible for breast screening and 79 screening centres in England. Wales has its own breast screening programme: Breast Test Wales. In 1993/94, 960 678 women aged 50–64 attended for screening.[11]

The Forrest Report recommended that a single assessment team should cover an eligible population of 41 150 women (one million population) in order to maintain sufficient multi-disciplinary expertise in both the assessment of mammographic abnormalities and the management of screen-detected cancers.[6]

There are 93 assessment units in England and Wales. Geographical access, population density and local purchasing decisions account for eligible populations ranging between 12 000 (Isle of Wight) and 130 000 (Greater Manchester).[43]

Funding of the service was based initially on three-yearly recall and the use of single-view mammography (oblique view).[6] All screening centres are now expected to provide two-view mammography (oblique and craniocaudal views) in the prevalent round.[45]

Family history of breast cancer

A family history of breast cancer is given by 20% of all women with breast cancer. An increasing demand for information on individual risk has been reported among young women with a family history.[46]

There has been a stream of experimental work aimed at characterizing and identifying genes responsible for breast cancer. The BRCA1 and BRCA2 genes are likely to cause the vast majority of genetically determined cases. One to six per 1000 women may carry BRCA1 or BRCA2 genes.[47] The BRCA1 gene has recently been cloned and with this comes the possibility of predictive genetic testing for carrier status.[48] However only 5% of all breast cancer cases are associated with highly penetrant dominant genes.[46]

Setting

Risk counselling is currently provided by GPs, clinicians and an increasing number of specialist genetic clinics. There are 18 such clinics in the UK.[49]

Site specific, familial breast cancer clinics are an alternative to general genetic clinics. These are multi-disciplinary involving surgeons, geneticists, radiologists and specialist nurses. They offer advice on individual risk, clinical examination, teach breast self awareness and may offer specific preventative interventions.[50]

Utilization

The Regional Family History Cancer Clinic based at the Royal Free Hospital saw 851 women between March 1988 and September 1990.[51] 58% of women attending were self-referrals. Of those seen 97% had a risk greater than that of the general population and 23% a specific familial breast cancer syndrome. The compliance rate among those offered screening was 83%.

Symptoms of breast cancer

Services for women presenting outside the screening service are often poorly co-ordinated. It is suggested that the symptomatic service should emulate the multi-disciplinary approach of the NHSBSP.

Setting

The majority of symptomatic women will initially attend their GP and be referred either to a general surgeon, a surgeon with an interest in breast diseases or a surgeon specializing in breast diseases.

Women may be seen in general surgical outpatient clinics, dedicated breast clinics or rapid diagnosis (one-stop) clinics. Rapid diagnosis clinics offer women consultation, investigation and diagnosis on the same day.

Diagnostic services include:

- breast imaging by mammography and/or ultrasound
- pathological assessment by FNAC, tru-cut biopsy and/or excision biopsy.

Some women will present with symptoms suggestive of metastatic breast cancer and require liver scans, bone scans and/or computed tomography (CT).

Utilization

Each year, one in 50 women consult their GP with a breast problem and approximately one in three of these are immediately referred for a surgical opinion.[52–54]

An audit of outpatient surgical workload in two provider units estimated that breast problems account for 20% of all new general surgical outpatient referrals and over 40% of follow-up visits.[17] One in five of the women referred did not require any investigation and an eighth of new referrals were diagnosed with breast cancer.

Women with breast cancer

The objectives of clinical management vary with the extent of the disease (Table 2).

Table 2: Objectives of clinical management

Subgroup	Objectives
DCIS	Local control of disease
Early breast cancer	Locoregional control Prolongation of disease-free and overall survival
Locally advanced breast cancer	Local disease control In some women, prolongation of overall survival
Metastatic breast cancer	Palliation

Ductal carcinoma *in situ*

Surgical management, mastectomy or breast conservation therapy (BCT), aims to achieve local control.[55] Mastectomy is the removal of the breast with some overlying skin, usually including the nipple, from the chest wall muscles. BCT involves either wide local excision (WLE), removal of the tumour with a 1 cm margin of normal tissue, or quadrantectomy, when a whole quadrant of the breast is excised.

Early breast cancer

Clinical management in women with early breast cancer aims to achieve locoregional control of disease and prolongation of disease-free and overall survival.[22]

Primary surgical treatment may be by mastectomy or BCT with post-operative radiotherapy. Axillary lymph nodes are surgically excised for pathological assessment. Disease in the axillary lymph nodes is treated by surgery or radiotherapy.[56]

Pathological assessment of the tumour and lymph nodes identifies women who would benefit from adjuvant therapy. Adjuvant therapy is administered with the aim of prolonging survival. Adjuvant therapies include chemotherapy, tamoxifen and ovarian ablation.

Ovarian ablation is the destruction of the hormone releasing function of the ovaries by surgery, radiotherapy or gonadotrophin releasing hormone analogue. Only the latter is reversible.

Women undergoing mastectomy require reconstructive surgery or breast prostheses. Reconstructive surgery may be undertaken at the time of the primary surgery or as a delayed procedure.[57,58]

Advanced breast cancer

Treatment strategies for locally advanced disease primarily aim to control local disease and include surgery, radiotherapy and systemic therapy.[59,60] In some women treatment also aims to prolong overall survival.

The management of women with disseminated breast cancer is palliative and aims to ameliorate and control distressing symptoms. Treatments include systemic therapy (chemotherapy or hormone therapy) and radiotherapy.

Approximately 40–70% of women with disseminated disease receive radiotherapy to relieve pain from bone metastases.[61] Orthopaedic intervention may be required to prevent fractures of the long bones or spine.

Setting

The needs of women with breast cancer extend beyond medical care. The clinical, social and psychological management of women during their illness requires a co-ordinated, multi-disciplinary approach involving surgeons, pathologists, clinical and medical oncologists, breast care nurses, psychiatrists, primary health care teams and other agencies from the statutory and voluntary sector.

Women with breast cancer are treated in acute provider units and/or specialist cancer hospitals. Surgery may be undertaken by general surgeons or surgeons interested in or specializing in breast diseases. Reconstructive surgery may be performed by breast surgeons with specific training or plastic surgeons. Pathologists with expertise in the assessment of the pathology of the breast are an essential component of the clinical team.

Breast care nurses can identify significant psychological morbidity,[62] provide information and advice on treatment options and fit breast prostheses.[63] Breast care nurses work within the acute care sector and/or the community.[64]

Radiotherapy requires specialist equipment and women needing radiotherapy are referred to a clinical oncologist in a specialist cancer centre.

Women requiring systemic therapy, e.g hormone therapy or chemotherapy, are usually referred to clinical or medical oncologists in specialist hospitals. Chemotherapy is also administered in acute provider units but this is not always under the guidance of an oncologist.[65]

The majority of women with breast cancer are followed-up after treatment by surgeons or oncologists. Schedules vary but typically may be once every three months for the first two years, every four months for the third and fourth year and then biannually. Women with advanced disease may be followed-up more frequently.

Utilization

Women with breast cancer accounted for 1% of all hospital episodes (46 008 admissions and 17 167 day cases) in the UK during 1991/92. The average length of stay was 8.3 days.[66]

Surgical

10 036 mastectomies (OPCS IV B27: total excision of the breast) and 13 036 BCTs (OPCS IV B28 other excision of the breast (excluding biopsies)) were undertaken for breast cancer. Almost 10% of BCT was performed as day cases.

These statistics should be interpreted with caution. Episodes relate to operations and not women; a woman may have more than one operation either because of bilateral disease or because of incomplete excision of the tumour.

Table 3 suggests there has been an increase in the frequency with which BCT is performed and this may, in part, be attributable to more small cancers detected by the NHSBSP.

It is not possible to identify the current level of breast reconstructive surgery from data collected routinely. Breast reconstructive surgery is not uniformly available in the NHS but an increase in demand from women undergoing mastectomy has been reported.[57]

Table 3: Temporal trends in operative procedures for women with breast cancer

Year	Mastectomy no. of episodes	BCT no. of episodes (% day case)	Ratio of mastectomy: BCT
1991/92	10 036	13 036 (9.4)	1 : 1.3
1990/91	9284	11 744 (8.0)	1 : 1.26
1989/90	9001	10 332 (7.7)	1 : 1.24

Specialist services

The majority of the 218.4 wte clinical and medical oncologists are based in specialist cancer centres.[67] There are 45 such centres in the UK.[68]

The trend toward greater use of BCT compounded by increased detection of small tumours by the NHSBSP will have a substantial impact on radiotherapy workload.[30,69]

Breast care nurses

In 1991 there were 170 breast care nurses employed in symptomatic and/or screening services in England and Wales.[64]

Summary

The key issues for purchasers are:

- quality assurance of the NHSBSP which was devolved to lead purchasers in 1996
- the investigation and treatment of women with breast cancer should be multi-disciplinary.

6 Effectiveness and cost-effectiveness

National Health Service Breast Screening Programme

Evidence of efficacy

Evidence accrued from randomized controlled trials (RCTs) suggests that mammographic screening can reduce mortality from breast cancer by between 25% and 30% in women aged 50 to 69.[70,71] There is insufficient evidence on the efficacy of screening in women over 70 as most trials had an upper age limit of 69.

Randomized controlled trials have failed to demonstrate a significant mortality reduction from the use of mammography in women aged 40–49 but none of these trials were designed to test this specific hypothesis and insufficient numbers in this age group were recruited. The sensitivity of mammography is lower in younger women. Tumours in this age group may be faster growing[72] and therefore younger women may benefit from more frequent screening. The benefit of annual screening in a cohort of women aged 40–41 at recruitment is currently being examined in a RCT (the UKCCCR Age Trial).

There is as yet no evidence of the efficacy of breast self-examination as a population-based screening test[73] but an intervention trial is ongoing in Russia.[74]

Costs

£55 million was initially invested by the Department of Health in establishing the NHSBSP with an additional £16 million developmental costs contributed from regional funds.[7]

In 1993 the revenue costs of the screening programme were £29 million: 90% was allocated for the purchase of breast screening by health authorities, £2 million to regional QA and the remainder to training and national initiatives including the national co-ordinating team.[10]

The Forrest Report calculated the cost-effectiveness of a breast screening programme using information from the Swedish Two Counties and Health Insurance Plan (HIP) trials and assuming:

- a 70% uptake of screening
- a three-year screening interval
- the use of single-view mammography.[6]

The estimate of £3500 per life–year saved (1983/84 prices) compared favourably with the cost-effectiveness of other health service interventions e.g. cervical screening and coronary artery bypass grafts.

Clarke *et al.* calculated the cost-effectiveness of breast screening using data from the Edinburgh Trial assuming a 70% compliance and a three-yearly screening schedule.[75] Their estimate of £8638 per life–year saved (1989 prices) was more than double the Forrest Report estimate. This difference may be due to the poorer outcome of the Edinburgh Trial compared to the Swedish Two Counties and HIP trials and to the inclusion of treatment costs in the calculation.

Family history of breast cancer

The management of young women with a family history of breast cancer remains problematic. Mammographic screening in this setting is of unproven value.

Prophylactic mastectomy is reserved for women with high risk of breast cancer but its psychological morbidity is unknown. Subcutaneous mastectomy leaves the overlying skin and nipple intact. It may give better cosmetic results but residual breast tissue can potentially undergo malignant change.

Women presenting with symptoms of breast cancer

Current opinion supports a combined modality approach in the assessment of symptomatic women.[76,77] This 'triple assessment' includes clinical examination, breast imaging (mammography and/or ultrasound) and either cytological (FNAC) or histological (tru-cut biopsy) assessment. Triple assessment aims to improve cancer detection rates while limiting the number of unnecessary surgical interventions. However in the presence of clinical uncertainty an excision biopsy is still considered mandatory. Inevitably improvements in sensitivity can only occur at the expense of reduced specificity.

The various estimates of sensitivity and specificity of diagnostic procedures are mainly derived from retrospective analyses (Table 4). The biases introduced by operator competence or experience and case selection may account for the wide variation in reported results.

Although excellent results from FNAC have been reported in some series, a recent review of 9533 consecutive FNACs suggests that results are heavily operator dependent; inadequate rates varied between 6–50% among 31 operators.[84] Errors in reporting may also reduce the effectiveness of FNAC.[85]

Rapid diagnosis (or one-stop) clinics have been introduced following concerns over diagnostic delay and frequency of hospital visits.[86] The costs and benefits of these clinics have not been assessed. Any change in the organization of services has implications for other aspects of the service. Potential disadvantages of rapid

Table 4: Sensitivity and specificity of diagnostic procedures[76–83]

Diagnostic procedure	Sensitivity (%)	Specificity (%)
Clinical examination	86–92	71–90
FNAC	79–99	93–100
Mammography	61–94	55–90
Ultrasound	82–97	84–95
Triple assessment		
clinical examination, FNAC and mammography	93 100	53
clinical examination, FNAC and ultrasound	100	61

diagnosis clinics include relaxation of referral criteria by GPs and increased psychological morbidity secondary to an expedited diagnosis of malignancy.

Routine use of bone, liver or CT scans to detect asymptomatic metastases is not recommended. Detection rates are low and false-positive rates high (7–9% and 22% respectively for bone scans).[87]

Women with breast cancer

Clinical management of DCIS

Mastectomy will cure 98–100% of women with symptomatic DCIS.[55]

Screen-detected asymptomatic DCIS is usually small and localized and there has been a marked shift towards the use of BCT to treat these lesions. However recurrences following BCT are common. In one series 25% of women had recurrences at ten years of which half were invasive.[88] There is increasing interest in identifying those subtypes of DCIS more likely to recur following BCT.[89]

The efficacy of post-operative radiotherapy and adjuvant hormone therapy in reducing recurrence rates following BCT is unproven. A randomized controlled trial under the auspices of the UKCCCR is currently evaluating the use of radiotherapy and/or tamoxifen in preventing subsequent invasion following wide local excision of DCIS.

It is generally considered unnecessary to sample axillary lymph nodes unless disease is extensive or multifocal.

Clinical management of early breast cancer

Clinical management of early breast cancer has four components:

1   primary treatment of the breast and axillary lymph nodes to gain locoregional control of disease
2   pathological staging to direct decisions on adjuvant therapy
3   adjuvant therapy to prolong disease-free and overall survival
4   routine follow-up.

Primary management – surgical treatment

Randomized controlled trials comparing BCT, axillary node dissection and post-operative radiotherapy with total mastectomy and axillary node dissection have demonstrated similar local recurrence-free and overall survival rates (Table 5). Breast conservation therapy is not always considered suitable for women with multifocal disease, large tumours, small breasts or when disease is beneath the nipple.

Table 5: Comparison of results from randomized controlled trials comparing mastectomy and breast conservation therapy

	Fisher et al.[90] Follow-up eight years (%)	Lichter et al.[91] Follow-up eight years (%)	Veronesi[8] Follow-up ten years (%)
Mastectomy			
disease-free survival	58	76	–
overall survival	71	79	76
BCT			
disease-free survival	59	78	–
overall survival	76	85	79

Primary management of the axilla

Treatment of the axilla, either by surgery (axillary node dissection or clearance) or by radiotherapy is effective in maintaining local control of disease.[92] However there is no convincing evidence of the superiority of any one of these modalities. Side-effects include lymphoedema, limited shoulder movement and inadvertent damage to the brachial plexus. There is some evidence that surgery and radiotherapy combined may increase side-effects without any additional benefit.[93]

Primary management of radiotherapy

Radiotherapy after BCT improves disease-free survival.[94] Routine post-operative radiotherapy following mastectomy has been shown to increase deaths related to cardiac causes.[95] However an updated overview of RCTs comparing survival following mastectomy alone with survival following mastectomy and post-operative radiotherapy has demonstrated that excess cardiac deaths may be offset by a reduction in breast cancer deaths and suggests a small but non-significant advantage from post-mastectomy radiotherapy after ten years of follow-up.[96]

Radiotherapy fractionation schedules for radical treatment following BCT vary in length between three to six weeks.[97] The cost per fraction of radiotherapy varies between £22 and £58.[98,99]

Pathological staging

Adequate pathological staging of early breast cancer is essential to direct adjuvant therapy. Both the tumour and axillary lymph nodes need to be assessed:

1 **assessment of tumour specimen** The histological type, grade and size of tumour provide important prognostic information. Incomplete excision of tumour may necessitate further operative intervention or radiotherapy.
2 **assessment of axillary lymph nodes**[56] Clinical examination is unreliable. Therefore surgical excision of axillary lymph nodes for pathological examination is essential. It is generally agreed that at least four lymph nodes should be available for examination to exclude metastases.

Surgical dissection or clearance, undertaken as part of the primary surgical treatment, usually provides sufficient lymph nodes to stage the axilla but the use of less radical axillary node sampling may reduce operative side-effects.[100] Two small RCTs have demonstrated that well performed axillary sampling is as effective as axillary dissection or clearance in obtaining sufficient lymph nodes for pathological assessment.[101,102] There is some concern that the excellent results of these trials may not be reproducible in all clinical settings.[103]

Adjuvant therapy

A meta-analysis of worldwide trials investigating adjuvant therapy in early breast cancer has produced imposing evidence of the effectiveness of these treatments in improving overall survival. The overview included 133 randomized trials involving 75 000 women.[9] Its conclusions were as follows.

- Tamoxifen
    a) tamoxifen therapy is effective in reducing recurrence and death from breast cancer particularly in women over 50 years of age
    b) tamoxifen therapy lasting at least two years is more effective than shorter term regimens.
- Chemotherapy
    a) chemotherapy is effective in reducing recurrence and death from breast cancer particularly in women under the age of 50
    b) women over 50 respond less well to chemotherapy
    c) chemotherapy regimens involving more than one drug are more effective than those involving single-agent drugs. Cyclophosphamide, methotrexate and fluorouracil (CMF) regimens were studied most often
    d) long-term courses (more than six months) do not confer any additional survival benefit.
- Ovarian ablation
    a) ovarian ablation is effective in reducing recurrence and death from breast cancer in women under 50.

Table 6 illustrates some of the results of the World Overview.[9,104] Estimates of effect are presented as annual odds of death. This is the probability of dying during a year divided by the probability of surviving the year. This can be translated into an absolute benefit and presented as the number of deaths prevented at ten years of follow-up per 100 women treated.

Table 6: Results from the Worldwide Overview of Adjuvant Trials

Adjuvant therapy	Reduction in annual odds of death (%)	Number of deaths prevented per hundred women treated at ten years of follow-up
Tamoxifen in women over 50 years	20	8
Chemotherapy in women under 50 years	25	10
Ovarian ablation in women under 50 years	28	11

Adjuvant therapy in women under 50

The use of adjuvant chemotherapy in premenopausal women is of proven value. Currently consensus opinion supports its routine use in women with node-positive disease.[105]

The absolute and relative benefit of multi-agent chemotherapy is greater in node-positive than node-negative women. The improvement in overall survival at ten years for node-positive women of all ages was 6.8% (46.6% vs 39.8%) compared to a 4% improvement in node-negative women (67.2% vs 63.2%).[9]

Treatment costs for node-positive premenopausal women receiving chemotherapy are between $4900 per quality adjusted life year (QALY) and $9200/QALY dependent on other risk factors (1989 prices).[106] Chemotherapy for node-negative premenopausal women costs $15 400/QALY (1991 prices).[107]

There are subgroups of high risk, node-negative women in whom chemotherapy may confer substantial survival advantage.[108] Many clinicians support adjuvant chemotherapy in node-negative women with high grade or large tumours.[39,108,109] Only one study has directly compared the effectiveness of chemotherapy and ovarian ablation in the management of premenopausal node-positive women.[110] It did not show a significant difference in survival but the power of the study was low and could not exclude a difference of 10%.

The Nottingham Prognostic Index combines information on several tumour characteristics to aid decisions on the requirement for adjuvant therapy.[111] Other prognostic indicators such as Cerb B2 oncogene, Capthesin D and S phase fraction have been suggested[39,112] but there is no evidence that these contribute sufficient additional prognostic information to support their use in routine clinical practice.

Adjuvant therapy in women over 50

The World Overview suggests that tamoxifen should be considered for node-positive and node-negative women over the age of 50.

Oestrogen and progesterone receptor status may be used to predict response to tamoxifen and other hormone therapies.[39] However even postmenopausal women with oestrogen receptor-poor tumours have a small but still significant survival advantage conferred by tamoxifen.[9]

The overview suggests that combining chemotherapy and tamoxifen (chemoendocrine therapy) may have a greater effect on mortality in women over 50 than tamoxifen alone. This is not based on RCTs directly comparing chemoendocrine therapy with tamoxifen alone but on indirect comparisons using the results of other trials. The results of RCTs of chemoendocrine therapy in postmenopausal women are awaited.

Adjuvant therapy in minimal risk tumours

Small (less than 1 cm) node-negative, low grade or special type (pure tubular or mucinous or papillary) tumours have an extremely good prognosis. They account for approximately 20% of screen-detected lesions.[40] The need for post-operative radiotherapy or adjuvant therapy in these patients[113,114] is being addressed by the British Association of Surgical Oncologists (BASO) II Trial.

Follow-up regimens

Women with early breast cancer may develop local recurrences (9% after ten years) or distant metastases and have a four-fold increased risk of developing cancer in the contralateral breast.[115,116] Post-operative mammographic surveillance is used to detect the following.

1   **Contralateral breast cancer** The increased risk of contralateral breast cancer probably justifies mammographic surveillance in this group of women. However the optimum screening interval is uncertain.
2   **Asymptomatic local recurrences** A difference in overall survival between women with clinically detected recurrences and those with asymptomatic screen-detected recurrences has not been consistently found.[117,118]

The role of post-operative mammographic surveillance needs to be further evaluated.

There is no evidence to support screening for asymptomatic distant metastases during routine follow-up. Two RCTs failed to demonstrate any added benefit, either in overall survival or quality of life, from the routine use of bone scans, liver scans and X-rays.[119,120]

Advanced disease

There are few large RCTs comparing treatment strategies in women presenting with advanced disease and there may be some reluctance amongst clinicians to recruit such patients into trials.[121] There are no trials comparing systemic therapy with supportive care alone in women with disseminated breast cancer and most clinicians would consider it unethical to undertake such a trial.

The mean cost of treating a patient with advanced disease is £7620 (1991 prices).[122]

Locally-advanced breast cancer

It has been suggested that chemotherapy in locally-advanced disease may prolong survival in some subgroups of women but comparisons of chemotherapy and local treatment e.g. surgery or radiotherapy with local treatment alone have produced inconsistent findings. The role of combined chemoendocrine therapy in this setting has not been clarified.[123,124]

Metastatic breast cancer

The management of women with metastatic disease is fairly uniform in the UK. The first-line drug of choice is tamoxifen. Other hormone therapies such as medroxyprogesterone acetate, megestrol acetate, gonadotrophin releasing hormone analogue, aminoglutethemide, androgens and ovarian ablation are used sequentially as breakthrough of disease occurs.[125,126]

Chemotherapy is usually offered when hormones fail. Trials do not demonstrate any benefit of multi-agent chemotherapy over single agent.[127]

High-dose chemotherapy followed by autologous bone marrow treatment or support with haemopoietic factors is used in some centres to treat metastatic disease. There have been no RCTs of this resource intensive treatment and treatment-related mortality is high.[128]

Palliative radiotherapy is useful in the treatment of bone, brain and skin metastases. The average cost per fraction of palliative radiotherapy for bone metastases at Mount Vernon Hospital was calculated to be £37 (1989 prices).[129] Randomized controlled trials have shown that short courses of radiotherapy (one or two fractions) are as effective as longer courses in ameliorating painful bone metastases.[130,131] The shorter regimens potentially represent substantial savings but some radiotherapists are concerned that the 12 week follow-up period of these studies limits their generalizability to breast cancer patients who may survive for several months after treatment. The results of a further RCT with longer follow-up are awaited.[132]

Psychosocial interventions

Psychological morbidity, detectable in 25–30% of women with breast cancer, may have a detrimental effect on treatment compliance.[133] Maguire et al. demonstrated in a RCT that a nurse counsellor was successful in identifying psychiatric morbidity in women undergoing mastectomy. Subsequent referral to a psychiatrist resulted in an overall lower level of morbidity in the intervention group a year later.[62] The cost of the nurse counsellor was offset by savings in psychiatric inpatient care and fewer days off work required by patient and carer.[134]

High levels of psychiatric morbidity have been demonstrated in women who have undergone mastectomy.[135] Women who undergo BCT have a better body image but levels of anxiety are still high.[136,137] Improved psychosexual wellbeing has been associated with breast reconstruction following mastectomy.[138]

There is no firm evidence to support the generally held opinion that offering women a choice of treatment reduces psychological distress. Over half of women with early breast cancer may wish to take a passive role in treatment decisions[139] and the communication style of the doctor may be more important than offering treatment choice.[140] Patients appear to value adequate information on diagnosis and treatment within the context of a caring physician–patient relationship.[141] There has been little formal evaluation of the best way of imparting information and current methods include leaflets, videotapes and written and taped recordings of consultations.[142]

Strength of recommendation

Table 7 summarizes the strength of intervention recommendation.

Table 7: The strength of intervention recommendation

Intervention	Strength of recommendation
Age at screening	
50–64 years	1/a
64–69 years	I/a
<50 years	I/d
>70 years	III/c
Screening interval period less than three yearly	I/b
Two-view mammography	I/b
Breast self-examination	II/c
Diagnostic procedures in assessment	II/b
Pre-operative bone/liver/CT scan	II/e
BCT and radiotherapy	I/a
Adjuvant therapy in early breast cancer	
chemotherapy in women under 50	I/a
ovarian ablation in women under 50	I/a
tamoxifen in women over 50	I/a
Breast care nurse counsellors	I/b
Intensive follow-up regimens	I/e

Key:
I well conducted RCT; II other studies; III opinions of respected authorities based on indirect evidence;
a good evidence for acceptance; b fair evidence for acceptance; c poor evidence for acceptance; d fair evidence for rejection; e good evidence for rejection

7 Models of care

Health gain may be maximized through:

- early detection by mammographic screening
- appropriate diagnosis and treatment of women with breast cancer.

National Health Service Breast Screening Programme

Population-based mammographic screening offers the best opportunity of reducing mortality from breast cancer. The cost-effectiveness of the programme will be influenced by the:

- age group invited for screening
- interval between screens
- sensitivity of the test
- compliance.

Age

Despite evidence from RCTs of the efficacy of breast screening in women aged up to 69,[81,82] women aged between 65 and 69 are not routinely invited for screening in this country. There were 12 591 breast cancers diagnosed in women over 65 in 1989.[12]

The Forrest Report suggested that screening would be inefficient in older women due to low compliance.[6] However 61% of Manchester women aged 65–74 responded to an invitation for screening.[143] The cancer detection rate in this population was 11.6 per 1000 screens.

A US economic analysis has shown that raising the screening age to 69 is more cost-effective than only screening women aged 50–64.[144] The model used data derived from the HIP trial and Breast Cancer Detection Demonstration Project and assumed biennial screening with annual clinical examination. A similar evaluation is now underway in the UK.[145]

Screening interval period

The NHSBSP is unique among population-based screening programmes in that the interval between screens is three years. The evidence adduced in support of breast screening effectiveness is mainly derived from trials with shorter screening intervals.

The first population-based report describing the incidence of interval cancers in the NHSBSP revealed that the rate of interval cancers in the third year after screening approaches that which would be expected in the absence of screening.[146] Similar results have been reported from other regional programmes.[147] These suggest that the screening interval may be too long.

The optimum screening interval remains uncertain. The United Kingdom Committee for Co ordinating Cancer Research (UKCCCR) frequency trial is comparing the benefits of yearly with three-yearly breast screening in a RCT involving 100 000 women. An economic analysis is incorporated in this study.

The cost-effectiveness of screening women aged 50–70 every two years has been shown to be comparable to screening women aged 50–65 every three years. This cost-effectiveness analysis, using a computer simulation model, was based on the results of the Dutch screening programme.[148]

Sensitivity of the test

There are two types of interval cancers; cancers present but not identified on previous screening examinations (false-negatives) or cancers which appear to have arisen *de novo* since the last screening examination (true intervals).

Although not all cancers are detectable by mammographic screening improvement in the sensitivity of the test may identify some cancers which would otherwise have been missed and hence lead to further reductions in the incidence of interval cancers.

It has been suggested that the sensitivity of the screening test can be further improved by optimizing the optical density of the mammographic film,[149] by two radiologists independently reading the mammogram (double reading)[150] and by employing two-view mammography.[151] The NHS Executive has instructed purchasers to fund the first and third of these initiatives.[55]

A RCT suggests that two-view mammography may increase the cancer detection rate in the prevalence round of screening.[152]

Compliance

Programme effectiveness will be adversely effected by low compliance.[153] Factors which may influence compliance include the following.

- **Accuracy of FHSA registers** One of the main reasons for non-attendance at screening is non-invitation due to inaccuracies in the FHSA database.[154]
- **Method of invitation** RCTs have demonstrated that invitation policy can influence compliance. Williams and Vessey demonstrated the superiority of pre-allocated appointments[155] and others have shown the effectiveness of personalized letters of invitation.[156]
- **Accessibility of primary screening facilities** The location of the screening unit may affect uptake.[157] A survey of the Lothian mobile unit in 1988 showed that it cost women 89 pence for every mile travelled to attend for screening and that 'access costs' were directly associated with the uptake of screening.[158]
- **Acceptability of screening** There is no evidence that the screening programme increases psychological morbidity among women invited for screening.[159,160] 90% of screened women will re-attend for further screening; women who do not are more likely to view the previous experience of screening negatively.[161] The majority of women with screen-detected abnormalities will have a benign diagnosis (false-positive). These healthy women undergo unnecessary investigation and occasionally treatment with the possibility of resultant physical and psychological morbidity.[162] Therefore it is important to keep the false-positive rate low. Concerns have been expressed about uptake among ethnic minorities. A RCT of pre-screening visits from linkworkers failed to demonstrate a beneficial effect on subsequent uptake of invitation.[163]

There is a need for more intervention trials of strategies designed to improve uptake, particularly amongst those reinvited for screening.

Diagnosis and treatment

The appropriate management of women with early breast cancer offers additional opportunities to reduce mortality and morbidity.

Variations in quality of care

Comparison of international and inter-regional relative survival rates for breast cancer have raised concerns over poor treatment outcomes in this country (Figure 5). A number of studies suggest that some women in the UK may be receiving less than optimum care.

Chouillet *et al.* found that of 334 women with breast cancer resident in four RHAs and treated in 81 hospitals, only 46% had undergone axillary node surgery and only 47% of premenopausal women had received chemotherapy.[164] The study predated the World Overview of randomized trials of adjuvant therapy.[9]

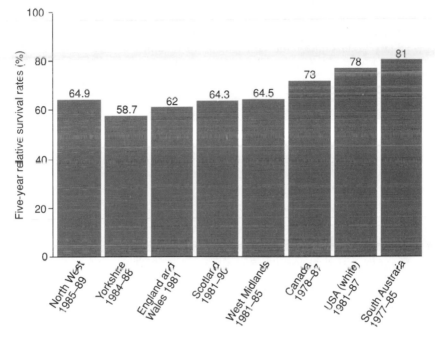

Figure 5: International variations in survival from breast cancer.

(Source: various cancer registries.[31–38])

A population-based audit of the management of 27,216 new cases of breast cancer registered in one RHA between 1978 and 1992 has reported interdistrict variations in the uptake of radiotherapy following surgery and in the use of adjuvant therapies.[165]

A questionnaire survey of surgeons in 1990 showed a marked shift towards BCT as treatment of choice in women with early breast cancer.[69,166,167] However 34% of surgeons would not routinely refer women undergoing breast conservation surgery for radiotherapy and only 74% of surgeons had access to a breast care nurse.

Impact of breast cancer services on outcome

It is important to identify the attributes of a service which may adversely affect the survival of women with breast cancer. Three have been extensively investigated.

Delay in diagnosis

There is no convincing evidence supporting the proposition that delays in diagnosis or referral of the magnitude routinely experienced within the NHS adversely influence survival.[168–170]

Type of hospital

Evidence to support a beneficial impact of specialist hospitals on survival of women with breast cancer is equivocal. Two studies in Italy and Australia have failed to demonstrate a significant difference in survival between women attending private institutions compared to public hospitals.[171,172] Although Karjalainen did find a better survival among Finnish women with breast cancer resident in districts with a university teaching hospital with radiotherapy facilities, this was confined to women with advanced disease.[173]

Lee-Feldstein *et al.* demonstrated a significantly better survival among US women with breast cancer treated in large community hospitals compared to those treated in smaller community and Health Maintenance Organisation hospitals even after adjustment for other factors known to influence survival.[174]

Basnett *et al.* showed that women resident in a London teaching hospital district were more likely to undergo BCT, axillary node surgery and adjuvant chemotherapy.[175] The women in the non-teaching hospital district had a higher risk of death even after adjustment for age and stage at presentation. The conclusions of this study are limited by the small study size and the short period of follow-up.

Workload of consultant surgeons

It is more likely that it is the competence of the treating surgeon which influences survival rather than the type of hospital attended.

There exists a strong belief that only those surgeons with a significant caseload of women have the skills necessary to manage breast cancer.[176] Hand *et al.* reported a significant association between failure to deliver radiotherapy for early breast cancer and number of cases treated.[177]

Uncertainty exists as to the volume of new cases necessary to maintain competence but a notional minimum figure of 50 has been suggested.[178] A population-based audit of breast cancer in Yorkshire has demonstrated that survival was better among women treated by surgeons who had a caseload in excess of 30 breast cancers a year.[179]

In one region with approximately 2000 breast cancer registrations per year analysis of Korner Episode System data for 1992/93 showed that women with breast cancer undergoing surgery were treated in 25 different hospitals. There were only seven consultants in the region treating more than 50 patients (unpublished data).

A Policy Framework for Commissioning Cancer Services

A national Expert Advisory Group was established to consider the organization of cancer care in England and Wales. The report of this group to the Chief Medical Officers of England and Wales, *A Policy Framework for Commissioning Cancer Services*[2] heralds a major reorganization of cancer services. Purchasing authorities will be responsible for securing uniform access to high quality services for their population.

The report recommends a model of care based on the following three levels of service provision.

1 **Primary care** Primary care teams are involved in the initial assessment and referral of patients and in providing ongoing practical and emotional support to patients within the community.
2 **Designated cancer units** Each cancer unit would be responsible for the clinical management of a common cancer, such as breast cancer and would have a lead consultant responsible for co-ordinating care, site-specific specialists and input from non-surgical oncologists.
3 **Cancer centres** These centres would provide specialist services to support cancer units. They would serve a population of between two-thirds of a million to a million and would provide radiotherapy services, specialist diagnostic services, management of rare cancers and intensive chemotherapy regimens.

The report emphasizes the importance of a holistic approach to cancer care from referral through assessment and treatment to palliative care. It stresses integration between primary care, acute providers and specialist services and the co-ordination of surgical and non-surgical expertise with the appropriate specialist backing from support services in radiology, pathology, nursing and palliative care. Key themes in the strategy are adherence to treatment protocols, development of local guidelines on referral practice, clinical audit and continuing medical education.

Levels of service provision

The following section outlines the service requirements of a notional HA with a female population of 150 000 and an age–sex structure similar to that in England and Wales.

OPCS estimates of the incidence of breast cancer in England and Wales for 1992[180] suggest that 172 new breast cancer cases would be expected in this HA per annum; 32 would be screen-detected (Figure 6) and 140 would present symptomatically.

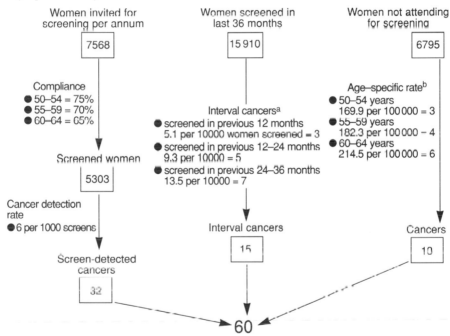

Figure 6: Source of breast cancers detected in the age group eligible for screening. Notional health authority. Population eligible for screening = 22 705.[a] Assuming NWR BSP interval cancer rates.[146] [b] Assuming 1986 OPCS age-specific incidence rates.

The stage distribution of the 172 breast cancer cases occurring in the notional HA has been estimated using 1992 data supplied by the East Anglian Cancer Registry.[10] The proportion of women with stage I high grade tumours has been estimated using unpublished data held by the North Western Regional Cancer Registry. Operative rates were derived from analysis of the Hospital Episode System. These data have been used to suggest a possible treatment profile for these 172 cases (Figure 7).

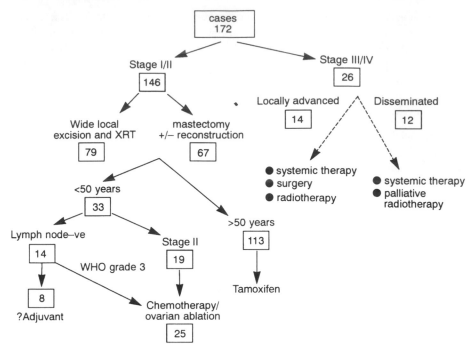

Figure 7: Treatment profile for breast cancer in notional health authority.

Resource implications for notional health authority

The resource implications for this notional HA which follow from the diagnosis and management of these screen-detected and symptomatic cases are now outlined.

Women attending the National Health Service Breast Screening Programme

Manpower requirements have been estimated by the Forrest Working Party and the NHSBSP for the minimum eligible population of a screening centre.[6,42,181,182]

The notional HA alone would not be large enough to support a screening centre. Its pro-rata contribution to the costs of a screening centre is outlined in Table 8.

Table 8: Manpower requirements for notional health authority

	Manpower recommendations	Notional HA (22 705 eligible women)
Radiologist	0.4 wte/ 41 150 eligible population	0.2 wte
Radiographer	4 wte/ 41 150 eligible population	2.2 wte
Surgeon	0.3 wte/ 41 150 eligible population	0.15 wte
Pathologist	0.2 wte/ 41 150 eligible population	0.1 wte
Clerical	3 wte/ 41 150 eligible population	1.5 wte
Medical physics	1 wte/ 15 screening sets	0.1 wte

Women presenting with symptoms suggestive of breast cancer

Resource requirements for diagnostic services are driven by the number of women referred with a breast-related problem of whom, it must be stressed, only a small proportion will have breast cancer.

It has been estimated that for every breast cancer there are seven or eight new referrals of women with other breast problems.[16,17] If the notional HA generates 140 new cases of symptomatic breast cancer the total number of new referrals to the symptomatic service will be 1120–1260.

An audit of the workload of one consultant undertaking all the breast work within a DGH with a catchment population of 212 000 found that outpatient referrals for breast problems constituted 60% of the consultant's workload (approximately 800 referrals) and 20% of the operative workload.[183] The consultant's workload was in excess of that suggested by the Royal College of Surgeons[184] and the authors concluded that one wte consultant breast surgeon is required per 1000 new referrals. This assumption requires validation.

Summary

The key issues for purchasers are:

- the optimum scheduling of screening visits has yet to be determined
- there is variable service provision for the assessment and treatment of women with breast cancer outside of the screening programme
- the report of the Expert Advisory Group has major implications for the provision of local breast cancer services.

8 Outcome measures

National Health Service Breast Screening Programme

The impact of screening on mortality may not be apparent for at least a decade after its implementation.[29] Four interim measures of programme effectiveness have been suggested:

1 compliance
2 cancer detection rate
3 interval cancers
4 characteristics of screen–detected cancers.

Compliance

The minimum standard for the NHSBSP is an uptake of 70% among women invited for screening. The uptake of primary screening in 1993/94 was 72.1%; this varied from 62% in North West Thames to 79% in East Anglia.[44]

Cancer detection rate

The cancer detection rate is the number of screen-detected cancers per 1000 screens in the eligible population.

The minimum standard for the NHSBSP is five cancers per 1000 screens in the prevalence round and 3.5 per 1000 in the incident round. The overall cancer detection rate for the NHSBSP in 1993/94 was 5.1 per 1000 screens: 5.7 per 1000 in the prevalence round and 3.8 per 1000 in the incident round.[44]

Interval cancers

An interval cancer is a cancer occurring in a woman between screens (see page 369). The NHSBSP standards are 2–3, 4–5 and 7–8 interval cancers per 10 000 screens for the first 12 months, 12–24 months and 24–36 months respectively after screening.

The interval cancer rate in the North Western Regional Breast Screening Programme was 5.1, 9.3 and 13.5 per 10 000 screens at 12, 12–24 and 24–36 months respectively after screening.[146] These rates are substantially higher than the NHSBSP targets.

The NHSBSP standards are currently being revised.

Characteristics of screen-detected cancers

It is hoped that screening will lead to the detection of a higher proportion of prognostically favourable tumours. Generally women with grade 3 tumours have a poor prognosis but this is markedly improved if the tumour is less than 15 mm. Data from the Swedish Two Counties Trial suggests that over 30% of grade 3 tumours should be less than 15 mm.[40]

Analysis of pathology reports from women with screen-detected cancer in the North Western Regional Breast Screening Programme between 1 March 1988 and 31 March 1992 has shown that over 30% of invasive grade 3 tumours were less than 15 mm (unpublished data).

Diagnosis and treatment

There are no routine indicators used to assess the quality, effectiveness and efficiency of diagnostic and treatment services. Standards for the symptomatic service have been set by the Cancer Relief Macmillan Fund[185] and the British Association of Surgical Oncologists.[176]

The following list of audit topics may be helpful in assessing the quality of breast cancer diagnostic and treatment services. Their provenance can be found in the previous discussion on service provision and effectiveness.

Although delays in diagnosis, referral and treatment routinely experienced by women in the NHS are unlikely to effect outcome, they are important QA issues.

The Cancer Relief Macmillan Fund suggests the following standard: 'a firm diagnosis within four weeks of being referred to a hospital by a general practitioner'.[185]

The Joint Committee for Clinical Oncology has set national standards for waiting times for post-operative radiotherapy for early breast cancer of four weeks and for palliative radiotherapy of 48 hours.[186]

Breast imaging

Topics suitable for audit include:

- availability and appropriate use of mammography and ultrasound for the investigation of symptomatic women
- technical performance of diagnostic mammography sets; these are not subject to the strict external QA guidelines found in the NHSBSP.

Adequacy of fine-needle aspiration cytology

Inadequate rates have been shown to vary considerably between operators.

Intraoperative frozen biopsies

Intraoperative frozen biopsies to diagnose clinically suspicious lesions are rarely necessary and are undesirable because they limit the involvement of women in treatment decisions.

Adequacy of pathology reporting

Pathology reports of breast cancer specimens should include, wherever appropriate, a description of:

- histological type, size and grade of tumour
- the adequacy of excision margins.

The rate and adequacy of axillary node surgery

The frequency with which axillary lymph nodes are sampled in premenopausal women is an important indicator of the quality of surgical management. At least four nodes should be available for assessment.

Rate of referral for radiotherapy following BCT

All appropriate women should be referred for radiotherapy following BCT. The need for radiotherapy in 'minimal risk' tumours will be clarified by ongoing trials.

Rate of referral for consideration of adjuvant therapy

All women with high risk early breast cancer should be offered adjuvant therapy. All premenopausal node-positive women should be offered chemotherapy.

Training and qualification of breast care nurses

A survey of breast care nurses in the UK revealed that a significant proportion may not have received recognized training in counselling skills or in oncology.[64]

Screening for asymptomatic metastases

The routine use of liver/bone/CT scans and X-rays in preoperative staging and follow-up regimens is not recommended.

9 Targets

Breast cancer is a key target area in The Health of the Nation.[1] The target is 'To reduce the death rate from breast cancer in the population invited for screening by at least 25% by the year 2000 (baseline 1990)'. A third of breast cancer deaths occur in this age group.[12]

National Health Service Breast Screening Programme

The Health of the Nation target coincides with the target set by the NHSBSP.

Diagnosis and treatment

There are no official targets.

Summary

The key issues for purchasers are:

- the Health of the Nation target is 'To reduce the death rate from breast cancer in the population invited for screening by at least 25% by the year 2000 (baseline 1990)'
- there are four key interim measures for evaluating the success of the NHSBSP
  a) compliance
  b) cancer detection rate
  c) interval cancer rate
  d) characteristics of screen-detected cancers
- there are QA standards for the NHSBSP
- there are a number of areas where clinical audit can be used to assess the quality of local symptomatic services.

10 Information and research

Information

Cancer registries

The importance of cancer registries has been emphasized by the report of the Expert Advisory Group.[2] Cancer registration data allow for:

- description of the burden of disease in the population
- evaluation of the effectiveness of the screening programme
- population-based investigations of variation in the clinical management of breast cancer.

Extent of disease at presentation has not in the past been collected routinely by many cancer registries but is now part of the minimum data set. This will enable cancer registries to contribute more extensively to the evaluation of the screening programme and of diagnostic and therapeutic strategies provided in defined populations.

Changes in the structure of RHAs will result in cancer registry contracts being devolved to lead purchasers after 1996.

National Health Service Breast Screening Programme

Information on the achievement of NHSBSP standards is available at national, regional and screening office level. There are some limitations to the current method of collating screening data particularly in providing district level information and in linking screening related events for individual women. The system is currently being improved.

Hospital information systems

Accurate estimates of resources used in diagnosis and treatment of breast cancer are currently limited by a lack of routinely available hospital activity data and financial information. This may improve following the implementation of the outpatient minimum data set and health care resource groups for radiotherapy.[187]

Research priorities

Primary prevention

There are no proven strategies for the primary prevention of breast cancer although a number are currently under investigation.

Tamoxifen has been shown to reduce the risk of a woman developing a second primary cancer in the contralateral breast by 39%.[9] Randomized controlled trials to assess the effectiveness of tamoxifen in reducing breast cancer in women at increased risk because of a family history or previous breast disease are currently underway in the UK, Europe and the US.[188,189]

Tamoxifen may also reduce the risk of heart disease and osteoporosis but concerns have been expressed following the increased risk of endometrial cancer observed in the ongoing trials of tamoxifen regimens in women with breast cancer.[190]

Family history clinics

The availability of predictive genetic testing following the cloning of the BRCA1 gene has major implications for purchasers.

Predictive genetic testing is a potentially resource intensive intervention for which the likely demand for services is difficult to predict. While it has been shown that the majority of first degree relatives of women with breast cancer may express an interest in undergoing genetic testing, experience with testing for Huntington's disease has demonstrated that interest is not always followed by demand.[191]

In addition there are ethical, social and public health implications to predictive genetic testing. Effective management options for young women found to be at high risk of breast cancer are not available. The acceptability and long-term psychosexual impact of prophylactic mastectomy and the psychosocial effects of awareness of carrier status are unknown. It is imperative that predictive genetic testing is fully evaluated before it enters routine use.

Screening policy

Issues that remain to be resolved include the cost-effectiveness of raising the age limit of screening or reducing the screening interval to two years.

Breast imaging

New techniques for imaging the breast are being developed. They include magnetic resonance imaging (MRI) and digital mammography.[192]

The usefulness of MRI in the diagnosis of symptomatic breast cancer, identification of recurrences following BCT and monitoring of response to systemic therapy is currently being assessed. At present MRI remains primarily a research tool.

Digital mammography is being evaluated as a screening test and in the localization of impalpable tumours. There is no evidence as yet of the superiority of this technique over conventional mammography although it may provide opportunity for cost savings from the reduced storage space required for optical discs. A full health technology assessment is needed before it is introduced routinely.

Systemic therapy in breast cancer

The World Overview provided valuable information on the role of adjuvant therapy in early breast cancer.[9] However a number of important clinical questions remain, some of which may be addressed by ongoing trials.[193–198] The results of the third World Overview with 15 years of follow-up of trials of adjuvant therapy are also awaited.

- There is a need to clarify which subgroups of node-negative women would benefit from adjuvant chemotherapy (or ovarian ablation). A number of trials are currently ongoing.
- The World Overview suggested that prolonged use of tamoxifen for at least five years may confer additional survival benefit over regimens of two years or less. No firm conclusion could be drawn as the sample size was small and estimates were considered unreliable. Confirmation of the benefit of prolonged use of tamoxifen is awaited from various trials.
- Cyclophosphamide, methotrexate and fluorouracil is the most commonly used regimen in this country. The addition of adriamycin to multi-agent regimens has gained favour with some clinicians. Optimum chemotherapeutic regimens remain to be clarified.
- The role of chemoendocrine therapy in postmenopausal women and of endocrine therapy in premenopausal women also remains to be clarified by ongoing trials.
- Primary treatment with chemotherapy or tamoxifen prior to surgery (neoadjuvant therapy) is an alternative management strategy which aims to downstage large breast tumours and facilitate BCT.[199] The results of ongoing RCTs are awaited.
- A subgroup of high-risk women with ten or more involved lymph nodes has been identified. High-dose chemotherapy with autologous bone marrow transplant or support with haemopoietic factors has been suggested for this group. This resource intensive therapy has a high case mortality rate. Randomized controlled trials are ongoing.[128]

The role of systemic therapy in advanced disease is even less clear and an overview of published trials could aid rational clinical management decisions. Paclitaxel (taxol) is a new chemotherapeutic agent which has been shown in non-randomized studies to reduce symptomatology in women with metastatic breast cancer.[200,201] There is as yet no evidence from RCTs of it superiority over conventional chemotherapeutic agents.

Radiotherapy schedules

Treatment schedules for radical radiotherapy vary from three to six weeks. This variation appears to reflect training and institutional policy rather than patient factors.[107] Shorter regimens can potentially reduce waiting times and costs. The morbidity of the different schedules is not known and urgent evaluation is required.

Breast cancer in the elderly

Over half of all breast cancers occur in women aged over 70. Advanced disease at presentation is more common in older women (Table 9).

Table 9: Stage of presentation by age

	Less than 50 years (%)	50–64 years (%)	65 years and over (%)
Stages I and II	86	88	69
Stages III and IV	14	12	31

Source: East Anglian Cancer Registry[19]

The relative survival of women with breast cancer in the UK decreases markedly with age. This age differential is not seen in the US and may reflect a reluctance in this country to deliver radical treatment either because of greater comorbidity in older women or the need to ration resources (Figure 8). This is a cause for concern because the average life expectancies of women aged 75 and 85 in England and Wales are 11.2 and 6.1 years respectively.

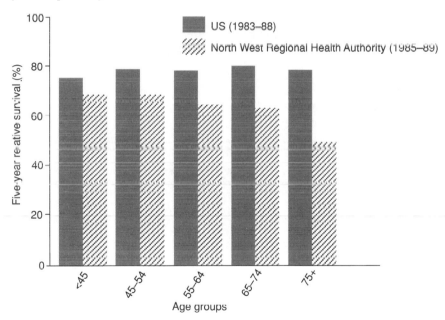

Figure 8: International comparison of age-specific survival from breast cancer.
(Sources: North Western Regional Cancer Registry, Surveillance Epidemiology and End Results programme.[32])

Some clinicians have favoured the use of tamoxifen alone in elderly women with operable tumours. One RCT demonstrated no difference in disease-free survival between elderly women treated with tamoxifen alone and those treated by surgery.[202] However a subsequent RCT comparing tamoxifen alone with tamoxifen and surgery did demonstrate an increased locoregional recurrence rate in the tamoxifen only group.[203,204] This strategy is no longer recommended.

Elderly women are a heterogenous group. Some will benefit from management regimens at present reserved for younger women. Further evaluation of treatment regimens are required in this age group.

Summary

The key issues for purchasers are:

- information
  a) cancer registration data are essential for evaluation of the screening programme and monitoring of the quality of breast cancer services
  b) there is a paucity of hospital activity and costing information on symptomatic cancer services
- research
  a) current research into lowering the age limit for screening and the primary prevention of breast cancer using tamoxifen may have significant implications for purchasers
  b) the cost-effectiveness of raising the age of the screening programme and reducing the interval of call/recall needs early evaluation
  c) predictive genetic testing has major public health implications and should be fully evaluated before introduction into routine clinical use
  d) more attention should be focused on improving the survival of elderly women with breast cancer
  e) clarification of management strategies requires the recruitment of women into breast cancer trials. This has major resource implications for provider units.

Appendix I Relevant coding classifications

ICD 9

International statistical classification of diseases: injuries and causes of death. Ninth revision.

174	malignant neoplasia of the female breast (excludes: skin of breast)
174.0	nipple and areola
174.1	central portion
174.2	upper inner quadrant
174.3	lower inner quadrant
174.4	upper outer quadrant
174.5	lower outer quadrant
174.6	axillary tail
174.8	other
174.9	breast unspecified
233.0	ductal carcinoma *in situ*

ICD 0

International classification of diseases for oncology.

174	malignant neoplasia of the female breast (excludes: skin of breast)
174.0	nipple and areolae
174.1	central portion
174.2	upper inner quadrant
174.3	lower inner quadrant
174.4	upper outer quadrant
174.5	lower outer quadrant
174.6	axillary tail
174.8	inner breast
	lower breast
	midline of breast
	outer breast
	upper breast
174.9	female breast NOS
233.0	ductal carcinoma *in situ*

behaviour code /3 malignant /2 *in situ*

ICD 10

Tenth revision.

C50	malignant neoplasia of breast (excludes: skin of breast)
C50.0	nipple and areolae
C50.1	central portion of breast

C50.2	upper inner quadrant of breast
C50.3	lower inner quadrant of breast
C50.4	upper outer quadrant of breast
C50.5	lower outer quadrant of breast
C50.6	axillary tail of breast
C50.8	overlapping lesion of breast
C50.9	breast unspecified

ICD 0

Second edition.

C50	breast (excludes: skin of breast)
C50.0	nipple and areolae
C50.1	central portion of breast
C50.2	upper inner quadrant of breast
C50.3	lower inner quadrant of breast
C50.4	upper outer quadrant of breast
C50.5	lower outer quadrant of breast
C50.6	axillary tail of breast
C50.8	overlapping lesion of breast
	inner breast
	lower breast
	midline of breast
	outer breast
	upper breast
C50.9	breast NOS mammary gland

behaviour code /2 *in situ* /3 malignant neoplasia

Diagnostic related groups

DRG	Description of group
257	Total mastectomy for malignancy with CC
258	Total mastectomy for malignancy W/O CC
259	Subtotal mastectomy for malignancy with CC
260	Subtotal mastectomy for malignancy W/O CC
268	Skin, subcutaneous tissue and breast plastic procedures
274	Malignant breast disorders with CC
275	Malignant breast disorders without CC
409	Radiotherapy
410	Chemotherapy

CC = complications or comorbidity

Appendix II Staging classifications

Clinical staging

- **Stage 0** CIS only.
- **Stage I** Tumour 2 cm or less in greatest dimension, no metastasis
- **Stage IIA** Tumour less than 2 cm in greatest dimension, metastasis to movable ipsilateral axillary lymph node(s), no distant metastasis; or tumour more than 2 cm but not more than 5 cm in greatest dimension, no metastasis.
- **Stage IIB** Tumour more than 2 cm but not more than 5 cm in greatest dimension, metastasis to movable ipsilateral axillary lymph node(s); or tumour more than 5 cm in greatest dimension, no metastasis.
- **Stage IIIA** Tumour of any size, metastasis to ipsilateral lymph node(s) fixed to one another or to other structures, no distant metastasis.
- **Stage IIIB** Tumour of any size with direct extension to chest wall or skin, metastasis to ipsilateral lymph nodes, no distant metastasis; or any type of tumour, metastasis to ipsilateral mammary lymph node(s), no distant metastasis.
- **Stage IV** Tumour of any size, with or without lymph node(s) involvement, but with distant metastasis.

TNM staging

The TNM system, in which T defines primary tumour, N regional lymph nodes and M distant metastasis.
Primary tumour (T) is further sub-divided into:

T0	No evidence of primary tumour
Tis	Carcinoma *in situ*
T1	Tumour 2 cm or less in greatest dimension
T2	Tumour more than 2 cm but not more than 5 cm in greatest dimension
T3	Tumour more than 5 cm in greatest dimension
T4	Tumour of any size with direct extension to chest wall or skin

Regional lymph nodes (N) are sub-divided into:

N0	No regional lymph node metastasis
N1	Metastasis to movable ipsilateral axillary lymph node(s)
N2	Metastasis to ipsilateral axillary lymph node(s) fixed to one another or to other structures
N3	Metastasis to ipsilateral internal mammary lymph nodes

Distant metastases (M) are sub-divided into:

M0	No distant metastasis
M1	Distant metastasis (includes metastasis to ipsilateral supraclavicular lymph nodes)

Appendix III Age-specific incidence rates for breast cancer

Age group (years)	Rate per 100 000 population
Under 1	0.6
1–4	0.1
5–9	0.1
10–14	0.1
15–19	0.2
20–24	0.2
25–29	1.2
30–34	24.6
35–39	57.3
40–44	105.5
45–49	160.4
50–54	181.1
55–59	214.7
60–64	257.5
65–69	253.4
70–74	254.4
75–79	274.5
80–84	285.0
85 and over	356.0

Source: OPCS Cancer Registration (1989) Series MB1, No. 22

Appendix IV National Health Service Breast Screening Programme

Objective	Criteria	Acceptable standard	Achievable standard
To maximize the number of eligible women attending for screening	Proportion of eligible women who attend for screening	70% of women to be invited for screening	75%
To maximize the number of cancers detected	The rate of cancers detected in eligible women invited and screened (including CIS)	Greater than 50 in 10 000 (1st screen) Greater than 35 in 10 000 (routine re screen)	60 per 10 000 (1st screen)
To maximize the number of small cancers	The proportion of invasive cancers equal to or less than 10 mm in diameter detected in eligible women invited and screened	15 in 10 000	
To achieve optimum image quality	a) High contrast spatial resolution b) Minimal detectable contrast (approx.) 5–6 mm detail, 0.5 mm detail	10 lp/mm 1% 5%	
To limit radiation dose	Average glandular dose per film to average breast using a grid	Less than 2 mGy	
To minimize the number of women undergoing repeat films	Number of repeated examinations	Less than 3% of total examinations	Less than 2%
To minimize the number of women referred for further tests	Onward referral assessment	Less than 7% of women screened	5% first screen 3% routine re-screen
To minimize the number of unnecessary invasive procedures	a) Malignant to benign biopsy ratio b) PPV c) Benign biopsy rate	1:1 50% Less than 50 per 10 000 (first screen) Less than 35 per 10 000 (routine re-screen)	1.5:1 60% Less than 40 per 10 000 (first screen)
To minimize the number of cancers in women screened between screening episodes	The proportion of cancers presenting in screened women in the subsequent 12 months after screening	Not more than three per 10 000 women screened	

References

1 *The Health of the Nation: A Strategy for Health in England.* London: HMSO, 1992.
2 Report of the Expert Advisory Group to the Chief Medical Officers of England and Wales. *A Policy Framework for Commissioning Cancer Services.* London: HMSO, 1995.
3 CRC Cancer Factsheet No. 6. *Breast Cancer.* CRC Promotions Ltd, 1991.
4 OPCS *Mortality Statistics; General. England and Wales. 1992.* Series DH. No. 27. London: HMSO, 1993.
5 Carter CL, Allen C, Henson DE. Relation of tumour size, lymph node status and survival in 24 740 breast cancer cases. *Cancer* 1989; **63**: 181–7.
6 *Breast cancer screening.* Report to the Health Ministers of England, Wales, Scotland and N. Ireland. Working group chaired by Sir Patrick Forrest. London: HMSO, 1986.
7 *Cervical and Breast Screening in England.* Report by the Comptroller and Auditor General. London: HMSO, 1992.
8 Veronesi U, Saccozzi R, Del Vecchio M. Comparing radical mastectomy with quadrantectomy, axillary dissection and radiation in patients with small cancer of the breast. *NEJM* 1981; **305**: 6–11.
9 Early breast cancer trialists' collaborative group. Systemic treatment of early breast cancer by hormonal, cytotoxic or immune therapy. *Lancet* 1992; **339**: 1–15; 71–84.
10 NHSBSP. *A response to the functions and manpower review.* December 1993.
11 *Hospital Episode Statistics Vol. 2 1991/92.* Department of Health. London: HMSO, 1995.
12 *Cancer statistics registrations England and Wales.* OPCS Series MB1 No. 22 1989. HMSO, 1995.
13 Gough DB, Donohue JH, Evans MM *et al.* A 50 year experience of male breast cancer: is outcome changing? *Surg Oncol* 1993; **2**: 325–33.
14 Thompson WD. Genetic epidemiology of breast cancer. *Cancer Supplement* 1994; **74(1)**: 279–87.
15 Dixon JM, Mansel RE. Symptoms, assessment and guidelines for referral. *BMJ* 1995; **309**: 722–6.
16 Barclay M, Carter D, Horrobin JM *et al.* Patterns of presentation of breast disease over ten years in a specialised clinic. *Health Bulletin* 1991; **41/4**: 229–36.
17 Dawson C, Reece Smith H, Lancashire MJ *et al.* Breast disease and the general surgeon: I referral of patients with breast problems. *Annal Surg Oncol* 1993; **73**: 79–86.
18 Information supplied by Wessex Cancer Intelligence Unit, 1994.
19 Information supplied by East Anglian Cancer Registry, 1994.
20 Van Dongen, Holland R, Peterseis JL *et al.* Ductal carcinoma in situ of the breast; second EORTC Consensus Meeting. *Eur J Cancer* 1992; **28**: 626–9.
21 Evans AJ, Wilson ARM, Pinder SE *et al.* Ductal carcinoma in situ: imaging, pathology and treatment. *Imaging* 1994; **6**: 171–4.
22 Harris J, Lippman ME, Veronesi U *et al.* Breast cancer. *NEJM* 1992; **6**: 390–8.
23 Kamby C. The pattern of metastases in human breast cancer: methodological aspects and influence of prognostic factors. *Cancer Treatment Review* 1990; **17**: 37–61.
24 Fentiman IS, Cuzick J, Millis RR *et al.* Which patients are cured of breast cancer? *BMJ.* 1984; **289**: 1108–11.
25 OPCS. *Mortality statistics: cause. England and Wales 1992.* Series DH2 No. 19. London: HMSO, 1993.
26 Pat Prior. Personal communication, 1995.
27 Garfinkel L, Buring C, Heath C *et al.* Changing trends: An overview of breast cancer incidence and mortality. *Cancer Supplement* 1994; **74(1)**: 222–7.
28 Beral V, Herman C, Reeves G *et al.* Sudden fall in breast cancer death rates in England and Wales. *Letter to Lancet*, June 24, 1995.

29 Day NE, Williams DRR, Khaw KT. Breast cancer screening programmes; the development of a monitoring and evaluation system. *Br J Cancer* 1987; **59**: 954–8.

30 Forman D, Rider L (eds). *Cancer in Yorkshire. 3 Breast Cancer*. Leeds: Yorkshire Cancer Organisation, 1995.

31 Woodman CBJ, Wilson S, Hare L *et al. Cancer in the North Western Region*. Manchester: Centre for Cancer Epidemiology, 1993.

32 Miller BA, Ries LAG, Hankey BF *et al.* (eds) *Cancer Statistics Review, 1973–1989*. National Cancer Institute NIH Publ. No. 92–2789.

33 Joslin C, Rider L, Round C *et al. Yorkshire Cancer Registry Report for Year 1991 including cancer statistics for 1984–1988*. Yorkshire Regional Cancer Organisation, 1991.

34 Woodman CBJ, Wilson S, Prior P *et al. Cancer in The West Midlands Region 1981–88*. West Midlands Regional Cancer Registry, 1989.

35 Giles GG, Armstrong BK, Smith LR. *Cancer in Australia 1982*. Cancer Statistics Publications No.1. Australian Association of Cancer Registries and Australian Institute of Health.

36 Black RJ, Sharp L, Kendick SW. *Trends in cancer survival in Scotland 1968–90*. Information and Statistics Division. Edinburgh: National Health Service in Scotland, 1993.

37 Cancer Research Campaign. *Survival – England and Wales*. Factsheet 9.1. CRC Promotions Ltd, 1988.

38 National Institute of Canada. *Canadian Cancer Stastics 1991*. Toronto, Canada, 1991.

39 Gasparin G, Pozza F, Harris AL. Evaluating the potential usefulness of new prognostic and predictive indicators in node-negative breast cancer patients. *JNCI* 1993; **85(15)**: 1206–19.

40 Tabar L, Gunnar F, Duffey SW *et al.* Update of Swedish Two County programme of mammographic screening for breast cancer. Breast imaging: current status and future directions. *Radiol Clin North Am*. 1992; **1**: 187–209.

41 Pathology reporting in breast cancer screening. Royal College of Pathologists Working Group. *J Clin Pathol* 1991; **44**: 710–25 .

42 *Quality assurance guidelines for medical physics services*. NHSBSP, 1995.

43 *Statistics supplied by the Cancer Screening Evaluation Unit*, Institute of Cancer Research.

44 DH Statistics Division 2B. *Breast cancer screening. 1993–4*. Summary information from Form KC62. England. London: DOH, 1995.

45 NHSE EL(95)7. London: HMSO.

46 Evans D, Fentiman I, McPherson K *et al.* Familial breast cancer. *BMJ* 1994; **308**: 183–7.

47 Porter DE, Steel CM, Cohen BB. Genetic linkage analysis applied to unaffected women from families with breast cancer can discriminate high from low risk individuals. *Br J Surg* 1993; **80**: 1381–5

48 Miki Y, Swensen J, Shattuck-Eidens D *et al.* A strong candidate for the breast and ovarian cancer susceptibility gene BRCA1. *Science* 1994; **266**: 66–71.

49 Gareth Evans. Personal communication, 1995.

50 Ponder BJA. Setting up and running a familial cancer clinic. *Br Med Bull.* 1994; **50(3)**: 732–45.

51 Houtston RS, Lemoine L, McCarter E *et al.* Screening and genetic counselling in relatives of patients with breast cancer in a family cancer clinic. *J Med Genetics* 1992; **29**: 691–4.

52 McCormick A, Fleming D, Charlton J. *Morbidity statistics from General Practice. Fourth National Study 1991–2*. OPCS. Series MB5 No. 3. London: HMSO, 1995.

53 Roberts MM, Elton RA, Robinson SE *et al.* Consultations for breast disease in general practice and hospital referral patterns. *Br J Surg* 1987; **74**: 1020–2.

54 Nichols S, Wales WC, Wheeler MJ. Management of female breast disease by Southampton general practitioners. *Br Med J* 1980; **281**: 1450–3

55 Holland PA, Bundred NJ. The management of ductal carcinoma in situ. *The Breast* 1994; **3**: 1–2.

56 Sacks N, Barr L, Allan S *et al.* The role of axillary dissection in operable breast cancer. *The Breast* 1992; **1**: 41–9.

57 Watson JD, Sainsbury JRC, Dixon JM. Breast reconstruction after surgery. *BMJ* 1995; **310**: 117–21.

58 Dixon JM. Breast reconstruction. *Br J Surg* 1995; **82**: 865–6.

59 Hortobagyi G. Multidisciplinary management of advanced primary and metastatic breast cancer. *Cancer Supplement* 1994; **74(1)**: 416–23.

60 Rubens RD. Improving treatment for advanced breast cancer. *Cancer Surveys*. 1993; **18**: 199–207.

61 Coleman RE, Rubens RD. The clinical course of bone metastases in breast cancer. *Br J Cancer* 1987; **55**: 61–6.

62 Maguire P, Tait A, Brooke M *et al*. Effect of counselling on the psychiatric morbidity associated with mastectomy. *BMJ* 1980; **281**: 1454–6.

63 Royal College of Nursing. *Standards of care for breast care nursing*. 1994.

64 Tait A. *Breast cancer nursing*. A report to Cancer Relief Macmillan Fund, 1994.

65 Rees GJ, Deutsch GP, Dunlop PRC *et al*. Royal College of Radiologists' survey. Clinical oncology services to District General Hospitals: Report of a Working Party of the Royal College of Radiologists. *Clin Oncol* 1991; **3**: 41–5.

66 Hospital Episode System data supplied by the Department of Health, 1995.

67 Association of Cancer Physicians: *Review of the Pattern of Cancer Services in England and Wales*. ACP, 1994.

68 *Summary of radiotherapy machine activity. England. Financial year 1992/3*. DOH statistics Division 2. London: HMSO, 1993.

69 Morris J, Farmes A, Royle G. Recent changes in surgical management of T1/2 breast cancer in England. *Eur J Cancer* 1992; **28a(10)**: 1709–12.

70 Fletcher S W, Black W, Harris R *et al*. Report of the International workshop on screening for breast cancer. *JNCI* 1993; **85(20)**: 1644–56.

71 Nystrom L, Rutqvist LE, Wall S *et al*. Breast cancer screening with mammography: overview of Swedish randomised trials. *Lancet* 1993; **341**: 973–8.

72 Peer PGM. Age dependent growth rate of primary breast cancer. *Cancer* 1993; **71(11)**: 3547–51.

73 Ellman R, Moss SM, Coleman D *et al*. Breast self examination programmes in the early detection of breast cancer: 10 year findings. *Br J Cancer* 1993; **68**: 208–12.

74 Semiglazov V F. Study of the role of breast self examination in the reduction of mortality from breast cancer. *Eur J Cancer* 1993; **29a(14)**: 2039–46.

75 Clarke PR, Fraser NM. *Economic analysis of screening for breast cancer*. Report for Scottish Home and Health Department, 1991.

76 Donegan W. Evaluation of a palpable breast mass. *New Eng J Med* 1992; **327(13)**: 937–42.

77 Hermansen C, Poulsen HS, Jensen J *et al*. Diagnostic reliability of combined physical examination, mammography and fine needle puncture ('triple test') in breast lumps. A prospective study. *Cancer* 1987; **60**: 1866–71.

78 Hardy JR, Powles TJ, Judson I *et al*. How many tests are required in the diagnosis of palpable breast abnormalities? *Clin Oncol* 1990; **21**: 48–52.

79 Edeiken S. Mammography and palpable breast cancer. *Cancer* 1988; **61**: 263–5.

80 Perre CI, Koot CM, de Hooge *et al*. The value of ultrasound in the evaluation of palpable breast tumours. A prospective study of 400 cases. *Eur J Surg Oncol* 1994; **20**: 637–40.

81 Dixon JM, Mansel RE. Symptoms, assessment and guidelines for referral. *BMJ* 1994; **309**: 722–6.

82 Wilkinson EJ, Schuette CM, Ferrier CM *et al*. Fine needle aspiration of breast masses. *Acta Cytologica* 1989; **33(5)**: 613–9.

83 Dixon JM, Anderson TJ, Lamb J *et al*. Fine needle aspiration cytology in relationship to clinical examination and mammography in the diagnosis of a solid mass. *Br J Surgery* 1984; **71**: 593–6.

84 Ciatto S. Fine needle aspiration cytology of the breast: review of 9533 consecutive cases of breast cancer. *The Breast* 1993; **2**: 87–90.

85 Wells CA. Quality assurance in breast cancer screening cytology. A review of the literature and a report to the UK National Scheme. *Eur J Cancer* 1995: **31a(2)**: 273–80.

86 Gui GP, Allum WH, Perry NM *et al.* Clinical audit of a specialist symptomatic breast clinic. *J R Soc Med.* 1995; **88**: 330–3.

87 Ciatto S, Cariaggi P, Bulgaresi P *et al.* Preoperative staging of primary breast cancer. A multicentre study. *Cancer* 1988; **61**: 1038–40.

88 Fisher B, Constantino J, Redmond C *et al.* Lumpectomy compared with lumpectomy and radiation therapy for treatment of intraductal breast cancer. *NEJM* 1993: **328**: 1582–6.

89 Silverstein MJ, Poller DN, Waisman JR *et al.* Prognostic classification of breast ductal carcinoma in situ. *Lancet* 1995; **345**: 1154–7.

90 Fisher B, Redmond C, Poisson R *et al.* Eight year results of a randomised clinical trial comparing total mastectomy and lumpectomy with or without irradiation in the treatment of breast cancer. *New Engl J Med* 1989; **32**: 822–8.

91 Lichter AS, Lippman ME, Danforth DN *et al.* Mastectomy vs breast conserving therapy in the treatment of stage I and II carcinoma of the breast: a randomised trial of the National Cancer Institute. *J Clin Oncol* 1992; **10**: 976–83.

92 Cabanes PA , Salmon RJ, Vilos JR. Value of axillary dissection in addition to lumpectomy and radiotherapy in early breast cancer. *Lancet* 1992; **339**: 1245–8.

93 Forrest APM, Everington D, McDonald C *et al.* The Edinburgh randomised trial of axillary sampling or clearance after mastectomy. *Br J Surg* 1995; **82**: 1504–8.

94 Veronesi U. Radiotherapy and breast preserving surgery in women with localised cancer of the breast. *New Eng J Med* 1993; **328:22**: 1587–91.

95 Haybittle JL, Brinkley D, Houghton J *et al.* Postoperative radiotherapy and late mortality: evidence from the Cancer Research Campaign trial for early breast cancer. *BMJ* 1989; **298**: 1611–4.

96 Cuzick J, Stewart H, Rutqvist L *et al.* Cause-specific mortality in long term survivors of breast cancer who participated in trials of radiotherapy. *J Clin Oncol* 1994; **12**: 447–53

97 Priestman T, Bullimore JA, Godden TP *et al.* The Royal College of Radiologists' fractionation survey. *Clin Oncol* 1989; **1**: 39–46.

98 Penn CRH. Megavoltage irradiation in a DGH remote from a main oncology centre: The Torbay Experience Reviewed. *Clin Oncol* 1992; **4**: 108–13.

99 Goddard M, Hutton J. *Cost of radiotherapy.* York: University of York, 1988.

100 Christensen SB, Lundgren E. Sequelae of axillary dissection vs axillary sampling with or without radiotherapy. *Acta Chir Scand* 1989; **155**: 515–20

101 Steele RJC, Forrest APM, Gibson T *et al.* The efficacy of lower axillary sampling in obtaining lymph node status in breast cancer: a controlled randomised trial. *Br J Surg* 1988; **72**: 368–9.

102 Christensen SB, Jansson C. Axillary biopsy compared with dissection in the staging of axillary lymph nodes in operable breast cancer. *Eur J Surg* 1993; **159**: 159–60.

103 Bundred NJ, Morgan DAL, Dixon JM. Management of regional nodes in breast cancer. *BMJ* 1995; **309**: 1222–5.

104 Gelber RD, Goldhirsch A, Coates AS. Adjuvant therapy for breast cancer: understanding the overview. *J Clin Oncol* 1993; **11(3)**: 580–5.

105 Consensus Development Conference: treatment of primary breast cancer. *BMJ* 1986; **293**: 946–7.

106 Smith TJ, Hillner B. The efficacy and cost effectiveness of adjuvant therapy in early breast cancer in premenopausal women. *J Clin Oncol* 1993; **1(4)**: 771–6

107 Hillner B, Smith TJ. Efficacy and cost effectiveness of adjuvant chemotherapy in women with node-negative breast cancer. *New Eng J Med* 1991; **324**: 160–8.

108 Glick JH, Gelbe RD, Goldhirsch A *et al.* Adjuvant therapy of primary breast cancer. 4th International Conference On Adjuvant Therapy of Breast Cancer. St Gallen Switzerland. *Annal Oncol* 1992; **3**: 801–7.

109 Harris J, Lippman M, Veronesi U *et al.* Breast cancer (third of three parts). *NEJM* 1992; **327**: 473–9.

110 Scottish Cancer Trials Breast Group and ICRF Breast Unit, Guys Hospital, London. Adjuvant ovarian ablation vs. CMF chemotherapy in premenopausal women with pathological stage II breast carcinoma: the Scottish Trial. *Lancet* 1993; **341**: 1293–8.

111 Galea M H, Blamey R W, Elston C E *et al.* The Nottingham Prognostic Index in primary breast cancer. *Breast Cancer Res Treat* 1992; **22**: 207–19.

112 Ravdin P. A practical view of prognostic factors for staging, adjuvant treatment planning and as baseline studies for possible future therapy. *Haem Oncol Clinics North Am* 1994; **81(1)**: 197–211.

113 Clark R. Randomised clinical trial to assess the effectiveness of breast irradiation following lumpectomy and axillary dissection for node negative breast cancer. *JNCI.* 1992; **84(9)**: 683–9.

114 Stewart H. South East Scottish trial of local therapy in node-negative breast cancer. *The Breast* 1994; **(3)**: 31–9.

115 Sarrazin MG, Arriagada R, Contessa G *et al.* Ten year results of a randomised control trial comparing conservation therapy to mastectomy in early breast cancer. *Radiotherap Oncol* 1989; **14**: 177–84.

116 McPherson K, Steel CM, Dixon JM. Breast cancer – epidemiology, risk factors and genetics. *BMJ* 1995; **309**: 1003–4.

117 Barr L, Skene A, Fish S *et al.* Post treatment mammography following the breast conserving treatment of breast cancer: is it of value? *The Breast* 1993; **2**: 253–4.

118 Orel SG, Fowble BL, Solin LJ. Breast cancer recurrence after lumpectomy and radiation therapy for early disease: prognostic significance of detection method. *Radiology* 1993; **188**: 189–94.

119 Del Turco MR, Palli D, Cariddi A *et al.* Intensive diagnostic follow up after treatment of primary breast cancer. A randomised control trial. *JAMA* 1994; **271(20)**: 1593–97.

120 Givio Investigators. Impact of follow up testing on survival and health related quality of life in Breast Cancer Patients. *JAMA* 1994; **271(20)**: 1587–92.

121 Ingle J N. Principles of therapy in advanced breast cancer. *Haem Oncol Clinics North Am* 1989; **3(4)**: 743–62.

122 Richards M. Advanced breast cancer: use of resources and cost implications. *Br J Cancer* 1993; **67**: 856–60.

123 Perez CA. Management of locally advanced carcinoma of the breast. *Cancer Supplement* 1994; **74 (1)**: 453–65.

124 Piccart MJ, Kerger J, Tomiak E *et al.* Systemic treatment for locally advanced breast cancer; what we still need to learn after a decade of multimodality clinical trials. *Eur J Cancer* 1992; **28(2/3)**: 667–72.

125 Glauber JG. The changing role of hormonal therapy in advanced breast cancer. *Seminars Oncol* 1992; **19(3)**: 308–16.

126 Parrazzini F, Colli E, Scatigna M *et al.* Treatment with tamoxifen and progestins for metastatic breast cancer in postmenopausal women: A quantitative review of published randomised controlled trials. *Oncol* 1993; **50**: 483–9.

127 Clavel M, Catimel G. Breast cancer: chemotherapy in the treatment of advanced disease. *Eur J Cancer* 1993; **29a(4)**: 598–604.

128 Triozzi, PL. Autologous bone marrow and peripheral blood progenitor transplant for breast cancer. *Lancet* 1994; **344**: 418–9.

129 Goddard M, Maher EJ, Hutton J *et al.* Palliative radiotherapy-counting the costs of changing practice. *Health Policy* 1991; **17**: 243–56.

130 Price P, Hoskin PJ, Easton D *et al.* Prospective randomised controlled trial of single and multifractionation radiotherapy schedule in the treatment of painful bony metastases. *Radiotherap Oncol* 1986; **6**: 247–55.

131 Tong D. The palliation of symptomatic osseous metastases. *Cancer* 1982; **50**: 893–97.

132 Barton R, Hoskins P, Yarnold Y. Radiotherapy for bone pain: is a single fraction good enough? *Clin Oncol* 1994; **6**: 354–5.

133 Pinder K, Ramirez A, Black E *et al.* Psychiatric disorder in patients with advanced breast cancer: Prevalence and associated factors. *Eur J Cancer.* 1993; **29a**: 524–7.

134 Maguire P, Pentol A, Allen D *et al.* Cost of counselling women who undergo mastectomy. *BMJ* 1982; **284**: 1933–5.

135 Maguire P *et al.* Psychiatric problems in the year after mastectomy. *BMJ* 1978; (ii): 963–5.

136 Morris J, Rolde G. Choice of surgery for early breast cancer: pre- and post-operative levels of clinical anxiety and depression in patients and their husbands. *Br J Surgery* 1987; **74**: 1017–19.

137 Fallowfield L, Baum M, Maguire GP. Effects of breast conservation on psychological morbidity associated with diagnosis and treatment of early breast cancer. *BMJ* 1994; **293**: 1331–4.

138 Schain WS. Breast reconstruction. Update of psychological and pragmatic factors. *Cancer Supplement* 1991; **68**: 1170–4.

139 Luker K, Leinster S *et al. Preferences for information and decision making in women newly diagnosed with breast cancer.* Final report. Liverpool: Liverpool Research and Development Unit, University of Liverpool, Department of Nursing, 1993.

140 Fallowfield L, Hall A, Maguire P *et al.* Psychological effects of being offered a choice of surgery for breast cancer. *BMJ* 1994; **309**: 448.

141 Roberts CS, Cox CE, Reintgen DS *et al.* Influence of physician communication on newly diagnosed breast cancer patients, psychological adjustment and decision making. *Cancer Supplement* 1994; **74**: 337–41.

142 Richards MA, Ramirez A, Degner LF *et al.* Offering choice of treatments to patients with cancer. *Eur J Cancer* 1995; **31a**: 112–16.

143 Hobbs P, Kay C, Friedman E. Response by women age 65–79 to an invitation for screening for breast cancer by mammography; a pilot study. *BMJ* 1990; **301**: 1314–6.

144 Brown M. Economic considerations in breast cancer screening in older women. *Geronto* 1992; **47**: 51–8.

145 Threlfall A. Personal communication, 1995.

146 Woodman CBJ, Threlfall AJ, Doggis CMR *et al.* Is the three year breast screening interval too long? Occurrence of interval cancers in the NHS breast screening programmes' NWR *BMJ* 1995; **319**: 224–6.

147 Day N, McCann J, Camilleri-Ferrante C *et al.* Monitoring interval cancers in breast screening programmes: the East Anglian experience. *J Med Screening* 1995; **2**: 180–5.

148 de Konig HJ, van Ineveld BM, van Oortmarssen GJ *et al.* Breast cancer screening and cost effectiveness; policy alternatives, quality of life considerations and the possible impact of uncertain factors. *Int J Cancer* 1991; **49**: 531–7.

149 Young KC, Wallis MG, Ramsdale ML. Mammographic film density and detection of small breast cancers. *Clin Radiol* 1994; **49**: 461–5.

150 Anderson EDC, Muir BB, Walsh JS *et al.* The efficacy of double reading mammograms in breast screening. *Clin Radiol* 1994; **49**: 248–51.

151 van Dijck JAAM, Verbeek ALM, Hendriks JHCL. One view vs two view mammography in baseline screening for breast cancer: a review. *Br J Radiol* 1992; **65**: 971–6.

152 UKCCCR multicentre randomised controlled trial of one and two view mammography in breast cancer screening. *BMJ* 1995; **311**: 1189–93.

153 Knox E. Evaluation of a proposed breast cancer screening regimen. *BMJ* 1988; **297**: 650–4.

154 McEwan J, King E, Bickler G. Attendance and non-attendance for breast screening service. *BMJ* 1989; **294**: 104–6.

155 Williams E, Vessey M. A randomised trial of two strategies offering women mobile breast cancer screening. *BMJ* 1989; **298**: 158–9.

156 Irwig L. A randomised trial of general practitioner written invitations to encourage attendance at screening mammography. *Comm Health Studies* 1990; **XIV(4)**: 357–63.

157 Haiart DL, Mckenzie L, Henderson J *et al.* Mobile breast screening: factors affecting uptake efforts to increase response and acceptability. *Public Health* 1990; **104**: 239–42.

158 Henderson J, Mckenzie L, Haiart D. Uptake of a mobile screening project: implications for a breast screening service. Discussion paper 04/88. Aberdeen: University of Aberdeen, Health Economics Research Unit.

159 Walker LG, Cordiner CM, Gilbert FJ. How distressing is attendance for routine breast screening? *Psycho Oncol* 1994; **3**: 299–304.

160 Dean C, Roberts MM, French K *et al.* Psychological morbidity after screening for breast cancer. *J Epid Comm Health* 1986; **40**: 71–2.

161 Orton M, Fitzpatrick R, Fuller A *et al.* Factors affecting women's response to an invitation to attend for a second breast cancer screening examination. *Br J Gen Pract* 1991; **41**: 320–3.

162 Hurley SF. The benefits and risks of mammographic screening for breast cancer. *Epidemiol Rev* 1992; **(14)**: 103–30.

163 Hoare T, Thomas C, Bradley S *et al.* Can the uptake of breast screening by Asian women be increased? A randomised controlled trial of a linkworker intervention. *J Pub Health Med* 1994; **16(2)**: 179–185.

164 Chouillet AM, Bell C, Hiscox J. Management of breast cancer in South East England. *BMJ* 1994; **308**: 168–71.

165 Sainsbury J, Rider L, Smith A *et al.* Does it matter where you live? Treatment variation for breast cancer in Yorkshire. *BJ Cancer* 1995; **71**: 1275–8.

166 Gazet JC, Rainsbury R, Ford HT *et al.* Survey of treatment of primary breast cancer in Great Britain. *BMJ* 1985; **290**: 1793–5.

167 Morris J. Changes in surgical management in early breast cancer in England. *J R Soc Med* 1989; **82**: 12–14.

168 Hainsworth P J, Henderson MA, Bennett RC. Delayed presentation in breast cancer: relationship to tumour stage and survival. *The Breast* 1993; **2**: 37–41.

169 Porta M, Gallen M, Malats. Influence of 'diagnostic delay' upon cancer survival: an analysis of five tumour sites. *J Epid Comm Health* 1991; **45(3)**: 225–30.

170 Jones RVH, Dungeon TA. Time between presentation and treatment of six common cancers: a study in Devon. *Br J Gen Pract* 1992; **42**: 419–22.

171 Bofetta P, Merletti F, Winkelman R *et al.* Survival of breast cancer patients from Piedmont Italy. *Cancer Causes Control* 1993; **4**: 209–15.

172 Bonnet A, Roder D, Esterman A. Case survival rates for infiltrating ductal carcinomas by category of hospital of diagnosis in S Australia. *Med J Aust* 1991: **154**; 695–7.

173 Karjalainen S. Geographical variation in cancer patient survival in Finland: chance, confounding or effect of treatment? *J Epid Comm Health* 1990; **44**: 210–4.

174 Lee-Feldstein A, Anton Culver A, Feldstein PJ. Treatment differences and other prognostic factors related to breast cancer survival. *JAMA* 1994; **271(15)**; 1163–68.

175 Basnett I, Gill M, Tobias JS. Variations in breast cancer management between teaching and non-teaching district. *Eur J Cancer* 1992; **28a (12)**: 1945–50.

176 The breast surgeons group of the British Association of Surgical Oncology. *Guidelines for surgeons involved in the management of symptomatic breast disease in the UK*, 1994.

177 Hand R, Sene S, Imperato J. Hospital variables associated with quality of care for breast cancer patients. *JAMA* 1991; **266(24)**: 3429–32.

178 British Breast Group. *The provision of breast services in the UK: the advantage of specialist breast units.* Report of a working party of the British Breast Group. Edinburgh: Churchill Livingstone, 1995.

179 Sainsbury R, Howard B, Rider L *et al.* Influence of clinician workload and patterns of treatment on survival from breast cancer. *Lancet* 1995; **345**: 1265–70

180 OPCS estimates of cancer incidence 1992 (unpublished).

181 *Radiographers' working practices.*1990/91, NHSBSP, 1992.

182 *Draft guidelines for surgeons.* NHSBSP, 1991.

183 Lewis WG, Donaldson KI, Sainsbury JRC. Breast surgery: a manageable specialty in the DGH? *The Breast* 1994; **3**: 24–6

184 The Royal College of Surgeons of England. *The General surgical workload and providers/purchaser contract. Notes for guidance.* December 1990.

185 *Breast cancer. How to help yourself.* Cancer Relief Macmillan Fund. May 1994.

186 Joint Council for Clinical Oncology. *Improving quality control in cancer care.* March 1993.

187 Read G. Radiotherapy in a District General Hospital. *Clin Oncol* 1994; **6**: 349–51

188 Friedman MA, Trimble EL, Abrams JS. Tamoxifen: trials, tribulations and trade offs. *JNCI* 1994, **86(7)**: 3–4.

189 Jordan VC. Tamoxifen for breast cancer prevention. *Proc Soc Exp Biol Med* 1995; **208(2)**: 144–9.

190 Fisher B, Costantino JP, Redmond CK *et al.* Endometrial cancer in tamoxifen treated breast cancer patients: findings from the National Surgical Adjuvant Breast and Bowel Project NSABP B14. *JNCI* 1994; **86(7)**: 527–37.

191 Lerman C, Daly M, Masny A, Balshem A. Attitudes about genetic testing for Breast and Ovarian Cancer susceptibility. *J Clin Oncol* 1994; **12(4)**: 843–50.

192 Adler DD, Wahl RL. New methods for imaging the breast: techniques, findings and potential. *AJR* 1995; **164**: 19–30.

193 Wood CDC. Current trials and future directions of the Eastern Cooperative Oncology Group breast cancer committee. *Cancer Supplement* 1994; **74(3)**: 1132–4.

194 Wood CDC. Progress from clinical trials on breast cancer. *Cancer Supplement* 1994; **74(9)**: 2606–9.

195 Osborne CK. Current trials and future directions of the South West Oncology group breast cancer committee *Cancer Supplement* 1994; **74(3)**: 1994.

196 Burt AM. The UKCCCR Adjuvant Breast Cancer (ABC) trial. *Clin Oncol* 1994; **6**: 209–10.

197 Cuzick J, Mossman J, Stewart H. Co-operative breast cancer trials organized by the United Kingdom Coordinating Committee on Cancer Research. *Cancer Supplement* 1994; **74**: 1160–3.

198 Stewart HJ. Open randomised trials in the management of primary breast cancer. *Eur J Surgl Oncol* 1995; **21**: 223–37.

199 Powles TJ, Hickish TF, Ashley SE *et al.* Randomised controlled trial of chemoendocrine therapy started before or after surgery for treatment of primary breast cancer. *J Clin Oncol* 1995; **13(3)**: 547–52.

200 Hortobagyi GN, Holmes FA, Thenault RL *et al.* Use of taxol (paclitaxel) in breast cancer. *Oncology* 1994; **51(1)**: 29–32.

201 Rowinsky EK, Donehower RC. Paclitaxel(taxol). *NEJM.* 1995; **332(15)**: 1004–14.

202 Gazet JC, Ford HT, Coombes RC *et al.* Prospective randomised trial of tamoxifen vs surgery in elderly patients with breast cancer. *Eur J Surg Oncol* 1984; **20**: 207–14.

203 Dixon JM. Treatment of elderly patients with breast cancer. *BMJ* 1992; **304**: 996–7.

204 Bates T, Riley DC, Houghton J *et al.* Breast cancer in elderly women: a Cancer Research Campaign trial comparing treatment with tamoxifen and optimal surgery with tamoxifen alone. *Br J Surg* 1991; **78**: 591.

Acknowledgements

We are extremely grateful to the following for their comments on earlier drafts: Mr Andrew Baildam; Mr Brian McGee; Dr Penelope Hopwood; Dr Gareth Evans; Dr Anthony Howell; Dr Ellis Friedman; Dr Caroline Boggis.

We are also grateful to the Statistical Unit of the Department of Health who provided us with additional information.

The final text and the conclusions are the responsibility of the authors.

7 Genitourinary Medicine Services

A Renton, S Hawkes, M Hickman, E Claydon, H Ward, D Taylor-Robinson

1 Summary

This chapter addresses the need for genitourinary medicine (GUM) services, the promotion of sexual health and diagnosis and treatment of sexually transmitted diseases (STDs), excluding HIV and AIDS.

Sexually transmitted diseases – categories and definitions

- A wide range of conditions present to GUM clinics. These conditions may be classified according to the symptoms and signs (syndromically), according to causative agents (for infectious STDs) and according to the long-term sequelae of the conditions.
- The most useful existing classification scheme is that used to report clinic activity to the Department of Health on the KC60 statistical return. This scheme uses information describing syndromic features and causative organisms to classify cases. The scheme is especially useful for infectious conditions. However a substantial proportion of individuals presenting to GUM services do not have an infectious condition. These individuals may be attending, for example with psychosexual problems, or merely for a check-up. Although within some clinics there is provision for allocating separate KC60 codes to different non-infectious conditions and thus disaggregating this important area of activity, these codes vary from clinic to clinic.

Incidence and prevalence of genitourinary conditions and risk behaviours for acquisition of sexually transmitted infections

- The principal source of information on the frequency and occurrence of STDs is derived from a statistical return from GUM clinics to the DOH (KC60). Other possible information sources are described – but none offer data that can be used at a local level.
- Allocation of individuals attending STD clinics to district of residence data is not easy as the KC60 does not record district, and because extensive cross-boundary flows may occur. The paucity of information attributable to district populations is highlighted throughout this chapter and urgently needs to be addressed.
- During 1993/94 over 45 000 new episodes were recorded at 225 STD clinics in England and Wales – corresponding to one in 50 of the population aged 16–64.
- Most GUM clinics are small – over half record less than 1500 episodes a year and 90% recording less than 5000. There is considerable variation in attendance rates between regions, with the highest rate in clinics located in the North Thames RHAs, approximately three times that found in the West Midlands. While the majority of DHAs have one local GUM clinic, there are still a few districts without a GUM clinic. The difference between regions varies less generally for the viral and chronic infections, such as genital

warts and herpes simplex virus. Very large differences occur between DHAs in rates of initial contacts. However these largely reflect differences in the location of clinics.

- About one-third of all new contacts in GUM clinics are classified as D category under the KC60 scheme. This represents individuals attending for one or more of the many different services or problems catered for by GUM services, such as counselling, treatment of rare conditions, sexual health screening, or family planning. It is important therefore that providers are aware of the different types of services offered by the local GUM clinic and of which types are included in the 'catch-all codes' in order to interpret the activity data. The breakdown of GUM clinic activity in the UK in 1990/91 is shown in Figure 1.

Proportion of all first contacts by STD group

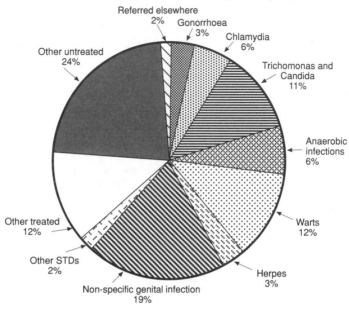

Figure 1: Breakdown of GUM clinic activity in the UK in 1990–91 across KC60 categories.

- The reported incidence of STDs has changed markedly over time. Gonococcal infections were declining in importance over the period 1976 to 1986, the decline accelerating in 1985/86. It is important to note that the fall in gonorrhoea pre-dated recognition of HIV infection. In women *Trichomonas vaginalis* infections also declined. Over the same period the number of diagnoses of genital warts or genital herpes increased substantially. Several explanations can be offered for these trends, including improved diagnosis and treatment of bacterial STDs, changes in sexual behaviour and greater ascertainment of asymptomatic disease. However the extent to which these different explanations account for the observed trends is not known.

- Sexually transmitted diseases mostly affect young people with the bulk of cases occurring in women aged 16–24 years and in men aged 20–29 years. In women the rates of initial contacts among those below 16 years (age of legal consent) are higher than rates in women over 45 years. It follows therefore that GUM services must be acceptable to young sexually active people and that other services sought by young people need to provide advice and information on sexual health and the availability of GUM services.

- People with STDs presenting to GUM clinics may represent the tip of the iceberg of sexually transmitted infection. Unfortunately most available prevalence surveys have small sample sizes and the samples were not selected randomly from the population. They do suggest however that young age is associated with an increased risk of infection and that the difference between asymptomatic and symptomatic infection can be large. Of course not all asymptomatic infection will lead to complications but clearly if untreated the probability of transmission to others remains. Further investigation of STD prevalence via the use of local surveys is needed.

Services available

- Good GUM services remain the cornerstone of any strategy aiming to treat and prevent STDs. These services are based on three key principles:
  a) that they should be open access
  b) free at the point of delivery
  c) confidential.
- Although GUM services represent the principal place of management of people with genitourinary problems, such people may also be managed in a variety of other settings within the health service such as by their general practitioner (GP), ante-natal or family planning clinics. It is necessary to develop a sexual health strategy that encompasses different services and aims to improve co-ordination and collaboration between them. At present there is no method for assessing what proportions of STDs are treated in GUM clinics.
- By now most if not all districts should have a local GUM clinic, or be opening one shortly. If not then need is almost certainly being unmet and serious consideration should be given now to funding a new GUM clinic.
- The central pillars of the GUM service have traditionally been the provision of facilities for the early diagnosis and treatment of individuals with sexually transmitted infections and the contact tracing and appropriate management of their sexual partners. The decline in the relative incidence of the curable bacterial STDs and the increased occurrence of chronic and incurable STDs has been accompanied by an expanding emphasis on primary prevention.
- Key elements of primary prevention within GUM clinics include:
  a) health education and the promotion of healthy sexual lifestyles
  b) provision of condoms
  c) contact tracing services and the provision of appropriate diagnostic and treatment facilities for those contacts traced
  d) the provision of hepatitis B vaccination for appropriate groups.
  All clinic staff must have a role in prevention and health promotion activities although these activities are a particular responsibility of health advisors.
- Key elements of clinical provision within GUM clinics include:
  a) appropriate mix of trained staff
  b) on-site diagnostic laboratory services for instant diagnosis of some GU conditions
  c) access to a microbiological service for diagnosis that requires confirmation and cannot be carried out in the clinic laboratory
  d) facilities and drugs for treatment
  e) contact tracing and follow-up services
  f) provision for referral to other specialties.
  In addition facilities for the management of women with abnormal smears, psychosexual services and contraceptive advice are increasingly being offered within GUM services.
- Many sexually transmitted infections may be asymptomatic and may lead to serious sequelae associated with chronic infection. Therefore the role of the GUM service in screening self-referred individuals who may be asymptomatic but perceive themselves to be at risk of infection is very important.

Effectiveness of services

- Existing evidence for the effectiveness of STD interventions relates primarily to the efficacy of drug treatments which is in general of high quality. Very little information is available on the effectiveness of other key activities involved in the control of STDs such as contact tracing and health education. One exception is hepatitis B vaccination where there is good evidence for its effectiveness, although it is apparently not reaching those at greatest risk.

Models of care

- There is one basic model of care that covers the whole of GUM services in the UK; the provision in each district of at least one specialist GUM clinic within an acute unit or, less frequently, attached to a community unit.
- In recent years there has been a shift away from a disease based approach (which underpins GUM) towards the broader concept of sexual health. This shift has yet to be fully reflected in the provision of services. A few districts have integrated sexual health services where GUM, family planning, termination of pregnancy, psychosexual counselling and related services are provided in one clinic. In other areas there is no unified service but greater links are being established between community gynaecology and GUM. Family planning clinics can also provide screening for sexually transmitted organisms, such as *Chlamydia trachromatis*.
- There is a clear case for better planning of services and liaison between sectors. Primary prevention including health education, condom distribution and hepatitis B vaccination is carried out within GUM clinics but also needs to be co-ordinated across other services within the district. This reflects the widening role of GUM into sexual health which must be carried forward into district models of care where either GUM clinics are integrated with other sites in the delivery of services, or the management of sexual health services is integrated through common protocols and shared care schemes.
- The potential role of GUM services in wider community based screening for STDs needs to be considered. In the first instance questions relating to the potential value of extending screening beyond individuals who present themselves to clinics will need to be addressed at the national rather than district level.

Outcome measures and targets

- National targets for a reduction in gonorrhoea incidence were set in the Government's strategy The Health of the Nation and have been achieved.
- Further development of appropriate outcome measures and targets will require the enhancement of surveillance and information systems from GUM clinics and laboratories. The installation of GUM clinic computers provides the opportunity for collating data at a population level and several regions are piloting new information systems.

Information and research priorities

- Information systems require further development to allow geographical attribution of individuals with STD infections.
- Currently little is known about the amount of STDs diagnosed and treated outside GUM. This must change as districts develop more integrated sexual health services and more extensive screening of people in other settings is carried out.
- Information derived from clinic activity will need to be supplemented by the findings of new sample surveys which establish the prevalence of STDs in different populations.

- Studies are needed into the benefits and effectiveness of selected preventive interventions, including population screening or universal screening for STDs in asymptomatic women.
- Models of shared care and education and the cost-effectiveness of treating chronic viral STDs (excluding HIV) outside GUM clinics needs to be assessed.
- Hepatitis B is currently the only sexually transmitted virus for which an effective vaccine is available but there is evidence that coverage is low. Studies are required to explain why vaccination is not reaching those people who are at highest risk of infection, and to make practicable proposals on how this can be changed.
- Sexual health services are becoming integrated. It is important to establish what role GUM physicians have in the education of other health care workers in the recognition of STDs and the development of local algorithms for the management of STDs outside GUM clinics. Also whether there is scope for managing chronic STDs in primary care with the advice of GUM consultants, following a similar model of other chronic diseases.

2 Introduction

Genitourinary medicine is one part of the services concerned with the sexual health of the population and is one of the key Health of the Nation areas. Sexual health like the WHO definition of health is not merely the absence of disease and any definition must recognize both the positive and negative consequences of sexual activity. Sexual health can be regarded as:

the enjoyment of sexual activity of one's choice without causing or suffering physical or mental harm.

The undesired results of sexual activity include unwanted pregnancies and the transmission of STDs, which if untreated can have long-term consequences such as infertility, ectopic pregnancy and genital cancers.

Health authorities implementing the Health of the Nation strategy will need to plan integrated and complementary services and to develop alliances to promote sexual health across traditional boundaries. Genitourinary medicine services will play a key role within this strategy and it is important to be aware that:

- an integrated sexual health services package incorporates other health care providers (e.g. family planning, obstetrics and gynaecology, general practice), local government (e.g. health education in schools and management of social services homes) and voluntary organizations (e.g. provision and targeting of sex education in the population)
- complementarity between GUM and other sexual health services must be a primary concern of those commissioning services.

Though the models of care section focuses on sexual health services, the role of non-GUM services in the delivery of sexual health must be the subject of other needs assessment exercises. Moreover planning the future delivery of sexual health services has been addressed by a joint working group.

GUM services have a split role and responsibilities. First they have a responsibility for the alleviation of disease in individuals. Second they fulfil an important public health function to control sexually transmitted infections in the population, through the rapid diagnosis and treatment of symptomatic individuals, screening and treating individuals for asymptomatic infection, contact tracing, diagnosis and treatment of infection in sexual partners and provision of health education materials and advice on prevention. Third they may adopt a further responsibility for promoting and improving the sexual health of the population, through the provision of psychosocial counselling of sexual health problems and family planning.

A brief description of STDs, still the cornerstone of GUM clinics, follows.

3 Categories and definitions

The linkage of sex and disease has a long history, with lurid descriptions of the consequences of amorous excesses going back to the middle ages, if not antiquity.[1] Popular names for STDs can be equally ancient, for instance 'clap' referring to a 'certain inward heat and excoriation of the urethra' was coined in the late 14th century. Most historical descriptions and sexually transmitted epidemics can be attributed to gonorrhoea or syphilis. Further advances in the definition of STDs and their effective treatment have gone hand in hand with the development of microbiological techniques.

Sexually transmitted disease are described in three ways.

- Level 1 Acute clinical symptoms – early signs of infection.
- Level 2 Infectious organisms – causative agent.
- Level 3 Complications – long-term sequalae.

First the clinical symptoms of patients presenting to GUM services fall into a few well recognized types or syndromes (Table 1). These may be caused by a number of infectious agents, or may be due to non-infectious causes. Deciding the correct treatment for a patient often will require the microbiological diagnosis or exclusion of possible causes.

Table 1: Common symptoms presenting to genitourinary medicine services

Syndrome	Description
Vulvovaginitis	inflammation, irritation in the vagina or vulval area with or without discharge
Urethritis in men	urethral irritation with or without discharge and pain on passing urine
Genital ulceration/erosion	internal or external
Genital warts	internal or external
Pelvic pain (pelvic inflammatory disease (PID))	with or without vaginal discharge, cervical motion, tenderness and toxic features (e.g. malaise, fever)

Second sexually transmitted infections are not always symptomatic and may only be discovered through microbiological screening. Some infectious agents can be transmitted through other routes, in particular intravenously. The main causative microorganisms are shown in Table 2.

Table 2: Important sexually transmitted pathogenic organisms

Type of organism	Name (disease)
Bacteria	*Treponema pallidum* (syphilis)
	Neisseria gonorrhoeae
	Chlamydia trachomatis
Viruses	*Herpes simplex*
	Human papilloma (warts)
	Hepatitis B
Ectoparasites	*Phthirus pubis* (crab louse)
	Sarcoptes scabiei (scabies)
Protozoa	*Trichomonas vaginalis*
Fungus	*Candida albicans*

In addition STDs may lead to chronic symptoms or complications if untreated. The main complications which may also have a non-infectious cause are shown in Box 1.

Box 1: Common long-term complications of STDs

- Tubal infertility
- Miscarriage
- Ectopic pregnancy
- Ano-genital cancer
- Chronic hepatitis

A more complete list of STD organisms, together with a description of the common features of acute infection and chronic sequelae, is given in Appendix VI.

Classification of presenting conditions

The principal source of information on GUM clinic activity and STD incidence in England and Wales combines data on syndrome, organism, plus treatment of suspected disease (i.e. clinical diagnosis without microbiological confirmation). Known as the KC60 it is a statistical return made quarterly to the DOH from each GUM clinic. An abridged list of the main conditions are shown in Table 3. A complete list with the recent revisions is shown in Appendix II.

If a patient is admitted into hospital with an STD or genitourinary condition the diagnosis will be coded under the ICD classification system. The hospital information system (IIS) will be less useful for assessing the STD related health service activity because only a small fraction is dealt with in the inpatient setting. A list of relevant ICD 10 codes is given in Appendix I, in the event that health care commissioners or providers wish to monitor GU related hospital inpatient activity.

Much of the information presented on the frequency of occurrence of these infections in section 4 will be based on this summary KC60 classification. The KC60 also provides data on whether selected STDs were acquired homosexually. However not all GUM clinics submit data on acquisition and a review of those that did submit data found it to be highly variable and unlikely to be accurate. The KC60 data on homosexual acquisition, therefore, have not been used. Commissioners and providers wishing to monitor STDs by sexual acquisition will need to review data quality in their local GUM clinic and establish the policy on sexual history taking and routine data collection.

Table 3: The KC60 classification of STD workload

KC60 code	Condition	Description[a]	Intensity[b]
A1–9	Syphilis	genital ulcers plus complex multi-system chronic sequelae	3
B1.1–4a,5	Gonorrhoea	urethritis in men, vulvovaginitis in women	1
C4a–e	Chlamydia	cervicitis and vulvovaginitis in women (though usually asymptomatic), urethritis in men	1
C4h–i	Non-specific genital infection	urethritis of unknown cause in men only (though Chlamydia may not be tested for)	1
C6a, C7a	Trichomonas and Candidosis	vulvovaginitis	1
C6b–c,7b	Vaginosis and other anaerobic infections	mostly vulvovaginitis (some infection in men)	1
B1.4b–c, C4f–g	Pelvic inflammatory disease (PID)	pelvic pain with or without discharge of gonoccocal, chlamydial or unknown origin	3
C11a–b	Genital warts		2
C10a–b	Herpes simplex	ulceration	2
C13a–b	Hepatitis	serologically confirmed	3
C1–3, C5, C8–9[c]	Other specific STDs and complications	ulcers, infestation and other complications	1/2
D2	Any other condition requiring treatment		
D3	Other episode not requiring treatment		
D4	Other conditions referred elsewhere		

[a] See Table 1.

[b] 'Intensity' refers to service need: 1 on the spot diagnosis, antibiotic treatment, and contact tracing; 2 multiple outpatient visits; 3 may require inpatient management.

[c] Chancroid, donovanosis, scabies, pediculosis, LGV (lymphogranuloma venereum) or sexually acquired arthritis.

4 Incidence and prevalence of genitourinary conditions and risk behaviours for acquisition of sexually transmitted infections

In 1993/94 over 45 000 new episodes were recorded at 225 GUM clinics in England and Wales. Roughly this corresponds to one in 50 of the 16–64 year-old population attending a GUM clinic. Even though over one-third of people who attend are found not to have a STD, treatable STDs at GUM clinics represent only the tip of the iceberg of sexually transmitted infections. Most GUM clinics are small – with over half recording less than 1500 episodes a year and 90% recording less than 5000. The number of GUM clinics in each RHA is shown in Table 4 on page 408. Inner-city DHAs can have two or three local GUM clinics (which provide a service to a much wider population). While the majority of DHAs have one local GUM clinic, there are still a few districts without one.

Sources of information

There are several other sources of data that may allow an estimation of the incidence or prevalence of genitourinary conditions in the population. Unfortunately the value and interest to commissioners and providers may be only in working on improving them.

- Department of Health KC60 returns on GUM clinic activity.
- Department of Health KH09 returns on GUM clinic activity.
- Special prevalence surveys.
- Public Health Laboratory Service (PHLS) laboratory reporting systems.
- General practice morbidity data.

All GUM clinics are required to report numbers of initial contacts with patients by diagnostic group on a quarterly basis. The figures are used to estimate the number of incident cases occurring in the population. The baseline data do not refer to individuals. A patient may have several episodes recorded at one time corresponding to separate STDs or complications and may have the same STD episode recorded throughout the year corresponding to re-infections.

Aggregate data from this reporting system are published by the DOH and commented on by the Communicable Diseases Surveillance Centre (CDSC). No useful breakdowns of these data have been available below the national level (apart from regional total STD clinic attendances) to date. District of residence data are not collected by the KC60. Cross-boundary flows in GUM service utilization, between health agencies and regions, can be considerable and currently are not possible to track. It is not possible therefore to reach a valid assessment of the actual disease burden falling on any particular district population. In addition there is evidence of variation between clinics in how cases are recorded and classified.

Nationally however the KC60 data represent the most useful and comprehensive information available on the occurrence of GU problems in the population. Districts wishing to gain a wider appreciation of the size and nature of the burden of genitourinary disease in their locality should request clinics within their geographical areas to provide copies of KC60 returns and should work collaboratively with the clinics, and neighbouring health agencies to interpret these data. The continuing implementation of the recommendation of the Monks' Report[2] that GUM clinic information be computerized will provide new opportunities for enhancing information available for needs assessment and planning of GUM services.

Genitourinary conditions seen in GUM clinics in the UK

Analysis is primarily at the national level and by RHA of report (not residence). It aims to show the range of information which is available and the magnitude of the problem. Estimates of incidence applicable directly to local populations are not available.

The distribution of initial contacts has changed markedly over time. Figures 2 and 3 show the trends in number of total attendances at GUM clinics in the UK between 1976 and 1992 for males and females.

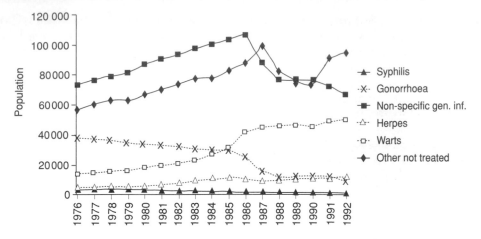

Figure 2: Initial contacts seen in GUM clinics in the UK 1976–92: selected diagnoses: male.

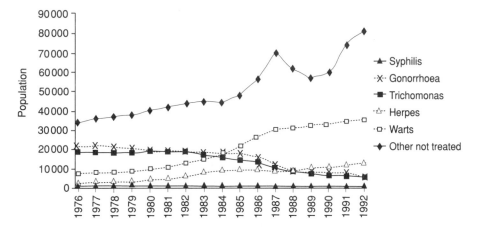

Figure 3: Initial contacts seen in GUM clinics in the UK 1976–92: selected diagnoses: female.

Infectious syphilis is very rare. Gonococcal infections were declining in importance over the period 1976 to 1986 and the decline accelerated in 1985/86. In women trichomoniasis infections also declined. Over the same period the number of initial contacts in whom a diagnosis of genital warts or genital herpes was made increased substantially. Concomitant increases in non-specific genital infection in males (mainly non-gonococcal urethritis) and patients attending with other conditions for which no treatment was required also increased.

Several explanations can be offered for these trends. Bacterial STDs can be controlled effectively through the early diagnosis and effective treatment of index cases and their sexual partners. It may be therefore that improved clinical services throughout the 1970s led to a reduction in the average duration of infectivity of this group of STDs with a consequent decline in incidence. In addition bacterial STDs have declined in incidence as a consequence of changes in sexual behaviour within the population, in particular in response to AIDS awareness, and campaigns promoting safer sex. Indeed this notion has been enshrined within the Health of the Nation strategy setting a target for a reduction in gonorrhoea incidence within the population. This target was set, not to reflect the public health importance of gonorrhoea itself, but because gonorrhoea incidence nationally was measurable, and in the belief that gonorrhoea incidence provided a good indicator of underlying 'unsafe' sexual behaviour within the population. It is important to note that the beginnings of the decline in gonorrhoea predated the recognition of AIDS/HIV infection by several years, although the response to the latter may be responsible for the acceleration in decline.

The apparent rise in incidence of warts and genital herpes over the time period is clearly not explicable by a move towards safer sex within the population. Initial contacts with untreated non-STD conditions show a similar pattern suggesting that at least for some of these diseases the increase might be accounted for by ascertainment of asymptomatic disease among the increasing overall number of attenders, a feature of greater access to GUM services. Attendance increased by roughly 50% in men over the time period and effectively doubled in women. However an increase in attendance of the order of 50–75% may not explain entirely the four- to five-fold increase in genital warts or the rise in genital herpes seen over the period, although it may explain the increase in non-gonococcal urethritis.

Two further explanations have been offered for the rise in incidence of the viral STDs. First that the different STDs are associated with different types of sexual behaviour, which if they change in frequency will not have any significant effect on the occurrence of other STDs. Second that the viral diseases are in an epidemic phase and have not yet reached a stable endemic equilibrium incidence within the population. The extent to which these different explanations account for the observed trends is not known.

Incidence estimates for genitourinary conditions based on GUM clinic attendance

Estimates of the crude incidence of the important KC60 based groupings of genitourinary conditions averaged for the years 1990 and 1991 are shown in Table 4. An overall attendance rate of over 2% (one in 50) is seen for men and women aged 16–64 years in the UK in 1991 and 1992. There is considerable variation in attendance rates between regions, with the highest rate in clinics located in the North Thames RHAs, approximately three times that found in the West Midlands. It is important to remember that variations between RHAs reflect cross-boundary flow, the number of clinics located within the region and differences in diagnostic or coding practice. The difference between regions varies less for the viral and chronic infections, such as genital warts and herpes simplex virus. The relative frequency of the different conditions in the UK is shown in Figure 1, page 398.

Two of the largest categories of patients are those classified as having other untreated conditions, or treated for any reason other than those classified in the STD categories. Thus one-third of all new contacts in GUM clinics are unspecified, though they could refer to the many different services or problems catered for by GUM, such as counselling, treatment of rare conditions, sexual health screening, family planning, etc. It is important therefore that providers are aware of the different types of services offered by the local GUM clinic and of which are included in the 'catch-all codes' in order to interpret the activity data.

The most common specific diagnoses (excluding non-specific genital infections in men) are candidal infection and warts. In the case of chlamydiae infection it is important to appreciate that the proportion of initial contacts to whom this diagnosis is assigned will be greatly influenced by the availability and extent of testing for *Chlamydia trachomatis* in clinics.

Variation between districts within regions

It is difficult on the basis of current knowledge to explain the observed regional variation. It may reflect real differences in the geographic incidence of specific STDs. Alternatively regional differences may reflect differences in the availability and location of clinics, or health seeking behaviour across the country. Very large differences occur between DHAs in rates of initial contacts. This is shown for a single RHA in Table 5 and largely reflect differences in access and clinic location. The differences cannot be used to reflect differences in population incidence of STD; although STD incidence is likely to be geographically heterogenous it is not possible to say by how much.

Table 4: Initial contacts by KC60 diagnosis per 100 000 population aged 16–64 in 1990/91

KC60 grouping	UK	N Thames East	N Thames West	S Thames East	S Thames West	E Anglia	Mersey	Northern	N Western	Oxford	S Western	Trent	Western	W Midlands	Yorkshire
No. of GUM clinics	205	20	15	18	11	9	10	14	20	10	15	16	12	21	14
Syphilis	1	2	3	3	2	0	1	1	1	1	1	1	0	1	1
Gonorrhoea	65	136	111	115	36	24	25	29	62	49	47	66	34	49	65
Chlamydia	125	182	125	174	72	87	77	109	131	112	140	158	105	116	100
Trichomonas and Candida	240	508	438	382	227	184	101	136	130	289	152	228	242	128	169
Anaerobic infections	139	196	182	260	142	108˙	70	86	81	164	108	202	120	79	111
Warts	267	399	355	337	219	246	229	226	224	257	238	303	266	169	241
Herpes	70	122	149	101	64	59	37	34	42	64	64	70	82	31	50
Non-specific genital infection	421	794	955	708	433	367	233	237	213	367	271	367	324	206	355
Other specific STDs	51	105	97	84	54	30	39	32	25	37	28	59	39	24	54
Other treated conditions	260	505	657	261	239	163	243	77	170	582	124	251	166	98	130
Other untreated conditions	498	1020	967	695	357	489	423	330	297	482	345	472	432	280	342
Other referred elsewhere	36	89	91	55	36	30	19	43	10	36	18	35	17	16	9
All conditions	2173	4058	4130	3175	1881	1787	1497	1340	1386	2440	1536	2212	1827	1197	1627

Table 5: Initial contacts rates per 100 000 population aged 16–64, for a single RHA and highest and lowest district rates (average for years 1990 and 1991)

	Males			Females		
KC60 grouping	Average RHA rate per 100 000	Highest district rate per 100 000	Lowest district rate per 100 000	Average RHA rate per 100 000	Highest district rate per 100 000	Lowest district rate per 100 000
Gonorrhoea (excluding epidemiological treatment)	131	626	3	58	200	2
Non-specific genital infection	829	2867	18	–	–	–
Warts (first attack)	209	782	33	170	528	41
Herpes (first attack)	75	366	2	73	285	3
Pediculosis and scabies	55	234	1	18	62	0
Other untreated	1083	6256	69	868	4310	46
All conditions	4392	6558	165	3528	7304	186

Districts with relatively low contact rates will need to establish whether these rates reflect problems of access. In addition districts will have to collaborate with their neighbours and the nearest inner-city GUM clinics in order to establish the distribution of clinics serving their population.

Age distribution of initial contacts

The age distribution of individuals with new episodes of STDs is shown in Table 6. A characteristic pattern is seen: the bulk of cases in women occurs in those aged 16–24 years. In men the distribution is shifted to the right by about five years; the bulk of cases occurring in those aged 20–29. In women the rates of initial contacts among those below 16 years (age of legal consent) are higher than the rates in women over 45 years, for all the diagnoses shown.

This has important implications for service configuration. Genitourinary medicine services must be acceptable and accessible to young sexually active people. Equally services sought by young people such as school nurses, primary health care team, family planning, accident and emergency (A and E) and social services, need to be co-ordinated in order to advise individuals (who may still be at school) of the availability of GUM services and to encourage them to attend clinics where appropriate.

Table 6: Age-specific rates per 100 000: initial contacts with GUM services by diagnosis in the UK 1990/91

Infection	Females						Males					
	rate per 100 000						rate per 100 000					
	<16	16–19	20–24	25–34	35–44	>=45	<16	16–19	20–24	25–34	35–44	>=45
Syphilis	0.2	0.6	1.7	1.1	0.5	0.1	0.1	0.7	2.1	2.9	1.3	0.0
Gonorrhoea	7.7	156.0	128.0	43.0	7.2	0.6	3.0	101.0	216.0	126.0	26.9	0.4
Herpes (first attack)	5.0	105.0	136.0	62.9	17.5	2.6	0.9	28.0	97.7	73.3	28.0	5.1
Warts (first attack)	19.7	549.0	514.0	160.0	41.2	5.6	4.9	219.0	624.0	286.0	72.5	12.6
Chlamydia	17.4	393.0	380.0	113.0	18.5	1.8	2.5	123.0	294.0	151.0	35.6	4.7

Clearly the age specific rates of STD occurrence in the peak age groups are several times that for the whole population aged 16–64. Because the KC60 data are contact rather than person based, it is difficult to estimate the incidence rate of any STD. However there is little doubt that it exceeds 1% per year. The data are not generalizable to individual districts, nor are they available for individual DHAs.

KH09 data

As with other outpatient clinics, GUM clinics collect information on the number of clinic sessions held and the total number of attendances: the KH09 statistical return. KH09 could serve to interpret the KC60 activity between clinics, for example, by comparing the ratio of total KC60 contacts to the overall number of attendances. However in a recent study commissioned by the DOH and carried out by the Policy Studies Institute[3] there were many problems found in comparing KH09 data between clinics. Clinic sessions were defined in different ways: some recorded male and female clinics running concurrently as one session, whilst others recorded it as two clinic sessions and in some clinics telephone consultations were included in the overall workload returns. When districts are assessing the workload of clinics in their area it will be imperative for them to know the method by which the workload is measured before valid comparisons can be made. The KH09 for GUM clinics is not published separately but aggregated with other hospital outpatient returns. Districts therefore must arrange with their local providers for access to this data source.

Sexually transmitted diseases prevalence surveys

While KC60 data provide reasonable estimates of the incidence of symptomatic disease, they provide little information on the population incidence and prevalence of total infection (asymptomatic and symptomatic) with sexually transmitted pathogens. Estimates of STD prevalence in a district can be gleaned from information already collected in *ad hoc* surveys of STD prevalence which have been carried out both in STD clinic and non-clinic settings. The results of the most recent of these surveys are presented in Table 7.

It cannot be assumed that these figures are universally valid since the sample sizes are small and not randomly selected from the population but it is of note that many of the surveys give very similar prevalence rates for the asymptomatic carriage of sexually transmitted pathogens. The most common finding in all the surveys is that young age is associated with an increased risk of infection, with the highest prevalence consistently found in young sexually active teenagers.

The difference between asymptomatic and symptomatic infection can be large, suggesting that a very large proportion of the total burden of sexually transmitted infection may remain undiagnosed and asymptomatic. For example approximately 20 000 incident cases of *Chlamydia trachomatis* infection are recorded in the UK annually. Even if it is assumed that all chlamydial infections diagnosed in the clinics occur in women aged 16–30, the figure still represents only three per 1000 women, which in turn represents only 6% of the total caseload (if we assume 5% of women are infected).

Of course not all asymptomatic infection will leading to complications but clearly if untreated the probability of transmission to others remains. Further investigation of STD prevalence via the use of local surveys is needed.

Laboratory reports

Other measures of the prevalence of STDs in a particular district can be compiled from laboratory reports. The only STD which is notifiable under the infectious disease legislation is ophthalmia neonatorum. This was commonly caused by gonococcal disease, transmitted vertically from the mother to child, starting as conjunctivitis in the new born and sometimes leading to blindness. During the 19th century ophthalmia neonatorum occurred in 1 to 15% of infants born in US and European hospitals. However the district prevalence rates for this condition now are so low as to be meaningless for planning services, or for monitoring the prevalence of STDs.

There is a system of voluntary reporting of laboratory data to the PHLS Communicable Disease Surveillance Centre (CDSC) and through the 53 area and regional laboratories which constitute the Public Health Laboratory Service. These collect data on the prevalence of extra-genital *N. gonorrhoeae* and together with the Gonococcus Reference Unit at Bristol carry out specialized typing of strains of gonococci and determine resistance patterns. It must be remembered however that this is a voluntary reporting system and it is recognized that the data set is incomplete and does not refer to district populations. In a recent survey of one region only half of the eligible NHS laboratories reported regularly to the CDSC and samples from one-third of the GUM clinics were tested at laboratories which did not report at all (unpublished).

However steps are being taken to improve laboratory reporting by developing and implementing electronic means of capturing the relevant data from the pathology computer and transferring it to the CDSC (M Catchpole, personal communication). In 1995 the PHLS STD/HIV/AIDS Committee recommended that all gonococcal infection diagnosed by laboratories be reported to the CDSC, in order to provide a more complete picture. The success of this initiative however will depend on the programme to introduce a computerized reporting system.

The data are used by the CDSC in their reports on the epidemiology of STDs nationally. It is not published on a regular basis by area of report, though the CDSC can provide data to individual districts.

Table 7: Summary of results from recent STD prevalence surveys

Investigator	Year	Setting	Sample	Organism	Prevalence (%)
Ridgway et al.[4]	1983	University College Hospital, London	89 women attending for termination of pregnancy	Chlamydia Gonorrhoea Candida	8 1 18
Southgate et al.[5]	1983	General Practice in East London	248 women attending their GP who required a speculum vaginal examination	Chlamydia Gonorrhoea	8 2
Wood et al.[6]	1984	Antenatal clinic, Liverpool	252 women attending for their first clinic visit	Chlamydia	7
Edet[7]	1988–90	Chatham, Kent	1611 gynaecological patients	Chlamydia (all ages) <25 26–29 >30	6 10 5 4
Fish et al.[8]	1985	University College Hospital, London	1267 gynaecological patients	Chlamydia (all ages) 16–20 21–25 26–30 >31	4 15 7 3 1
Longhurst et al.[9]	1987	Inner-city general practice	169 premenopausal women who required a pelvic examination	Chlamydia	11
Macauley et al.[10]	1989	Manchester	452 women attending family planning clinics	Chlamydia Gonorrhoea Trichomonas Bacterial vaginosis Candida	7 3 10 9 15
Preece et al.[11]	1988–89	Wolverhampton	3309 women in labour attending an obstetric unit	Chlamydia <20 20–24 25–29 >30	15 8 4 2

Smith et al.[12] | 1991 | Colposcopy clinic and general practice | 101 women attending colposcopy clinic; 197 women attending GP for cervical smear

Organism	Colposcopy	General practice
Chlamydia	6	12
Gonorrhoea	–	1
Trichomonas	1	3
Candida	9	17

Investigator	Year	Setting	Sample	Organism	Prevalence (%)
Blackwell et al.[13]	1993	Swansea	400 women attending for a termination	Chlamydia Trichomonas Bacterial vaginosis Candida	8 1 28 24

Thin et al.[14] | 1986–87 | London GUM and Swansea GUM | 121 adolescents (11–18 years) in London and 95 in Swansea

Organism	Boys (%) London	Boys (%) Swansea	Girls (%) London	Girls (%) Swansea
Chlamydia	0	18	8	9
Gonorrhoea	23	18	17	8
Trichomonas	2	0	7	0
Bacterial vaginosis	–	–	13	26
Candida	9	18	15	19
Non-specific general infection	49	26	25	16
Herpes	4	2	0	0
Warts	11	16	5	20
PID	–	–	8	0

Maini et al.[15] | 1989–91 | London GUM clinic | Analysis of all urethral and cervical cultures

Organism	Men Homo	Men Hetero	Women
Chlamydia	5	3	1
Gonorrhoea	1	6	5
Non-specific	10	18	–

Investigator	Year	Setting	Sample	Organism	Prevalence (%)
Dimian et al.[16]	1990	London GUM clinic	363 women	Chlamydia Gonorrhoea Trichomonas Candida Gardnerella Herpes Warts	9 6 9 3 2 4 10

Districts should check whether their local laboratories are contributing to this surveillance system and identify how much infection is diagnosed outside the local GUM clinic.

The PHLS is currently implementing a system of sentinel surveillance for STDs. At present this involves just three clinics (two in London and one in Sheffield) but there are plans to extend and expand this to 15 clinics in 1996/97. This surveillance system may provide useful data on the epidemiology of sexually transmitted infections in England and Wales and will be available for district planners to use when assessing GUM service requirements in their area. The CDSC is also planning to set up a collaborative system to monitor the incidence and distribution of congenital syphilis in England and Wales.

General practice morbidity survey

The Office of Population, Censuses and Surveys (OPCS) has recently published preliminary findings from a national survey on patient visits to GPs.[17] This survey takes place once a decade, the most recent being November 1991 to end of October 1992, in 60 volunteer practices in England and Wales. The results are published as numbers of patients consulting per 1000 person–years at risk. The rates for diseases which may be sexually transmitted were 0.6 for syphilis and other venereal diseases, 8.1 for herpes simplex infections and 31 for candidasis.

Whilst it is difficult to comment in detail on these figures, as they are not specific for individual conditions, it would appear that GPs see a substantial number of women whom they diagnose as having candidal infection (thrush) and not many other sexually transmitted diseases. The OPCS will publish further details of the study and its results, including tables of prevalence, incidence and service utilization for the whole study population and for people with different socioeconomic characteristics.

The CDSC in collaboration with the Royal College of General Practitioners is currently looking more closely at the presentation and management of people with STDs in general practice. Through a nationwide network of GPs who are collaborating in this research, information will be available on the specific rates of presentation, and diagnoses and management strategies used by GPs. The results of this survey will be published by the CDSC.

Sexual behaviour surveys

The final source of information relevant to GUM service provision is provided by the surveys of sexual behaviour. The recently published National Survey on Sexual Attitudes and Lifestyles (NSSAL)[18] has, for the first time, provided epidemiologists and planners with detailed information on the sexual behaviour of the UK population. It is planned that information from the NSSAL survey will be presented to district health authorities by standard area in 1995/96 for their own assessments of need.

As shown in Table 8 on average men report more partners than women, and men and women living in Greater London tend to report larger numbers of partners. If 'risk of STD acquisition' is defined as having had more than one partner then about 15% of males and 10% of females aged 16–59 are at risk.

In Table 9 the distribution of reported numbers of lifetime sexual partners is presented; there again being a remarkable similarity across the regions, apart from Greater London. If we define 'lifetime risk of STD acquisition' as having had more than two lifetime partners, then about 50% of males and 40% of females might be deemed to be at risk.

Table 8: Distribution of number of sex partners in previous year of respondents to NSSAL: broken down by standard region

Region	Males							Females						
	n	0	1	2	3–4	5–9	10+	n	0	1	2	3–4	5–9	10+
	%			%				%			%			
Northern	427	11	77	5	5	1	1	565	15	80	4	1	0	0
North Western	857	11	74	9	3	2	0	1165	14	81	4	1	0	0
Yorkshire/Humberside	638	13	73	8	4	2	0	869	12	82	4	2	0	0
West Midlands	761	12	76	7	3	1	0	904	15	79	5	1	0	0
East Midlands	603	11	76	8	4	1	0	673	11	80	7	2	0	0
East Anglia	316	15	76	5	3	0	1	358	12	83	3	2	0	0
South Western	622	12	76	7	6	0	0	793	10	81	6	2	0	0
South Eastern	1715	12	74	10	3	1	0	1975	14	79	5	1	0	0
Greater London	1059	13	65	11	7	3	1	1243	16	75	5	3	1	0

Table 9: Distribution of lifetime number of sex partners of respondents to NSSAL

Region	Males							Females						
	n	0	1	2	3–4	5–9	10+	n	0	1	2	3–4	5–9	10+
	%			%				%			%			
Northern	426	6	22	9	24	16	24	565	6	50	18	13	10	3
North Western	854	5	21	9	19	20	26	1165	5	41	19	19	11	4
Yorkshire/Humberside	636	7	20	11	20	18	24	866	5	40	17	18	14	6
West Midlands	759	8	21	12	19	19	21	902	7	40	15	20	13	5
East Midlands	600	6	24	13	13	19	24	674	5	39	19	19	12	6
East Anglia	316	7	24	14	14	19	21	358	6	44	16	15	14	5
South Western	621	5	22	9	19	21	24	791	3	38	17	19	15	8
South Eastern	1704	6	20	10	18	23	23	1969	6	37	16	20	14	8
Greater London	1053	6	13	11	18	19	34	1240	7	28	15	18	18	14

Table 10 shows the number and proportion of respondents in the sample in each standard region who reported ever having attended a GUM clinic. The figures are shown for the whole sample and separately for those individuals who reported more than two partners in the previous year and more than five lifetime partners. It can be seen that larger proportions of individuals with larger numbers of partners report having attended a GUM clinic at least once, though the proportion only reaches greater than one in four for people living in Greater London. Differences between regions in GUM clinic attendance are likely to represent differences in availability and accessibility of services, which should be noted and acted upon by those commissioning and delivering services.

Table 10: Number and percentage of respondents to NSSAL who report ever having attended a GUM clinic: by standard region and number of sex partners in defined periods

Standard region	All respondents				Respondents with > = two partners in last 12 months				Respondents with > = five partners in lifetime			
	Males		Females		Males		Females		Males		Females	
Region	n	%	n	%	n	%	n	%	n	%	n	%
North	20	(5)	8	(2)	4	(10	0	(0)	19	(11)	5	(7)
North West	48	(6)	40	(4)	15	(12)	7	(11)	38	(9)	19	(11)
Yorks/Humberside	52	(8)	47	(5)	12	(15)	10	(21)	45	(17)	37	(22)
West Midlands	43	(6)	34	(4)	10	(12)	2	(3)	37	(12)	20	(13)
East Midlands	46	(8)	33	(5)	15	(20)	11	(17)	39	(15)	18	(15)
East Anglia	19	(6)	16	(4)	4	(13)	1	(8)	18	(15)	7	(11)
South Western	52	(9)	45	(6)	13	(17)	8	(12)	42	(15)	26	(14)
South Eastern	144	(9)	107	(5)	40	(17)	20	(15)	108	(14)	68	(16)
Greater London	155	(16)	159	(14)	63	(27)	29	(24)	137	(24)	114	(30)

There are marked differences by age, with both older and younger subjects less likely to have attended. Only a relatively small proportion of young people aged 16–19 reporting at least five partners have attended a GUM clinic (6% in men, 11% in women). Districts need to assess the risk of asymptomatic infection among these individuals and to consider whether positive efforts to encourage these individuals to be screened may be appropriate.

5 Services available

The principles and history of GUM service provision are described briefly in section 7 and the effectiveness of these services are reviewed in section 6. Patients with genitourinary problems are managed in a variety of settings within the health service, though the GUM clinic department is the main one. Some people will seek advice or treatment from their GP, an ante-natal clinic or family planning clinic. Hence there is a need to develop a sexual health strategy which encompasses different services and aims to improve co-ordination and collaboration between them. At present there is no method for assessing the proportion of STDs treated in GUM clinics.

In 1988 the DOH published the Report of the Working Group to Examine Workloads in Genitourinary Medicine Clinics – known as the Monks Report.[2] The terms of reference of the working group were:

to examine current and forecast workloads in GUM clinics ... to recommend any action which may need to be taken on manpower (including nursing manpower), training, resources and accommodation.

The recommendations of the Monks report are given in Appendix III. The key recommendations are that:

- any person presenting with a new clinical problem suggestive of a sexually transmitted disease or who considers himself or herself to have been in contact with such a disease should be seen on the day of presentation or failing that on the next occasion the clinic is open
- there must be GUM ... provision in every district. Districts lacking a clinic should be able to call on a nominated GUM consultant.

Following publication of the Monks report the DOH has issued yearly executive letters which request health authorities to give an update of progress in implementing the recommendations of the report.

By now most if not all districts should have a local GUM clinic, or be opening one shortly. If not then need is being almost certainly unmet and serious consideration should be given now to funding a new GUM clinic.

In 1990/91 the DOH commissioned a second study carried out by staff from the Policy Studies Institute.[5] Both reports found considerable variations in the work done by members of staff in different clinics and no clear guidelines with respect to working roles. The main recommendations of the second study are given in Appendix IV. The ability of staff to fulfil the multiple functions within GUM will vary widely depending on the patient workload, clinic opening hours and number of trained staff within each department.

The size of individual clinics varies enormously between districts. However because services are open access and little is known about the population prevalence of STDs, it is not possible to determine the appropriate size, or 'norms' of a local service. Instead districts need to obtain knowledge about their own local services and determine where else their population seek treatment and advice for STDs before comparing service provision with other commissioning agencies.

The basic facilities which should be on offer within every clinic follow.

Primary prevention

The epidemiological shift away from curable STDs and towards the diagnosis of a greater number of chronic and incurable viral infections has been accompanied by the realization that a mainstay of public policy towards these diseases should be primary prevention. Thus it has been recognized that education about sexual health plays a vital role in promoting sexual wellbeing and hence in avoiding the risks posed by unsafe sexual activity.

Education is carried out by both local health promotion departments and within clinic settings (especially by health advisers). While in an ideal world every health care professional in a GUM clinic will endeavour to incorporate messages about primary prevention and safer sexual practice time constraints often preclude this. As a result most GUM departments currently employ health advisers whose principal role is generally split between providing education and information to patients, with contact tracing and counselling. A review of the work undertaken by health advisers found that:

- many had received no training in GUM related topics
- increasing amounts of their time is being spent on HIV-related issues (mainly pre- and post-test counselling but also in dealing with HIV-positive patients in some clinics) thus leaving less time for discussing other STDs or for partner notification work.

However the work of health advisers and the primary prevention services offered by GUM departments should encompass the following.

Health education

This is aimed primarily at the provision of information about health risks and their prevention through the development of an individual's skills in making choices and hence changing sexual behaviour and activity.[19] Promotion of safer sexual activity and the maintenance of healthier lifestyles are messages that health advisers must make available and acceptable to all sections of the client population. Depending on the demographic mix of the local population, health education material will need to be targeted specifically at certain groups who are either at potentially higher risk of STDs or less likely to utilize services effectively. Some groups, who may need special consideration include:

- gay men and men who have sex with men
- injecting drug-users
- adolescents and young people
- commercial sex workers (male and female)
- people from ethnic minority groups.

Clearly health education is not limited just to those people who present to GUM clinics but is also targeted at those who may be at higher risk of infection and reluctant to attend GUM clinics (or asymptomatic and hence unaware of their STD). While the majority of work in the area of promoting safer sexual practices in the general community and increasing the uptake of sexual health screening facilities, is carried out by people in health promotion departments, health advisers from GUM clinics also play a significant role in this area. In a number of districts health advisers go out into the community, for example into schools and youth groups and either undertake health education themselves or are involved in the education of peer educators in each community.

Provision of free condoms

The question of resource allocation to establish and maintain this service is something which often requires negotiation at a local level as it can become a significant part of the purchasing budget of a clinic.

Hepatitis B vaccination

At present (1997) hepatitis B virus is the only sexually transmitted pathogen against which there is a safe and effective vaccination (although currently there is research on the development of vaccines against both *Chlamydia* and *Herpes simplex* virus). In 1983 Adler *et al.*[20] concluded that screening and vaccination of homosexual men against hepatitis B is cost-effective in reducing the incidence of the disease and its potentially lethal sequelae. In 1989 a survey by Loke *et al.*[21] found that of 121 clinics in the UK, 81% offered screening for hepatitis B surface antigen but only 30% were able to offer the vaccine itself. Each district should assess the prevalence and uptake of hepatitis B screening and *et al.*.Avaccination programmes in its own area.

Contact tracing

Largescale programmes for contact tracing (partner notification) for STDs have been in operation in the UK for over 40 years[22] with the intention of:

- preventing re-infection of the index case
- controlling community spread (as it allows the identification and treatment of asymptomatic and pre-symptomatic individuals who otherwise may not seek treatment)
- providing health education about STDs to the individual.

A description of partner notifications is provided by the World Health Organization. Recently there has been a concerted shift of emphasis from provider to patient referral, i.e. it is the index patients themselves who are encouraged to notify their sexual contacts.

Secondary prevention

This is defined as work to halt the progression of a disease once it is established. In GUM this involves the early detection and early diagnosis of an infection followed by prompt and effective treatment in order to:

- reduce the incidence of STD complications
- reduce the prevalence of STDs in the community.

Case finding and screening

The control of STDs depends heavily on the screening of persons (especially women) for the diagnosis of asymptomatic infections. The relatively large number of people infected asymptomatically also emphasizes the need to co-ordinate screening between different services. The benefits and effectiveness of screening programmes for STDs are discussed in section 6.

Clinical management of presenting STDs

Diagnosis of STDs

When a patient visits a GUM clinic complaining of new symptoms or requesting a sexual health check-up she or he can often expect a preliminary diagnosis to be given on the day of attendance. Genitourinary medicine clinics are equipped with diagnostic facilities on site, mostly using microscopy. In general it is the nursing staff who carry out microscopy but in some clinics it is the medical staff or MLSOs specifically employed for this task. To increase both the sensitivity and specificity of rates of diagnosis, each clinic must also have access to a pathology laboratory with microbiology, serology and virology. Many clinics will use also the services of immunologists.

The diagnostic facilities required for the detection of sexually transmissible pathogens are outlined in Appendix VII, along with the approximate cost of diagnostic tests for each pathogen. It should be recognized that within the laboratory services there are several tiers of facilities available. Those outlined in the appendix include both the general facilities required at district level and the more sophisticated facilities which may be necessary for confirming a diagnosis. The latter will not be cost-effective to run in every district laboratory but it is recommended that district laboratories have the means to contract services from more specialized laboratories for the effective and correct management of individual cases. It must also be recognized that the specialist laboratories offer access to a range of advice from experts in the field, such as consultant virologists.

The field of diagnostics is constantly expanding and changing. New developments will reach commercial and hence widespread use in the near future, such as screening tools for *Chlamydia trachomatis*. Though the cost of these new diagnostic techniques is likely to fall with increasingly widespread use, district planners should take into consideration the possibility of purchasing improved diagnostic techniques and services when planning future budgets. Advice can be obtained from the consultant in communicable diseases and local hospital microbiologists and virologists.

Treatment of STDs

Treatment may be given at the time of the presenting visit. The value of epidemiological treatment (i.e. providing treatment before a diagnosis is established microbiologically or serologically) is based on a number of factors:[23]

- risk of infection being present
- seriousness of the disease
- difficulty of diagnosis
- effectiveness of treatment available
- any side-effects of treatment
- likelihood of spread if not treated
- facilities available for observation.

For a large number of patients treatment regimens will be delayed until the diagnosis is confirmed and therefore a follow-up visit is required.

Treatment of women with abnormal cervical smears

The role of cervical screening programmes in reducing the incidence of cervical cancer is a widely debated issue[24] but targeting women at higher risk is thought to be successful in decreasing the incidence of cervical carcinoma.[25] Women attending GUM clinics will have usually put themselves at risk of acquiring a STD and may therefore also be at risk of cervical carcinoma associated with the presence of sexually acquired papilloma viruses, which cause genital warts.[26,27] The GUM clinic thus provides an ideal environment for opportunistic screening of women at higher risk from cervical cancer in the population.

The management of women with cervical smear abnormalities will depend usually on the grade of abnormality and local management guidelines. Most clinics will refer women with an abnormal smear for a colposcopic examination. Colposcopy is a specialized service allowing magnification and inspection of the cervix. In some clinics this procedure can be carried out on site, while at other clinics it may be necessary to refer patients to other departments (usually gynaecology). Many women will be treated definitively at the time of their colposcopy with laser therapy, electrocoagulation or cryosurgery, which also may be on site.

Psychosexual services

Patients attending for the diagnosis and treatment of STDs may require support, treatment or counselling for psychosexual conditions. The number of trained psychosexual physicians in a district is likely to be small. Therefore if the service is not based in the local GUM clinic, adequate access to psychosexual services needs to be established by the commissioner and local GUM physicians. There are two main treatment modalities within psychosexual medicine: drug treatment and/or psychotherapy.

Contraceptive services

The number of GUM clinics offering these services is gradually increasing as part of a move towards the provision of a holistic sexual health service. However it is important to know whether the service is being offered in an appropriate and acceptable way, through collaboration and review by the family planning service and commissioners.

Services at other sites

The majority of STD services is provided within GUM clinics but there is increasing recognition of the role of other health care providers in the provision of STD services and of the opportunity for GUM clinics to provide other services apart from STD treatment. The role of GUM staff in providing services away from their usual clinic sites is under review in many districts and several are currently implementing innovative models of service provision for client groups who are perceived to currently under-utilize existing service networks. It is also important to recognize that many patients who initially present to GUM clinics will require referral to other departments within the hospital, such as dermatology, gynaecology and urology.

Cost of GUM problems

The structure and components of the costs to society arising from GUM conditions are complex and there is scant information available. They involve not only the direct costs associated with the provision of GUM services directed towards the prevention, diagnosis and management of acute GU conditions but also the costs of management of the serious sequelae of infection which may arise through untreated STDs and the attendant social and economic costs associated with loss of economic activity.

Direct costs of GUM services

There is no published literature on the direct costs of providing GUM services in England and Wales. While all districts included data on GUM funding in their AIDS (Control) Act reports, there is little consistency in the way the data are presented and they should be treated with extreme caution. Not all reports break down funding into mainstream (i.e. general capitation), HIV treatment and care and prevention funding; nor are the costs allocated to the different services provided by the GUM clinics. It is not possible therefore to compare funding levels across different hospitals and commissioning agencies at present.

This situation is unlikely to change until the commissioning agencies themselves encourage the GUM clinics to compile better cost data, as part of their local service specifications and business plans.

Estimating cost per attendance

Data have been obtained from two clinics which allow an estimation of some of the direct costs for 1993/94. These are summarized in Table 11.

Table 11: Cost of two GUM clinic services

Costs	Clinic 1	Clinic 2
Laboratory	186 217	40 626
Drugs	52 600	40 583
Staff	336 200	214 298
Other direct	52 600	20 000
Central overheads @ 40% staff	134 480	85 719
Total cost	762 097	401 226

The costs are indicative only but they suggest that there may be extensive differences in the cost of GUM services between clinics. This makes it all the more important that commissioners obtain detailed cost data and a breakdown of the services offered and activity generated for the purpose of assessing value for money, which we are not in a position to judge here.

Cost to health service of untreated STDs

Inadequate or non-treatment of STDs can have major implications at both the individual and societal levels. Sexually transmitted diseases tend to affect people at a young age. Any assessment of the cost to society of untreated STDs must take into account the loss of productivity and the costs of continuing care. Also the potential physical and psychological consequences of the major complications will affect the infected person and his/her partner, family and children.

However very few cost–benefit analyses have been carried out. One infection that has been assessed in terms of the cost to the health service is that caused by *Chlamydia trachomatis*, which is presented here as an example of the potential cost of untreated STDs versus that of providing a screening service.

Chlamydia trachomatis has the highest prevalence of any diagnosed bacterial sexually transmitted pathogen in the UK. Estimates of current prevalence range from 3 to 8% in asymptomatic populations to over 10% in GUM clinic attenders (Table 7). The potential sequelae of untreated infection are pelvic inflammatory disease (PID), chronic pelvic pain, infection of the cervix (cervicitis), tubal infertility, ectopic pregnancy and neonatal conjunctivitis and pneumonia.

Costs of morbidity associated with *Chlamydia trachomatis* (CT) infection

There have been a number of studies carried out, primarily in the US, which have sought to estimate the costs of CT-associated morbidity and the potential benefits of screening.[13,28–35] There has been some difference of opinion on the interpretation of the results of these studies. Broadly screening programmes among young women are expected to be cost-efficient (to the health service) when the prevalence is above 5%. The advantages or disadvantages to the screened and treated women have not been determined and the value of screening for improving health gain needs to be addressed more thoroughly.

In Table 12 descriptive epidemiological findings with the costs derived from one of the studies in the US[28] are applied to an 'untargeted' screening programme in a region. The assumptions made are as follows:

- all women aged 16–39 are screened (700 000)
- 75% of true-positives are identified and all women identified are treated and cured
- prevalence of CT is 5%
- incidence of PID in untreated women equals 11.5% per annum; 25% of PID treated in hospital; 12.5% of women with PID develop tubal infertility, 1% of women with PID experience subsequent ectopic pregnancy
- 15% of women with undetected CT develop chronic pain
- 10% of babies from infected mothers develop conjunctivitis and 10% develop pneumonia.

Under these assumptions there is a small negative cost to the health service if screening was carried out. Clearly the cost would increase if the screening programme failed to cover all women and the treatment of CT was not 100% successful. Similarly the cost of not screening would be greater if the prevalence of CT was higher than 5% and the incidence of complications was higher. The decision by DHAs on whether to introduce universal screening must wait until it has been fully evaluated.

Table 12: Indicative costs of screening or not screening women aged 16–39 in North Thames (West)

	Number of women	Cost (no screening) (£)	Cost (screening) (£)
Action and gynaecological consequences			
Population women (aged 16–39)	700 000		
Infected with Chlamydia (5% prevalence)	35000		
Detected by screening (75%)	26250		
Tested			4 900 000
Treated			394 000
Trace and treat partner			525 000
Annual CT-related PID cases – 1006			
Treated as an inpatient	1000	1 000 000	250 000
Treated as an outpatient	3000	270 000	67500
Chronic pelvic pain	5250	2 400 000	600 000
Cervicitis	6000	300 000	75000
Tubal infertility (involuntary)	500	2 000 000	500 000
Sub-total		5 970 000	7 311 500
Obstetric consequences			
Live births	44700		
Live births to mother with CT	4470		
Chlamydial conjunctivitis	447	20000	5000
Neonatal CT pneumonia	447	200 000	50000
Ectopic pregnancy	44	88000	22000
Abortions (aged 11–49)	18460		
Post-abortion PID			
Treated as an inpatient	81	81000	20250
Treated as an outpatient	242	21780	5445
Post-abortion infertility (involuntary)	32	64000	16000
Sub-total		474 780	118 695
Total		6 444 780	7 430 195

6 Effectiveness of services

Scientific peer-reviewed literature on the effectiveness of STD interventions is directed at the efficacy of therapeutic interventions, with much less on the effectiveness of other key activities involved in the control of STDs, such as contact tracing. Data on the cost-effectiveness of specific interventions are meagre also. Definitions of the gradings for the strength of recommendations (A–E) and quality of evidence (I–III) are given in the introduction to the needs assessments series.

Current drugs in use

The treatment of bacterial STDs is a constantly changing field because of the swift development of antibiotic resistance (especially against gonorrhoea) and the development of new drugs. The drugs most commonly in use are given in the Appendix VIII together with a ranking of their level of effectiveness. There are a number of treatment regimens and interventions for each condition. Choice of drug depends not just on local antibiotic resistance patterns but also on the characteristics of the patient (for example, history of drug allergy, pregnancy or lactation and perceived level of compliance).

The decline in the prevalence of bacterial STDs has been accompanied by a steady increase in the number of viral STDs diagnosed.[36] The treatment of chronic viral STDs has become a greater part of the workload of each clinic.

Prevention programmes

The cost-effectiveness of preventing the spread of STDs has not been widely investigated.[37,38] Resources devoted to prevention are small in comparison to both the costs of treatment and the secondary impact of sexually transmitted infections. It is also not known whether the balance of funds between prevention, treatment and research is equitably and effectively distributed.[39]

Health education (AIII)

The effectiveness of barrier methods in preventing the transmission of STDs is shown in Table 13.[40–42]

Table 13: Effectiveness of barrier methods

Method	Mechanism	Efficacy
Condom (male)	protects sexual partner from direct contact with body fluids	reduces risk of gonorrhoea, HSV, genital ulcers, PID, HIV, HBV, *C. trachomatis*
Condom (female)	protects sexual partner from direct contact with body fluids	*in vitro* studies show it is impermeable to HIV; not tested for other STDs
Spermicide	chemically inactivates infectious agents	inactivates gonococci, *T. pallidum*, *T. vaginalis*, HSV, ureaplasmas
Diaphragm/spermicide	mechanical barrier, covers cervix	appears to decrease risk of acquiring gonorrhoea and PID

Part of the consistency of use will depend on availability and behaviour change, both of which can be addressed by GUM clinics. Surveys of sexual behaviour have shown that sexual lifestyles in some communities have been modified.[43,44] For outcome indicators of health education interventions districts might consider:

- the number of patients presenting to a clinic who have been treated previously for a different infection (who presumably, continued to have unsafe sex)
- *ad hoc* sexual behaviour surveys in clinics to assess changes in sexual behaviour pre- and post- counselling
- patient views on the effectiveness of different health education strategies appropriate to individual communities.

Unfortunately in contrast to drug treatment the effectiveness of health education is a very difficult process to measure, though its benefits may be far reaching.

Hepatitis B vaccination programme

Hepatitis B virus (HBV) has higher prevalence rates in certain at-risk groups: homosexual men, commercial sex workers, injecting drug-users and persons of south-east Asian or African origin (where the disease is endemic). 2–10% of those infected will become chronic carriers of the virus[45] and will be at future risk of chronic hepatitis, cirrhosis and hepatocellular carcinoma. Hepatitis B vaccine is effective in preventing infection in those individuals who produce specific antibodies after immunization.[46] The vaccine is given as a course at zero, one and six months with a follow-up blood test to check that sufficient antibodies are being produced after the end of the course. The vaccine is effective for at least five years in most patients.

Hepatitis B virus infection is currently the only sexually transmitted viral infection for which an effective vaccine is available but it is apparently not reaching those people who are at highest risk of infection.[47]

Case finding and screening

Screening for STD leads to prompt treatment of the affected individual and thus has the potential to reduce the size of the disease pool and the risk of transmission to third parties. The challenge is how to reach women of child-bearing age who may be infected asymptomatically. Screening programmes can either be selective or universal.[29,48]

Syphilis (AII-2)

All pregnant women are screened routinely for syphilis and the current prevalence of syphilis in women of child-bearing age is low. A study in 1985[49] in which the costs of screening were compared with the avoided costs of caring for affected infants or the effects of increased rates of stillbirth and neonatal deaths showed that the screening programme was cost-effective even when the prevalence of syphilis infection was extremely low.

Chlamydia trachomatis (BII-2)

Screening programmes for *Chlamydia trachomatis* have been assessed in a variety of settings in both the US and the UK. A study in Swansea [13] compared the cost of screening and prophylactic treatment for all women attending for termination of pregnancy with the cost of treating the well-recognized sequelae of undiagnosed chlamydial infection in these women. Overall 8% of the women were infected with *C. trachomatis* and there was a high incidence of chlamydia-associated pelvic infection requiring treatment (including hospital admission). The estimated costs of hospital admissions for complications of chlamydial infection were more than double the cost of providing routine screening and prophylactic treatment. Similarly work in Scandinavia[35] showed that pre-termination screening and treatment was cost-effective when the prevalence of chlamydial infection in the population was 4.3% or higher.

In order to decide locally the best policy for targeting screening it is essential to assess the prevalence of *C. trachomatis* in defined populations (e.g. women attending family planning clinics, ante-natal clinics and gynaecology outpatients) and which women are most at risk. This work is of particular importance because the benefits of universal screening are unproven.

Partner notification (AII-2)

Partner notification developed as part of routine case management in order to assist in the control of these infections in the population. The recognition that much disease was asymptomatic, particularly in women, led to the need for 'case finding' to identify and treat individuals who may otherwise develop serious sequelae, to reduce reinfection in the index patient and to prevent further transmission in the population.

- **Does partner notification contribute to the control of STD in the population?** 'Evidence' to support the common sense supposition that good partner notification must improve the control of STD in the population is largely unavailable for two reasons. First a lack of carefully designed studies. Second the fact that partner notification is only one part of a control programme and it is difficult to distinguish its contribution from that of, for example, free treatment, antibiotic therapy, health education, changes in contraceptive norms and secular trends in sexual behaviour. An additional problem is that a good partner notification scheme will improve case finding, and therefore routine surveillance systems are likely to show an increase in the rate of infection.[50]

  The specific contribution of partner notification to STD control is difficult to measure because it occurs invariably alongside other aspects of a control programme. Sweden, for example, has an aggressive partner notification programme rooted in legislation for gonorrhoea, syphilis and more recently chlamydia. How much of the decline in gonorrhoea is due to partner notification is therefore hard to determine.[51] Talbot explored the relationship between two measures of 'efficiency' in contact tracing and the incidence of gonorrhoea in the population in Sheffield.[52] There was no correlation between the incidence of gonorrhoea and either the mean infectious patient days (between start of contact tracing and attendance of contacts), or percentage of 'source' contacts brought to examination within 30 days, something described in the article as a paradox.

  It is easier to show that where new infections, or new strains of a pathogen in an endemic infection, appear in a community causing distinct outbreaks, partner notification can play an important role in control. In an outbreak of infectious syphilis in Alberta in the mid-1980s, Romanowski reported that: 'contact tracing played an important role in controlling the outbreak with 16% of men and 45% of women being diagnosed and treated as a result of this activity.'[53] While it is difficult to find empirical evidence of a causal relationship between partner notification activities and declining rates of STD in the population, epidemiological models may be able to indicate the likely impact.[54] A broader 'ethnographic' approach to partner notification, working with groups of people linked socially and sexually, can locate members of the 'core' group that are sustaining the disease in the population.[55]

- **Does partner notification improve patient management through reducing repeat infection?** There is some evidence to support this. In an observational study of contact tracing for *C. trachomatis* in Sweden, 10.2% of women who had no partner notification were found to be reinfected (within the 3–15 months follow-up period).[56] The reinfection rate was lower in those who had patient referral accompanied by health worker verification that the contact had attended (4.8%). These data must be interpreted with care as they are based on a review of routine practice over a ten-year period and it is probable that the patients receiving different types of contact management were not comparable. While the data suggest that the provision of scripts for male partners of women with chlamydial infection may be effective in some populations (with a low rate of transmission perhaps), they do not permit further identification of the chain of transmission. It also goes against the principles of most GUM practice (diagnosis before treatment, test for other STDs, follow-up to ensure clinical and microbiological cure, trace contacts and investigate).

- **Does partner notification identify previously unrecognized cases of infection and, through treatment, prevent the development of serious sequelae?** The result of almost all studies of partner notification show that the prevalence of infection in traced partners is higher than in the general, or clinic, population. This reason alone makes partner notification a useful method of case finding within a control programme.

  Burgess reported in 1963 that 342 (27%) of 1248 'VD' contacts were found to have an infection, of whom only 31 were already having treatment prior to contact tracing.[57] Early discussions of the importance of partner notification concentrated on asymptomatic infection in women, but asymptomatic infection in men, while less common, may play an equally important role in sustaining infection in the population. Studies of male sexual contacts of women with PID show relatively high levels of asymptomatic disease – in one study 59% of 86 gonorrhoea-positive male partners (of women with PID) were asymptomatic.[58] This and other findings suggest that there may be as much male as female untreated disease which partner notification could help identify and treat.

- **What are the most effective methods of partner notification?** A review by Oxman identifies comparative studies and reveals the lack of good randomized controlled trials, though there are various observational studies which provide some 'evidence' of relative effectiveness.[59]

- **Is provider referral better than patient referral in ensuring that contacts are informed and screened?** Observations in many reviews indicate that provider referral achieves a higher rate of attendance than patient referral, in some studies fewer contacts are reported.[59]

- **Do trained health advisers obtain better outcomes from partner notification than doctors or nurses?** The early reports of contact tracing showed an increase in the attendance of contacts if a trained 'VD social worker' carried out the interview and the follow-up.[60] However the comparison is usually between doctors issuing contact slips and social workers or health advisers carrying out more intensive investigation and follow-up. Potterat supports this argument, adding that trained ethnographers also can achieve good results in bringing contacts and others who are at risk into the clinic.[54] Clearly doctors and nurses, if they are to support trained health advisors, need training to recognize that a contact slip alone is not enough. In one study of contact tracing for ocular chlamydial infection, without health advisers, 87% of partners who were given appointments attended and reportedly 67% of those given contact slips attended other clinics.[61]

7 Models of care

The basic model of GUM service provision

There is one basic model of care that covers the whole of GUM services in the UK, namely the provision in each district of at least one specialist GUM clinic within an acute unit or, less frequently, attached to a community unit.

The clinics are based on the following key principles:

- services are open access and self-referral
- services and treatment are free at the point of delivery
- patients receive a confidential service.

These principles have guided the provision of services since 1916, when a network of clinics was established following a report of the Royal Commission on Venereal Diseases.[1] The Commission recommended that county and borough councils provide free and confidential treatment for patients at convenient hours. These recommendations were translated into law by the Venereal Diseases Act of 1917[62] and reaffirmed in 1988 by the Report of the Working Group to examine workloads in GUM clinics (the Monks Report)[2] and a subsequent NHS Executive Circular.

The clinics are run by specialists in GUM together with trained nurses and health advisers and have a combined role of providing clinical care for those who present to them and a public health role in relation to case finding and disease control in the population through partner notification, outreach programmes and health promotion programmes in the local community.

The minimum level of provision is one clinic per district, though some urban districts, particularly in London may have several clinics. The large variation in GUM provision (several districts had no clinic at all at the time of the Monks report) is due to various historical factors, including the level of demand for services locally. However the relationship of the numbers of clinics to the need of the population as expressed in rates of STDs in the population is difficult to measure, as much of the information on population STD rates is inferred from the workload of these clinics. In general as the number of clinics and clinic sessions increases, so the number of cases of STD identified will also rise.

The NSSAL data show higher rates of STD attendance, particularly in London but this is associated with higher levels of risk behaviour. Indeed that survey suggests that only a minority of people at risk of STD (defined by recent sexual behaviour) attend clinics and therefore there may be considerable unmet need.

Greater provision of GUM services will be needed in:

- districts with higher rates of STD
- districts with greater proportions of the population which are likely to be at increased risk of STDs (e.g. gay men, tourists, migrant workers and other migrants, prostitutes, injecting drug users, young homeless).

In general these occur in larger urban areas, in addition to ports and some tourist areas. Ideally each district should have a profile of the local population and be able to describe sections of the population at increased risk and ensure that the GUM services meet their needs. At the very least each district should ensure local GUM provision.

A broader model of sexual health service provision

While the general model outlined above is common to all districts, it does not cover all GUM care. Patients with STDs and related problems may present and be managed in a number of other sectors of the health service. As outlined in section 4, GPs see an unknown number of cases of STD and other patients present to family planning services and specialists in gynaecology, urology, A and E, dermatology, infectious diseases, general medicine and mental health.

In recent years there has been a shift away from a disease based approach (which underpins GUM) towards the broader concept of 'sexual health'. This was initiated in health promotion work, where there is an obvious overlap between the prevention of STD/HIV and the prevention of unplanned pregnancy.

This shift has yet to be fully reflected in the provision of services. A few districts have integrated 'sexual health' services where GUM, family planning, termination of pregnancy, psychosexual counselling and related services are provided in one clinic. In other areas there is no unified service but greater links are being established between community gynaecology and GUM. Many GUM clinics now provide some contraceptive services and some family planning clinics (FPCs) provide screening for sexually transmitted infections, such as chlamydial infection.

Full integration into a sexual health service, as exists in parts of Australia for example, is controversial but there is a clear case for better planning of services and liaison between sectors.

Two models are proposed as follows.

1 The integration of sexual health services, with a specialist sexual health clinic providing a full range of sexual health services under one roof. This would need to be linked to satellite clinics (current family planning clinics) where part of the service is provided closer to the local population with easy referral into the specialist centre. The sexual health clinic would remain open access, self-referral and free. This would require the inclusion of consultants in GUM and community gynaecology in the senior staff and the management of such a clinic would have to be located appropriately (in acute or community sector).

The aim would be to make the service more convenient for patients (they would no longer need to visit different sites) and potentially reduce the stigma of the 'special clinic'.

2   The maintenance of GUM and family planning as distinct services (physically, managerially and professionally) but with a far greater level of integration, including reciprocal clinics at the other site(s), development of common protocols specifying indications for referral and standards of management for conditions seen in both settings.

The role of general practitioners

As outlined in previous sections, GPs see an unknown but probably relatively large, number of patients with STDs. They also provide a large proportion of family planning services to patients. The standard of care provided for STD in primary care is unlikely to be the same as in specialist clinics, given the lack of facilities for diagnosis, knowledge about current effective treatments and opportunities for partner notification. However many patients will continue to present initially to their GPs and may prefer not to attend the local GUM (or sexual health) clinic. In order to promote good standards of practice, GPs should be involved with genitourinary physicians in the development of guidelines for diagnosis and management of common conditions, including the provision of partner notification and indications for referral to specialist services.

Commissioning and the role of specialists in public health

GUM services should continue to be core funded and open access and therefore should be excluded from GP 'total fundholding'. In each district a forum of GUM, family planning and GPs should be established to enable the integration of services and develop common guidelines and audit tools for improving standards of care. Public health specialists should play a lead role in initiating this discussion in an attempt to reduce problems of 'territoriality'.

As GUM deals primarily with infectious disease it is important that the perspective of control is maintained in the planning of services, specifically the involvement of public health specialists in the commissioning agencies, including the CCDC.

Commissioning agencies should consider contracting out some control (e.g. partner notification and outreach programmes) and health promotion (e.g. work with at risk populations and in schools) initiatives, to local GUM services, using the skills of the health professionals. They should also develop guidelines for the reporting and management of patients diagnosed with STDs outside of GUM clinics where responsibilities are statutarily defined. This will be increasingly important as more screening (e.g. for *C. trachomatis*) takes place in general practice, family planning and gynaecology clinics.

Resources

The proposals above have not been costed as they are dependent on the extent of provision in any locality and cost of GUM care is difficult to separate from HIV and AIDS care in many places. There is no *a priori* reason why a shift to more integrated services, including a fully integrated sexual health service, should involve greater recurrent expenditure, although some areas would need initial capital investment. The further expansion of existing services must go hand in hand with work to improve information on the extent of STDs in the population and where the local population is currently being diagnosed and treated for STDs.

8 Outcome measures and targets

Health of the Nation

The Government's targets for sexual health[63,64] outline the following objectives for STDs:

- to reduce the incidence of STDs
- to develop further and strengthen monitoring and surveillance
- to provide effective services for diagnosis and treatment of STDs.

The specific target applies to gonorrhoea:

To reduce the incidence of gonorrhoea among men and women aged 15–64 by at least 20% by 1995 (from 61 new cases per 100 000 population in 1990 to no more than 49 cases per 100 000).

In response to these objectives the Association for Genitourinary Medicine (AGUM) produced a document *Goals, indicators and targets for the management of sexually transmitted diseases: guidelines for purchasers and others.* Recommendations from their guidelines are shown in Appendix IX as they give the most comprehensive guide to setting and measuring structure, process and outcome targets for GUM services.

The most important barrier to measuring outcomes, or informing the commissioning process lies with the current method of collecting GUM clinic data (section 9).

9 Information and research priorities

Problems with GUM clinic information

The KC60 is the primary source of information on STDs in the UK and was used as the baseline for the Health of the Nation targets on gonorrhoea. Though one of the most comprehensive routine systems in Europe, it has several shortcomings. First it cannot provide data by place of residence. Second there is heterogeneity in the way the KC60s are compiled, in terms of the case definitions and attribution of new episodes. Third it does not reflect the true activity levels of GUM clinics. As a form of reporting the KC60 fails to capture and exploit much of the information already recorded in local provider units which would be of value for commissioning and ignores the IT developments occurring in most provider units. Taken together the above create major problems for district population based commissioning and describing the local epidemiology of sexually transmissible infections. In addition it makes the identification of denominators for the calculation of incidence and prevalence rates almost impossible.

KC60 GUM clinic returns report each new episode as a case. Multiple STDs are common and a person may have multiple episodes of different STDs during any reporting period. In addition for the chronic STDs, misclassification of follow-up visits as new episodes may bias the figures considerably in an upward direction.

Towards a solution

The primary responsibility for service development lies with the individual commissioning agencies. However the key features of the epidemiology of sexual health and patterns of sexual health service utilization make it essential that an information strategy be co-ordinated over a larger geographical area than the DHA. People with sexually transmitted infections regularly cross administrative boundaries in their use of services (and in the course of their sexual activities). Therefore local surveillance and needs assessment initiatives cannot be relied upon solely for planning sexual health services.

Current developments in the contract minimum data set will not be extended at this present time to GUM clinics. This is partly because many GUM clinics remain separate from hospital information systems and partly because of concerns over confidentiality and VD legislation.[62] At least two RHAs have begun to collate data on STDs across GUM clinics (West Midlands and S Thames East), though largely for epidemiological purposes, they have not been explicitly involved with service development or commissioning. The computerization of GUM clinics does provide the opportunity of improving routine data. A further pilot study in North Thames aims to provide information both for public health surveillance and commissioning.

Non-GUM STDs

Currently little is known about the number of STDs diagnosed and treated outside GUM. This must change as districts develop integrated sexual health services and more extensive screening of people in other settings is carried out. For this reason districts should examine laboratory reporting with the view to improving its coverage and use the data to monitor overall numbers of STDs, positive rates by source of request and provide a sampling frame for clinical audit of the management of specific STDs.

National, regional and local studies of prevalence and incidence rates of STDs

There is a gap between the information obtained from GUM clinics on people presenting for screening and/or treatment and the information obtained from population surveys of STDs, often on self-selected or serial samples from hospital clinics. Several areas require further work:

- examining how the current surveys could be generalized for use by district populations
- establishing the level of infection diagnosed and treated by GUM clinics, in order to set targets and inform the commissioning of GUM
- commissioning new population surveys which could establish the population levels of STDs in different populations in the UK that can be used for planning by DHAs.

Is gonorrhoea the best marker for sexual activity?

The national Health of the Nation target for reducing the incidence of gonorrhoea by at least 20% has already been met. Before setting new targets, which have a crucial influence on the research and development agenda, it is necessary to be sure that gonorrhoea trends are sensitive to changes in sexual behaviour. This in turn relates to HIV incidence and whether other sexually transmitted infections or a range of such infections (such as chlamydial or herpes simplex virus) would not be better indicators of the level of risk and behaviour change in the population.

Studies into costing and the cost-effectiveness of GUM services

There are no reliable studies on the costs of different ways of delivering specialist services for the treatment of STDs. These are required to inform the development of commissioning sexual health services, in particular the diagnosis and treatment of STDs in other settings (primary care, obstetrics and gynaecology, casualty, family planning) and the treatment of chronic conditions. In addition the variation in the costs of GUM clinics can be addressed only by assessing the different costs and components of the service.

Studies into the benefits and effectiveness of selected or universal screening for STDs in asymptomatic women

Of particular importance is genital chlamydial infection which may present the greatest health burden of a sexually transmissible infection in the UK (excluding HIV infection). It is unlikely that the findings from studies in the US and other European countries can be transposed to the UK. Therefore largescale intervention must wait until properly designed population trials of screening have been carried out in the UK.

Models of shared care and education

Sexual health services are becoming integrated. It is important therefore to establish what role GUM physicians have in the education of other health care workers in the recognition of STDs and the development of local algorithms for the management of STDs outside GUM clinics. Also whether there is scope for managing chronic STDs in primary care with the advice of GUM consultants, following a similar model of other chronic diseases.

Develop surveillance of STDs from GUM clinics and laboratories

Throughout this chapter it has been emphasized that there is a paucity of data for commissioning agencies to make informed choices over service development. It is essential that studies are started with the aim of improving the routine STD/GUM data available to all DHAs (in addition to sentinel surveillance initiatives which serve a national agenda) from both GUM clinics and laboratories. Of course an important part of any evaluation will be to show the added value of improved surveillance on policy.

Audit of hepatitis B vaccination

Hepatitis B virus infection is currently the only sexually transmitted infection for which an effective vaccine is available. Studies are needed in order to understand why vaccination is not reaching those people who are at highest risk of infection and to make practicable proposals on how this can be changed.

Appendix I ICD codes for GUM-related conditions (excluding HIV/AIDS and neoplasia)

ICD 9

Herpes simplex	054.0–054.9
Viral hepatitis	070.0–070.9
Molluscum contagiosum	078.0
Viral warts	078.1
Congenital syphilis	090.0–090.9
Early syphilis, symptomatic	091.0–091.9
Early syphilis, latent	092.0–092.9
Cardiovascular syphilis	093.0–093.9
Neurosyphilis	094.0–094.9
Other forms of late syphilis, with symptoms	095
Late syphilis, latent	096
Other and unspecified syphilis	097.0–097.9
Gonococcal infections	098.0–098.8
Chancroid	099.0
Lymphogranuloma venereum	099.1
Granuloma inguinale	099.2
Reiter's disease	099.3
Other non-gonococcal urethritis	099.4
Candidiasis	112.0–112.9
Trichomoniasis	131.0–131.9
Pediculosis and phthirus infestation	132.0–132.9
Scabies	133.0
Inflammatory diseases of prostate	601.0–601.9
Orchitis and epididymitis	604.0–604.9
Disorders of penis	607.0–607.9
Other diseases of male genital organs	608.0–608.9
Acute salpingitis and oophoritis	614.0
Chronic salpingitis and oophoritis	614.1
Salpingitis or oophoritis, not subacute, acute or chronic	614.2
Inflammatory diseases of uterus	615.0–615.9
Inflammatory disease of cervix, vagina and vulva	616.0–616.9
Malposition of uterus	621.6
Non-inflammatory disorders of cervix	622.0–622.9
Non-inflammatory disorders of vagina	623.0–623.9
Non-inflammatory disorders of vulva and perineum	624.0–624.9
Pain and other symptoms associated with female genital organs	625.0–625.9

ICD 10

Congenital syphilis	A50
Early syphilis	A51
Late syphilis	A52

Other and unspecified syphilis	A53
Gonococcal infection	A54
Chlamydial lymphogranuloma	A55
Other sexually transmitted chlamydial diseases	A56
Chancroid	A57
Granuloma inguinale	A58
Trichomoniasis	A59
Anogenital herpes viral infection	A60
Other predominantly sexually transmitted diseases (nec)	A63
Unspecified sexually transmitted disease	A64
Molluscum contagiosum	B08.1
Acute hepatitis A	B15
Acute hepatitis B	B16
Other acute viral hepatitis	B17
Chronic viral hepatitis	B18
Unspecified viral hepatitis	B19
Malignant neoplasm of vulva	C51
Malignant neoplasm of vagina	C52
Malignant neoplasm of cervix uteri	C53
Malignant neoplasm of corpus uteri	C54
Malignant neoplasm of uterus, part unspecified	C55
Malignant neoplasm of penis	C60
Malignant neoplasm of prostate	C61
Malignant neoplasm of testis	C62
Malignant neoplasm of other and unspecified male genital organs	C63
Benign neoplasm of vulva	D28.0
Benign neoplasm of vagina	D28.1
Benign neoplasm of male genital organs	D29
Hyperplasia of prostate	N40
Inflammatory diseases of prostate	N41
Hydrocele and spermatocele	N43
Torsion of testis	N44
Orchitis and epididymitis	N45
Male infertility	N46
Redundant prepuce, phimosis and paraphimosis	N47
Other disorders of penis	N48
Inflammatory disorders of male genital organs (nec)	N49
Other disorders of male genital organs	N50
Salpingitis and oophoritis	N70
Inflammatory disease of uterus, except cervix	N71
Inflammatory disease of cervix uteri	N72
Other female pelvic inflammatory diseases	N73
Diseases of Bartholin's gland	N75
Other inflammation of vagina and vulva	N76
Polyp of female genital tract	N84
Other non-inflammatory disorders of uterus, except cervix	N85
Erosion and extropion of cervix uteri	N86
Dysplasia of cervix uteri	N87

Other non-inflammatory disorders of cervix uteri N88

Other non-inflammatory disorders of vagina N89

Other non-inflammatory disorder of vulva and perineum N90

Other abnormal uterine and vaginal bleeding N93

Pain and other conditions associated with female genital organs and menstrual cycle N94

Special screening examination for infections with a predominantly sexual mode of transmission Z11

Special screening examination for neoplasm of cervix Z12

Contact with and exposure to infections with a predominantly sexual mode of transmission Z20

Carrier of infections predominantly sexually transmitted Z22

Need for immunization against viral hepatitis Z24.6

Contraceptive management Z30

Appendix II Summary list of KC60 codes

Current codes

Syphilis (primary)	A1
Syphilis (secondary)	A2
Syphilis (latent in first two years of infection)	A3
Syphilis (cardiovascular)	A4
Syphilis (of the nervous system)	A5
Syphilis (all other late/latent stages)	A6
Syphilis (congenital aged under two years)	A7
Syphilis (congenital aged two years and over)	A8
Syphilis – epidemiologically treated	A9
Gonorrhoea (lower genitourinary tract)	B1.1
Gonorrhoea (mouth and throat)	B1.2
Gonorrhoea (eye infections, adult)	B1.3
Gonorrhoea (upper GU tract) excluding PID and epididymitis	B1.4a
Gonorrhoea PID/epididymitis	B1.4b
Gonorrhoea and chlamydial PID/epididymitis	B1.4c
Gonorrhoea (systemic complications)	B1.5
Gonorrhoea (pre-pubertal infections)	B2
Gonorrhoea (ophthalmia neonatorum)	B3
Gonorrhoea – epidemiologically treated	B4
Chancroid	C1
Herpes simplex (primary infection)	C10A
Herpes simplex (recurrent infection)	C10B
Herpes simplex (primary or recurrent?)	C10C
Warts (first attack), sexually acquired	C11A
Warts (recurrence), sexually acquired	C11B
Warts (first attack/recurrence?)	C11C
Hepatitis B (antigen positive)	C13A
Hepatitis (other viral)	C13B
Lymphogranuloma venereum	C2
Granuloma inguinale	C3
Post-pubertal uncomplicated Chlamydia	C4A
Other complicated Chlamydia	C4B
Pre-pubertal Chlamydia	C4C
Chlamydial ophthalmia neonatorum	C4D
Chlamydia – epidemiologically treated	C4E
Chlamydial PID/epididymitis	C4F
Non-specific PID/epididymitis	C4G
NSU (Chlamydia negative, or not known)	C4H
Non-specific genital infection (NSGI)	C7B
NSGI with arthritis	C5
Trichomoniasis	C6A
Bacterial/anaerobic vaginosis	C6B
Other vaginosis/vaginitis/balanitis	C6C

Candidiasis	C7A
Scabies	C8
Pediculosis pubis	C9
Other treponemal diseases treated	D1
Previously treated conditions requiring further treatment	D2.2
Epidemiologically treated conditions	D2/3
Dermatological conditions requiring treatment	D2/4
Herpes simplex (not sexually acquired)	D2/5
Ulceration	D2/6
Carcinoma	D2/7
Urinary infection/urethral syndrome	D2/8
Psychosexual problems	D2/9
Hepatitis (non-viral)/hep. B vaccination	D2/10
Enteric pathogens	
Bartholinitis	D2/12
Prostatitis	D2/13
Psychiatric/psychological	D2/16
Neurological	D2/17
Gynaecological	D2/18
Cardiological	D2/19
Renal	D2/20
Rheumatological	D2/21
Bartholin's cyst	D2/22
Behcet's disease	D2/23
Cervical erosion	D2/24
Erythroplasia of Queyrat	D2/25
Foreign body in vagina	D2/26
Haemorrhoids	D2/27
Hydrocoele	D2/28
Conjunctivitis	D2/29
Paraphimosis	D2/32
Pediculosis corporis	D2/33
Phimosis	D2/34
Plasma cell balanoposthitis	D2/35
Pregnancy	D2/36
Pyogenic infection	D2/37
Sebaceous cyst	D2/38
Undescended testicle(s)	D2/39
Lymphocele	D2/40
Peyronie's disease	D2/41
Cytological abnormality of cervix	D2/42
Venerophobia	D2/70
Dental	D2/72
Drug addiction	D2/73
Urological	D2/84
Anal fissure	D2/85
Other conditions not requiring treatment	D3
Other conditions referred elsewhere	D4

Appendix III Recommendations from the Monks report

Genitourinary medicine workloads

Recommendations

The following recommendations are addressed in particular to health authorities, both at district and at regional level and to the DOH. While some of them quite clearly call for action from only one of these bodies others require more than one body to take action. Moreover it is the team's view that the current situation, which demands an urgent response, has arisen to a large extent either because it is not clear who is responsible for some area of work or because the various people who are acknowledged to have responsibilities have not co-ordinated their efforts.

In the team's view therefore it would be useful for readers to consider all the recommendations carefully before dismissing any of them as being someone else's responsibility. However we have first listed five priority recommendations and then 13 further recommendations.

1 The GUM service must be designated as a priority.
2 Additional resources must be made available to implement the team's recommendations.
3 Ministers and the NHS should give a lead in developing this service.
4 Any person presenting with a new clinical problem suggestive of a sexually transmitted disease or who considers himself or herself to have been in contact with such a disease should be seen on the day of presentation or failing that on the next occasion the clinic is open.
5 There must be GUM provision in every district. Districts lacking a clinic should be able to call on a nominated GUM consultant from another district, until such time as they establish their own clinic.

Other recommendations.

6 GUM clinics should be situated in the general outpatient department of a district general hospital.
7 Clinics should be clearly signposted from all patient entrances to the hospital and use the title Genitourinary medicine department.
8 All areas where patients may wish to discuss confidential matters should be soundproof.
9 The individual roles of the doctor, nurse, health adviser, clerical and other staff should be examined, together with their interaction with the working of the whole GUM clinic.
10 Guidelines for staff requirements based on patient attendances and time required per patient should be established.
11 Staffing levels should then be reviewed and adjusted to give adequate time for each patient and allow for the change in the type of cases currently being seen.
12 Every clinic should have at least one health adviser. A certificate course for health advisers needs to be established, which will be run regularly and be of sufficient content and duration to cope with the complexities of health advising.
13 All clinics should have access to the support of clinical psychologists or psychiatrists.
14 New patients and repeat patients presenting with a new clinical problem, should be clinically examined by a doctor rather than a nurse.
15 Regions should be required to review the distribution of their main GUM services and improve distribution where required.

16 Additional funding should be made available to assist in the completion of the KC60 return. Districts should make funds available either for computerization or for increased clerical help. Computers should be compatible with those in other districts within each region.

17 All clinics should continue to provide comprehensive counselling for patients and clients.

18 In accordance with the recommendation of the Venereal Disease Regulations 1916,[1] arrangements should be made for some clinic sessions to be held after 5pm.

Appendix IV Policy implications and key findings from a study of work roles and responsibilities in GUM clinics

This study was carried out by the Policy Studies Institute and examined in detail the work roles and responsibilities of staff in 20 GUM clinics in the UK.[3] The policy implications of the key findings and recommendations of the researchers are listed as follows.

1 In developing GUM clinic services, there should be a fundamental review of the aims and objectives of the clinics themselves and of their place within the wider health service.

2 There should also be a review of the most appropriate skill mix within GUM clinics to meet the aims and objectives, with the recognition that GUM clinics are by no means homogenous in terms of the populations they serve, the conditions they see, the staff they can attract, the physical conditions in which they are housed and the areas of the country in which they are situated.

3 There is a need for a review at a national, regional and local level of the balance of work in GUM clinics between HIV/AIDS and other sexually transmitted diseases. The nature of the work should be assessed and measures taken to ensure that the appropriate staff time is spent equitably.

4 It is essential to institute a reliable statistical basis by which the workload of GUM clinics can be measured so that accurate forecasting and strategic planning can be developed.

5 There is a need for a clearer understanding and assessment of what constitutes workloads in GUM clinics.

6 There is an urgent need for a review of workload measurements. This should cover both sets of Korner returns – the KH09 and the KC60.

7 The KH09 review should aim for a clearer definition of clinic sessions, cancelled clinic sessions, attendances, non-attendances, telephone consultations, etc. There is a need to be able to measure (a) the number of individuals attending the clinic in any one year, (b) the number of occasions on which each individual attends the clinic and (c) the number of 'threshold crossings' in any one year. There is also a need to be able to make proper distinctions between new and old patients.

8 The KC60 review should determine the nature of the information currently required, and should recognize the present wide anomalies and inconsistencies in allocating codes in GUM clinics.

9 Both reviews should examine the process by which data are collected and collated, with special attention to how diagnostic coding of conditions is recorded, supervised and checked in GUM clinics. There is a need for guidance and agreement on the level and type of staff who should be responsible for the allocation of the diagnostic codes. All diagnostic coding should be checked by the senior doctor.

10 Guidelines should be compiled and issued to aid the understanding of the requirements of the statistical returns and to facilitate collection and collation of the data. They should include clearer definitions of component categories. The guidance should cover both the KH09 and KC60 requirements in one document.

11 A basis is needed for a more accurate audit of the workload of the clinic as a whole, as well as the workload of the different types of staff and individual members of staff.

12 Individual clinics must be able to audit their work with reference to regional needs and national policy.

13 A review is needed of the skills in GUM clinics and the numbers and types of staff needed to fulfil these roles. There is a need for leadership in designating these skills and for assessing the skill mix required.

14 All staff employed in GUM clinics should have job descriptions. These should be drawn up in consultation with staff in post and with their professional managers, and regularly reviewed and revised as necessary. The job descriptions should reflect the demands and the 'culture' of the clinic and the post.

15 There is a clear need to provide proper clerical and administrative support for medical, nursing and health advising staff to avoid inappropriate use of their skills.

16 There is an urgent need to review the recruitment, retention, training and support of reception staff in some clinics.

17 The personal and professional development of all staff in GUM clinics is a high priority. Training and continuing education should be offered and maintained. There should be recognition of particular skills and aptitudes which should be developed fully. The value of interdisciplinary courses should be acknowledged.

18 A comprehensive audit and activity analysis is required of the tasks carried out by individual members of staff.

19 A system of individual performance review should be instituted for all staff.

20 The study indicated a need for a clear management structure within each GUM clinic, however small and whatever the local conditions. The relationship between this management structure and the wider hospital or community context within which it is placed should be made explicit.

21 The research showed the need for clear lines of management and professional accountability for all types of staff in GUM clinics. Staff should be made aware of the identity of the managers to whom they are both managerially and professionally accountable.

22 Professional staff should be professionally accountable to suitably qualified managers from the same professional discipline.

23 The study indicated a need for a designated clinic manager to take charge of all routine administrative and day-to-day needs of running a GUM clinic, and for a designated 'business' manager of audit, performance measurement, finance and organizational matters such as business plans.

24 The study underlined the need for a clinical director to be responsible for the clinical policy and supervision of the clinic. It is unlikely that any consultant can supervise more than two clinics adequately.

25 Adequate soundproofing of all parts of the clinic is essential to ensure confidentiality.

26 Adequate space is necessary to ensure that staff can carry out their designated responsibilities.

27 There is a need to review and rationalize the counselling work undertaken within GUM clinics. All staff should be made aware of the policy of the clinic on counselling in connection with different conditions, the definition of counselling and the respective functions of all staff as far as counselling is concerned. The differences between advice, information and counselling should be made clear to all staff.

28 The role of GUM staff, not only in controlling the spread of infection but also in creating and maintaining sexual health in the population by means of education and health promotion, both within the clinics and in the wider community, should be developed.

29 The role of GUM clinic staff in giving education in sex and personal relationships and about contraception, especially to young people, should be developed. Young people are noted for wanting 'one door to knock on' and every opportunity should be taken to give contraceptive advice and information to people who are clearly 'at risk', not only from infection but also from unwanted pregnancies.

30 Questions regarding the supply of condoms by GUM clinics should be reviewed as a matter of urgency.

31 The unique role of GUM clinics in relation to the sexual health of the nation should be recognized. The contact they have with sexually active people should be used as a basis from which to develop their services and to maximize their contribution. Encouragement should be given to GUM clinics to extend the boundaries of their work. The provision by GUM clinics of treatment and advice in areas closely related to sexual health should be encouraged, given the necessary training and expertise among staff.

32 Close and continuing links should be fostered with all professionals and agencies who may refer patients to GUM clinics and to whom GUM clinics may refer. Issues of confidentiality, which are of paramount importance to GUM clinic staff should be discussed as a matter of routine with all external agencies.

33 There is a need to conduct research into the views and experience of patients using GUM clinics. Many of the issues examined in the study need to be looked at through the eyes of the consumer.

Appendix V Genitourinary syndromes, aetiologies and complications

The majority of patients present describing one of a number of symptoms which can be classified within a syndromic approach. The major syndromes and their aetiologies are listed as follows.

Vaginal discharge

- **Infective causes**
  Candida albicans
  Trichomonas vaginalis
  Gardnerella vaginalis
  Anaerobic organisms
  Chlamydia trachomatis
  Neisseria gonorrhoeae
  Cervical *Herpes genitalis*
  Syphilis (*Treponema pallidum*)
  Toxic shock syndrome
  Mycoplasmas
  Haemolytic streptococci

- **Non-infective**
  Cervical ectropion
  Cervical polyps
  Retained products
  Trauma
  Allergy

Urethral discharge

- **Infective causes**
  Neisseria gonorrhoea
  Chlamydia trachomatis
  Ureaplasma urealyticum
  Trichomonas vaginalis
  Candida albicans
  Other bacteria – *E. coli*, Proteus

- **Non-infective**
  Intraurethral lesions – syphilis, herpes, warts
  Physical or chemical trauma
  Allergy
  Non-specific causes

Genital ulceration/erosion

- **Infective causes**
  Herpes genitalis
  Syphilis
  Chancroid
  Granuloma inguinale
  Lymphogranuloma venereum
  Candida albicans
  Trichomonas vaginalis
  Scabies
  Folliculitis
  TB

- **Non-infective**
  Reiter's syndrome
  Leukoplakia
  Carcinoma
  Lichen sclerosis et atrophicus
  Balanitis xerotica obliterans
  Bechcets syndroms
  Erythema multiforme
  Stevens-Johnson syndrome

Complications

- Pelvic inflammatory disease
- Tubal infertility
- Ectopic pregnancy
- Miscarriage, premature delivery
- Fetal and perinatal morbidity and mortality
- Ano-genital carcinomas
- Chronic hepatitis, hepatoma
- Neurological and cardiovascular disease

Appendix VI Acute presentation and complications of sexually transmitted pathogens

Organism	Acute presentation	Complications/chronic sequelae
BACTERIA		
1 *Treponema pallidum* (syphilis)	1 Syphilitic chancre (ulcer) 2 Secondary syphilis – systemic illness with fever, malaise, adenopathy and rash.	1 Tertiary syphilis – gummas – cardiovascular damage – neurological: meningitis tabes dorsalis, general paresis – congenital: miscarriage stillbirth Neonatal death Child infected (early and late complications)
2 *Neisseria gonorrhoeae* (gonorrhoea)	**Men** Urethral discharge Dysuria Acute prostatitis Pharyngitis Acute epididymitis Disseminated infection (arthritis-dermatitis syndrome) Conjunctivitis	**Men** Chronic prostatitis Lymphangitis and urethral stricture Infertility
	Women Vaginal discharge Dysuria Intermenstrual bleeding Menorrhagia Pharyngitis Rectal infection (usually asymptomatic) Disseminated infection Perihepatitis Abscess of Bartholin's gland	**Women** Acute salpingitis (PID) leading to: infertility, ectopic pregnancy Complications of pregnancy/ delivery spontaneous abortion – premature rupture of membranes – acute chorioamnionitis – infection of other mucosal sites – arthritis
3 *Chlamydia trachomatis* A	**Men** Urethral discharge Prostatitis Proctitis Reiter's syndrome Conjunctivitis	**Men** Infertility

		Women	Women
		Cervicitis – discharge Urethritis Abscess of Bartholin's gland Endometritis Perihepatitis Salpingitis	PID – leading to: infertility, ectopic pregnancy Possible – spontaneous abortion – prematurity – amnionitis Puerperal infection Post-abortion salpingitis Ophthalmia neonatorum
Chlamydia trachomatis	**B**	Lymphogranuloma venereum Primary: genital papule or ulcer Secondary: i. inguinal syndrome lymphadenitis with bubo formation ii. Anogenitorectal syndrome – acute haemorrhagic proctitis Other: Urethritis Cervicitis Salpingitis Parametritis Conjunctivitis Regional lymphadenitis Meningitis	 Genital elephantiasis Genital ulcers and fistulas/ Rectal stricture Perirectal abscesses Anal fistula Frozen pelvis Scarring
4 *Haemophilus ducreyi* (chancroid)		Genital ulcer inguinal bubo ± dysuria pain on defaecation rectal bleeding dyspareunia vaginal discharge urethritis	Genital fistulas
5 *Calymmatobacterium granulomatis* (donovanosis)		Genital ulceration Tissue lymphoedema Involvement of distal sites – lesions on head, liver, thorax and bones	Tissue destruction Residual scarring and fibrosis
6 Genital mycoplasmas (*Mycoplasma hominis, Ureaplasma* *urealyticum, Mycoplasma genitalum*)		**Men** Urethritis Prostatitis Epididymitis Reiter's disease	Decreased fertility

	Women	Disorders of reproduction:
	Bartholin's abscess	Chorioamnionitis
	Viginitis (bacterial vaginosis)	Low birth weight
	PID (possible)	[Possible: spontaneous
	Endomyometritis (post-abortion)	abortion]
	Endometritis – postpartum fever	
7 Enteric bacterial pathogens (Shigella, Salmonella and Campylobacter)	Bacillary dysentery Acute gastroenteritis Systemic invasion: septicaemia	Persistent infection asymptomatic carrier state

VIRUSES

8 Herpes simplex	Primary attack – genital ulcers – cervicitis – systemic symptoms – vaginal/urethral discharge – dysuria – pharyngitis	Primary attack – central nervous system involvement (meningitis, radiculopathy, myelitis) – extragenital lesions – direct extension of disease PID Pelvic cellulitis Suppurative lymphadentis **Recurrent attacks** Generally more mild than primary attack **Effects in pregnancy** spontaneous abortion premature delivery (mainly with primary attack) Intrapartum transmission
9 Human papilloma	Anogenital warts	Association with cancers of cervix, vulva, penis, anus
10 *Molluscum contagiosum*	Papular skin lesions	Bacterial superinfection of lesions Molluscum dermatitis
11 Viral hepatitides	Hepatitis A – acute hepatitis	Hepatitis A Fulminant hepatitis (0.1–0.2% mortality rate)
	Hepatitis B – acute hepatitis – asymptomatic (majority) – serum-sickness-like syndrome	Hepatitis B Acute hepatic failure (75% mort.) Persistent carrier state – chronic persistent hepatitis

Hepatitis C
— asymptomatic infection
— acute hepatitis
— chronic persistent hepatitis
— chronic active hepatitis
— cirrhosis
— hepatocellular carcinoma

— chronic active hepatitis
— cirrhosis
— hepatocellular carcinoma

ECTOPARASITES

12 *Phthirus pubis*

Pubic lice

Secondary bacterial infection of lesions

13 *Sarcoptes scabiei*

Scabies

PROTOZOAN INFECTIONS

14 *Trichomonas vaginalis*

Vaginal discharge
Urethral discharge
Dysuria
Vaginal pruritis

15 Intestinal protozoa
(*Giardia lamblia*)

Diarrhoea
Upper abdominal pain

Malabsorption
Bloating and flatulence

Entamoeba histolytica

Acute recto colitis
Symptomatic non-invasive
infection

Chronic non-dysenteric
intestinal disease
Toxic megacolon
Fulminant colitis and
performation
Amoeboma
Perianal ulceration
Liver abscess ± peritonitis,
empyema pericarditis, lung/
brain abscess
Anogenital fistulae/ulcers

FUNGAL INFECTIONS

16 *Candida albicans*

Vaginal discharge
Urethral discharge
Acute pruritis
Dysuria

Recurrent and chronic
vulvovaginal candidiasis
Dyspareunia

Appendix VII Diagnostic techniques and their approximate costs

Organism	On-site diagnosis	Central reference laboratory
1 *N. gonorrhoeae*	Direct smear, with Gram stain	Culture and isolation (£2) Screen for B-lactamase Antibiotic susceptibility Antigen detection Serological testing
2 *C. trachomatis*		Antigen detection (£6.20–£10.40) (1) Direct immunofluorescence staining of smears (£8.30–£20.90) (2) Enzyme immunoassay (£10.00)
3 *T. pallidum*	Darkfield microscopy	Definitive serological tests for syphilis (£4) Rapid plasma reagin card test
4 *M. hominis*		Culture and isolation Antibiotic susceptibility
5 *G. vaginalis*	Wet mount, Gram stain	
6 *T. vaginalis*	West mount	Culture and isolation
7 *C. albicans*	Direct smear	Culture and isolation
8 *H. ducreyi*		Culture and isolation (variable success) PCR (experimental)
9 Herpes simplex virus	Clinical	Virus culture (£20–£30) EIA (£10) Antigen detection
10 *Molluscum contagiosum*	Clinical	
11 Hepatitis A virus		Antibody screen (£4–£6.80)
12 Hepatitis B virus		Serology for screening (£20–£30) pre-immunization acute hepatitis (£27.50) carrier status (£26.80)
13 Hepatitis C virus		Antibody screen (£4–£6.80)
14 Human papilloma virus		Clinical cytology of PAP smear (£6.80–£10.80) (histopathology) DNA detection

Appendix VIII Current STD treatment guidelines

Disease treatment	Treatment effectiveness (reference) [grade of evidence]
1 Chancroid – Azithromycin 1 g or Ceftriaxone 250 mg im (no resistance yet reported) – Erythromycin 500 mg qds × 7/7	High[65-67]; [A]
2 HSV – Acyclovir 200 mg × 5 × 7/7 (1st attack) – Topical treatment with acyclovir is substantially less effective, and its use is discouraged – Supressive treatment in those with frequent (> 6 yr) episodes	Treatment effective in first attack but probably does not reduce the % of persons who subsequently develop clinical recurrences. Will need i.v. treatment for those with severe infections (e.g. aseptic meningitis)[68]; [A]
3 LGV – Doxycycline 100 mg bd × 21/7 – Erythromycin 500 mg qds × 21/7 – Sulfisoxazole 500 mg qds × 21/7	Medium-High[69,70]; [A]
4 Syphilis – Parenteral penicillin – Doxycycline 100 mg bd × 2/52 – Tetracycline 500 mg qds × 2/52 non-pregnant allergic patients	High (may be reduced in immunosuppressed); [A]
5 Non-gonococcal urethritis – Doxycycline 100 mg bd × 7/7 – Erythromycin 500 mg qds × 7/7	Moderate in non-chlamydial NGU[71]; [A]
6 Chlamydia – Doxycycline 100 mg bd × 7/7 – or Azithromycin 1 g stat – or Erythromycin 500 mg qds × 7/7 – or Ofloxacin 300 mg bd × 7/7	High[69–71]; [A]

7 Gonococcal infections
 	
– **Uncomplicated**: Amoxycillin 3 g stat. plus
             Probenecid
             Ceftriaxone 125 mg im
– Cefixime   400 mg o
– Ciprofloxacin   500 mg o
– Ofloxacin   400 mg o
– **Pharyngeal**: Ceftriaxone   125 mg
          Ciprofloxacin 500 mg
	High, but need access to antibiotic sensitivity testing[72]; [A]

8 **Bacterial vaginosis**
  (MTZ = metronidazole)
  – MTZ 500 mg bd × 7/7
  – MTZ 2 g stat
  – Clindamycin cream 2% (5 g) pv × 7/7
  – MTZ gel 0:75% (5 g) pv × 5/7
  – Clindaymcin 300 mg bd × 7/7

Moderate -> High[72,73]
[B – reservations over long-term effectivcness]

9 **Trichomonas vaginalis**

  – MTZ 2 g
  – MTZ 500 mg bd × 7/7

IIigh[72]; [A]

10 **Vulvovaginal candidiasis**

  – Clotrimazole 1% (5 g) pv × 7–14/7
  Clotrimazole 100 mg tab pv × 7/7
  Clotrimazole 100 mg tab bd pv × 3/7
  Clotrimazole 500 mg tab × 1.
  or miconazole *or* terconazole

Acute attack – 70–90% cure rate with topical
treatment;[73]
[B] – rccurrent attacks may require prolonged
treatment as prophylaxis

11 **PID**

  – Cefoxitin 2 g iv qds *plus* doxy 100 mg bd
  – Clindamycin 900 mg tab iv *plus* gentamycin 1.5
  mg/kg tds
  Ceftriaxone 250 mg im or cefoxitin 2 gm
  (+ probenecid) plus doxy 100 mg bd × 14/7
  – Ofloxacin 100 mg bd × 14/7, plus Clindamycin 450
  mg qds *or* MTZ 500 bd × 14/7

Good results with respect to eradication of
organisms and clinical recovery if treatment started
early.[74,75]
[B – questions over prevention of sequelae]

12 **Epididymitis**

  – Ceftriaxone 250 mg stat (im)
  – plus Doxycycline 100 mg bd × 10/7
  – Ofloxacin 300 mg bd × 10/7

[B]

13 **HPV**

Poor to moderatc[76]

  – cryotherapy
  – podophyllin 10–25%
  – podofilox 0.5%
  – TCA 80–90%
  – electrocautery/other surgery

[B]
[B]
[A/B]
[B]
[B/C]

14 **HBV**

  – Management depends on clinical presentation

15 **Ectoparasitic infections**

  – Lindane 1%
  – Permcthrin 1%
  – Pyrethrin with piperonyl butoxide

High, if used according to instructions;[65] [B]

16 **Scabies**

  – Permethrin 5%
  – Lindane 1%

High, if used according to instructions;[65] [B]

See [66]

Appendix IX Goals, indicators and targets for the management of STDs

Indicators

Indicators	Examples of source of data (for UK)
1 Nos of GUM clinics	AIDS Control Act Reports
2 Nos of GUM clinics with health advisors	AIDS Control Act Reports
3 Nos of new infections	KC60
4 Total attendance	KH09
5 Nos of complications in OPs	KC60
6 Nos of complications admitted, e.g. PID	ICD codes

Data needed in GUM clinics and simple to collect

1 Speed of referral – interval between patient's realization of need to attend and actual attendance (self-referrals, contacts, GP and other referrals to be considered separately).
2 Use of condoms (two surveys outside GUM clinics have already provided some data).
3 Efficacy of partner notification: numbers named, numbers attending, numbers infected, speed with which contacts attend (for source and secondary contacts).

Data needed but more difficult to collect

1 Level of knowledge of sexual behaviour, pregnancy, efficacy of condoms, STDs and HIV infection in the population in general and especially in teenagers and GUM clinic patients. Surveys such as the National Survey of Sexual Attitudes and Lifestyles, surveys by the HEA, and the General Household Survey provide some information.
2 Attitudes to attending GUM clinics, e.g. is attendance:
   'Just like any other hospital department?', 'anonymous and confidential?', 'best place to discuss personal matters such as sex?'.
3 Demographic and epidemiological data on those individuals who present repeatedly to GUM clinics with fresh episodes of infection.

Indicators within GUM clinics

1 Locations of clinic, signposting and access.
2 Ease of first visit, i.e. walk-in or by appointment.
3 If by appointment, delay in obtaining appointment.
4 Within-clinic waiting time for first visit.
5 Appointment or walk-in for subsequent visit.
6 If follow-up by appointment, delay in obtaining appointment.
7 Within-clinic waiting time for subsequent visits.
8 Total time for visit, i.e. time from leaving home or work to time of arriving back.
9 Responsiveness of staff, especially regarding discussion of diagnosis and treatment.
10 Layout, decor, lighting, furnishings, reading material and facilities for small children.

11 Provision of 24-hour information service including staff on call and a recorded telephone message.

12 Patient and staff satisfaction with hospital, e.g. location, transport, facilities, signposting, cleanliness, layout, cafeteria facilities, standard of toilets, and for patients, responsiveness of non-GUM clinical staff.

13 Time to written reponse to referral letters.

14 Efficacy in diagnosis, e.g.
   - agreement between Gram stain and culture for urethral gonorrhoea in men
   - proportion of cases of uncomplicated gonorrhoea in women diagnosed at first or subsequent visit
   - chlamydia detection techniques and rates.

15 Efficacy of treatment, e.g.
   - antibiotic resistance patterns of gonococci and cure rates for first-line treatment of uncomplicated gonorrhoea
   - therapy for uncomplicated chlamydial infection, NSU and NSGI
   - indications for oral acyclovir
   - use of epidemiological treatment.

16 Management of STD in other facilities, e.g. general practice and gynaecology departments.

17 Counselling, e.g. in herpes, warts.

18 Provision of psychosexual/clinical psychology services.

Targets

Educational

1 GUM to be involved in alliances with other health educators in setting targets for health education on the following:
   - school leavers knowledge, including:
     a) names of common STDs
     b) methods of catching and spreading, and avoiding STDs
     c) need for early medical care of STDs
     d) safe and safer sex, and value of condoms
     e) relationship skills
     f) where and how to obtain information locally.

2 Information as above to be available to all GUM clinic attenders before discharge from clinic, plus more detailed information on their own conditions as appropriate (targets to be set locally).

3 The establishment of a formal training course for health advisors in STD.

4 Following the establishment of new course (or courses) for nurses working in GUM – at least 50% of GUM nurses to have attended an appropriate specialist course.

5 All clerical staff to receive training on confidentiality and departmental procedures before starting work in a GUM clinic.

6 All members of GUM clinic staff to receive continuing education (details to be agreed locally) every year.

7 Target – all GUM budgets to include provision for training for all clinic staff.

Process targets

1 Family accessible GUM clinic/GUM provision for residents of every district should continue to be a priority within the NHS. In addition clinics to be open for a minimum of two days each week – 95% after three years, but higher regional and local targets might be considered. (This target is based on the districts in 1988; review may be needed with amalgamation of districts.)

2   Early morning/evening clinics should be available if there is a need, provided adequate resources are available to maintain the quality of service.

3   Follow-up visits to be arranged on a day:
    – suitable for medical care and
    – convenient for patient.

Outcome targets

1   Overall to reduce uncomplicated gonorrhoea reported from GUM clinics to 49 cases per 100 000 of the population aged 15–64 years in three years. Local targets to be agreed and regional targets may be considered.

2   Overall to reduce uncomplicated chlamydial infection reported from GUM clinics to 100 cases per 100 000 of the population aged 15–64 years in three years. Local targets to be agreed and regional targets may be considered.

3   Maintain the number of cases of congenital syphilis in England and Wales under the age of two years at not more than two per year.

4   All clinics to make KC60 returns within time limits set by health departments to allow more timely national KC60 publication.

5   Hepatitis B immunization to be available for all GUM clinical staff and for patients in at risk behaviour groups.

6   In collaboration with GPs and other services to ensure that cervical screening is available in accordance with national guidelines. In collaboration with other services to ensure that women have ready access to a colposcopy service with a maximum waiting time of eight weeks for a first appointment – local targets may be set to improve on this.

References

1 Royal Commission on Veneral Diseases. London: HMSO, 1916.

2 Department of Health. *Report of the working group to examine workloads in genitourinary medicine clinics.* London: Department of Health, 1988.

3 Allen I, Hogg D. *Work roles and responsibilities in GUM clinics.* London: Policy Studies Institute, 1993.

4 Ridgway GL, Mumtaz G, Stephens RA *et al.* Therapeutic abortion and chlamydial infection. *BMJ* 1983; **286**: 1478–9.

5 Southgate LJ, Treharne JD, Forsey T. *Chlamydia trachomatis* and *Neisseria gonorrhoeae* infections in women attending inner city general practices. *BMJ* 1983; **287**: 879–81.

6 Wood PL, Hobson D, Rees E. Genital infection with *Chlamydia trachomatis* in women attending an antenatal clinic. *B J Obs Gynae* 1984; **91**: 1171–6.

7 Edet EE. The prevalence of *Chlamydia trachomatis. C. trachomatis* infection among gynaecological patients. *BJCP* 1993; **47**: 21–2.

8 Fish ANJ, Fairweather DVI, Oriel JD *et al. Chlamydia trachomatis* infection in a gynaecology clinic population: identification of high-risk groups and the value of contact tracing. *Eur Obs Gynae Reprod Biol* 1989; **31**: 67–74.

9 Longhurst HJ, Flower N, Thomas BJ *et al.* A simple method for the detection of *Chlamydia trachomatis* infections in general practice. *JRCGP* 1987; **37**: 255–6.

10 Macauley ME, Riordan T, James JM *et al.* A prospective study of genital infections in a family-planning clinic. *Epidemiol Infect* 1990; **104**: 55–61.

11 Preece PM, Ades A, Thompson RG *et al. Chlamydia trachomatis* infection in late pregnancy: a prospective study. *Paed Perinatal Epid* 1989; **3**: 268–77.

12 Smith JR, Murdoch J, Carrington D *et al.* Prevalence of *Chlamydia trachomatis* infection in women having cervical smear tests. *BMJ* 1991; **302**: 82–4.

13 Blackwell A, Thomas PD, Wareham K *et al.* Health gains from screening for infections of the lower genital tract in women attending for TOP. *Lancet* 1993; **342**: 206–10.

14 Thin RN, Whatley JD, Blackwell AL. STD and contraception in adolescents *Genitourin Med* 1989; **65**: 157–60.

15 Maini M, French P, Prince M *et al.* Urethritis due to *Neisseria meningitidis* in a London GUM clinic population *Int J STD & AIDS* 1992; **3**: 423–5.

16 Dimian C, Nayagam M, Bradbeer C. The association between STDs and inflammatory cervical cytology. *Genitourin Med* 1992; **68**: 305–6.

17 *Morbidity statistics from General Practice, 1991/92* . MB5 94/1. London: OPCS publications (HMSO), 1993.

18 Johnson AM, Wadsworth J, Wellings K *et al. Sexual Attitudes & Lifestyles.* London: Blackwell Scientific Publications, 1994.

19 Curtis H. Sexual Health and Health promotion. In *Promoting Sexual Health* (ed. H Curtis). London: BMA foundation for AIDS & Health Education Authority, 1991.

20 Adler MW, Belsey EM, McCutchan JA *et al.* Should homosexuals be vaccinated against hepatitis B virus?: cost and benefit assessment. *BMJ* 1983; **286**: 1621–4.

21 Loke RHT, Murray-Lyon IM, Balachandron T *et al.* Screening for hepatitis B and vaccination of homosexual men. *BMJ* 1989; **298**: 234–5.

22 Department of Health guidelines. *Guidance on partner notification for HIV infection.* London: Department of Health, HMSO, 1992.

23 Rothenberg RB, Potterat JJ. Strategies for management of sex partners. In *Sexually Transmitted Diseases* (eds KK Holmes *et al.*). 2nd edn. New York: McGraw-Hill, 1990.

24 McCormick JS. Cervical smears: a questionable practice? *Lancet* 1989; **2**: 207–9.

25 IARC Working group. Screening for cervical cancer: duration of low risk after negative results of cervical cytology and its implication for screening policies. *BMJ* 1986; **293**: 659–64.

26 zur Hansen H, Schneider A. The role of papillomaviruses in human anogenital cancer. In: *The Papovauiridae Vol. 2: the papillomaviruses* (eds NP Salzmann, PM Howley). New York: Plenum, 1987, pp. 245–63.

27 Dalgleish AG. Viruses and cancer. *Bri Med Bull* 1991; **47 (1)**: 21–46.

28 Trachtenberg AI, Washington E, Halldorson S. A cost-based decision analysis for Chlamydia screening in California FPCs. *Obs Gynae* 1988; **71**: 101–8.

29 Handsfield HH, Jasman LL, Roberts PL. Criteria for selective screening for *Chlamydia trachomatis* infection in women attending family planning clinics. *JAMA* 1986; **255**: 1730–4.

30 Humphreys JT, Henneberry JF, Rickard RS *et al.* Cost-benefit analysis of selective screening criteria for *Chlamydia trachomatis* infection in women attending Colorado family planning clinics. *Sex Transm Dis* 1992; **19**: 47–53.

31 Weinstock HS, Bolan GA, Kohn R *et al. Chlamydia trachomatis* infection in women: a need for universal screening in high prevalence populations? *Am J Epid* 1992; **135**: 41–7.

32 Randolph AG, Washington AE. Screening for *Chlamydia trachomatis* in adolescent males: A cost-based decision analysis. *Am J Pub Hlth* 1990; **80**: 545–50.

33 Nettleman MD, Jones RB. Cost-effectiveness of screening women at moderate risk for general infections caused by *Chlamydia trachomatis. JAMA* 1988; **260**: 207–13.

34 Buhaug H, Skjeldestad FE, Backe B *et al.* Cost-effectiveness of testing for chlamydial infections in asymptomatic women. *Med.Care* 1989; **27**: 833–41.

35 Skjeldestad FE, Tuveng J, Solberg AG *et al.* Induced abortion: *Chlamydia trachomatis* and postabortal complications: a cost-benefit analysis. *Acta Obstet Gynecol Scand* 1988; **67**: 525–9.

36 Department of Health. *New cases seen at NHS GUM clinics in England.* Summary information from form KC60. 1992 annual figures. London: Department of Health, 1992.

37 Scitovsky A, Over M. AIDS: Costs of care in the developed and developing world. *AIDS* 1988; **2 (suppl.1)**: 571–81.

38 Scitovsky A, Rice D. Estimates of the direct and indirect costs of AIDS in the US, 1985, 1986 and 1991. *Public Health Reports* 1987; **102**: 5–17.

39 Godfrey C, Tolley K, Drummond M. The economics of promoting sexual health. In *Promoting Sexual Health* (ed. H Curtis). London: BMA foundation for AIDS & HEA.

40 Drew WL, Blair M, Miner RC *et al.* Evaluation of the virus permeability of a new condom for women. *Sex Transm Dis* 1990; **17**: 110–12.

41 Stone KM, Grimes DA, Magder S. Primary prevention of STDs. *JAMA* 1986; **255**: 1763–6.

42 MMWR Update: Barrier protection against HIV infection and other STDs. *MMWR* 1993; **42**: 589–97.

43 Winkelstein W, Samuel M, Padian NS *et al.* The San Francisco men's health study. III Reduction in HIV transmission among homosexual–bisexual men 1982–1986. *Am J Public Health* 1987; **76**: 685–9.

44 Johnson AM, Gill ON. Evidence for recent changes in sexual behaviour in homosexual men in England & Wales. *Philos Trans R Soc Lond* 1989; **325**: 153–61.

45 Leman SM, Newbold JE. Viral hepatitis. In *Sexually Transmitted Diseases* (eds KK Holmes *et al.*). 2nd edn. London: McGraw-Hill, 1990.

46 Schultz KF, Murphy FK, Patamasucon P *et al.* Congenital syphilis. In *Sexually Transmitted Diseases* (eds KK Holmes *et al.*). 2nd edn. New York: McGraw-Hill, 1990.

47 Department of Health. *Immunisation against infectous disease.* London: HMSO, 1992.

48 Sellors JW, Pickard L, Gafni A. Effectiveness and efficiency of selective vs. universal screening for chlamydial infection in sexually active young women. *Arch Intern Med* 1992; **152**: 1837–44.

49 Williams K. Screening for syphilis in pregnancy: an assessment of the costs and benefits. *Comm Med* 1985; **7**: 37–42.

50 Wigfield S. 7 years of uninterrupted contact tracing: the Tyneside scheme. *Brit J Vener Dis* 1972; **48**: 37–50.

51 Gonorrhoea and Syphilis in Sweden – past and present. *Scand J Infect Dis* 1990; **69**: 69–76.

52 Talbot MD. The relationship between incidence of gonorrhoea in Sheffield and efficiency of contact tracing: a paradox? *Genitourin Med* 1986; **62**: 377–9.

53 Romanowski B, Sutherland R, Love EJ *et al.* Epidemiology of an outbreak of infectious syphilis in Alberta. *Int J STD AIDS* 1991; **2**: 424–7.

54 Potterat JJ, Meheus A, Gallwey J. Partner notification: operational considerations. *Int J STD AIDS* 1991; **2**: 411–15.

55 York JA, Hethcote HW, Nold A. Dynamics and control of the transmission of gonorrhoea. *Sex Trans Dis* 1978; **5(2)**: 51–5.

56 Ramstedt K, Forssman L, Johannisson G. Contact tracing in the control of genital *Chlamydia trachomatis* infection. *Int J STD AIDS* 1991; **2**: 116–18.

57 Burgess JA. A contact-tracing procedure. *Brit J Vener Dis* 1963; **39**: 113–15.

58 Potterat JJ, Phillips L, Rothenburg RB *et al.* Gonococcal pelvic inflammatory disease: case-finding observations. *Am J Obstet Gynecol* 1980; **138**: 1101–4.

59 Oxman AD, Scott EA, Sellors JW *et al.* Partner notification for sexually transmitted diseases: an overview of the evidence. *Can J Public Hlth* 1994; **85**: S41–7.

60 Dunlop EMC, Lamb AM, King DM. Improved tracing of contacts of heterosexual men with gonorrhoea. *Brit J Vener Dis* 1971; **47**: 192–5.

61 Patel HC, Viswalingam ND, Goh BT. Chlamydial ocular infection: efficacy of partner notification by patient referral. Int J STD AIDS 1994; **5**: 244–7.

62 *Veneral Diseases Act, 1917.* NHS (Venereal Diseases) Regulations, 1974.

63 Department of Health. *AIDS and HIV: service objectives 1990/91.* Annex to EL (90) P/30. London: Department of Health, Feb 1990.

64 Department of Health. *HIV/AIDS and sexual health.* Key area handbook for the health of the nation. London: Department of Health, 1993.

65 Holmes KK, Mordh P-A, Sparling PF *et al.* (eds) *Sexually Transmitted Diseases.* 2nd edn. New York: McGraw-Hill Publications, 1990.

66 MMWR 1993 STD Treatment guidelines. *MMWR* 1993; **42**: 1–102.

67 Ronald AR, Corey L, McCutchan JA *et al.* Evaluation of new anti-infective drugs for the treatment of chancroid. *Clin Infect Dis* 1992; **15 (Suppl. 1)**: S108–14.

68 Corey L, McCutchan JA, Ronald AR *et al.* Evaluation of new anti-infective drugs for the treatment of genital infections due to Herpes simplex virus. *Clin Infect Dis* 1992; **15 (Suppl. 1)**: S99–107.

69 Handsfield HH, McCutchan JA, Corey L *et al.* Evaluation of new anti-infective drugs for the treatment of uncomplicated gonorrhea in adults and adolescents. *Clin Infect Dis* 1992; **15 (Suppl. 1)**: S123–130.

70 Handsfield HH, Ronald AR, Corey L, McCutchan JA. Evaluation of new anti-infective drugs for the treatment of sexually transmitted chlamydial infections and related clinical syndromes. *Clin Infect Dis* 1992; **15(Suppl. 1)**: S131–9.

71 Bowie WR. Effective treatment of urethritis. A practical guide. *Drugs* 1992; **44(2)**: 207–15.

72 McCutchon JA, Ronald AR, Corey L *et al.* Evaluation of new anti-infective drugs for the treatment of vaginal infections. *Clin Infect Dis* 1992; **15 (Suppl. 1)**: S115–22.

73 Sweet RL. New approaches for the treatment of bacterial vaginosis. *Am J Obstet Gynecol* 1993; **169(2)**: 479–82.

74 Westrom L, Mardh P-A. Acute Pelvic Inflammatory Diseases. In *Sexually Transmitted Diseases*(eds KK Holmes *et al.*).(2nd edn). New York: McGraw-Hill, 1990.

75 Cates W, Rolfs RT, Aral SO. Sexually transmitted diseases, PID and infertility: an epidemiologic update. *Epidemiol Re* 1990; **12**: 199–220.

76 Holmes KK, Mordh P-A, Sparling PF *et al.* (eds) *Sexually Transmitted Diseases.* 2nd edn. New York: McGraw-Hill Publications, 1990.

8 Gynaecology

CDA Wolfe

1 Summary

Introduction and statement of the problem

Gynaecology is the specialty concerned with diseases of women, which excludes breast disease, in the UK. The gynaecology service encompasses a range of preventive, medical and surgical interventions in primary and secondary care settings. Gynaecological symptoms and conditions may be managed exclusively in primary care or with additional secondary care provided by a number of specialty departments. For genital tract infections, excluding human immunodeficiency virus (HIV), women may be referred to genitourinary medicine and family planning departments as well as gynaecology and acute abdominal pain referred to general surgery. This chapter provides a framework for assessing the needs for the major components of the service and the scope for shifts in service provision from the secondary to primary care sector, inpatient to day case surgery and conventional to minimal access surgery (MAS) which are all major purchaser and provider issues.

This assessment relies on the 1991/92 morbidity survey from general practice and 1993/94 hospital episode statistics for the UK. Data are presented by international classification of disease (ICD) category with the equivalent Office of Population and Censuses and Surveys (version 4R) surgical operation codes (OPCS4R). The health care resource grouping (HRG) data for the same time period have been analysed but there are reservations over data quality. The categories of the gynaecological service have been grouped into 13 groups mirroring broad pathological and health service groupings which closely reflect important ICD codes as follows:

- subfertility
- pelvic inflammatory disease (PID)
- lower genital tract infections
- endometriosis
- menopause
- urinary incontinence/utero-vaginal prolapse
- menstrual disorders
- pelvic pain
- premenstrual syndrome
- ectopic pregnancy
- early pregnancy loss
- genital tract cancer – secondary prevention
- genital tract cancer.

Termination of pregnancy and subfertility have been considered in another needs assessment.[1]

Incidence and prevalence

- The overall burden of gynaecological disease is not estimable as studies of incidence and prevalence, especially in the UK have not been undertaken.
- The most prevalent conditions include menstrual disorders, pelvic pain, early pregnancy loss, urinary incontinence, menopause and lower genital tract infections (Table 4, page 478).
- There are problems of case definition and diagnosis with several conditions: silent PID, endometriosis, pelvic pain, premenstrual syndrome.

Services available

- In primary care gynaecology accounts for some 1500 consultations per 10 000 female population and 2250 consultations per 10 000 women–years at risk. A further 500 women consult per 10 000 women–years at risk with 700 consultations per 10 000 women – years at risk for candida and trichomoniasis infections of the genital tract. Over the past ten years there has been a doubling of the reports of genitourinary diseases and a 150% increase in consultations for menopausal symptoms.
- The main reasons for consultation in primary care in order of magnitude are:
  a) candidiasis
  b) disorders of menstruation
  c) menopause
  d) pelvic pain
  e) PID.
- A typical gynaecological secondary care service consists of general and specialist outpatient clinics including colposcopy, cancer and subfertility, and inpatient gynaecological beds, the majority of inpatients receiving an operation. Because of directives from the Department of Health there is an expanding day case surgery service. It is estimated that between 25–40% of hospital episodes are non-elective. Up to 17% of all gynaecological surgery is performed outside scheduled operating theatre sessions.
- In secondary care there are no routine data on outpatient activity. There are 7000 ordinary admissions per 100 000 female population for the main gynaecological ICD codes, of which 2000 are for gynaecology and 5000 for pregnancy related disorders relevant to the gynaecological service.
- The main non-pregnancy related reasons for admission are:
  a) disorders of menstruation
  b) non-inflammatory disorders of the cervix (mainly preinvasive lesions of the cervix)
  c) genital prolapse
  d) the menopause.
- This assessment estimates there to be 1.7 ordinary cases to every day case. The number of bed days for gynaecology equates to 1.5% of all beds and 4% of the acute sector beds.
- The operative intervention rate is estimated at 3000 per 100 000 females over the age of 15. The major operative categories are:
  a) dilatation and curettage (D&C)
  b) evacuation of the retained products of conception (ERPC)
  c) hysterectomy
  d) laparoscopy
  e) prolapse operations
  f) operations of the vagina and cervix.
  It is estimated that 37% of all procedures are undertaken as day cases.

- A Scottish needs assessment estimated that gynaecological services cost in the region of £15 million for a female population of nearly half a million, of which 73% was for inpatient care.
- The balance between services provided in primary and secondary care varies between districts and is dependent on local expertise and resources. Secondary care gynaecological services impinge on services in primary care, community gynaecological services provided in reproductive health departments and services provided in genitourinary medicine (GUM) departments.
- The main areas of overlap in service provision are in the diagnosis and treatment of PID, lower genital tract infection, the menopause, pelvic pain and the medical management of menstrual disorders.

Effectiveness of services

- There is no strong evidence on which to base decisions on how gynaecological services should be delivered in totality, or the optimum balance of care between primary and secondary care sectors, or between specialties in secondary care for certain conditions.
- There is very little evidence on the longer term outcome of MAS for gynaecological conditions.
- Although the resource implications of the increased use of day surgery are established, the benefits to women in terms of quality of care remain unevaluated.

The evidence of effectiveness for the sub-categories is outlined here but a full review is presented in section 6.

- As with much of medicine, gynaecological practice is in the main not based on evidence based medicine and this is particularly so for surgical procedures. More recently evaluations, often unrandomized, of new technologies for MAS have been undertaken but there is evidence that implementation of these techniques by departments, before evidence is available, has occurred.

Subfertility

- The average maternity rate of *in vitro* fertilization (IVF) is 12% per treatment cycle.[2] Effectiveness is reduced in clinics treating women over the age of 35.
- There is no evidence of increased effectiveness overall of IVF over gamete intra-fallopian transfer (GIFT).
- There is currently no effective treatment for male infertility and the main success in treating male infertility is by artificial inception by donor (AID).

Pelvic inflammatory disease and lower genital tract infections

- Strategies for detection and screening have been incomplete in the UK[3] although there is evidence from Sweden that widespread screening for chlamydia has virtually eradicated the disease.[4] In primary care the routine testing of women for chlamydia in younger women in the UK has been shown to be cost-effective.[5]
- A meta-analysis of trials of antibiotics for the treatment of PID indicated there was a lack of uniformity among studies regarding diagnosis, care and follow-up. Pooled cure rates ranged from 75–94%, with Doxycycline and Metronidazole being the least effective regimen. They concluded that clinical treatment of acute PID is likely to be inappropriate in many women and inadequate for chlamydia in much of the remainder.
- Bacterial vaginosis has a 75% cure rate at one month using a combination of Metronidazole and Clindamycin.[6]

Endometriosis

- Most regimens to treat endometriosis have not been shown to be effective. The most commonly prescribed drugs, Danazol and leutinizing hormone releasing hormone (LHRH) are costly but equally effective in relieving symptoms.
- With regard to fertility all treatments, medical and surgical, appear to be ineffective but assisted conception techniques appear to be successful.[7]

Menopause

- The effectiveness of hormone replacement therapy (HRT) in reducing the incidence of the long-term risks associated with the menopause such as osteoporosis and cardiovascular disease remain unclear. The effect of the newer preparations and different methods of administration on longer term outcome have not been assessed.
- Trial evidence has demonstrated that HRT relieves symptoms effectively.[8]
- Reductions of up to 20% in cardiovascular disease have been observed in cohort studies using older preparations.[9]
- Trials have shown that after ten years of HRT use bone loss is substantially prevented[10,11] but protection is reduced once HRT is stopped.
- Decision analysis studies have demonstrated the potential benefits of HRT but many assumptions are made. Roche and Vessey[12] consider the benefits in terms of reduced mortality and treatment costs are greater for women who have had a hysterectomy receiving unopposed oestrogen therapy than for women with a uterus receiving combined therapy, with a net gain to the NHS of £137 per woman being suggested if women who have had a hysterectomy are treated with oestrogen therapy.

Urinary incontinence/utero-vaginal prolapse – stress incontinence

- The success of pelvic floor re-education varies from 60–90% but when compared with surgery physiotherapy compares poorly.[13]
- No single operation could be offered to all women in all situations as a first choice.[14]
- Colposuspension and sling operations appeared to be the most effective procedures.
- There is no trial evidence to support or refute the use of repair of prolapse operations.

Menstrual disorders

- The effectiveness of D&C in the management of menstrual disorders in younger women has been questioned and the use of alternative outpatient endometrial sampling techniques has been shown to be effective.
- There is trial evidence that certain medical treatments of menstrual disorders can be effective. Minimal access surgery alternatives to invasive abdominal operations have been assessed by trial but the longer term benefits are not established and whilst both procedures continue to be carried out in units the financial benefits of MAS will be lost. The long-term advantages of transcervical resection of the edometrium (TCRE) are not established although TCRE appears to be cost-effective in the short term.[15] The use of laparoscopically assisted vaginal hysterectomy (LAVH) has been shown to be cost-effective in the short term.[16]

Pelvic pain

- There is insufficient evidence of the effectiveness of therapies to enable guidelines to be established.[17]

Premenstrual syndrome (PMS)

- The use of stress management, relaxation techniques, exercise and dietary change including oil of evening primrose oil supplementation, although often helping women with mild symptoms has not been shown to be effective in trials.[18]

Ectopic pregnancy

- There is fair evidence to recommend that operative laparoscopy be used in some ectopic pregnancies.[19]

Early pregnancy loss

- The evidence that progestational agents are effective at reducing recurrent miscarriage is inconclusive.
- Mifepristone is an effective antiprogestational agent for evacuating the contents of the uterus but its use for miscarriage remains to be assessed.[20,21]

Genital tract cancer – secondary prevention

- There is no trial evidence to support screening for cervical cancer but evidence that in countries where screening has been co-ordinated centrally mortality from the disease has fallen.
- The use of certain local ablative therapies for cervical intraepithelial neoplasia has been shown to be effective, especially large loop excision of the transformation zone (LLETZ).
- There is no evidence that screening for ovarian or endometrial cancers is effective.

Genital tract cancer

- There is generally no trial evidence to support the current surgical procedures undertaken for the various gynaecological cancers.
- For ovarian cancer the use of platinum based therapy in combination with other agents probably improves survival.
- The use of platinum as adjuvant therapy in women with persistent or recurrent cervical cancer has a response rate of 30%.[22]

Models of care

- The overall models of care that are developed locally will be dependent on those factors analysed at a national level in this chapter and include the need for the service, the current patterns of service and scope to move towards those practices identified as being both effective, cost-effective and acceptable to women.
- A needs assessment group comprising gynaecologists, general practitioners (GPs), nurses, public health physicians and local users of the service, along with information and health economics support should identify the necessary information on which to base decisions on the models of service to be provided.
- The areas purchasers should be concerned with will be determined locally but could include patient information, monitoring patient satisfaction, shifts in service provision: secondary to primary care, inpatient to day case surgery, conventional to MAS, development of guidelines and development of tertiary level services.

- Information provision should be co-ordinated across the levels of care and between specialties.
- The written provision of information on any diagnostic or therapeutic intervention is particularly relevant when it involves the genital tract as the implications for a woman's sexuality and femininity of the interventions need to be discussed, e.g. abnormal smear results, hysterectomy, removal of ovaries.
- Assessment of patient satisfaction should be an integral component of any service or intervention evaluation.
- Evaluation of shifts of service to primary care is required as their cost effectiveness has not been established. One of the aims of such a shift is to reduce duplication across the sectors and guideline development is integral to this process. The conditions where a shift in service provision to primary care could be considered include:
  a) the initial management of subfertility and follow-up after
     management in secondary care
  b) the prevention and management of PID and lower genital tract infections
  c) the management of the menopause
  d) the medical management of incontinence
  e) the initial management of menstrual disturbance
  f) the management of chronic pelvic pain and PMS
  g) the follow-up of an abnormal smear.
- National targets for day case surgery have been set and adapted locally. To achieve these targets dedicated day case facilities are required with skilled staff to enable efficient use of theatre time and the appropriate support for women. Current targets are set for D&C, laparoscopy and termination of pregnancy.
- The replacement of D&C with hysteroscopic sampling or vabra or pipelle endometrial sampling techniques provides the service with increased flexibility in that not only can the proportion of women having day care be increased but the procedures can be performed in outpatient clinics.
- The development of see and treat clinics for diagnostic and therapeutic procedures has the advantage of reducing waiting list times along with reducing patient anxiety. The service does require specialist training and the back up of appropriate resuscitation facilities. The procedures that could be undertaken include colposcopy and ablative therapy for preinvasive lesions of the cervix, the diagnosis of menstrual disorders with hysteroscopy or other endometrial sampling techniques, minor procedures of the cervix and vagina such as cervical polypectomy and the use of vaginal ultrasound for the diagnosis of pelvic pathology.
- Although early pregnancy assessment units have not been assessed for their cost-effectiveness, the development of a specialist service where women can be directly referred from primary care for both diagnosis and management without the need to involve accident and emergency (A and E) or ultrasound services would reduce duplication and probably provide a more sympathetic service.
- The Royal College of Obstetricians and Gynaecologists has produced guidelines for training in MAS that require integration into local accreditation programmes.[23] Few gynaecological MAS procedures have been subject to rigorous clinical and economic evaluation and purchasers should consider specifying in contracts that new MAS techniques may only be used within an evaluative framework. Whilst MAS is not the major intervention for a particular condition the benefits to the service in terms of reduced lengths of stay will not be realized. The main areas where MAS has a significant role and where a shift could be implemented are in emergency surgery[24] and alternatives to hysterectomy.
- The aim of guidelines for management and referral is to provide a seamless service across sectors and between specialties and require ownership from all the relevant health care professionals. An outline of the models of care that could be developed using guidelines is described on page 462.

Subfertility

- A comprehensive subfertility service for a population of 100 000 will result in around 100 referrals and cost around £300 000 per year, including the additional costs for neonatal care. The total cost to the NHS which also includes administrative and accommodation overheads and the extra neonatal intensive care costs has been estimated to be just under £900 000 (1992 prices).[2]
- Guidelines should be developed to increase primary care involvement in the preliminary diagnosis of subfertility. Subfertility clinics in secondary care should be provided in a dedicated clinic with support of relevant investigative services including radiology and reproductive endocrinology. It is estimated that there be at least one secondary care service per 500 000 population and one tertiary centre per 2 million population. Tertiary centres should offer donor insemination, ovulation induction, tubal surgery, IVF and have links with endocrine laboratories.

Pelvic inflammatory disease/lower genital tract infections

- Investment in preventive strategies for lower genital tract infections may be the most cost-effective way to reduce eventual upper genital tract infection, including PID and subsequent tubal surgery. Multi-agency collaboration is a strategy advocated in the Health of the Nation *Key Area Handbook* to tackle this issue.[25]

Menopause

- Whether women are seen in general practice, gynaecological outpatients or a specialist clinic the principles of management remain the same. It is considered that hospital clinics could not cope with the information and therapy needs of the population. Important elements of the service include information provision and monitoring of symptoms. Guidelines for referral to secondary care should be developed and such centres should be involved in clinical trials of the effectiveness of HRT.

Urinary incontinence/utero-vaginal prolapse

- Guidelines for investigation in primary care and referral to secondary care should be developed. Colposuspension and sling operations have the best cure rates for stress incontinence. There is a place for tertiary referral centres for complex cases and repeat operations where expertise and a high volume of surgery for such women exists.
- Support from continence advisors has been advocated. The Scottish Needs Assessment Programme estimated that five physiotherapists be employed to develop management of urinary incontinence for a female population of 500 000.[26] There is no conclusive evidence however that physiotherapy is effective and there are problems with the monitoring of improvement of symptoms whilst receiving therapy.

Menstrual disorders

- The development of guidelines for the investigation and medical management of menstrual disorders in primary care is required as this disorder is the most prevalent condition seen in both primary and secondary care.
- Criteria for the use of D&C should be developed and a shift of service to hysteroscopy or other endometrial sampling techniques agreed. A local shift from total abdominal hysterectomy (TAH) to TCRE should be agreed and patients undergoing such procedures as LAVH enrolled into clinical trials as the evidence for their use is not strong.

Ectopic pregnancy/early pregnancy loss

- The ability of GPs to perform pregnancy tests to exclude the possibility of an ectopic pregnancy or miscarriage should be considered. A service which includes the routine use of ultrasound scanning in the management of a possible ectopic pregnancy is required. Referral to an early pregnancy assessment unit with diagnostic tests and skilled personnel appears to be efficient but their effectiveness has not been proven. Training of gynaecologists using the RCOG guidelines will reduce the requirement for removal of the ectopic pregnancy by laparotomy and units should have targets set to manage a high proportion of ectopic pregnancies by laparoscopy.

Genital tract cancer – secondary prevention

- The NHS cervical screening programme has published guidelines for the management of the screening programme generally.[27] The Health of the Nation *Key Area Handbook* on cancer provides useful checklists on the various elements of a successful programme (Appendix VI). These include a defined target programme, screening the female population at 3–5 year intervals, personal invitations to women and a health education programme, quality of the cervical smear test and follow-up of abnormal smears and implementation of treatment (fail-safe protocols).
- The latter is within the remit of the gynaecological service in conjunction with the cervical screening programme locally. There are guidelines on fail-safe action for GPs, clinics, laboratories, the FHSA and the programme manager.[28] Salfield and Sharp estimated the need for diagnostic colposcopies at 1300 per 100 000 women but this estimate requires local adaptation depending on the policy for colposcopy for cervical intraepithelial neoplasia (CIN) 1.[29] They estimated there would be 600 treatment and 2000 follow-up sessions per 100 000 women.
- The colposcopy service requires dedicated clinic space with the facilities for 'see and treat' sessions under local anaesthetic. The guidelines for follow-up need to be developed with the screening programme group and involve local GPs and cytology nurses.

Genital tract cancer

- Although there is little trial evidence for the management of gynaecological cancers, the expert advisory group on cancer has recommended that there be a concentration of oncology services.[30] Gynaecological cancers require multi-disciplinary management and guidelines for the staging, management and follow-up need to involve health care professionals in the cancer units/centres and specialist nurses in primary care.

Outcome measures

There are outcome measures that are suggested for each of the sub-categories of the service but the development of health-related outcome measures in gynaecology is poor.

Targets

The models of care outline the shifts in service that are required but due to variations in the current levels of service provision it would not be sensible to set targets apart from at a local level. Targets could be set for development of guidelines for the shift of services to primary care, the use of day case surgery and MAS and the development of tertiary level services such as cancer centres. Specific targets can be set in line with national strategies for various sub-categories.

Information

This assessment has relied on the routine morbidity returns from selected general practices in 1992/93 along with hospital episode statistics (HES) data and its regrouping as HRGs from the UK for the financial year 1993/94. As there is no linkage between primary and secondary level care the referral patterns to secondary care can not be assessed and this is information required when developing guidelines across the sectors. There appears to be no easy way of estimating the elective/emergency split or proportion of day cases for gynaecology. Local provider unit databases usually produce these data for contract monitoring and purchasers require these categories for monitoring the shifts in service provision.

The quality of these data has been a cause for concern and the use of HES data to produce HRGs appears to have confused the situation further. The training of relevant clerical and health care professional staff to code diagnoses and operations accurately and completely is central to the type of data required to produce HRGs.

Provider units will need to record not only day case/elective splits but also 'see and treat' episodes. The development of gynaecology outpatient audit systems should facilitate the collection of such data and provide important information on the case-mix in the outpatient setting which is currently not recorded.

2 Introduction and statement of the problem

This section outlines the aims of the assessment, describes the setting and content of gynaecology services in primary and secondary care settings and outlines the 13 headings under which the gynaecology service will be considered. The relevance of day case and MAS will be discussed.

Introduction

Gynaecology is the specialty concerned with diseases of women, which now excludes breast disease, in the UK. It has developed in a short period of time from a specialty dealing in a compartmentalized way with disorders of menstruation, urinary problems and genital tract prolapse and the treatment of cancer to one managing the problems of women in a more holistic way and encompassing all aspects of their sexual and reproductive lives. Gynaecological complaints are amongst the most common presenting to GPs and gynaecological disease accounts for nearly 5% of hospital activity within the NHS and a considerable proportion of activity in the private sector. Because of the wide range of preventive, medical and surgical services encompassed under the term gynaecology this assessment:

- provides a framework for assessing the needs for the major components of the gynaecological service
- assesses the scope for shifts in service provision from:
  a) the secondary to primary care sector.
  b) inpatient to day case surgery.
  c) conventional surgery to MAS.

Gynaecological disease prevention, diagnosis and management can be considered to occur at a variety of levels (Box 1).

Box 1: Levels of gynaecological service

- prevention
- secondary prevention
- primary care consultation
- primary care procedure
- outpatient consultation
- outpatient procedure
- day care procedure
- inpatient assessment
- inpatient procedure
- palliative care

Diagnosis and treatment are provided at both the primary and secondary care level, gynaecology accounting for some 1500 consultations per 100 000 female population in primary care[31] (Appendix II) and 7000 ordinary admissions per 100 000 female population into hospital in the UK[32] (Appendix III). However HRG data suggest a rate of nearly 3000 per 100 000 female population. The consultation rate in primary care excludes women who go to family planning clinics with a gynaecological condition and hence primary care data are an underestimate. It is also unclear whether this type of consultation is made more frequently by certain groups e.g. ethnic minorities.

In the secondary care setting gynaecological advice is usually provided by a consultant team with the relevant gynaecological nurse support. A typical gynaecological secondary care service consists of the following components (Box 2).

Box 2: Gynaecological services

- outpatient clinic activities
- colposcopy service for cervical smear abnormalities
- inpatient admissions to gynaecology beds with the majority of patients receiving an operation
- day case admissions for surgical procedures
- emergency service for women attending the accident and emergency (A and E) department
- subfertility service

Regional centres provide specialist services for oncology and radiotherapy and advanced treatments for subfertility, such as IVF. Whether a hospital has a urodynamic service for women suffering from incontinence or clinics for problems relating to the menopause depends on the interests of the consultants. Psychosexual counselling may also be offered in some departments but is not considered further as no routine data are available.

It is unusual for individual consultants to provide only an obstetric service or a gynaecology service; the normal pattern is for each doctor to cover both services. The junior medical staff in larger departments may have separate duties during weekdays and when on call out of hours. In terms of the physical arrangements, the obstetric facilities (clinic accommodation, antenatal and postnatal wards, delivery suites, obstetric theatre and maternity nursery) in many hospitals are separate from the gynaecology facilities. The obstetric unit may be in a separate building adjacent to the main hospital building or even in a hospital in a different location. Over a third of hospital departments of obstetrics and gynaecology in England and Wales are on split sites.[33]

Gynaecological services are provided by specialists who also manage pregnancy and its complications. There is an arbitrary division of pregnancy into that managed by the gynaecological service and that by the obstetric service. This relates to early pregnancy loss during the first half of pregnancy, before viability of the fetus, which is managed in the gynaecological service. Termination of pregnancy has been considered in another needs assessment.[1]

Data sources

In total there were 2000 ordinary admissions to hospital per 100 000 women for non-pregnant conditions. Taking both the general practice survey consultation rate of 150 per 100 000 female population[31] and HES data together, this represents a ratio of eight women consulting in primary care for every ordinary admission. There were additionally 5000 admissions per 100 000 women for pregnancy-related gynaecological problems.

For the purposes of this assessment gynaecological activity has been divided to mirror both physiological and pathological processes and current service provision, relevant to both purchasers and providers and will be dealt with in these groupings (Box 3).

Box 3: Sub-categories of gynaecological needs assessment

```
1 subfertility
2 pelvic inflammatory disease
3 lower genital tract infections
4 endometriosis
5 menopause
6 urinary incontinence/utero-vaginal prolapse
7 menstrual disorders
8 pelvic pain
9 premenstrual syndrome
10 ectopic pregnancy
11 early pregnancy loss
12 genital tract cancer – secondary prevention
13 genital tract cancer
```

Family planning services and GU medicine are covered elsewhere in the series.

Day case and minimal access gynaecological surgery

In the 1990s there have been directives from the Department of Health and consequently purchasers to reduce the use of inpatient beds and expand the use of day surgery. There has also been a drive by providers to avail themselves of the emerging technologies for MAS. Both these initiatives affect the gynaecology service.

Day case

A day case is defined as an individual admitted to hospital for an elective admission, who is discharged home on the same day and who underwent an operation. Procedures recommended as suitable for day surgery are planned, clean surgical procedures which require a total operating time not exceeding 30 minutes. The advantages of day case surgery are that costs are lower, waiting lists reduced, risks of cross-infection and thrombotic complications are reduced and there is greater convenience for patients.

Targets for day case surgery

Targets have been set by regions and by the National Audit Office[34] and require local adaptation to take into account socio-economic circumstances and case-mix.

Procedure	upper quartile	optimistic
dilatation and curettage	73%	86%
laparoscopy and sterilization	16%	65%
termination of pregnancy	40%	70%

Gabbay and Francis used the Delphi study methodologies to assess what specialists considered the proportion of cases of a particular operation that could be undertaken as a day case.[35] This ranged from a median of 55% for cone biopsy to 70% for cervical polypectomy, D&C and incision of a Bartholins gland.

Minimal access surgery

- It has been forecast that MAS will account for up to 70% of surgical procedures within ten years.
- Few procedures have been subject to rigorous clinical and economic evaluations[36] and there is a need to develop evaluation methodologies. Sculpher discusses some of the controversies surrounding the introduction of new technologies.[37] There are two issues that require consideration:
  a) how does the cost of new technologies compare with that of existing technologies?
  b) what additional benefits, in terms of patient outcome are being generated by these technologies?

MAS includes procedures such as laparoscopy to replace conventional abdominal laparotomies and new therapies such as TCRE to replace hysterectomy. 50% of gynaecologists were using TCRE in 1991 although there was no evidence at that time that TCRE was as effective as hysterectomy at reducing menstrual symptoms.[38] The longer term follow-up of women undergoing MAS operations replacing hysterectomy requires the full benefits to be assessed. There may be short-term benefits such as reduced post-operative pain but disadvantages longer term, for example retreatment to relieve repeat symptoms. A lack of follow-up means that the overall outcome advantages are not established.

Adopting the patient as consumer perspective it is possible to see how MAS may influence surgical thresholds operating on people considered previously not to warrant it. This therefore influences the private individual's trade-off. The availability of MAS alternatives to hysterectomy, for example, has been widely publicized in the lay press and gynaecologists have claimed that a patient-led demand has been an important factor behind the rapid diffusion of these procedures.

The short-term impact of MAS is a shorter stay in hospital but there will be constraints on reducing the demand for hospital beds whilst MAS is not the key process and alternatives are still used. There has over recent years been a general reduction in post-operative length of stay.[39] In one region in the UK the average length of stay per episode in gynaecology fell from 5.1 days in 1975 to three in 1985.[40]

It may be argued that more widespread use of MAS is being superimposed on to a system already displaying a reduced need for hospital beds and that the additional savings resulting from MAS may not be as significant as is frequently claimed.

Although there may be decreased length of stay initially, readmission for further surgery[41] with an 11% repeat TCRE/hysterectomy rate needs to be taken into account. There is evidence that TCRE does reduce theatre time and requires fewer staff and less anaesthetic demand and overall operative costs are reduced.[15] There is a resource imposed in the transition to MAS. Clinicians at the foot of the learning curve are not as effective as more experienced clinicians in undertaking a new form of MAS.

The implications of MAS on community-based health services are not quantified. There is a need to move to multi-centre trials and have similar skills and experience in both arms of the trial. Incorporation of patient preference into the evaluations is important.[15]

3 Sub-categories

Gynaecological services divide into sub-categories which closely mirror important ICD codes. They are relevant to both purchasers and providers as they also reflect specific clinical services. This section considers 13 categories.

Subfertility (ICD 628)

An *Effective Health Care Bulletin*[42] and the family planning, abortion and fertility services needs assessment[1] have succinctly reviewed the evidence of the effectiveness of subfertility services and this needs assessment summarizes the findings and updates the literature. Two conditions; PID and endometriosis, although resulting in subfertility, are addressed under separate headings as they have other implications for the gynaecological service, infertility being the longer term outcome.

Subfertility can be defined as two or more years of involuntary failure to conceive. Of the subfertile couples 70% have not conceived before (primary subfertility) and 30% have conceived previously (secondary subfertility).[42]

Currently subfertility is diagnosed in both primary and secondary care settings with treatment usually being initiated in the secondary care setting and with the possibility of continued treatment in primary care.

Subfertility is associated with considerable social and mental distress.[43]

Pelvic inflammatory disease (ICD 614)

The term PID has come to represent clinically suspected endometritis and/or salpingitis that has not been objectively confirmed pathologically or visually.[44] Less than half of the cases of PID cause symptoms and produce visual salpingitis. Pelvic inflammatory disease can present to the GP or the A and E department staff as acute pelvic pain which requires urgent diagnosis and treatment or as chronic pelvic pain. Management can be undertaken by gynaecologists or GUM physicians in conjunction with primary care. Pelvic inflammatory disease is associated with a risk of infertility as a result of fallopian tube damage.

Chronic, subacute and/or latent endometrial infection may present in a large number of women, but a consensus definition of the clinically subtle infections is lacking and the magnitude of the problem is unknown.

Lower genital tract infections (ICD 616)

Vaginal discharge is a common presenting complaint in both primary and secondary care settings and like PID is managed by primary care, GUM and gynaecology. Vaginal discharge can result from a variety of bacterial, parasitic, viral, atrophic and traumatic causes which are often difficult to differentiate clinically from physiological causes of excessive vaginal discharge. The organisms which are most commonly associated with vaginal discharge include *Candida albicans*, *Trichomonas vaginalis*, *Gardnarella vaginalis*, gram negative rods, *Chlamydia trachomatis*, Herpes and wart virus infections. Bacterial vaginitis is a common lower genital tract infection and women with it have 100–1000 times more virulent bacteria per ml of vaginal flora than women without this infection and it is associated with postpartum and post-hysterectomy infection.

Bartholins cysts and abscesses are a relatively common gynaecological emergency and arise as an obstruction to the duct of the Bartholins gland and present as either labial swellings or acutely as abscesses.

Endometriosis (ICD 617)

Endometriosis is a condition in which there is functional endometrium outside the uterine cavity. The disease process is usually limited to the pelvis and clinical manifestations include pain, dyspareunia, menstrual disorders, subfertility and the presence of pelvic masses. The disease remains a mystery in terms of aetiology and pathogenesis. Whether it is a cause or consequence of childlessness also remains the subject of debate.[45]

Menopause (ICD 627)

Menopause literally means cessation of menstruation and the WHO suggests it be defined as the permanent cessation of menstruation resulting from loss of ovarian follicular activity whereas the climacteric includes the period immediately prior to the menopause and at least the first year after the menopause.

The main reason for contact with a GP and referral to the gynaecological services is for advice and management of symptoms associated with the menopause which may be menopause specific or confounded by age and other conditions. The most characteristic symptoms are hot flushes, night sweats, palpitations, headaches, vaginal dryness and dyspareunia.[46] The main chronic diseases associated with the menopause are osteoporotic bone disease and atherosclerotic cardiovascular disease.

Hormone replacement therapy increases levels of circulating oestrogens that fall at the menopause as a result of the loss of ovarian follicular activity and it is possible that some of the risks and benefits of HRT are secondary to these changes.[47] The geographical and secular variations in many of the conditions traditionally associated with the menopause cannot be attributed to differences in the use of HRT or endogenous oestrogen levels and suggest that while the menopause may be a risk factor, there are other determinants which are likely to have a profound influence.[47]

Urinary incontinence/utero-vaginal prolapse (ICD 618)

Urinary incontinence is defined as a condition in which involuntary loss of urine is a social or hygienic problem and can be objectively demonstrated.

A National Institute of Health Consensus Conference in 1988 highlighted the magnitude of the problem of incontinence. It is not part of the normal ageing process, leads to stigmatization and social isolation and in the US more than half of those with incontinence have had no evaluation or treatment, most health care professionals are not taught about incontinence and ignore the problem and inadequate staffing of nursing homes prohibits proper treatment and contributes to neglect of residents.

The causes of incontinence are numerous and this assessment focuses on genuine stress incontinence and detrusor instability which are the mainstay of gynaecological involvement with female incontinence. The management of incontinence is obviously not solely within the remit of the gynaecologist – primary care, urology, general medicine and surgery being involved in managing the condition.

Utero–vaginal prolapse is predominantly a problem of middle and old age in women who have had children. The initial damage generally occurs during childbirth, with further potential for weakness of the pelvic floor occurring after the menopause.[48]

Menstrual disorders (ICD 626)

Menstrual disorders involve a range of physiological and pathological (benign and malignant) changes in the hypothalamic pituitary ovarian and genital tract axis. This assessment will focus on the generic management of the most prevalent conditions which influence the gynaecological service, i.e. menorrhagia. Menorrhagia is the excessive loss of menstrual blood.[49]

The main issues that remain unresolved are:

- the balance of management that can be undertaken in primary care without referral to the gynaecological outpatient department
- the balance between medical and surgical treatments
- the use of day case and MAS.

Some conditions that present as menstrual disorders are discussed elsewhere (e.g. endometriosis, PID, malignant neoplasms).

The other problem is that in routine practice there is rarely any objective measurement of menstrual loss

Pelvic pain (ICD 625)

Pelvic pain refers to lower abdominal pain that can occur during the reproductive years and includes both gynaecological and non-gynaecological causes. The gynaecological causes include PID, pelvic pathology such as benign and malignant ovarian cysts and fibroids, endometriosis and PMS.

The subjective nature of the label of pelvic pain means the epidemiology is unclear. Painful menstruation can either be primary, which is more common in younger women, or secondary to other pelvic pathologies such as PID, endometriosis and fibroids and represent another symptom of diseases whose management is discussed elsewhere. The term 'severe pain requiring time off work' has been used to classify the pelvic pain syndrome and is estimated to occur in 3–10% of young women and is the primary cause for these women to visit their GPs. The label pelvic pain now tends to be reserved for the 60–70% of patients with lower abdominal pain who apparently have negative gynaecological laparoscopy.[50] There is some evidence that this is associated with pelvic congestion.[51]

Premenstrual syndrome

The epidemiology of PMS is unclear as symptoms can be diverse and duration and timing in relation to the menstrual cycle variable. Budeiri *et al.* reviewing the literature estimated that 199 symptoms and signs, along with 65 different assessment questionnaires have been employed in the study of PMS.[52] There is little conclusive information on the aetiology or treatment of PMS, although it attracts significant media attention. Premenstrual syndrome is of importance in the needs assessment of gynaecology as the label is recognized and services provided although the extent to which need, demand and supply of services is addressed by the NHS must remain an assumption.

Ectopic pregnancy (ICD 633)

Ectopic pregnancy is the siting of a pregnancy outside the uterine cavity, the most common site being the fallopian tube. By virtue of its site, as pregnancy advances the surrounding anatomical structure can not support the growing pregnancy and the ectopic pregnancy causes acute pain and often severe haemorrhage which may result in maternal death or severe morbidity.

Early pregnancy loss (ICD 630, 631, 632, 634)

Recurrent miscarriage

Recurrent miscarriage is defined as the loss of three or more consecutive pregnancies before 20 weeks gestation.[53] The aetiology is not fully understood and causes include infection, medical disorders, chromosomal abnormalities in the fetus, parental translocations and structural abnormalities of the genital tract.[54] Recently interest has focused on the immunologically mediated miscarriage and the role of 'blocking' antibodies.[54] An association with polycystic ovary syndrome is found with 80% of women with recurrent miscarriage.[55]

Miscarriage

Miscarriage is defined as loss of pregnancy before viability and the WHO definition has a weight cut-off of less than 500 g.

Genital tract cancer – secondary prevention

Cervix (ICD 233.1)

Squamous cell carcinoma, which accounts for 95% of cervical tumours, occurs most commonly at the squamo-columnar junction of the cervix and is characterized by a disordered morphology of the squamous epithelium which, by virtue of its site, is accessible for exfoliate cytology. Premalignant changes in cervical cytology are usually present and detectable for several years before an invasive lesion becomes clinically evident (the lead time). The dilemma is that the natural history of an abnormal smear is still not fully established with many minor abnormalities regressing over time and not requiring treatment.[56] Dyskariotic cells are derived from the surface epithelium of the cervix with cervical intraepithelial neoplasia (CIN) or invasive disease. Cervical intraepithelial neoplasia ranges from I (mild), II (moderate) to III (severe/carcinoma *in situ*).

Cervical cancer presents with local symptoms such as vaginal bleeding or discharge. The disease progresses locally and involves the ureters, bladder and rectum in later stages. Death is often associated with ureteric obstruction.

Screening aims to detect CIN-I–III lesions and early asymptomatic invasive lesions (stage 1), which if appropriately treated have a good prognosis. The management of abnormal smears involves primary care, family planning services, GUM departments and the gynaecological colposcopy services.

Other sites

There are no defined pre-invasive stages for cancers of the ovary and endometrium. Ovarian cancer has less than a 35% five-year survival rate as it is usually asymptomatic until widely disseminated. Methods to detect ovarian cancer at an early stage have been investigated as five-year survival is then as high as 85%.[57] There are currently national screening programmes for cervical and breast cancers and suggestion that screening for ovarian and endometrial cancers using ultrasound and CA 125 measurements are a possibility.[58–60] There are criteria for any potential screening programme that should be considered before implementation.[61] The disease needs to be of public health importance which ovarian cancer could be considered to be. The natural history should be known which is not clear for ovarian or endometrial cancer and diagnosis should be feasible which it is in both cases.

Genital tract cancer (ICD 182, 183, 186)

Three gynaecological cancers: cervix, uterus and ovary are among the ten most common malignancies in women and are managed by the gynaecological service along with radiotherapists and oncologists as appropriate. There is debate as to where the management of cancers should be sited and the role of cancer centres for gynaecological cancers. Other gynaecological cancers are rarer and not considered in this assessment (vulva, vagina, fallopian tube) but the principles discussed for the main sites are relevant for these cancers.

4 Incidence and prevalence

This section estimates the incidence and prevalence rates and hence potential for services needs for gynaecological conditions. The denominators are given wherever possible for the relevant female population e.g. reproductive age group (15–44 years).

Introduction

There are no data on the overall incidence or prevalence of gynaecological conditions. This section provides some estimates based mainly on specific research studies and therefore these data have to be interpreted with caution. It is not possible to give incidence/prevalence rates by age group for most conditions. Table 1 details broad estimates of incidence/prevalence.

Sub-categories

Subfertility

At any point in time the proportion of women of childbearing age experiencing subfertility is between 9–14%.[12,62] A health authority with a population of 100 000 with 18 400 women aged 20–44 with an established subfertility service may expect around 92 (0.5%) new consultant referrals each year and this demand is likely to increase due to trends towards later first pregnancies and an increasing number of remarriages and will be sensitive to changes of some sexually transmitted diseases. Demand is increasing due to raised public awareness of treatment possibilities.[63]

Pelvic inflammatory disease

The commonest organisms implicated in tubal occlusion are *Chlamydia trachomatis*, *Neisseria gonorrhoea* and anaerobic bacteria frequently associated with bacterial vaginosis. Infections with *N. gonorrhoea* and *C. trachomatis* are estimated to produce PID in 10–50% of cases. An epidemiological review[65] indicated the limited impact prompt treatment would have on subfertility rates because of:

1   the role of silent PID, which accounts for more than half of the tubal occlusion found in most clinical series of infertile couples
2   the failure to show that any current PID treatment regimens have a positive impact on future fertility.

Table 1: Incidence and prevalence of sub-categories (see text for full details of how estimates were calculated)

Sub-category	Incidence	Prevalence (females)
1 Subfertility	92/100 000 (0.5%) (total population M+F)	9–14% (age 15–44)
2 PID-Chlamydia	19/1000 (persons aged 15–59 attending GUM clinics)	5–12% (age 15–44)
3 Lower genital tract infection		4–28% (age 15+)
4 Endometriosis		1.3% (age 25–29)–8.1% (age 40–45)
5 Menopause		18% total population
6 Urinary incontinence		women (45+) attending menopause clinics 6–13% objective evidence 3–8%
7 Menstrual disorders – menorrhagia		20% (age 15–44)
8 Pelvic pain	10% females (aged 15+)	25% (age 15+)
9 Premenstrual syndrome		20–95% (age 15–44) 5% severe
10 Ectopic pregnancy	12/100 maternities 9/1000 pregnancies	
11 Early pregnancy loss – spontaneous miscarriage	12% clinically recognizable pregnancies	
– recurrent miscarriage	0.8–1% clinically recognizable pregnancies	
12 Cancer-2^0 prevention		
– cervix CIN III	53/100 000 females	
13 Cancer – cervix	17/100 000 females	
– uterus	15/100 000 females	
– ovary	20/100 000 females	

Taylor-Robinson estimates, conservatively, that genital and associated infections and their sequelae cost the UK at least £50 million a year for diagnosis and treatment.[3]

Chlamydia infections occur twice as frequently as gonorrhoea in most populations studied.[65] Serotypes D and K of *C. trachomatis* are causes of sexually transmitted disease and are an important cause of morbidity. Such infection cause up to half of all mucopurulent or follicular cervicitis and in developed countries up to 60% of PID.[66] There are only a few prevalence studies in general practice, gynaecology or antenatal clinic settings. In these 5–12% of women of child bearing age have been found to be infected.[67–70]

The organisms that lead to chronic PID and subfertility are those isolated from women often referred to GUM or gynaecology departments and include gonorrhoea and chlamydia which are reported in KC60 returns in England and Wales.[36] The trends of reporting are downwards but represent incomplete data. In 1992 just under 9000 cases of gonorrhoea and 66 000 cases of non-specific genital infection including chlamydia were reported.

Ashton *et al.* estimated the incidence of sexually transmitted diseases (met need based on GUM returns KC60) for both men and women in a reference population of 100 000 to be 1140.[1] The annual rate was 19 per 1000 population aged 15–59. A further 10% are treated outside GUM clinics. Some sexually transmitted diseases may go on to affect about 10–50% of cases although it is difficult to make estimates.

The use of intrauterine contraceptive devices (IUCD) by women in non-mutually monogamous relationships has been linked to higher than expected levels of genital tract infection and this also leads to tubal problems later.[71]

Lower genital tract infections

The prevalence of vaginitis ranges from 4% in asymptomatic college students to 10–28% in gynaecology and termination of pregnancy clinics.[72–74] Risk factors include being caucasian, prior pregnancy, IUCD, post-hysterectomy and abortion. Approximately 5–10% of women who complain of vaginal discharge have no pathological cause identified.

Endometriosis

Endometriosis is a common cause of gynaecological morbidity with an estimated prevalence of between 2.5–3.3%.[75] In a family planning cohort in the UK Vessey *et al.* estimated the prevalence rates to increase from 0.13 per 1000 woman–years in 25–29 year olds to 0.81 in 40–45 year olds.[76] A definitive diagnosis can only be made by laparoscopy or laparotomy and the prevalence of endometriosis at laparoscopy has been estimated at 1–2% of women of reproductive age.[77]

Menopause

The median age of the menopause in western women is 50 years, ranging from 35–59 years. Nutritional status and smoking are the main factors determining the age of the menopause. With increased life expectancy it is estimated that 18% of the population is postmenopausal. Most women will be postmenopausal for one-third of their life.

Symptoms

The main reason for contact with the health services is for treatment of symptoms associated with the menopause which may be menopause specific or confounded by age or other conditions. The most characteristic symptoms are hot flushes, night sweats, palpitations and headaches and it has been suggested that at least 80% of women are affected. Psychological symptoms are reported increasingly in the perimenopausal period and in a western survey affected 25% of women. Vaginal dryness, atrophic vaginitis and dyspareunia are said to be universal menopausal problems.[46]

Chronic diseases associated with menopause

The incidence of most chronic diseases increases with age and osteoporotic bone disease and atherosclerotic cardiovascular disease are two major causes of morbidity in women which have been suggested to be exacerbated by the menopause. However the two- to three-fold secular increase in the last 30 years in osteoporotic hip fractures in the UK can not be attributed to any changes in the age at menopause, or to changes in HRT[78] and geographical variations in many of the conditions traditionally associated with the menopause suggest that while the menopause may be a factor there are other determinants which are likely to have a more profound influence. It is therefore not clear how much these conditions can be remedied by HRT. The hormonal epidemiology of the menopause has mainly been determined in studies of western women and extrapolation to ethnic minorities is problematic. Exogenous factors, in particular diet, have been suggested to play a role in determining sex hormone levels and should be considered when devising preventive programmes.[47] The influence of diet, physical exercise and smoking on hormonal status is incompletely understood.

Cardiovascular disease

There were nearly 68 500 female deaths from myocardial infarction in England and Wales in 1992.[79]

Osteoporosis

Bone resorption is increased and cortical bone in the peripheral skeleton is lost at a rate of approximately 1% per annum. Rates of loss of vertebral trabecular bone are much higher; approximately 5–6% per annum during the early postmenopausal years and about half of all the bone loss that occurs in women may be attributed to the menopause. The incidence of fractures of the distal radius in women increases approximately 10–12-fold between the ages of 50 and 75. Approximately 25% of caucasian women have radiological evidence of vertebral compression by the age of 65. The incidence of femoral neck fracture doubles every five to seven years after the age of 70 and approximately 16–20% of women die as a consequence. HIPE data showed that over the age of 65, 82% of admissions for fractured neck of femur were in women of whom 83% were over 75.[80] Postmenopausal bone loss is insidious and causes no symptoms until fracture occurs, by which time it is too late to restore bone mass. There were over 900 deaths from fractured neck of femur in England and Wales in 1992.[79] Recent studies implicate physical activity, calcium nutrition and sex hormone status are the three most important determinants of peak bone mass.[81]

Urinary incontinence/utero-vaginal prolapse

A MORI poll in 1991 estimated 3.5 million and possibly 10 million people in the UK suffered from incontinence.[82] Thomas *et al.* estimated that one-third of women over the age of 35 were incontinent, twice each month or more. 85–90% of urinary incontinence is due to genuine stress incontinence or detrusor instability and it is not unusual for them to coexist. Versi and Cardozo estimated the incidence of a complaint of a poor stream or incomplete emptying in 5.6–13% of perimenopausal and postmenopausal women attending a menopause clinic.[84] Objective demonstration of an imbalance in micturition function, as measured by urodynamics is in the region of 3–8%.[84]

Genuine stress incontinence is associated with pregnancy, vaginal delivery and the menopause.[85] It is the involuntary urethral loss of urine without detrusor instability. Detrusor instability affects up to 10% of the population.

Estimates of the prevalence of prolapse are not available. Women who have a vaginal hysterectomy for prolapse may be coded simply as hysterectomy and the estimates of prolapse operations are an underestimate of the problem. Long lengths of labour and instrumental delivery are thought to be contributors to prolapse and with the advent of augmentation of labour and increasing caesarean section rates it is likely that the prevalence of prolapse will decline over the next few decades, although with increased life expectancy the number of menopausal women will increase and the effect this will have on prevalence rates is not known.[86]

Menstrual disorders

Menorrhagia is the excessive loss of menstrual blood and affects up to 20% of women in their reproductive years.[49] Excessive menstrual bleeding is the most common cause of iron deficiency in the UK affecting 20–25% of the fertile population.[87] It would appear that the upper limit of normal menstrual loss is between 60–80 ml.[88] Menorrhagia is however difficult to assess objectively in the absence of anaemia which is said to be present in 66% of women with menorrhagia.

In one population study 26% of those women with menstrual losses well within the normal range considered their periods heavy, whilst 40% of those with heavy losses considered their periods light.[49]

In those women over the age of 40 dysfunctional uterine bleeding (DUB) is the most common reason for a woman to consult her GP. Dysfunctional uterine bleeding is related to oestrogen withdrawl or hyperstimulation of the endometrium and represents 60% of cases. Specific gynaecological pathology (endometriosis, adenomyosis, fibroids (leiomyomata)) represents 35% and endocrine or haematological causes represent less than 5%.

Fibroids are present in 20% of the caucasian population with a three- to nine-fold increase in the African/Afro-Caribbean population over the age of 35. The proportion who develop menorrhagia varies from 17–61% with about 30% overall.[89]

Although the Oxford Family Planning Association Study is not representative of the UK female population data from this cohort have demonstrated that social class has a modest influence but parity and age (30–39 years) have strong influences on rates of menstrual disturbances (excluding fibroids).[90] Kuh and Stirling have reported socioeconomic variations in the risk of D&C and of hysterectomy are large.[91] They suggest lessening the socioeconomic gradient in risk of admission and surgery for diseases of the female genital tract, particularly for menstrual disorders, could have important resource implications.[91]

Pelvic pain

A survey by the RCOG revealed that 52% of laparoscopies were performed for pelvic pain.[92] Davies *et al.* estimated the incidence of pelvic pain syndrome to be 0.56–3.6 per 1000 women, with an average of 0.98 per 1000 women and the prevalence to be between 13.8–90 per 1000 women, with an average of 24.4. Using UK 1991 population estimates they calculated that this represents about 14 000 incident cases (7900–51 000) and 345 000 (195 200–272 800) prevalent cases.[93]

Premenstrual syndrome

Mild psychological symptoms occur in as many as 95% of women in the reproductive age range but only 5% will have severe symptoms that disrupt their lives. A diagnosis is not in the strictest sense possible, hence the prevalence estimates of between 20–95% of women of reproductive age are quoted.[18]

Ectopic pregnancy

The incidence of ectopic pregnancy appears to be rising in several industrialized countries especially with the advent of more sensitive pregnancy tests and ultrasound techniques. Factors which are associated with an increased incidence include tubal surgery, use of the progesterone-only pill, PID and the IUCD.[94] Ectopic pregnancy accounts for 10.3% ($n = 19$) of maternal deaths,[30] the main reason for death being haemorrhage. In a hospital-based series Norman estimated the incidence to be 11.9 per 1000 maternities and 9.1 per 1000 pregnancies (miscarriages and induced abortions plus total births).[95] Chow *et al.* estimate that in industrialized countries ectopic pregnancies account for 1.2–1.4% of all reported pregnancies.[96]

Ectopic pregnancy is more common in women of older age, lower parity and who have had a previous ectopic pregnancy with a three-fold increased risk of death from ectopic pregnancy amongst black compared with caucasian women.[94] 50% of ectopic pregnancies can be attributed to PID.[97]

Early pregnancy loss

Recurrent miscarriage

Observed frequencies of 0.8–1% of clinically recognizable pregnancies have been reported.[98]

Miscarriage

Spontaneous abortion is the commonest complication of pregnancy, affecting roughly one in four of all women who become pregnant.[99] The overall incidence of clinically recognizable spontaneous abortion before 20 weeks of gestation is approximately 12%.[100] The incidence of subclinical pregnancy loss may be as high as 60%.[101] Most early fetal losses are abnormal karyotypes but caffeine, alcohol and smoking have all been implicated in the past.

Genital tract cancer – secondary prevention

In the UK 4.5 million smears are performed annually of which 2.4% show mild dyskariosis and 3.4% are reported as showing borderline changes, although in younger women the borderline rate is about 4.9%.[102] There are no routine data collected on CIN I and II. Cancer registries collect data on CIN III/carcinoma *in situ* with registration rates of 53 per 100 000 females in the UK in 1986 with 13 609 registrations.[103] The standardized registration ratio varies significantly between region (36 in South West Thames to 134 in Yorkshire) but whether this is due to true incidence variations or registration differences is unclear.

Some postulate that as the CIN registration rate has been increasing in the UK mortality rates would have been even higher had cervical screening not been in place. This is probably true but the magnitude of the increasing incidence is not possible to calculate because the natural history of the disease is not fully understood and because the incidence trends of *in situ* lesions are also not clearly understood.[27]

Genital tract cancer (ICD 182, 183, 186)

The incidence of ovarian cancer (ICD 183) is approximately 20 per 100 000 with endometrial cancer (ICD 182) 15 and cervical cancer (ICD 186) 17.3.[104] The directly age standardized rates (World standard per 100 000 women) are 12.26 ovary, 8.7 endometrium and 13 cervix. Mortality data show significant variation in age standardized mortality ratios between district.[104] The overall mortality rates in the UK are 19.7 per 100 000 for ovary (including other adnexal tumours), 14.3 for endometrium and 16 for cervix.[104]

There were nearly 5200 cases of ovarian cancer in England and Wales in 1988. Ovarian cancer is predominantly a disease of older women, the incidence rising over the age of 30 to more than 50 per 100 000 in the over 65s. The regional standardized registration ratios indicate lower rates generally in the north but also in Oxford and South Western.[104]

Nearly 3800 new cases of cancer of the endometrium were registered in 1988 in England and Wales. Endometrial carcinoma is rare in women under 40 and the incidence rises to around 50 per 100 000 in 70–74 year olds.[104] Although there are significant differences in registration in the UK there is no obvious pattern in the standardized registration ratios.

There were nearly 4500 cases of cervical cancer in England and Wales in 1988. Carcinoma of the cervix is rare before the age of 20, peaks in incidence at 35–44 and then again at 60–64; over 90% of tumours being squamous cell carcinomas. In general the standardized registration ratio is higher in the north of England and lowest in the Thames regions. Although only 15.5% of cases occur in women under 35 it is the most common cancer in this age group, accounting for 25% of all new cancers.[104]

For all three cancers there is no significant overall trend in age-specific incidence rates over the past decade. However a study in the UK, adjusting for the hysterectomy rate, demonstrated an increased incidence of endometrial cancer of between 15–20%.[105] As the population ages the risk of endometrial cancer will increase but will be influenced by the use of oral contraceptive, HRT and hysterectomy rate. As large numbers of women with these exposures or attributes age into higher risk groups, age-specific rates are likely to fall.

International FIGO data[106] indicate considerable variation of survival by stage at each site (Table 2) which has a particular bearing on the current state of effectiveness of interventions.

Table 2: Disease stage at diagnosis[106]

	Stage I (%)	Stage II (%)	Stage III (%)	Stage IV (%)
Ovary	10	8	60	17
Endometrium	75	14	6	5
Cervix	35	35	25	5

The reasons for these variations in survival are reflected in the proportions of cases presenting at each stage (Table 3). England and Wales data indicate five-year survival rates overall of 30% ovary, 70% endometrium and 60% cervix.[104]

Table 3: Five-year survival rates[106]

FIGO stage	Ovary (%)	Endometrium (%)	Cervix (%)
I	85	75	78
II	50	57	57
III	25	30	31
IV	5	10.6	7.8
Overall	32.7	67.7	55

5 Services available

There are no national guidelines on what constitutes a typical gynaecological service, patterns of delivery having been built up over the years based on a combination of need, demand and supply. A typical district general hospital would employ at least three to four whole-time equivalent consultant obstetricians and gynaecologists. With the 'New Deal' the number of trainee medical staff has increased and such a unit may be supported by two to four middle grade staff (staff grade, senior registrar/registrar) and eight SHOs. Each consultant team would undertake one to two gynaecology outpatient sessions per week with two to three operating sessions. A gynaecology ward of 30 beds with day case facilities would be required for this workload.

Approximately 75% of the gynaecology budget is spent on hospital cases with only 25% on prevention and management in primary care.

Current service utilization using routine data sources is outlined below.

Primary care

Women with gynaecological symptoms may not consult a GP, preferring to self-medicate for such conditions as candida with over-the-counter (OTC) preparations from pharmacies.

Between the ages of 15 and 64 the consulting rate for women exceeds that for men, particularly for genitourinary disease. There has been a 103% increase in the prevalence of urogenital candida consultations between 1981 and 1982 and 1991 and 1992. Similarly a 154% increase in menopause/postmenopause consultations to 328 per 10 000 female–years at risk.[31]

- Overall 1500 women consult their GPs a year per 10 000 women–years at risk for gynaecological diseases including early pregnancy loss with 2250 consultations per 10 000 women–years at risk.
- A further 500 women consult per 10 000 women–years at risk with 700 consultations per 10 000 women–years at risk for candidiasis and trichomoniasis infections.
- Specific consultation rates are detailed in Appendix II. The main reasons for consultation in order of magnitude are outlined in Table 4.

Table 4: Main consultation categories in primary care[31]

Condition	ICD code	Patients consulting per 10 000 women–years at risk	Consultations per 10 000 women–years at risk
Candidiasis	112	521	690
Disorders of menstruation	626	449	676
Menopause/ postmenopause	627	328	583
Pain associated with female organs	625	278	394
Pelvic inflammatory disease	614–16	212	198

Outpatient facilities in secondary care

Gynaecology outpatients are usually separate from medical and surgical outpatient space. Gynaecological referrals are now not all seen in a general clinic, specialty clinics are common for the following categories of the service:

- termination of pregnancy
- colposcopy
- subfertility
- urogynaecology
- menopause
- oncology – combined clinics with oncologist and radiotherapist which may be in another department of the hospital.

There are no routinely collected data on use of gynaecological outpatients or the procedures undertaken in outpatients e.g. hysteroscopy, pipelle and vabra sampling of the endometrium.

Emergency facilities in secondary care

Unfortunately the published HES data do not provide an elective/emergency split.[32] The HRG data do split work into elective and emergency although the data across the specialty are not easily estimated. Of the 692 000 cases in the female reproductive system groups 167 500 (24%) were emergency admissions.

A survey in south London by the author indicates that around 40% of consultant episodes are emergency, of which 50% are for early pregnancy problems.

The model of referral, triage and management of emergencies is usually similar to medical and surgical specialties. There are changes to service provision that are emerging and which are discussed in the subsections. These include the development of early pregnancy assessment units for the management of problems of pregnancies under 20 weeks gestation. The increasing use of MAS requires operating theatres to be appropriately equipped and staff appropriately trained to provide the service.

Dowie indicated in his survey of gynaecology that most emergency operations were done outside normal theatre hours in six of the seven departments surveyed.[33] According to Korner statistics in 1987/88 17% of the total number of gynaecology cases in a London associate teaching hospital were operated on outside scheduled theatre session.

Appendix III, page 540 details the proportion of emergency cases by HRG category.

The main conditions and procedures are as follow.

- **Early pregnancy loss and threatened miscarriage** Evacuation of retained products of conception.
- **Ectopic pregnancy** Excisison of ectopic pregnancy laparoscopy/ laparotomy.
- **Ovarian cyst** Diagnostic and therapeutic laparoscopy/ laparotomy.
- **PID** Diagnostic and therapeutic laparoscopy.
- **Bartholin's abscess** Bartholin's cyst marsupialization.

It is not clear in the HRG data (Appendix III, page 540) what emergency diagnoses are considered in the category m 20, non-inflammatory diseases of vulva and vagina. Admissions for carcinoma of the ovary appear to be frequent as emergencies, probably with acute abdominal symptoms.

Ordinary and day case admissions into secondary care

The hospital episode statistics collect data on ordinary and day case admissions, operations and length of stay by ICD and surgical OPCS4R groupings[32] (see section 10). This assessment bases service availability on the UK data for the financial year 1993/94. Unfortunately no summary data are provided for gynaecology alone and either include breast disease or obstetric and pregnancy loss and general practice in one meaningless category.

Appendix III details the types of data available and the admissions and operations performed for the ICD and OPCS4R sub-categories of gynaecology. It is not possible to cross-tabulate operation by ICD code to assess the interventions undertaken for a particular pathology. Appendix III details the inpatients cases (ordinary and day case) by ICD.

There were a total of nearly 2000 cases per 100 000 female population aged over 15, with a further 5000 for pregnancy related disorders, totalling nearly 7000 per 100 000.

The most common categories are listed in Table 5 which are in contrast to the main categories seen in primary care (Table 4). Non-inflammatory disorders of the cervix mainly relate to precancerous lesions of the cervix.

Table 5: Main inpatient ICD 9 categories[32]

Condition	Number per 100 females
Disorders of menstruation	455
Non-inflammatory disorders of cervix	177
Genital prolapse	137
Menopause and postmenopause	117
Uterine leiomyoma	111

Appendix III details the admissions, splitting ordinary and day case admissions for the ICD sub-categories and bed days and lengths of stay. The proportion of ordinary to day cases for the main gynaecological categories is approximately 1.7 ordinary cases to one day case admission. The number of bed days equates to 1 300 000 days which is 1.5% of the total bed days in the UK and 4% of the acute sector according to HES data.

Appendix III lists the operations by OPCS4R codes with a total of 680 000 operations, equivalent to nearly 3000 per 100 000 females over the age of 15. The major operations are displayed in Table 6. Exploration of the vagina is a non-specific operation which relates to assessment of the vagina probably for postmenopausal bleeding.

Table 6: Main inpatient operations[32]

Condition	Number
Curettage of uterus	166 146
Other evacuation of contents of uterus	154 222
Abdominal excision of uterus	59 376
Endoscopic bilateral occlusion of fallopian tubes	50 969
Biopsy cervix uteri	23 031
Diagnostic endoscopic examination of uterus	21 853
Prolapse operations (P22 and 23)	21 248
Exploration of vagina	20 538
Destruction of lesions of cervix uteri	19 622

Appendix III details the operation by OPCS4R shortlist and splits ordinary and day cases and bed days. The proportion of ordinary to day cases varies by type of operation as does the use of bed days. Details of the waiting times in 1993/94 in the UK by main ICD categories and certain operation types are also given. There is significant regional variation. Appendix III also details the HRG data for 1993/94 in the UK. Overall 37% of the surgical admissions were treated as day cases. The accuracy of the data on ectopic pregnancy and termination of pregnancy are questionable as there appear to be a large number of admissions without operation.

Overall gynaecological service assessment

There are no routine data which provide overall cost/resource information for a gynaecology service. An example of how such data can be generated is provided by the Scottish Forum for Public Health Medicine.

The Scottish Forum for Public Health Medicine estimated that £15 000 000 per annum was spent for a female population of nearly 500 000 – 73% on hospital expenditure.[26] The costings (average cost in 1992) for each procedure involved (Table 7) and a programme budget based on activity were produced. Approximate proportions of the budget for each aspect of the service identified are outlined in Table 8.

Table 7: Average costs of gynaecology procedures[26]

Procedure	Elective (el)/ emergency (em)/day case	Cost (£)
Outpatient clinics		127
Inpatient day case		129
Inpatient case		104
Colposcopy		115
Smear		11
Hysterectomy	el	1241
Hysterectomy	em	1628
Vaginal repair	el	1568
Vaginal repair	em	2279
Hysteroscopy	all	231
D&C	el	404
D&C	em	597
D&C	day case	231
Open sterilization	el	838
Laparoscopy/lap. sterilization	el	447
Laparoscopy/lap. sterilization	em	640
Laparoscopy/lap. sterilization	day case	231
Termination of pregnancy	el/em	431
Termination of pregnancy	day case	231
Other operations	el	666
Other operations	em	808
Other operations	day case	231

Services available – sub-categories

All consultation rates in primary and secondary care are detailed in Appendices II and III respectively.

Subfertility

Initial investigations in primary or secondary care settings will result in a broad diagnosis in about 70% of patients. There is little uniformity in the diagnostic criteria and service availability used for diagnosing patients. In the secondary care setting subfertility is managed in both general gynaecology and specialist clinics.

The HES operative data are difficult to interpret as a range of diagnostic (diagnostic endoscopic examination of uterus (Q 18), curettage of uterus (Q10) and therapeutic operations (open myomectomy

Table 8: Programme budget for gynaecology services; proportion for each element of the service

Group	Unable to group (%)	Bleeding (%)	Cancers (%)	Inflammatory diseases (%)	Benign tumours (%)	Menopausal symptoms (%)	Incontinence (%)	Prolapse (%)	TOP (%)	Sterilization (%)	Infertility (%)	Others (%)	Total (%)
Prevention			13.00										13.00
Primary care	1.4					9.00	1.1				1.2	1.00	13.7
OP clinics	15.3		3.00										18.3
OP procedures			1.3										1.3
Day case surgery		0.8	0.1	0.1	0.02	0.3	0.2	–	2.5	0.6	0.3	1.7	6.62
IP surgery		5.2	2.9	2.7	2.00	1.7	1.4	12.00	5.5	3.00	2.00	7.5	45.9
IP no surgery		0.4	0.7	2.7	0.01	0.05	0.04	0.2	0.2		0.02	4.7	9.02
IP terminal care			0.2									0.03	0.23

OP = outpatient, IP = inpatient

(Q09), therapeutic endoscopic operations on uterus (Q17), open reversal of female sterilization (Q29)) interventions may be employed for subfertility.

- The IVF/GIFT rates are not available from HES.
- The waiting times for subfertility admission are on average 101 days, median 64 (Appendix III).

Pelvic inflammatory disease

Pelvic inflammatory disease is managed acutely in A and E departments and electively in gynaecology and GUM outpatient clinics.

Appendix III details the HES data for PID: salpingitis and oophoritis (ICD 614.0–614.2), inflammatory diseases of pelvic cellular tissue and peritoneum (ICD 614.3–614.9), inflammatory diseases of uterus, vagina and vulva (ICD 615, 616). The combined inpatient rates equate to 160 per 100 000 women aged over 15. It is not possible to interpret the operation codes as the interventions that are possible for PID are not specific. They include diagnostic procedures such as laparoscopy and therapeutic procedures which include laparoscopy and laparotomy with a variety of specific surgical procedures to relieve the sequelae of PID such as salpingolysis.

Buchanan and Vesssey showed that in the UK between 1975–85 the incidence of hospitalization for PID rose by 28%.[107] This increase occurred for both acute and chronic PID and was greatest in women in their 20s. The mean length of stay fell to four days in 1985 and the use of laporoscopy increased steadily over the time period to 54%. In a 6.5–8.5 years follow-up study this group showed that women discharged after a diagnosis of PID were nearly ten times more likely to be admitted for gynaecological pain, five and a half times more likely to be admitted for endometriosis, eight times more likely to be admitted for hysterectomy and nearly ten times more likely to be admitted with an ectopic pregnancy.[108]

HES data indicate the mean lengths of stay to be between three to six and six days, with a median of between two to six days for the sub-categories of PID.

Lower genital tract infection

Lower genital tract infections are managed in both gynaecology and GUM outpatient clinics. They may also be managed by self-medication in primary care with OTC preparations such as canestan. The HES data are only relevant for operations of the Bartholin's gland with an operation rate of 23 per 100 000 female population aged over 15, of which 20% were day cases.

There are no clinic attendance data for chlamydial infection prior to 1988. Large increases were seen between 1978 and 1986 in the number of attendances for non-specific genital infection of which 50% were thought to be due to *Chlamydia trachomatis*. Clinic returns in 1988 indicated 120 cases of chlamydial infection per 100 000 population aged 15–64. The 1992 returns indicate the number of new cases of trichomoniasis has declined to a rate of nearly 50 per 100 000 female population aged 15–44.[36]

The number of new cases of candidiasis recorded in GUM clinics has remained at about 60 000 per year since 1983.[36]

Endometriosis

The disease has no separate code in the general practice survey or HES data. In the US it is estimated that there were 18 hospital admissions for endometriosis per 100 000 women aged 15–44 in 1980 but the proportion of diagnostic and therapeutic procedures was not clear and readmissions were not considered.[109]

Menopause

Despite several active, predominantly teaching hospital, menopause clinics most of the care for menopause problems and prescription of HRT is clearly based in primary care.

A study in Oxfordshire indicated that there is a low overall use of HRT in the general postmenopausal population despite the recent media coverage of its benefits in the prevention of osteoporosis and subsequent fractures.[110] There is considerable uncertainty among GPs as to the balance of beneficial and harmful effects of HRT in the long term, particularly relating to its use for prevention of osteoporosis and cardiovascular disease. Most doctors would be prepared to participate in randomized controlled trials to determine the long-term effects of this increasingly widely used treatment.[111] The authors found that about 9% of women aged 40–64 were prescribed HRT. A study of perimenopausal women showed considerable interest (more than 75%) among perimenopausal women in taking HRT to prevent osteoporosis.[112] In a survey of women attending a general practice 59% of respondents wished to have more information about HRT and 80% more information about the menopause before its onset.[113]

Urinary incontinence/utero-vaginal prolapse

The general practice survey collects information on consultations for utero-vaginal prolapse, which is associated with incontinence, and genitourinary problems (Appendix II). Although genitourinary problems are not specific for incontinence (also includes eneuresis, bedwetting) it is the only category which reflects the burden of the condition and is not useful when considering the need for gynaecological services.

The specific operations undertaken for incontinence (m codes, Appendix IV) total nearly 7500 equating to 32 operations per 100 000 female population aged over 15.

The majority of women complaining of urge or stress incontinence are seen in general gynaecology outpatient clinics. There are specific urogynaecology clinics, more often in teaching hospitals.

The overall admission rate equates to a rate of nearly 140 per 100 000 females aged over 15 years.

- Prolapse procedures utilize 242 000 bed days with a mean length of stay of eight days, median six.[32]
- Repair of prolapse operations occur at a rate of 100 per 100 000 women aged over 15.
- The mean waiting time for admission was 147 days, median 105.

Menstrual disorders

Coulter et al. estimated 21% of gynaecology referrals in the mid 1980s in Oxfordshire were for menstrual disorders with significant variations in practice referral rates.[114]

The Effective Health Care report on the management of menorrhagia indicated that there is considerable variation in practice and uncertainty about the most appropriate management strategies.[115] A total of 822 000 prescriptions were issued in the UK in 1993 to 345 000 women for menorrhagia at an annual cost of £7.12 million and the most commonly prescribed drugs are norethisterone (38%), mefenamic acid (27%), combined oral contraceptive (11%); with tranexamic acid, the most effective drug, only prescribed in 5% of women.[115]

The possible operations undertaken for menstrual disorders include diagnostic – dilation of cervix uteri (D&C) and endoscopic examinations of the uterus and therapeutic – abdominal excision of uterus (hysterectomy (TAH)), vaginal excision of the uterus and open myomectomy endoscopic operations on the uterus (Appendix III).

HES data are difficult to interpret for menstrual disorders. The hospital admission rate for uterine leiomyomata of the uterus is 111 per 100 000 female population aged over 15. Disorders of menstruation accounted for a further 455 admissions per 100 000 female population aged over 15.

Coulter *et al.* demonstrated that although D&C rates declined in the US between 1977–90 they remained static in the UK, with a rate of 70 per 10 000 women in the UK compared with 11 in the US in 1988–90.[116] It was the most common procedure in the Oxford region; 40% of the women being under the age of 40 with a significant variation between districts and with day case rates varying from 22–82% (compared with National Audit Office targets of 86%). The problem with interpreting D&C rates is that the use of other outpatient endometrial sampling procedures, such as vabra and pipelle, are not recorded in HES data. In 1993/94 22 000 hysteroscopies were carried out in the UK, an increase of 22% on 1992/93.[32]

Hysterectomies are performed both abdominally and vaginally for a range of gynaecological conditions of which menstrual disorders contribute about half. Hysterectomy rates vary up to six-fold between countries, with the UK having a relatively low rate in the 1970s.[117] They showed that the variation was correlated in the UK with the number of GPs per 1000 population. 54% of the variation was accounted for by the number of GPs and whole-time equivalent gynaecologists. Coulter explored possible reasons for the variation in the hysterectomy rates: primary care interest in gynaecological conditions such as menorrhagia varies and hence referral rates to gynaecologists; patient's decision to consult their GP and gynaecologist's decision to operate also vary.[118]

In the Oxford survey more than 22% of women had undergone a hysterectomy. The problem with looking at hysterectomy rates is that they take no account of the proportion of women who have had the operation and are no longer at risk. Coulter *et al.* estimated that 60% of GP referrals for menorrhagia are treated within five years with a hysterectomy.[114]

Coulter *et al.* suggested that the referral rates from general practice were an important determinant of resource use and she demonstrated that as many as 43% of patients referred to gynaecology outpatient departments had presented to their GPs less than a month previously. Gath *et al.* commented that the prevalence of perceived menstrual problems is much higher than the number of women who actually consult their GPs about them.[119] Coulter *et al.* estimated hysterectomy rates to be on the increase with levels of 30 per 10 000 women in 1989/90.[116]

Pelvic pain

It has been estimated that one-third of gynaecological clinic presentations are for pelvic pain.[120] Pelvic pain consumes significant health care resources.[93] The lifetime costs are estimated to be £770 per woman. Total annual costs are estimated at £158.4 million, i.e. 0.6% of the NHS budget at 1990/91 prices.

The general practice survey data are difficult to interpret as women will present with pelvic pain associated with specific gynaecological conditions, non-gynaecological conditions as well as the pelvic pain syndrome.

Premenstrual syndrome

There are no routine data, although surveys suggest nearly all women suffer from symptoms but only 5% have severe symptoms, probably requiring at least an outpatient opinion and further investigations such as laparoscopy.

Ectopic pregnancy

Ectopic pregnancies can miscarry spontaneously or resorb, thereby either not presenting to the service at all or presenting to A and E departments as a miscarriage. Those women that present to A and E or the GP with pain, bleeding and shock are the most likely to be labelled as having an ectopic pregnancy.

The operative interventions are not specific to ectopic pregnancy and include therapeutic endoscopic operations on the uterus (Q17) and unilateral excision of adnexa of uterus (Q23).

Early pregnancy loss

Surgical evacuation of the uterus accounts for around three-quarters of emergency gynaecological operations. Data from the HES indicate that there were 1 170 192 inpatient cases equating to 5000 per 100 000 female population aged over 15.

Gilling-Smith *et al.* surveyed A and E departments in England and Wales to assess how women with bleeding in pregnancy were managed.[121] Although 88 (94%) of the 94 departments dealt with bleeding in early pregnancy, only 64 (73%) of these had gynaecologists on site. Of the 86 departments with ultrasound facilities on site, 40 (47%) could not obtain an ultrasound scan outside normal working hours. Nine (56%) of the 16 departments that did not stock either ergometrine or oxytocin had no gynaecology staff on site.

Recurrent miscarriage problems may be dealt with in general gynaecology outpatient clinics or specialist/research centres but there are no data to quantify how many such clinics exist.

Genital tract cancer – secondary prevention

Cervix

Recent Korner KC53 and KC61 (pathology laboratory activity) data (1991/92) indicate that the number of smears performed has increased to 4.5 million a year in the UK.[25]

The follow-up of 'abnormal' smears and implementation of treatment (fail-safe protocols) is the area of the screening service which affects the gynaecological service (Appendix VI). This will involve the gynaecology outpatient services and colposcopy in particular, along with treatment both as inpatients and day cases.

Data from the HES indicate an admission rate of 84 per 100 000 female population aged over 15 for carcinoma *in situ*.

Genital tract cancer

A woman will usually present to her GP in the first instance and the data show consultation rates of ten per 10 000 patients.[31] There were 38 712 inpatient admissions, equating to a rate of nearly 500 per 100 000 females aged over 15. It is not possible to break this down further into surgical procedures, other therapies, recurrences, progression or palliative care. From the operation codes it is not possible to assess which procedures were performed for gynaecological cancer.

Day case and minimal access gynaecological surgery

There are striking differences between units in terms of the use of day surgery and targets based on the proportions of specific procedures undertaken as day cases would need to take into account the same procedures undertaken in outpatient departments (e.g. colposcopy, cervical laser treatment, endometrial sampling). The case severity and presence of comorbidities may influence these proportions and should be adjusted for in any comparison.

Henderson *et al.* showed that the proportion of D&Cs performed as day cases varied from 1–43%. The same group also showed that the proportion of women being treated as day cases increased from 16% in 1976 to 26% in 1985.[122] Explaining within country variations Morgan and Beech suggest that the following factors be taken into consideration:

- characteristics of the patient e.g. age, severity
- characteristics of the health care systems e.g. supply of beds and staffing levels
- clinical practice style e.g. surgical technique and anaesthesia
- organization of hospital care e.g. availability of theatres.[123]

A recent small audit of day case surgery indicated that with the recent changes to anaesthetic practice, despite considerable morbidity after their return home, only 8% of patients said they would have preferred an overnight stay.[124]

Data from the HES shown in Table 9 indicate the proportions of common gynaecological procedures performed as day cases (Appendix III). The HRG data suggest 34% of gynaecological procedures are undertaken as day cases (Appendix III).

Table 9: Proportion of cases performed as day case procedures

Operation	%
Bartholin's abscess/cyst	13
D&C	44
ERPC	35
Diagnostic endoscopy	55
Therapeutic endoscopy	15

The National Audit Office estimated that 70% of the existing day case and inpatient waiting lists could be treated by day case surgery. The problems in its implementation are:

- lack of information to assess performance
- lack of specialist facilities
- inappropriate and insufficient use of existing facilities
- poor management
- clinicians' preference for traditional approaches
- disincentives for managers to prescribe change.[34]

Of the top ten day case procedures two were gynaecological: termination of pregnancy (3%) and D&C (5%).

6 Effectiveness of services

The evidence of effectiveness of aspects of the gynaecological service is reviewed here. The section is not intended as a complete, extensive review of all areas but provides purchasers with the balance of evidence for the various components of the service.

There have been Effectiveness Health Care Bulletins for two aspects of the service; subfertility[42] and menorrhagia[115] and the evidence for the other areas has been sourced from literature searches and review articles.

As with many other specialties in medicine the overall evidence of effectiveness of current interventions is not good. There are no evaluations of a complete gynaecological service and therefore models have to be built up using the components suggested in section 7. The National Perinatal Epidemiology Unit was set up to undertake rigorous trials and evaluations in the field of obstetrics and has done much to promote evidence-based medicine in the specialty. Gynaecologists should therefore be aware of the need for trials to assess their practice.

The evidence to support surgical procedures is generally weak, although trials of the newer developments in MAS have been undertaken. However procedures still slip into routine practice before evidence of effectiveness is available.

For the medical management of gynaecological conditions trials have often been small and outcome assessed poorly and the ethos of multicentre trials needs to be generated. Despite evidence of effective, cheap drugs for the management of menorrhagia, practitioners still prescribe ineffective and more expensive drugs.

Subfertility

Active and sensitive provision of information and support are important components of a high quality subfertility service. Stress is reduced in those couples who feel involved in and in control of their treatment (A-III).[125] The role of counselling has not been shown to be effective.

Assisted conception techniques include artificial insemination, IVF-ET (*in vitro* fertilization and embryo transfer) and GIFT (gamete intra-fallopian transfer). In 1990 the average pregnancy rate with IVF-ET was 17% per treatment cycle.[2] This translates into an average maternity rate of 12% (per treatment cycle) and 14% per couple treated because some couples have more than one cycle. The average number of treatment cycles per patient in 1990 in the UK was 1.16[2] and three cycles is considered by experts to be a reasonable limit. There is no evidence of increased effectiveness overall of IVF-ET over GIFT.

The effectiveness of IVF is reduced if the sperm used is of poor quality; effectiveness is also influenced by maternal age (AIII).[2] *In vitro* fertilization clinics providing a service for women aged over 35 have lower than average success rates.[2] Fetal abnormality occurs but not at statistically different levels to unassisted conceptions.[126] Maternal mortality and morbidity data are not available but recommendations that multiple pregnancies should be avoided have been made (AIII).[2]

The problem that is managed least successfully in terms of conceptions has been that of poor sperm quality or function; there is currently no completely effective treatment for male infertility. The administration of systemic corticosteroids to the 10% of men thought to have an immunological basis to their sterility is of doubtful efficacy and treatment may produce unpleasant and often unacceptable side-effects.[42,127] The main success in managing male infertility is by artificial insemination by donor (AID) and the provision of donor insemination should be an integral part of a district infertility service. There will also be a small demand for this service for the partners of males who are HIV positive and wish to conceive. There may be an increased need for AID, as the extent of male infertility becomes clinically recognized.

Medical treatments for ovulatory dysfunction caused by hyperprolactinaemia or hypothalamic amenorrhoea appear to be very effective at re-establishing fertility to normal levels (AII-2).[128]

There is a significant level of spontaneous pregnancy among untreated women with endometriosis and medical and surgical treatments have been shown to be ineffective. For couples who have failed to conceive, where mild or moderate endometriosis is implicated, assisted conception techniques appear to be successful (AII-2).

Assisted conception techniques appear the most effective treatment for unexplained subfertility (AII-1). Medical treatments may have some effect upon maternity rates and these require further investigation.

Pelvic inflammatory disease

Health education as it is currently provided in the school system is thought to have little influence upon sexual and contraceptive behaviour of young people and hence on PID.[129]

The use of barrier methods of contraception by those not in mutually monogamous relationships is an important part of any strategy to reduce PID and secondary infertility caused by sexually transmitted diseases (AIII).

Apart from primary prevention early diagnosis and treatment of sexually transmitted diseases plays an important part in reducing their incidence by shortening the time during which people can pass on infection to others (AIII). Strategies for detection and screening have been haphazard, so that the identification of infected individuals, with or without symptoms has been incomplete.[3] In Sweden a programme of widespread screening for chlamydial infection has virtually eradicated the disease.[4] There is evidence however that a small increase in 15–19 year olds may herald a resurgence and the differences between the Swedish population and that in the UK may mean such a reduction would not be seen in this country. High risk screening of women undergoing termination of pregnancy has been suggested as a more cost-effective way forward (BII-2).[130] In primary care it has been modelled that a routine test for chlamydial infection in asymptomatic 18–24 year old women during gynaecological examination was found to be cost-effective but this was not the case for older women (BIV).[5]

Chlamydia trachomatis can be diagnosed from swabs detecting endocervical chlamydial antigens and serum chlamydial antibodies but the woman may not present as she is often asymptomatic. The tests are expensive. A ligase chain reaction assay of urine to diagnose *Chlamydia trachomatis* has been shown to be highly effective for its detection in urine from women with or without symptoms of chlamydial genitourinary tract infection.[131] Standard regimens of tetracyclines, doxycycline or erythromycin appear to be effective against chlamydia in most circumstances (AI).[132] A meta-analysis of trials of antibiotics to treat PID indicated there was a lack of uniformity among studies regarding diagnosis, care and follow-up. Pooled cure rates ranged from 75–94%. Doxycycline and metronidazole was the least effective regimen (75% cure rate). Ciprofloxacin was the cheapest.[133] They concluded that clinical treatment of acute PID is still likely to be wholly inappropriate in many women and suboptimal in a high proportion of the remainder.

Lower gonital tract infections

Health promotion initiates should be in line with local strategies for the Health of the Nation targets.[134]

Contact tracing should become a matter of routine for all diagnosed cases of sexually transmitted disease.

Appropriate antimicrobial therapy is effective for chlamydial infection with cure rates of 80–90% (AI). Bacterial vaginosis can be treated with oral metronidazole and clindamycin intravaginal creams, with 75% being disease free one month after treatment (AI)[6] but whether a single dose or seven-day course is more cost-effective is unclear.

Bartholin's abscesses can either be surgically marsupialized or incised. Andersen *et al.* (AI) compared marsupialization with incision and curettage and primary suture of the abscess under antibiotic cover in a prospective trial of 32 patients.[135] The time for healing was significantly less in the suturing group than the marsupialization group, with the same length of stay.

Endometriosis

The aetiology and natural history of endometriosis is not known and thus most regimens have not been shown to be effective in the long term, hence the whole spectrum of strategies employed. Currently clear recommendations for treatment of endometriosis in symptomatic women can be made.[45] Medical treatment works only temporarily with the disease recurring once stimulation by ovarian steroids returns.[136] Endometriosis is more common in subfertile women and women with pelvic pain and logically these should be the main indications for treatment.[45] None of the trials show that medical treatment improves fertility.[45]

Hormonal treatment of symptomatic endometriosis is less of an issue if pain interferes with quality of life. As treatment is expensive and with side-effects the therapy should be contingent on the goals of treatment for each patient. Several modalities can be employed in managing the patient with endometriosis but the ultimate selection is determined by evaluating a number of criteria including age, extent of disease, severity of symptom and pain.

Treatment with progestogens alone has apparently been successful but they are prescribed less frequently than the androgenic steroid danazol.[137] Danazol reduces breakthrough bleeding but there is no evidence that pregnancy rates are any higher with this drug than progestogens.[138] A newer approach is ovarian suppression with luteinizing hormone releasing hormone (LHRH) analogues. However both danazol and LHRH are costly and have limitations for long-term use. Large multicentre trials of GnRH and danazol show equal effectiveness in relieving symptoms and resolving visible endometriotic lesions (AI).[139,140] Both preparations have side-effects that need to be considered when managing patients.

All medical approaches seem to offer relief of symptoms but the optimum duration of treatment is not clear and the relative merits in terms of pregnancy rates, disease eradication, side-effects and long-term benefits or disadvantages have yet to be compared with each other, with surgical methods and, in mild cases, with placebo.

For women wanting to become pregnant surgical intervention is indicated in those with moderate or severe disease associated with ovarian fixation, peritubal adhesions, or ovarian endometriomas (BIII). If surgery is indicated electrodiathermy is the conventional method with laser a more expensive alternative but one which allows treatment at the same procedure as diagnosis (BIII).[141] Comparison of conservative surgery with medical treatment or expectant management has shown no difference in the outcome in women with mild or even moderate endometriosis.[137,142,143] Likewise a combined surgical and medical approach seems to offer no advantage in mild disease, although it is the method most favoured in advanced cases.[137,142,143]

The *Effective Health Care Bulletin* on the management of subfertility states that there is a significant level of spontaneous pregnancy among untreated women with endometriosis. Medical treatments have been shown to be ineffective. Surgical treatments also appear ineffective. For couples who have failed to conceive naturally assisted conception techniques appear successful (AII-2).[42]

The debate about management continues and results of large trials on which to base rational management are awaited. Although there is a move to minimally invasive techniques for the treatment of endometriosis their effectiveness remains to be confirmed in controlled clinical trials.

A study in Leeds suggested that if a patient has a recurrence of endometriosis it may be possible for the GP to initiate retreatment with the same or alternative medication prior to a revaluation by the gynaecological team (CIII).[144] Surveillance and continuing prescription in primary care is required after hospital management.

Menopause and hormone replacement therapy

This assessment is predominantly concerned with the effectiveness of the gynaecological services. The debate over the effectiveness of HRT on chronic diseases such as osteoporosis, breast cancer and cardiovascular disease continues and only an outline is provided here but it is important to ensure that where menopause services are provided, information and management strategies incorporate consideration of the longer term benefits of HRT.

Symptoms

Placebo-controlled trials have shown consistently that HRT relieves flushes, sweats and the symptoms of lower genital tract atrophy and most have reported beneficial psychological effects (AI).[8]

Cardiovascular disease

Meade and Berra reviewing 12 retrospective case-control studies suggested that HRT reduced coronary risk by about 25% but little or no effect was seen for stroke (AII-2).[9] Reviewing the ten prospective cohort studies reductions of 20% for cardiovascular disease and 15% for stroke were observed (AII-2). There are no comparable data of treatment with patches or implants. It is not known whether opposed oestrogen therapy diminishes these beneficial effects as progesterone reduces the HDL cholesterol-raising effect of oestrogen. In the prospective studies notably the nurses study in the US it is not clear how much of the observed reduced risk is due to a selection bias of healthier women to the study. Posthuma *et al.* suggest that unintended selection of relatively healthy women for oestrogen therapy may have influenced the reported beneficial effect of oestrogen therapy on cardiovascular disease and it is unclear how much of the cardioprotection is due to this selection.[145]

Osteoporosis

Screening

Law *et al.* reviewed the studies using bone density measurements in women with hip fracture and age-matched controls and confirmed that it is a poor screening test.[80]

No simple cost-effective screening test is available. An *Effective Health Care Bulletin*[7] stated that there have been no scientific trials assessing the effectiveness of population bone screening programmes in preventing fractures in elderly women. The bulletin suggests that bone density measurements are poor at identifying which women will go on to have a fracture in later life. Less than a quarter of women are likely to attend for screening and take HRT over a long period of time. It is likely that a bone screening programme will lead to the prevention of no more than 5% of fractures in elderly women. Given current evidence it would be inadvisable to establish a routine population-based bone screening programme for menopausal women with the aim of preventing fractures.

A report of the Department of Health's Advisory Group on Osteoporosis recommends the use of bone density measurement in individual clinical decision-making in certain high risk groups.[146]

The only randomized controlled trial of exercise in premenopausal women showed that exercise significantly increases the mineral density of the young female skeleton (AI).[147]

Randomized controlled trials of up to ten years in duration have shown that oestrogen replacement substantially or totally prevents postmenopausal bone loss as have observational studies and bone loss is prevented for as long as treatment is maintained (AI).[10,11] The effect of oestrogen/progesterone preparations on the incidence of fractures has not yet been assessed but a preventive effect is likely because the combination prevents rapid postmenopausal bone loss in the same way as oestrogen alone.

The conclusions in the review by Law *et al.* are that increasing physical activity is the most important strategy for reducing the hip fracture rate and this would half the rate (AIII).[80] Similarly a reduction in smoking premenopausally can reduce the risk by a quarter. Although HRT more than halves the risk of fracture, once stopped the protection is reduced thereby reducing its utility. If it were to be beneficial it would need to be continued indefinitely from the onset of the menopause. In postmenopausal women with low bone density, bone loss can be slowed or prevented by exercise along with calcium supplementation or oestrogen/progesterone replacement (AI).[148] How long therapy needs to be continued to have an impact on fractures is unclear.

Overall benefits

A non-quantitative epidemiological overview of oestrogen replacement therapy with or without progestogens concluded that the benefits outweigh the risk.[149] A quantitative analysis came to similar conclusions for women after hysterectomy and women at high risk of cardiovascular disease.[150] Gorsky *et al.* evaluated the relative risks and benefits of exogenous oestrogen use among women entering the climacteric and considered oestrogen use for relief of symptoms or prevention of disease.[151]

Decision analysis was used to assess the value of HRT in a hypothetical cohort of 10 000 women assumed to be aged 50 years and health outcomes were extrapolated to age 75. The health benefits of postmenopausal oestrogen replacement were found to exceed the health risks incurred. The study assumes universal compliance with HRT and much of the data was derived from the nurses study in the US and may not be representative of the UK situation. Khaw illustrated the estimated changes in annual rates of certain menopause related events of ten years HRT (Table 10).[47]

Table 10: Illustrative estimated changes in annual rates[a] by ten-year age group in England and Wales associated with hormone replacement therapy (HRT) unopposed oestrogen or combined with progestogen for ten days a month, for ten years (Source:[47])

	Heart disease	Stroke	Breast cancer	Uterine cancer	Hip fracture	Net balance of events
Estimated annual rates per 100 000 by age group						
45–54 years	30	17	62	2	18	
55–64 years	171	60	101	8	66	
65–74 years	600	243	135	16	231	
75+ years	2419	1938	259	34	1480	
Unopposed oestrogen						
Relative risk	0.6	0.8	1.2	4.0	0.5	
Change in annual rates per 100 000 by age group						
45–54 years	−12	−3	+12	+8	−9	−4
55–64 years	−68	−12	+20	+32	−33	−61
65–74 years	−240	−49	+27	+64	−126	−324
75+ years	−968	−388	+52	+136	−740	−1908
Oestrogen with progestogen						
Relative risk	0.8	0.9	1.3	1.0	0.5	
Change in annual rates per 100 000 by age group						
45–54 years	−6	−2	+18	0	−9	−1
55–64 years	−34	−6	+30	0	−33	−43
65–74 years	−120	−24	+41	0	−126	−229
75+ years	−484	194	+78	0	−740	−134

[a] Ischaemic heart disease, cerebrovascular disease, breast cancer, endometrial cancer mortality rates from OPCS; hip fracture estimated incidence rates from HIPE data

Mode of delivery

The oestradiol patch is an alternative to oral oestrogens for women with menopause symptoms. It should be combined with an oral progestogen for women who have not had a hysterectomy. The theoretical advantage of the transdermal route is of unproven clinical benefit and the contraindications are the same as for oral HRT. Patches are not yet indicated for preventing osteoporosis and are more expensive than other oestrogen preparations. It is still not yet known whether transdermal oestradiol will protect against ischaemic heart disease in the way that ovarian or oral oestrogen does. Subcutaneous oestrogen is more effective than oral oestrogen in preventing osteoporosis, probably owing to the more physiological (premenopausal) serum oestradiol concentrations achieved. Subcutaneous oestrogen also avoids problems of compliance that occur with oral treatment.[152] Progestogen-releasing intrauterine systems can also be used to deliver progestogen direct to the endometrium in women who still have a uterus.

Cost-effectiveness

In the US Weinstein and Tosteson, using some assumptions, showed that oestrogen replacement therapy was found to be cost-effective with rates ranging between $9130 and $12 620 per additional life saved.[153] For women who have not had a hysterectomy ten- and 15-year courses of oestrogen combined with progesterone have been evaluated. The baseline assumptions were that breast cancer incidence and ischaemic heart disease deaths were unaffected and the study did not take into account the occurrence of fractures of the wrist or vertebrae. Under these assumptions combined therapy was more costly, with ratios ranging from $86 100 to $88 500.

Unless combined therapy is found to confer protection against IHD the most cost-effective strategies for women with no prior hysterectomy may involve screening perimenopausal women to detect women at highest risk of hip fracture followed by selective treatment. In a UK analysis Roche and Vessey concluded that the benefits in terms of reduced mortality and treatment costs are greater for women without a uterus receiving unopposed oestrogen therapy than for women with a uterus receiving combined therapy.[12] Indeed a net cost to the NHS of £137 per woman is suggested if hysterectomized women are treated with oestrogen therapy (Table 11).

Table 11: Average cost per woman treated for 15 years and followed up until age 79

Costs	ORT (£)	O+P (£)
Direct costs:		
Drug	110	453
Monitoring	117	117
Indirect costs:		
Breast cancer	13	13
Ischaemic heart disease	(18)	(9)
Cerebrovascular disease	(65)	(33)
Fractured neck of femur	(20)	(20)
Total cost	137	521

Figures in paranthesis are savings. All costs are discounted at 5% per annum.[12]

ORT = oestrogen replacement therapy.

O+P = oestrogen plus progesterone.

Coulter has estimated that 20% of the female population in the UK will have had a hysterectomy by the age of 50 and thus a strategy aimed at this group alone would have major public health implications.[118] As Weinstein and Tosteson indicate all conclusions from such analyses must be regarded as highly speculative because of the vast uncertainty that surrounds the possible effects of oestrogen and progesterone on heart disease.[153] In terms of cost-effectiveness they conclude that HRT compares favourably with other accepted health care interventions. Daly et al. similarly concluded that long-term prophylactic treatment of hysterectomized women and treatment of symptomatic women with a uterus compare favourably with other accepted health care interventions.[154] They estimated the cost per QALY to range from £700 for ten years of treatment with oestrogen alone HRT for women with mild menopausal symptoms to £6200 for combined therapy for women with mild symptoms.

Grady et al. estimated life expectancies and risks of certain sentinel events in groups: women without risk, women with cardiovascular disease and women at risk of breast cancer, fractured neck of femur, or cardiovascular disease.[150] Assumptions had to be made for the long-term effect of combined therapy. In the first optimistic setting addition of a progesterone to the oestrogen regimen was assumed not to change the relative risk of disease from oestrogen, except to prevent the increased risk of endometrial cancer. In the second more pessimistic scenario addition of progesterone was assumed to provide only two-thirds of the cardiovascular risk reduction while the relative risk of breast cancer was increased. Women who had undergone a hysterectomy had about the same change in life probability of disease and life expectancy as that of women with no special risk using combined therapy under optimistic assumptions. However because these women do not need to take progesterone the estimates are less certain.

Side-effects

The risk of endometrial cancer brought about by oestrogen can be virtually eliminated by cyclical treatment with progesterones.[155] Pooled data on the risk of breast cancer show a modestly increased relative risk of about 1.3 for 15 years of oestrogen use[156] but there is sufficient concern over the potential risk that largescale trials are proposed to estimate the risk of cancer with HRT.

Urinary incontinence/utero-vaginal prolapse

Stress incontinence

First-line investigations that can be performed in primary care include microscopy and culture of urine to exclude an infective cause of incontinence and the maintenance of a fluid balance chart which enables the clinician to obtain a better understanding of the problem.[157] The overlap of symptomatology between stress incontinence and detrusor instability is such as to make a diagnosis impossible without resource to urodynamic studies. Videocysto-urethrography may help with difficult cases. There is a poor correlation between clinical diagnosis and urodynamic diagnosis.[158] Urodynamic investigations are of three types:

1   simple and non-invasive (e.g. pad tests and frequency/volume charts), suitable for primary care
2   basic urodynamics suitable for district general hospitals
3   complex urodynamics suitable for a tertiary referral centre.

Conservative treatment is of use for those women with mild symptoms or with comorbidities but the majority will require surgery. Simple measures such as providing explanations, use of intravaginal tampons and sponges have been advocated (BIII).[157] Physiotherapists are treating considerable numbers of patients with stress incontinence but the efficacy data are still required to enable rationalization of resources to cater for the whole population.[159] There is no satisfactory method of measuring pelvic floor function and of monitoring progress during treatment. The success of pelvic floor re-education varies from 60–90% but when compared to surgery (Burch colposuspension) physiotherapy compares poorly.[13] In the study by Mantle and Versi all physiotherapy departments surveyed offered pelvic floor exercises and 93% inferential therapy.[159]

Hilton suggested the use of an algorithm to influence decision making with regard to incontinence which includes looking at predisposing factors, precipitating factors, conservative measures, urodynamic testing and, if stress incontinence is demonstrated, types of treatment.[160]

Jarvis reviewed the six common surgical procedures in over 200 studies and concluded that no single operation could be offered to all women in all situations as a first choice.[14] Only seven RCTs were identified and there is a need to have clearly defined inclusion and exclusion criteria and objective follow-up measures. The procedures with a continence rate of over 85% were the Marshall-Marchetti-Krantz operation, colposuspension, endoscopic bladder neck suspensions and bladder sling operations with only the colposuspension (87–92%) and sling operations (89–99%) having higher confidence intervals. For recurrent stress incontinence only colposuspension, endoscopic bladder neck suspension and sling operations had continence rates in excess of 80%.

There has been long debate over whether coincidental hysterectomy influences the incidence of continence when performed at the same time as the continence operation. Jarvis has pointed to the limited evidence on this that greater objective cure rates have been observed for genuine stress with hysterectomy than bladder buttress without.[14]

Detrusor instability

It is necessary to make the diagnosis urodynamically. Many drugs, including HRT, have been used to treat detrusor instability but none are universally successful and none shown to be effective. Surgical interventions range from urethral dilation followed by otis sphincterotomy to intermittent self-catheterization.[161] Habit retraining in the form of bladder drill, biofeedback, hypnotherapy and acupuncture have been successfully used and improve symptoms in up to 80% of women but not in the trial setting (CIII). Severe symptoms usually require surgery and the 'clam' ileocystoplasty is amongst the more effective procedures[162] but side-effects are quite significant. Combined stress and detrusor incontinence is probably best treated with initial medical methods and followed by surgery.[163]

Utero-vaginal prolapse

The nature of the intervention depends on the presenting symptoms which include 'something coming down', urinary incontinence, discharge and bleeding. If urinary symptoms are present appropriate investigations should be undertaken.

Non-surgical therapies include HRT for mild degrees of prolapse, ring pessaries and pelvic floor exercises. There is no trial evidence of effectiveness.

The type of surgical operation depends on the degree of prolapse and associated symptoms but is commonly a variation on a vaginal hysterectomy and repair of the pelvic floor. Recurrence rates of up to 25% are quoted (BIII).[48]

Menstrual disorders

Diagnosis

The diagnosis of menstrual abnormalities and postmenopausal bleeding requires a structured history and examination, along with a scheme for investigations in order that the following broad categories of disorders can be distinguished:

- young women with oligomenorrhoea
- post-contraceptive pill amenorrhoea
- polycystic ovarian syndrome
- diseases of the hypothalamic pituitary ovarian axis
- endometrial cancer or changes associated with mucosal atrophy in postmenopausal women.

Most women under the age of 40 with menstrual problems present with heavy frequent periods and most suffer from dysfunctional uterine bleeding, with no gross pelvic disease found on examination or investigation. Endometrial hyperplasia and adenocarcinoma of the endometrium are rare in this age group.

Diagnostic techniques

Dilatation and curettage is a diagnostic test for endometrial pathology but its sensitivity under the age of 40 has been repeatedly questioned[164] and should be replaced by other methods of endometrial sampling in the main[116] but their effectiveness has not been compared with D&C. The newer diagnostic methods have generally been considered to be of higher patient acceptance. Dilatation and curettage is an important operating theatre resource utilizer.

Ample evidence now exists that D&C will not reliably detect submucous fibroids and hysteroscopy is currently the diagnostic method of choice (AII-2).[165] The RCOG has indicated that in women under the age of 40 it is unlikely that D&C will detect gross pelvic disease and advocates the use of hysteroscopy.[23] The vabra aspirator is more sensitive than the pipelle.[166] The pipelle and Novak curette are alternatives but may be less effective in detecting abnormality because less surface area is sampled. The hysteroscope visualizes the endometrium and is not only useful in diagnosis but also for treatment such as removal of polyps, resection of endometrium and submucous fibroid resection (BIII). De Jong *et al.* reported that outpatient hysteroscopy considerably reduces the need for hospital admission and can provide early investigation of a spectrum of gynaecological disorders.[167] However no randomized controlled trials have been carried out to compare endometrial sampling with D&C.

The diagnosis of fibroids is either made clinically on examination, with or without ultrasound imaging to differentiate uterine enlargement from other pelvic pathology. Scanning is estimated to have a sensitivity of 80%.[168] Further diagnostic procedures are rarely indicated but include laparoscopy or laparotomy.

Treatment

The effectiveness of reassurance and counselling in appropriate women is unknown.[115] The management of menstrual disorders is complicated by a variety of decisions based on age, reproductive status and severity of symptoms. Medical management aims to reduce the psychological sequelae of a hysterectomy but may not effectively control the symptoms. About 50% of women referred with perceived menorrhagia are depressed or anxious and might benefit from psychiatric treatment or counselling rather than gynaecological management.[169]

The Effective Health Care report details the trial evidence for the management of menorrhagia.[115] There were 31 RCTs of drug therapies which included objective measurement of menstrual loss and three randomized controlled trials of surgery, comparing hysterectomy with MAS techniques.

The general problems with the drug trials are:

- inconsistency of entry criteria
- inconsistency of reporting side-effects
- comparison of different doses in different trials
- poor baseline pre-treatment observations
- short length of follow-up
- inappropriate analysis of blood loss.

In general the evidence is only suggestive because insufficient RCTs directly compare the top ranking drugs. The costs of medical treatments vary from several pounds for the oral contraceptive to £25 for danazol for a five-cycle treatment with five days of bleeding.[170] Other drugs include non-steroidal anti-inflammatory drugs, anti-fibrinolytics and ethamyslate.

There are several effective treatments for menorrhagia, though there is no evidence for the effectiveness of the most commonly prescribed agents – progestogens, such as norethisterone.[171] A number of trials have shown only a 20% reduction in blood loss for menorrhagia of progestogens and their use as first-line agents should be questioned (AI).[172] There is objective evidence of efficacy of the combined oral contraceptive[173] and prostaglandin inhibitors[174] even in the presence of an IUCD[175] but not fibroids and anti-fibrinolytic agents[176] which may also be effective in cases of menorrhagia induced by IUCDs.[177] All these agents reduce menstrual loss by an average of 50%. The evidence suggests that tranexamic acid is the most effective and acceptable of the currently available drug treatments and mefenamic acid also appears effective (AI).[115]

Danazol and luteinizing hormone releasing hormone (LHRH) agonists may be even more effective and produce amenorrhoea but side-effects preclude their prolonged use (AI).[172,178] The newer agent gestrinone may prove to be better tolerated but be equally effective (AI)[179] even to the extent of reducing the size of fibroids.[180]

There is evidence that the hormone releasing intrauterine systems are effective but these are not yet licensed for use in the UK (AI).[115] This may well have the effect of moving more care to the community although currently they are not readily available for contraception.

The management of menorrhagia associated with fibroids with progesterone or prostaglandin synthetase inhibitors or oral contraceptives is not established. Recently analogues of LHRH have been used to suppress ovarian function and have objectively reduced the size of fibroids and relieved menstrual symptomatology in the short term[181] and probably represent an alternative to surgery for women with medical complications to surgery and for symptomatic women perimenopausally, although further trials are required

Surgery

Surgery includes myomectomy, abdominally or hysteroscopic resection[182] especially in younger women wishing to retain fertility or hysterectomy or endometrial ablation if the family is complete. About two-thirds of hysterectomies are performed for menorrhagia (BIII).

Preoperative gonadotrophin hormone releasing hormone (GnRh) has been shown in the trial setting to reduce peroperative blood loss and operative time.[183,184]

Hysterectomy

Hysterectomy has a morbidity rate as high as 43% of procedures[185] and a mortality rate of six per 10 000.[186] Hysterectomy has been associated with adverse psychological and sexual sequelae but the case for a specific post-hysterectomy syndrome is not proven.[187] Whilst most psychiatric and sexual problems after hysterectomy occur in women with pre-existing problems some new cases develop and there is a need to assess women's emotional as well as physical response to surgery and provide effective information.

Clarke et al. looked at the satisfaction with length of stay (LOS) after hysterectomy and indicated that shorter LOS did not reduce substantially the benefits of hysterectomy compared with longer LOS (more than six days), although there were cost savings of £155 a day in the short LOS group.[188] However a high proportion of women in this group identified that their LOS was too short. The longer LOS group also had better access to community services.

McKee and Wilson reporting the conclusions of a Royal Society of Medicine meeting on hysterectomy, indicated the following issues required consideration in purchaser/provider discussions:[189]

- lack of assessment of longer term outcomes after hysterectomy
- limited understanding of the means of assisting patient choice.

Coulter reported that two-thirds of women had no preference for the type of treatment. She suggested GPs should assess the symptom severity, quality of life and preference for treatment.

Alternatives to total abdominal hysterectomy

An abdominal hysterectomy takes 45–60 minutes to perform and women may need to remain in hospital for up to seven days with 9–11 weeks convalescence.[41,190]

Endometrial ablation can be performed by transcervical resection of the endometrium (TCRE), coagulation with a rollerball electrode, laser ablation or radiofrequency-induced thermal ablation. With laser ablation most patients are discharged after an overnight stay in hospital and return to full activities within ten days.[191] Rollerball coagulation takes about 25 minutes and most patients return to full activity within one week, with 30–40% of women becoming amenorrhoeic and 55–60% having reduced menstrual flows which is similar to the results of laser ablation and radiofrequency-induced thermal ablation.[191–193]

Dwyer *et al.* demonstrated reduced morbidity with TCRE compared with TAH (AI) with a follow-up period of four months at which point there was a 10% failure rate with TCRE. This trial had a 46% morbidity rate with TAH and 25% psychiatric morbidity rate which is similar to previous studies. There was less satisfaction with TCRE than TAH, although satisfaction levels were high (85% TCRE, 94% TAH). Sculpher *et al.* analysing the same trial data concluded that up to four months post-operation TCRE had a cost advantage over abdominal hysterectomy in terms of health service resource costs.[15] However given the fact that a group of women required retreatment due to resection failure and that follow-up was short the long-term cost and benefits of endometrial resection need to be evaluated before widespread diffusion is justified. The cost of TCRE was estimated at £560 (range £420–£1691) versus TAH at £1060 (range £826–£2278). These costings took no account of time off work which was four to five times longer after hysterectomy than TCRE. In another trial Gannon *et al.* concluded that for women with menorrhagia who have no pelvic pathology TCRE is a useful alternative to abdominal hysterectomy, with many short-term benefits (AI).[189] These studies did not compare TCRE with vaginal hysterectomy.

Pinion *et al.* compared TAH, TCRE and endometrial laser ablation in a trial of 204 women with DUB.[194] Hysteroscopic endometrial ablation was superior in terms of operative complications and post-operative recovery. Satisfaction after hysterectomy was significantly higher but between 70% and 90% of the women were satisfied with the outcome of hysteroscopic surgery. The hysteroscopic procedures were significantly shorter and lengths of stay shorter (7.5 days TAH, 2.5 days hysteroscopic) (AI). In a non-randomized study Magos *et al.* followed-up TCRE patients for up to 2.5 years.[195] Results were best in women aged over 35 years and 4% underwent hysterectomy at a later date and menstrual symptoms were improved in over 90% of patients (AII-2).

Transcervical resection of the endometrium requires extensive training.[196]

Laparoscopically assisted vaginal hysterectomy

An argument for performing oophorectomy at the time of hysterectomy has been put forward to prevent the occurrence of subsequent ovarian pathology, although this is debated vigorously and the issue of consent is crucial.[46] To reduce the morbidity and use of resources associated with TAH a laparoscopically assisted vaginal hysterectomy may allow a vaginal hysterectomy to be performed with removal of the ovaries laparoscopically. Hunter *et al.* reviewing the procedure undertaken on a case series concluded that LAVH can be successful in most women selected for the procedure and there appears to be rapid return to normal activities and work (CII-2).[197] Boike *et al.* reviewing the literature concluded that despite the reduced length of stay LAVH was more expensive but was a useful technique for converting some TAHs into vaginal procedures if adnexal procedures were indicated.[198] Raju and Auld in a trial of 80 women with uterine size of less than 14 weeks demonstrated reduced lengths of stay and subsequent costs with similar morbidity rates in LAVH patients.[16] The debate as to whether to perform a vaginal hysterectomy or LAVH is ongoing and depends on the evidence of effectiveness of prophylactic oophorectomy (BI). Summit *et al.* in the US compared LAVH with vaginal hysterectomy in an outpatient setting and concluded that other than LAVH being more expensive than simple vaginal hysterectomy the outcomes were comparable but the number of women in the trial was only 56 (BI).[199]

Stovall *et al.* have shown outpatient vaginal hysterectomy to be a safe and acceptable method of treatment for selected patients in an uncontrolled study of 35 patients (BII-2).[200] Clinch[201] described the reduction in length of stay in Belfast after vaginal hysterectomy from 6.6 days in 1986 to 3.4 in 1992, confirming the report of others[200] that early discharge is possible. However Clinch eluded to the problems in inner cities of return to hospital for post-operative complications.[201]

There are no trials comparing surgery with medical management for menorrhagia.

Pelvic pain

A Lancet editorial[17] indicated insufficient evidence of the effectiveness of therapies to enable guidelines for the management of pelvic pain to be established. In a single blind placebo controlled trial Reginald *et al.* showed that acute attacks of pelvic pain can be relieved by the intravenous administration of dihydroergotamine, which has been shown venographically to relieve congestion (BI).[50] Psychotherapy is said to be an important part of therapy. Farquar *et al.* showed in a double blind RCT that medroxyprogesterone with psychotherapy and pain counselling was superior to placebo (AI).[202] Pelvic pain associated with benign ovarian pathology such as torsion or haemorrhage into a cyst is effectively managed by surgery which incudes laparoscopy or laparotomy.

Premenstrual syndrome

The most effective therapy is abolition of the ovarian cycle by drugs or surgery but is only appropriate in severe cases and can be affected by the oral contraceptive, continuous progesterone, oestradiol patches and implants and gonadotrophin releasing hormone analogues. Treatment of women with moderate symptoms has not been properly evaluated in trials until recently . The use of stress management, relaxation techniques, exercise and dietary change including oil of evening primrose oil supplementation although often helping women with mild symptoms has not been shown to be effective in trials.[18] Neither has the use of progestogens or progesterone.

Ectopic pregnancy

Vaginal or abdominal ultrasound can exclude the possibility of an ectopic pregnancy by confirming an intrauterine pregnancy on the grounds that a combination of both intra- and extra-uterine pregnancies is extremely rare (1 per 30 000 pregnancies). Human chorionic gonadotrophin (HCG) estimation remains the primary biochemical diagnostic test used in the differential diagnosis of abdominal pain in women of reproductive age. The use of laparoscopy provides a positive diagnosis in more than 90% of cases and a falsely negative diagnosis in 3–4% of cases which tend to be early in pregnancy.[203] The confidential enquiry into maternal deaths[204] highlights the potential for a poor outcome if management is suboptimal, with 14 out of 19 cases during the period 1988–90 having had suboptimal care (AIII).

Magos *et al.*[24] suggested that most gynaecological emergencies including ectopic pregnancy that have traditionally been managed by laparotomy can be treated effectively by laparoscopy (BII-2).[205] Apart from the obvious advantage of avoiding large scars the patient faces less discomfort, reduced morbidity, a shorter stay in hospital and an earlier return to normal activities (DII-2).[24,206] Brumsted *et al.* compared laparoscopy and laparotomy for ectopic pregnancy and showed that post-operative analgesia requirements were reduced with laparoscopy.[207] Poorly controlled or uncontrolled series to assess the effectiveness of laparoscopic removal of the ectopic remain the order of the day and Grimes in a review of endoscopic management of ectopic pregnancy concluded that the quality of evidence was less than ideal but there was fair evidence to recommend that operative laparoscopy be used in some ectopic pregnancies (BII-2).[19]

Early pregnancy loss

Recurrent miscarriage

When assessing the efficacy of treatments for recurrent miscarriage it must be remembered that about 60% of these women will be successful in their next pregnancy without intervention.

Meta-analyses have been conducted which used multiple endpoints but Goldstein *et al.* showed no effect of progestational agents on 'normal' outcome (rather than a decrease of miscarriage alone) of high-risk pregnancies.[208] Daya *et al.* in another meta-analysis, found progesterone in early pregnancy useful but indicated that there is a need for a trial of women with biochemical evidence of luteal phase progesterone deficiency (BI).[209]

Cervical cerclage has not been shown to be effective for recurrent miscarriage.[210]

Miscarriage

Evacuation of the retained products of conception (ERPC) is an acceptable management to reduce blood loss and infection which currently accounts for about three-quarters of emergency gynaecological operations in the UK (AII-2).[211]

Pilot studies of medical abortion using the antiprogesterone Mifepristone and the new synthetic prostaglandins indicate these to be safe and effective methods of evacuating the uterus (AI).[20,212,213] These data would indicate the potential for decreasing surgical workload along with the associated surgical morbidity and releasing surgical beds. Medical abortion has been shown to be a satisfactory alternative to surgical vacuum extraction in the trial setting of women undergoing legal induced abortion (AI).[212] Both procedures were highly acceptable to women with preferences but over 50 days gestation the choice for surgical aspiration was greater. There will be women who require surgical evacuation for heavy bleeding and in some women prostaglandins are contraindicated.[214] There is no evidence that ERPC is effective when ultrasound indicates the uterine cavity is empty of retained products.

Current common practice is for admission through A and E to a gynaecology ward and/or straight to the operating theatre with a return to the ward prior to discharge. The concept of an early pregnancy assessment unit with direct access from primary care to diagnostic testing facilities such as pregnancy testing service, ultrasound and counselling services has been employed. These units reduce the need for out of hours operating but have not been formally evaluated (BIII).[215] (D Hamilton-Fairley, personal communication, 1994.)

Gilling-Smith *et al.* have shown that the use of management guidelines and the provision of advisory leaflets to patients on discharge significantly enhances the service provided to women with such bleeding both by improved diagnostic accuracy and by reducing the numbers of unnecessary admissions or referrals.[216]

Genital tract cancer – secondary prevention

Cervix

Premalignant changes in the cervical epithelium may be detected by cytology and the cervical smear meets many of the criteria of an effective screening modality but a randomized controlled trial of cervical screening has not been undertaken (AII-2). The fact that the natural history of preinvasive lesions is not known is the major drawback. The test is cheap and simple. The British Columbia cohort study estimated the sensitivity to be 78%, specificity 96% with a positive predictive value of 25%.[217] The disease is readily diagnosed histologically and there is successful treatment for early stage disease. The most persuasive evidence that screening for squamous cell cancer of the cervix is effective comes from comparison of the trends in incidence and mortality in populations which introduced mass screening with different intensities at different times. Since the mid 1960s mortality has declined in most developed countries but especially in those that have a highly developed screening programme for carcinoma of the cervix.[218] Mortality has declined to a lesser extent in countries where only a proportion of the population is screened formally, most women having a smear taken when they visit their doctor for another reason. As a randomized controlled trial of the effect of screening for cervical cancer on mortality was never undertaken it is impossible to decide whether the decline in mortality is due solely to the introduction of screening or due to improvements in socioeconomic status, changes in sexual habit or an increase in the hysterectomy rate. Macgregor *et al.* suggested that screening has been effective in reducing the incidence of and mortality from cervical cancer in North East Scotland as the incidence had fallen mainly in the well-screened age group of 40–69 years (AII-2 in Scotland).[219]

Follow-up of abnormal smears and implementation of treatment (fail-safe protocols)

Mild and moderate dyskaryosis will be identified in 1–2% of women screened and of these around 30% will have CIN III which was underestimated by the smear. The proportion of smears classified as borderline or mildly dyskaryotic may represent 4–5% of all smears. Because of the paucity of information available to determine unequivocally what the optimal management policy for mild and moderate dyskaryosis is the Aberdeen Birthright Project was set up to evaluate the safety and effectiveness of a cytology-based approach to the management of these degrees of abnormality.

The natural history of CIN I (mild dysplasia) remains unclear and the Europe Against Cancer Programme suggested each case needs to be decided on an individual basis.[220] Usually a repeat smear is recommended within six months. Alternatively two to three consecutive negative smears should be obtained within 12–18 months before the woman may be returned to routine screening. If a district policy is to simply observe CIN I then the local circumstances must be taken into consideration, including the undercall rate and the patient default rate. Until recently there has been no justification for managing mild dyskaryosis by immediate colposcopy, although a survey by the British Society of Colposcopy and Cervical Pathology found that half the respondents considered that a single mildly dyskaryotic smear should be referred for colposcopy.[221] Johnson *et al.* using decision analysis modelling estimated that repeating a smear after a mildly dyskaryotic report is almost as effective as an immediate refferal to a colposcopy unit.[222] However a conservative policy is not financially cheaper; an average of six additional smears are required to save each colposcopy referral.

Anxiety levels are high in women attending colposcopy clinics and information provision can allay womens' fears, although specific counselling techniques have not been shown to reduce anxiety any more than information provision alone.[223] (CDA Wolfe, personal communication, 1996.)

Over 90% of colposcopies take place in gynaecology departments. The role of colposcopy in GUM clinics needs to be researched[224] although reports have demonstrated that such clinics are feasible.[225] Advice from the NHS Executive to the Royal College of Obstetricians and Gynaecologists[226] on GP involvement in colposcopy indicates that training to a clinical assistant level is required and proper equipment and nursing back up is essential. Evidence must be available to demonstrate a particular GP will perform sufficient procedures to maintain professional expertise.

The International Agency for Research into Cancer study of screening histories comparing women who developed invasive cervical cancer with those that did not demonstrated that the relative protection against cervical cancer in women with two or more previously negative smears participating in centrally organized screening programmes is 15-fold in first year, 12-fold in second and eight-fold in the third year, indicating that screening is effective if coverage is high (AII-2).[227] Centrally organized programmes were more effective than uncoordinated screening. Case-control studies have illustrated similar relative protection for those who have had a smear less than three years previously.[228,229]

Cervical intraepithelial neoplasia is arbitrarily classified as CIN I, II or III but many pathologists consider it a continuum from mild at one end to undifferentiated at the other. There is general agreement that high grade (CIN III) lesions should be treated (AII-2) but the natural history and consequently management of lesser degrees of abnormality remains somewhat unclear. The NHS cervical screening programme does not recommend immediate colposcopy for CIN I. The results of the Aberdeen Birthright study conclude that cytological surveillance, although safe, is not an efficient strategy for managing women with mildly abnormal smears, although a detailed cost-effectiveness analysis has not been presented.[230] They suggest women with any degree of dyskaryosis in a smear should be referred for colposcopy as only one in four women with mild dyskariosis reverted to normal over the two-year study period. The other important finding of the Aberdeen study was that one-third of women with CIN III had an index smear showing mild dyskariosis and that one in eight women defaulted from follow-up. Routine colposcopy would lead to 30% more referrals but would reduce cytological surveillance. The remaining potential disadvantage of immediate referral is the risk of overtreatment.[231] Although large-loop excision of the transformation zone is safe and effective (AI)[232] unnecessary treatment should be avoided. Without data from other prospective studies we must rely on cross-sectional and retrospective studies. All large studies have suggested that cytological surveillance is safe both individually and at a poulation level.[233,234] The smears of up to half the women will return to normal without treatment. The semi-quantitative polymerase chain reaction may allow a distinction between high and low grade disease in women with mild cytological abnormalities but needs large population-based studies.[235]

There is currently no routine clinical role for cervicography in either primary cervical screening or in the further assessment of patients with abnormal cytology. Although there may be a role for cervicography in the surveillance of patients with mild dyskaryosis or borderline changes to reduce the frequency of referral for formal colposcopy this requires further evaluation.[28,236]

There is similarly no international agreement on the management of CIN II or III (moderate and severe dysplasia and carcinoma *in situ*) which constitute 1.5–2% of all smears. Colposcopy is indicated with biopsy of abnormal areas and treatment if CIN II or more is diagnosed.

CIN II or III can be treated either by local destructive therapy or conization of the cervix. Local treatment may be cryotherapy, heat coagulation, laser coagulation or loop excision. Conization may be by cold knife conization, electric cautery or laser. It is generally agreed that the method of treatment is not considered to be of particular importance with regard to outcome, provided the pathologist receives some material for examination.[28] The mode of treatment may have relevance when deciding service provision options. Large-loop excision of the transformation zone (LLETZ) has enabled the colposcopist to make a diagnosis and treatment at just one outpatient visit without the need for pre-treatment cervical biopsy (AI).[232,237] There has been some concern over the pathological interpretation of the margins of such a procedure.[238] A controlled trial of LLETZ versus carbon dioxide laser vapourization showed reduced operative time, post-operative haemorrhage and discomfort in the LLETZ group. There was no significant difference in CIN recurrence rates. There are reduced capital outlays for LLETZ treatment.[239] A randomized controlled trial concluded that outpatient loop diathermy excision is an equally effective, quicker, safer and more reliable excisional technique than laser excisional conistion (AI).[240]

Woodman *et al.* undertook a trial of women with human papilloma virus infection occurring alone or in association with CIN I or II.[241] Patients were randomized to carbon dioxide laser or nothing. They reported the short-term efficacy of laser but cautioned that the substantial rate of spontaneous regression (26% (CI 19–33)) within one year suggests that intervention is frequently unnecessary, although there was no long-term follow-up in this study, as in Aberdeen.

Close follow-up by repeat smear is essential after treatment for up to three years. Colposcopy is not essential but may enhance detection of persistent disease. Residual disease is detected in between 5–15% of treated women, depending on the technique used and the grade of CIN treated. The risk of new disease developing is between 2–5% and the risk of invasive cancer in the order of 0.2%.[242]

Other sites

Recent studies on self-selected women using transabdominal and transvaginal ultrasound, CA 125 and doppler ultrasound[58,60,243] do not provide evidence that screening the general population for ovarian cancer with the present state of knowledge and available technology is useful or cost-effective. Before implementing a population-based screening programme the acceptability and feasibility of such a service, along with evidence of the effectiveness of such a test on reducing the incidence and mortality from these conditions are required. Bourne *et al.* screening self-selected women with a family history (one or more first-degree relatives) of ovarian cancer had a false-positive rate of 5.2% and a predictive value of a positive screen result of 7.7%.[244] The odds against finding primary ovarian cancer were 12 to one. A register for families with ovarian cancer in two or more relatives has been established by the UKCCC. No evidence exists that those families with predisposition to BRCAI locus on chromosome 17q would benefit from screening although screening of affected relatives in multiple case families aged 25–70 should be performed which would only involve very few scans. Bourne *et al.* suggested that there is a potential for transvaginal pulsed doppler ultrasonography, particularly with colour flow imaging, in the detection of endometrial cancers.[59]

There is no trial evidence to support population screening for these diseases. A feasibility study of a randomized controlled trial of ovarian cancer screening among women attending a breast screening centre in Reading, UK showed an uptake of 82% of eligible women.[245] The results indicated that the expected odds of being affected given a positive result in the general population would be about 1 : 12. A full RCT of ovarian cancer screening with mortality as the end point is needed to assess this and a multicentre European trial is currently underway and in a second feasibility study in Copenhagen, Denmark, not linked to the breast screening programme, the uptake was 64% with abnormalities detected in 12% and a false-positive laparotomy rate of 2%. Scanning of high-risk women is more feasible but the effect on survival has not yet been established.

Genital tract cancer

In general gynaecological oncology clinical research has been conducted in uncontrolled, non-randomized studies, with short follow-up periods, although more recently efforts have been made to produce overviews of treatment regimens with the planning of large multicentre trials. As there are few data based on randomized controlled trials evidence from special advisory groups and review articles form the basis of these recommendations (BIII).

Staging of the disease is central to appropriate management. The majority of staging procedures are low cost such as full blood count, urea and electrolytes, chest X-ray and others of intermediate cost such as cystoscopy, barium enema, intravenous pyelogram, CT scan and possibly MRI scans.

Ovarian cancer

The management of ovarian cancer was the subject of review by a SMAC panel (III).[246]

Early symptoms are vague and diagnosis can only be confirmed by a staging laparotomy by a consultant gynaecologist with full staging procedures included in the operation. Finn *et al.* indicated that only 30% of tumours were adequately staged.[247] Mayer *et al.*[248] and Eisenkop *et al.*[249] suggest that patients staged and treated by a trained gynaecological oncologist in the US have increased survival compared with those managed by a non-specialist but control for other factors associated with oncological care was not considered.

The standard surgical procedure for the disease is total abdominal hysterectomy, bilateral salpingo-oophorectomy and omentectomy along with debulking of the tumour (BIII). Early stage disease (IA and IB) in which the tumour is well differentiated and removed completely requires no adjuvant therapy but if the tumour is greater than stage I or poorly differentiated, chemotherapy may be beneficial. Residual disease after surgery also responds to chemotherapy, particularly using platinum and its analogues, especially carboplatin but quality of life can be a major problem (AI). There are no gynaecology-specific quality of life measures to assess this aspect of therapy. Palliation is a major aspect of care.

Germ cell tumours in the younger age group respond to specialist chemotherapy with tumour marker control and should be treated in centres specializing in this field. Borderline tumours are another special group for which referral to a specialist unit is recommended. As 90% of ovarian tumours present with disease that might benefit from chemotherapy it is important to have patients entered into randomized controlled trials. Those patients who are curable by surgery and who do not require further adjuvant therapy have not been clearly defined. The United Kingdom Coordinating Committee on Cancer Research is currently co-ordinating trials of adjuvant therapy. The MRC gynaecological cancer working party[250] in its overview of available data on adjuvant therapy suggest trials of at least 700 patients will be required. The Advanced Ovarian Trialists Group[251] undertook an extensive meta-analysis which was inconclusive but suggested that survival was enhanced by immediate platinum-based therapy and that platinum in combination was better than single-agent platinum when used at the same dose (AI). Cisplatinum and carboplatin appeared equally effective. There is evidence that doxorubicin confers highly significant survival benefit compared with cyclophosphamide and cisplatin alone. There is now a large study comparing the combination of all three drugs with carboplatin alone (ICON-2) in patients with advanced disease. Incorporating paclitaxel into first line and chemotherapy improves the duration of progressive-free survival and of overall survival in women with incompletely reseded stage II and stage IV ovarian cancer.[252]

Gillis *et al.*[253] reported that data from three ovarian cancer data sets indicated better survival in teaching versus non-teaching units but what 'teaching constituted in terms of multi-disciplinary treatment' was not stated.

Grant *et al.* in a retrospective analysis of clinical histories stated that patients with ovarian cancer who are managed by a specialized gynaecology unit are more likely to have adequate initial surgery and a longer median survival time.[254]

An audit of the surgical management of ovarian cancer[255] indicated considerable variation in the management in one region with optimal cytoreduction infrequently being achieved with substantially worse five-year survival rates than in other series.

Endometrial cancer

The most common symptoms associated with endometrial cancer are irregular and postmenopausal bleeding. The use of vaginal ultrasound scanning, along with colour flow doppler studies are an increasingly used method for the exclusion of benign intrauterine pathology as less than 10% of postmenopausal bleeding is caused by endometrial cancer. If the scan is suggestive of an intrauterine pathology hysteroscopically guided endometrial biopsy, if possible under local anaesthetic, is a more sensitive diagnostic test than D&C.

The standard surgical treatment is total abdominal hysterectomy and there are claims that high energy radiation to the pelvic lymph glands reduces the recurrence rate (AII–2). The use of medroxyprogesterone acetate post-operatively is not indicated for women with disease confined to the endometrium with moderately to well differentiated tumour (AI).[256] Alternative agents such as tamoxifen have been shown to have modest activity. Women with poorly differentiated tumours or with extensive myometrial invasion should be considered for post-operative radiotherapy.

Cervical cancer

There is no uniformity in the UK in the diagnosis and management of microinvasive carcinoma of the cervix.[257] The frequency of recurrence, lymph node metastases and death is low and non-radical surgery appears to give satisfactory results (AII-2).[257] The procedures employed include cone biopsy and simple hysterectomy for women who have completed their family.

Those women with borderline 1a and 1b tumours, if fit for surgery, appear to benefit from a Wertheims hysterectomy which is essentially a hysterectomy with pelvic lymph node dissection and removal of a vaginal cuff. There is however no clear superior benefits of surgery over radiotherapy. Unfit patients and those with more advanced disease benefit from radiotherapy with or without adjuvant chemotherapy. In general until there is clinical trial evidence confirming the place of radiotherapy following surgery in node positive patients, clinicians may well continue to use it. Recurrence can be treated with chemotherapy or palliative radiotherapy. If recurrence occurs post-radiotherapy a Wertheims hysterectomy or pelvic exenteration for central recurrence could be considered. Cervical cancer is relatively resistant to chemotherapy but platinum based regimens have the greatest success with responses of 30% in patients with persistent or recurrent disease.[22]

Pelvic exenteration is used for cervix, vagina and vulval cancers and in specialist centres five-year survival rates are 50%. Although only about 6% of women treated for cervical cancer will experience a recurrence that is localized solely to the pelvis and are thus potentially curable by ultraradical surgery; few centres manage more than a handful of cases a year and cases should be referred to regional or supraregional oncology centres.[258]

7 Models of care

The needs of women for gynaecological services spans all sectors of the health service and currently there are no published evaluations of a model integrated service, or a model service specification.

This section identifies the main components that require incorporation into any strategy or service specification from patient information to the development of tertiary level services in order that an effective, efficient service is planned. The main considerations are patient information, monitoring patient satisfaction, shifts to primary care, day case surgery and MAS and guideline development for management of all level of services.

In each part consideration is given to both the content of the service and the training needs of health care professionals.

Although these models of service are based on the evidence of this assessment they are still only suggestions that require local adaptation and evaluation.

Overall gynaecological service assessment

Gynaecological services are provided in primary care and in hospital settings at secondary and tertiary levels. The involvement of gynaecology services spans primary prevention through to palliative care with a differing input from each sector in the range of activities. This assessment has examined the needs for services and the scope for shifts in service provision from the secondary to primary care sector, inpatient to day case surgery and conventional to MAS. There are no previous overall models of service from which to draw recommendations.

The overall models of care that are developed locally will be dependent on those factors analysed at a national level in this chapter and include the need for services, the current patterns of service and scope to move towards those practices identified as being both effective, cost-effective and acceptable to women. The development of these models will therefore be dependent on the ability to identify the needs (see section 10), assess current service provision (local corporate needs assessment and information) and to provide the training and resources required to deliver effective services.

A needs assessment group comprising gynaecologists, community gynaecologists, genitourinary medicine specialists, GPs, nurses, public health physicians and local users of the service, along with information and health economics support should identify the necessary information on which to base decisions on the service to be provided in both the primary and secondary care sector. This has been an approach taken in Scotland[26] which identified areas in which the service should change which included a shift to day case surgery, replacement of D&C with outpatient endometrial sampling techniques, developing urinary incontinence and gynaecological oncology services.

Components of service

Outlined in this section are the main components of service that should be considered. As with much of medicine gynaecological practice has not been developed using evidence-based medicine principles and recommendations have been made taking into account not only the often weak evidence of effectiveness but the views of practitioners and users of the service. The main components for consideration when developing models of service are listed in Box 4.

Box 4: Components to consider when developing services

- Patient information
- Monitoring patient satisfaction
- Shift to primary care
- Shift to day case and 'see and treat' surgery
- Shift to minimal access surgery
- Guidelines for management and referral by sub-category of the service including the development of tertiary level services

Information

Informing women about specific gynaecological conditions and their management, especially operative procedures and what to anticipate post-operatively, in a letter or leaflet, is necessary. These information leaflets should be co-ordinated across the levels of care, providing the same messages.

The RCOG has produced standards for communication for common surgical procedures and a series of patient leaflets on common gynaecological disorders. The Audit Committee consider communications vitally important and worthy of audit.[259]

Sensitive provision of information is considered an important component of the subfertility service and stress is reduced in those couples who feel involved in and in control of their treatment.[125]

Information regarding the prevention of lower genital tract infections and PID should be produced in conjunction with health education departments and GUM clinics and be in line with local Health of the Nation strategies.

Roberts[113] illustrated the need for more information provision for women about the menopause before its onset and about HRT.

Versi et al.[157] advocate the use of explanatory materials for women with urinary incontinence which could be developed in conjunction with the community incontinence advisors.

Many units have leaflets which discuss menstrual disturbances and their management. They provide information on the options for treatment and the effects of treatment. There are widely available books on hysterectomy for the lay public which address questions commonly asked by patients.

Gilling-Smith et al. showed that the use of advisory leaflets to patients on discharge from hospital significantly enhanced the service provided to women with miscarriage.[121]

Leaflets explaining what an abnormal smear means and how it is managed should be provided in colposcopy clinics and be written in conjunction with the local cervical cancer screening group. Information regarding cancer and palliative care should also be available and developed by the cancer centres in conjunction with services supporting women when they leave secondary care e.g. hospices and Macmillan nurses.

Monitoring patient satisfaction

In general within the NHS there are moves to monitor patient satisfaction with the service. The surveys need to have a representative sampling frame and a good response rate to be of benefit to those delivering care. The areas for questioning could include outpatient facilities, day case surgery, inpatient stay and follow up. Satisfaction surveys should be an integral part of any service or intervention evaluation.

Shift to primary care

Although there are initiatives to shift services to primary care the evidence for their cost-effectiveness is usually not available and evaluation of these shifts needs to be an integral part of contract specification. Shifts can either be to management in a community setting by community gynaecologists, often linked with reproductive health services, management by health care professionals in general practice or management by secondary care gynaecologists in primary care. The latter has become an increasing trend in districts with fundholding general practices but the evidence for their effectiveness is lacking and some consider them to be an inappropriate use of resource, few practices having enough patients to sustain outpatient clinics.

Any shift from secondary care should have the aim of providing a more co-ordinated service with reduced duplication of the process of care which currently occurs when care is split between sectors. The shift should be facilitated by the development of guidelines to increase the appropriateness of care. This assessment has estimated that for every eight women consulting in primary care only one ordinary admission is generated.

The main conditions seen in primary care are detailed in Table 4 and consist of those relating to the management of genital infection, menopause, menstrual disturbances and pelvic pain. Unfortunately routine data in secondary care outpatient clinics are not recorded and it is not clear, other than through local audits, which conditions are more likely to be referred to secondary care. The case-mix will vary from unit to unit depending on the skills in primary and secondary care settings but is broadly similar to that seen in primary care. The HES data confirm that menstrual disorders and the menopause are prevalent conditions along with non-inflammatory disorders of the cervix and utero-vaginal prolapse. The management of these conditions in primary care may reduce the need for referral to secondary care if it is effective or merely delay the need for secondary level intervention.

The conditions where a shift in service provision has scope include:

- initial management of subfertility, including endometriosis and follow-up after management in secondary care
- prevention and management of PID and lower genital tract infections
- management of the menopause
- medical management of incontinence
- initial management of menstrual disturbance
- management of chronic pelvic pain and PMS
- follow-up of abnormal smear results.

The shift of care to primary care has implications for GPs and practice nurses and until the opportunity costs of inpatient and community staff have been evaluated decisions should be deferred.[260] There are also considerable training issues to be identified for health care professionals in primary care.

Shift to day case and 'see and treat' surgery

The Audit Commission and local commissioning authorities targets for day surgery include a basket of gynaecological interventions: D&C, laparoscopy and sterilization and termination of pregnancy.

To achieve these targets dedicated day case facilities are required with skilled staff to enable the efficient use of theatre time and the appropriate support for women. Day case units need to improve management by developing an operational policy, adequate managerial control and good management information.[34]

As Morgan and Beech state the 'transferred costs' must not be overlooked when weighing up the benefits of short stay or day surgery.[123] Morgan and Beech state that the rationale for advocating a reduction in length of stay and increased use of day surgery is to increase efficiency by reducing the cost per case while maintaining quality of care.[123] Mechanisms to promote change in clinical practice styles include independent professional audit, peer review and clinical directorate involvement by clinicians. When assessing the level of resources released in hospitals from an expansion of day care, marginal costs rather than average costs are required. Day case surgery costs are typically 40–50% less, depending on the procedure, than inpatient treatment.[123] However the conclusions were based on studies in the 1970s and 25–30% may be a more realistic figure now, the majority of the difference being for the 'hotel' element.

The replacement of D&C with hysteroscopic sampling or vabra and pipelle endometrial sampling techniques provides the service with increased flexibility in that not only can the proportion of women having day care be increased but the procedures can be performed in outpatient clinics.

See and treat clinics for minor procedures have developed haphazardly but have the potential for reducing waiting times for procedures along with the concomitant reduction in anxiety for the woman. The service requires trained staff to operate the equipment along with training in resuscitation. The service could include diagnostic techniques such as colposcopy, hysteroscopy, endometrial sampling techniques and transvaginal ultrasound. Treatments could include those for cervical CIN and minor vaginal and cervical abnormalities such as cervical polypectomy.

The development of early pregnancy units have probably enabled women to be more efficiently diagnosed and treated.

Shift to minimal access surgery

It has been suggested by Royston *et al.*[261] that some form of accreditation after a recognized training scheme would go a long way towards allaying the fears of the public over MAS. Training will be costly but litigation should be reduced and the royal colleges should be responsible for maintaining standards of teaching on recognized courses, setting criteria for accreditation and supervising a national audit of all laparoscopic procedures. The RCOG report on training in gynaecological endoscopic surgery[23] indicates how the college proposes to establish a MAS training and certification committee which will formulate criteria certification for different levels of complexity of MAS which should be a prerequisite to practising in the area (Appendix V).

Subsequent to the MISTLETOE (minimally invasive surgical techniques, laser endothermal and electroresection) survey in 1993/94 by the RCOG guidelines for good practice have been reported[262] on behalf of the British Society of Gynaecological Endoscopy. These include procedures, follow-up and training issues.

Few procedures in gynaecological practice have been subject to rigorous clinical and economic evaluation and purchasers should specify that new techniques be used within an evaluative framework whether this be locally developed or as part of a multicentre trial.

Whilst MAS is not the major intervention for a particular condition the benefits to the service in terms of reduced lengths of stay will not be realized and as discussed in section 2 the benefits of MAS on reducing length of stay may not be as dramatic as claimed. The main areas where MAS has a significant role is in emergency surgery[24] and alternatives to hysterectomy.

Guidelines for management and referral for sub-categories of service

Specific models of care for the sub-categories of the service are detailed below. There should be a move towards combined, co-ordinated guidelines for the management of gynaecological conditions which should include the relevant health care professionals in secondary care along with primary care doctors, nurses and therapists. These guidelines can be audited and monitoring specified in the gynaecology contract. As outlined in the section on effectiveness the strength of evidence is often weak which does make guideline development problematic.

Subfertility

Although not specifically within the remit of the gynaecologist or the gynaecology service there is a need to reduce the prevalence of those risk factors associated with subfertility and for contracts to be placed with primary care, family planning units, gynaecology and GUM units for screening of and treatment of sexually transmitted diseases such as chlamydia which may account for up to 14% of subfertility.[263] The Health of the Nation targets should go some way to addressing this problem.[25]

The comprehensive subfertility service for a population of 100 000 will result in around 100 referrals and cost around £300 000 per year, including the additional costs for neonatal care. The total costs to the NHS, which also include administrative and accommodation overheads and the extra neonatal intensive care costs have been estimated to be just under £900 000 (1992 prices).[2]

District subfertility services should develop guidelines for referral and treatment with specialist tertiary centres in order to enhance the continuity and quality of care and to keep tight contractual control on activity and costs. Emslie *et al.* indicated through a randomized controlled trial that the receiving of guidelines led to improvements in the process of care of infertile couples within general practice.[264] This effect was enhanced when the guidelines were embedded in a structured infertility management sheet for each couple. The Royal

College of Obstetricians and Gynaecologists has also recently published guidelines for the specialist management of subfertility.[265] The document provides an overview of current practice in infertility with a statement of good practice.

Agreed protocols should be developed which include increased primary care involvement in semen analysis and mid-luteal progesterone estimations. In secondary care subfertility should have a dedicated clinic with allied facilities such as HSG, laparoscopy, semen analysis with the support of a reproductive endocrinology service. Those clinics offering donor insemination and ovulation induction require appropriate laboratory and scanning facilities.

Resources currently allocated to tubal surgery could be more efficiently used if reallocated to a more appropriate mix of tubal surgery for women with less severe disease and assisted conception for those with more severe pathologies.

Tertiary centres have a responsibility for referrals from primary and secondary care along with a role in the organizing and audit of regional services. They should offer donor insemination, ovulation induction, tubal surgery, IVF and have links with endocrine laboratories.

It is estimated there should be at least one secondary care clinic per 500 000 population and one tertiary centre per 2 million population.

Fertility services for people belonging to ethnic minorities should be based at centres which are near concentrations of ethnic populations. They should aim to meet fertility needs within the bounds of a person's culture. This service development will give specific practitioners with an interest in fertility the chance to develop a lead role in ethnic health care.[1]

Redmayne and Klein[266] discuss how IVF has become one of the few examples of explicit rationing with three of six purchasing authorities studied deciding against buying the service. The decisions reflected local factors such as the presence of local providers and the views of the public and health professionals. Purchasers should be cognizant that if services are not provided locally that access to out of district centres is feasible for couples. Bull and Lyons[267] describe how purchasing IVF services in East Sussex was developed. A district group drew up clinical policy to govern access to the service which included such factors as the couple being in a stable heterosexual relationship and having no living children and with a limitation of two cycles per couple.

Pelvic inflammatory disease and lower genital tract infection

Investments in prevention of lower genital tract sexually transmitted diseases may be the most cost-effective way to reduce eventual upper genital tract infection, including PID and subsequent tubal infertility. The Health of the Nation key area of sexually transmitted disease has targets relating to organisms relevant to PID and the *Key Area Handbook*[268] expands upon the strategies to be developed. It indicates the need for collaboration between all possible agencies involved with the at-risk population and includes GUM clinics, family planning services, primary health care teams, drug agencies, schools and other agencies, which presumably includes the gynaecology services.

Ashton *et al.* make specific recommendations for public education.[1]

Protocols for the management of acute and chronic PID should cover diagnostic serology and microbiology, diagnostic laparoscopy and appropriate antimicrobial therapy. A meta-analysis of trials of antibiotics to treat PID indicated there was a lack of uniformity among studies regarding diagnosis, care and follow-up. Pooled cure rates ranged from 75–94%. Doxycycline and metronidazole was the least effective regimen (75% cure rate). Ciprotoxalin was the cheapest.[133] Clinical treatment of acute PID is still likely to be inappropriate in many and inadequate for chlamydia in much of the remainder.

Endometriosis

It is difficult to assess the current state of service provision and hence the changes that could be suggested as endometriosis is not coded separately. Protocols should be developed between primary and secondary care sectors to enable the following to be possible:

- diagnosis is by laparoscopy, hence early referral from primary care to the secondary care sector is necessary
- treatment should be initiated by gynaecologists with re-prescription through primary care
- there is a place for follow-up of women in primary care as well as in the gynaecology department and shared protocols should be developed. These may be part of the protocol developed for the management of subfertility.

Menopause

Whether women are seen in general practice, gynaecological outpatients or a specialist menopause clinic the principles of management remain the same. Further investigation is rarely required prior to prescribing HRT. Women should be assessed about three months after commencing therapy. It is considered that the hospital clinics could not cope with the information and therapy needs of the population. These need to be given consideration of the development of menopause clinics in the community, particularly in family planning and well woman clinics.

The important elements of the service are adequacy of information and education, inclusion of the partner in decision making where appropriate and monitoring of menopausal symptoms.[267,269] Information from the Osteoporosis Society indicates that within the NHS there are nine clinics in London, all at teaching units and 23 in the rest of England, of which the majority are in teaching units. Criteria for referral to secondary care clinics should be developed and include women with an early menopause, increased risk of osteoporosis, cardiovascular disease and severe or uncontrollable symptoms. Such clinics should link with research activities such as multicentre clinical trials of therapy and basic research into the menopause.

Urinary incontinence/utero-vaginal prolapse

- **Primary care** An investigation protocol should be in place which includes history, examination, mid-stream urine analysis and the use of the pad test and frequency/volume charts.
- **Secondary care** Diagnosis should include urodynamic investigations to distinguish between stress incontinence and detrusor instability. The evidence for non-surgical interventions for stress incontinence is not strong but depending on the woman's wishes and fitness for surgery should be an available option. Colposuspension and sling operations have the best cure rates.

There should be consideration of referring complex cases and repeat operations to centres with facilities for more sophisticated investigations and with expertise and a high volume of surgery for such women.

Support from continence advisors should be available. The Scottish Needs Assessment Programme[26] estimated that five physiotherapists should be employed to develop the management of urinary incontinence for a female population of nearly 500 000. There is no conclusive evidence however that physiotherapy is effective and there are problems with the monitoring of improvement of symptoms whilst receiving therapy (see section 5).

Menstrual disorders

Guidelines for assessing menstrual disorders in primary and secondary care should be developed locally and include a structured history and estimation of haemoglobin or serum ferritin concentrations. Further endocrine investigations should be undertaken according to guidelines and completed as efficiently as is feasible. The development of guidelines for the medical management of menstrual disturbance in primary care would appear to be a priority. General practitioners should offer at least one course of effective drug therapy prior to referral for surgical treatment.[115] The cost implication in shifting prescribing habits from the use of norethisterone to tranexamic acid is estimated at 20% of the drug costs but as norethisterone is ineffective in the short term, money spent on it is wasted; in addition many women treated in this way would be referred for surgery. It is also estimated that if tranexamic acid were to replace all other drugs used there would be a net saving of at least 10% on the total drug bill for menorrhagia.[115] Drug use in primary care should be monitored to identify prescribing of relatively ineffective drugs.

Criteria for using D&C should be developed and a shift of service to hysteroscopy or other endometrial sampling techniques agreed. The increased use of day case services and see and treat clinics should be developed to enable the Audit Commission targets to be met.[34]

A shift from TAH to TCRE should be agreed. Patients undergoing such procedures as LAVH should be enrolled into trials as the evidence for their use is not established.

The Effective Health Care report[115] recommends that all options should be discussed with the woman, allowing her to make an informed choice.

Pelvic pain

Guidelines should be in place to exclude specific gynaecological conditions and non-gynaecological causes of pelvic pain.[270] Assessment should include laparoscopy. The trial evidence does not allow conclusions to be drawn on specific therapies but the need for adequate explanation and possibly counselling should be considered, particularly if hysterectomy is to be considered.

Premenstrual syndrome

Currently it is assumed that the majority of women with PMS are seen and treated in primary care. Given the current state of knowledge regarding the definition and treatment it seems to be appropriate for the majority of women. Referral to gynaecology clinics should enable the use of standardized diagnostic scales in the secondary care settings. Women should be treated following guidelines and entered into trials where appropriate.

Ectopic pregnancy and early pregnancy loss

Both in the US and UK failure of the pregnant woman with an ectopic pregnancy to seek medical attention contributes to the death rate. Protocols should be developed both in primary care, A and E and gynaecological departments for the diagnosis of ectopic pregnancy.

The ability of GPs to perform pregnancy tests to exclude the possibility of an ectopic pregnancy should be considered. All junior medical staff should be made aware of the possibility of an ectopic pregnancy in a woman of reproductive age who presents with pelvic pain or bleeding. Direct access to a diagnostic ultrasound scan is a priority which gynaecological departments should consider along with protocols for referral of women with miscarriage or possible ectopic pregnancy.

Referral to an early pregnancy assessment unit with diagnostic tests and skilled personnel appears to be efficient, although the cost-effectiveness of such a service has not been established.[214] (D Hamilton-Fairley, personal communication, 1996.)

Training of gynaecologists to perform laparoscopic surgery should be in line with RCOG recommendations for MAS training, with the aim of reducing the proportion of laparotomies performed for ectopic pregnancies (Appendix V).

Appropriate senior level anaesthetic support should be available for the resuscitation of these women.[203]

Appropriate support services should be available to advise the woman on future contraception and to cope with bereavement.

Cancer of the cervix – secondary prevention

The Royal Colleges of Pathologists, Obstetricians and Gynaecologists and General Practitioners issued guidelines for good practice when setting up cervical cancer screening programmes.[271] These have been updated by an NHS cervical screening programme working party.[27,272] The NHS Cervical Screening Programme national co-ordinating network was set up to co-ordinate and promote research, the development and co-ordination of educational and professional development for women and health care professionals, running the service and to promote measures which would improve the quality of the service and to develop information systems. A programme matrix has been developed which provides a framework to ensure a comprehensive programme is developed. Recommendations from these bodies along with salutary lessons that can be learnt from a case review of 100 cases of invasive cervical cancer[273] outline main areas the service should be concerned with of which gynaecology services are a part, particularly for the follow-up of abnormal smears, management of CIN and invasive disease. Also the Europe Against Cancer Programme has published guidelines for quality assurance in cervical cancer screening.[219]

The Health of the Nation *Key Area Handbook on Cancer*[268] provides useful checklists of the various elements of a successful screening programme and these are expanded on in this assessment (Appendix VI).

- **Defined target population** Based on accurate family health service authority (FHSA) registers which will allow a call/recall system to operate. In 1985 the Department of Health gave districts the responsibility of organizing computer management schemes in conjunction with the FHSA. In 1988 the age limits for inclusion in the system were changed to 20–64. Whilst the FHSA GP lists may be reasonably accurate in many parts of the country there are particular problems with inner cities where women with an increased risk of cervical carcinoma often reside. A study in an inner-city district has estimated that only 31% of those called for a smear by the FHSA fulfilled the criteria for being called.[274] The main reasons for not fulfilling the criteria were that the woman no longer lived at the address or that the address was incorrect, that she had had a smear in the last three years or was older than 65. Integral to the whole process of call/recall is the computerized age–sex register maintained by the FHSA which may not be of sufficiently high quality for this purpose in deprived inner-city areas with high mobility of the population. The mobile population is less likely to register with a GP and the GPs may fail to inform the FHSA of changes known to them. Recent Korner KC53[275] and KC61[102] (pathology laboratory activity) data (1991/92) indicate that the number of smears performed has increased to 4.5 million, with a response rate to screening of 48%.[275] This increase has an impact on gynaecology outpatients, colposcopy services and operating theatre utilization.
- **Screening the female population at three- to five-yearly intervals**[221] Screening takes place in the age group 20–64. The Department of Health[276] advised districts to screen women aged 20–64.

Elkind *et al.* reported that 50% of districts operated five yearly programmes, 29% three-yearly and 21% a combination of three- and five-yearly programmes.[272] The current coverage of screening is 80% in the target age group, with a considerable variation between regions from 64% in NE Thames to 88% in Trent and Wessex.[275] As 40% of deaths occur in women over the age of 65 it is necessary to put additional effort into ensuring that there is a good screening uptake by older women. There should also be no upper age limit for women who have never had a smear.

- **Personal invitation to women and health education** An invitation letter is considered fundamental to good coverage which gives the women a choice of location for the smear test. 86% of districts give this choice but only half state where these are.[272] Only 55% of districts include health leaflets routinely and very few ethnic minorities whose cultural and religious beliefs may not make the offer of screening acceptable are targeted. A randomized controlled trial has failed to show any benefit from counselling women with an abnormal smear result (CDA Wolfe, personal communication, 1996).

The importance of reducing risk factors associated with cervical cancer needs to be stressed to women. With advances in the knowledge of the disease and its aetiology, different information may be given by health care professionals in the future but at present discussion of barrier methods of contraception and the possible association of cervical cancer with heavy smoking is advisable. Education of doctors and patients is inadequate and there is a need for a sustained programme of public and professional learning aimed at ensuring that the potential benefits and requirements of an effective screening programme are appropriately understood. Education of the women at risk towards an understanding of the objectives of the programme is essential. This is clear from the high incidence of invasive cervical disease occurring in women who have never been screened.[272] Efforts must be directed to ensure that all women, including those of lower socioeconomic status, are offered screening programmes. Majeed *et al.* illustrated how routine data from FHSAs practice indicators of deprivation could explain over half the variation in cervical smear uptake rates in terms of census and FHSA data.[277] These variables may have a role in explaining variations in performance of practices and in producing adjusted measures of practice performance. Practices with a female partner had independent and significant effects on uptake rates.

- **Quality of the cervical smear test** There are two components to the false-negative rate of cervical smears. 10–15% of smears are reported as negative because either cells were not exfoliated or were not picked up by the person taking the smear.[56] This may be partly dependent on the type of spatula used to take the smear, certain designs being more appropriate in women with varying shapes of cervix. In a study comparing cytological results with colposcopic biopsy findings, Giles reported a 58% false-negative rate on cytology for small lesions (less than two quadrants of the cervix).[278] This observation is of importance as 6% of the general population have these lesions on smear.

The National Audit Office found that although laboratories were committed to the principles of external quality assessment, two of the three regions visited did not have it in place. They recommend that purchasers should specify laboratory fail-safe mechanisms in their service contracts and require regular reports on their performance.[279] Organization of training programmes, proficiency-testing and systems of quality control are needed. A uniform nomenclature for both cytology and histopathology is recommended.

- **Follow-up of abnormal smears and implementation of treatment (fail-safe protocols)** In the UK a disturbingly high proportion of women found to have abnormal smears have not been adequately investigated or treated.[280] Ellman and Chamberlain found that 13% of patients with invasive cancer were also not followed up. Elkind *et al.*[273] showed that 43% of district pathology laboratories highlight abnormal smear results for GPs and 93% of districts have fail-safe systems to ensure appropriate follow-up of abnormal smears. Every screening programme should designate an individual as responsible for its management. Protocols for the management of women with abnormal results should be drawn up. There are guidelines on fail-safe action[28] for GPs, clinics, laboratories, the FHSA and the programme manager.

Salfield and Sharp[29] have calculated the demand for colposcopy services based on:

- number of women screened
- clinical policy for the referral of women with non-negative smears

- the rate and category of non-negative smears
- clinical referrals to the service.

They estimated a demand of 1320 for diagnostic colposcopy per 100 000 women.
They then estimated demand for treatment dependent on:

- number of women having diagnostic colposcopies
- % discharged after one colposcopy assessment
- % discharged after follow-up colposcopy
- average number of attendances/woman for treatment: 156 cone biopsies, 39 inpatient laser treatments, 584 outpatient laser treatments.

If the average number of lasers/woman = 1.04 the total number of treatment sessions = 607. Demand for follow-up would be 2117.

Colposcopy services have in the main been added to existing gynaecological services and as such are not in purpose built environs. A colposcopy service should consider the following recommendations:

- adequate information provision about colposcopy and treatment prior to appointment in the clinic along with speedy communication of results and management plans
- dedicated space within the clinic for equipment and resuscitation
- a lead clinician and nurse. The clinic numbers should be high enough to maintain the skills of the staff and be in the region of 400 per year. Practitioners should have been on a colposcopy course
- a high proportion of treatments should occur as outpatients under local analgesia
- guidelines for follow-up and communication with primary care.

Genital tract cancer

Although there is no evidence from trials of gynaecological cancers the specialist reports and the expert advisory group on cancer[95] all advocate the concentration of oncology services. This would appear necessary on several counts. A critical number of cases of each type of gynaecological cancer would be referred to enable appropriate training of surgeons, radiotherapists, oncologists and nurse specialists. This quantity of work would also enable audit to occur and for patients to be routinely randomized to trials. Even within these centres there may not be the expertise to deal with the very rare tumours and the identification of supra-regional centres for referral should be in place e.g. chorionic carcinoma. Details of the expert advisory group on cancer's consultation document are outlined in Appendix VII as they will determine the model of service in the future, although local adaptations may be necessary.

The RCOG's subspecialty training committee advises on a number of subspecialties of which gynaecological oncology is one. They recommended services be concentrated at regional or sub-regional referral centres with gynaecologists, oncologists and radiotherapists working together as multi-disciplinary teams. Colorectal and urological surgical expertise should be available.

There is a need for patients to be randomized into trials and for clinicians to be aware of the trial options. Similarly the audit of a unit's gynaecological oncology performance should be undertaken. It will be necessary to specify in contracts that guidelines for gynaecological malignancy management be drawn up and audited. This has successfully been undertaken in South East Thames.[281]

8 Outcome measures

This section outlines possible areas for development of outcome indicators. There also needs to be development of proxy outcome measures in areas where the evidence of effectiveness is strong e.g. the proportion of D&Cs performed in women younger than 40 could be a marker for the management of menstrual disorders. The current outcome assessments include the following.

Subfertility, PID and lower genital tract infections

- The incidence and prevalence of sexually transmitted diseases would to some extent provide an indication of the effectiveness of preventive services. However as outlined in the section on PID, these data do not exist and routine statistics underestimate the met need and do not quantify the extent of sub-clinical PID. The use of DoH returns from GUM clinics indicates to a certain degree the need for services and the outcome of preventive strategies.[36]
- There are several outcome measures used by researchers and subfertility units but the most useful reproductive outcome for health care planners is the maternity rate, although it is rarely reported in the literature.[42] Purchasers should also take into account the characteristics of the women treated, the length of follow-up and number of treatment cycles.
- Measurement of mortality and morbidity associated with investigation and treatment for subfertility, conception and delivery should be in place, including perinatal and neonatal events (through the national Confidential Enquiry into Stillbirths and Deaths in Infancy (CESDI)).

Menopause

- The prescriptions for HRT per 1000 women aged over 50 would provide a guide to the uptake of services and the consequent benefit.
- Quality of life measures have been employed in assessing the effectiveness of HRT but require further development.[154]
- Routinely available mortality data for fractured neck of femur and cardiovascular disease are proxies for risk associated with the menopause.

Urinary incontinence/utero-vaginal prolapse

- There are problems with the subjective and objective measures used to monitor success of interventions. Subjective patient questionnaires, urethral closure pressure and the position of the bladder neck and proximal urethra within the abdominal cavity would be suitable measures at an individual patient level.

Menstrual disorders

- Menstrual disorders can result in physical, psychological and social impairment of women but surprisingly little is known about the benefits of the various treatments in terms of improved health.
- The SF-36 has been shown to be a valid and reliable measure of general health status in women with menorrhagia.[282] Ruta et al.[283] have developed a patient-administered questionnaire which is a valid,

reliable measure of health status. This tool can be used to guide selection for treatment and in the assessment of patient outcome following treatment.
- A pictorial blood loss assessment chart has been developed which holds promise of increasing the precision of assessment of the severity of menorrhagia.[284]

Ectopic pregnancy

- Ectopic pregnancy is strongly associated with PID, which in turn is related to sexually transmitted disease. The Health of the Nation targets, if achieved, will reduce the number of women at risk of ectopic pregnancy.
- The number of maternal deaths attributed to ectopic pregnancy reported to the Confidential Enquiry at a national level may provide indicators of substandard care.[204]

Genital tract cancer – secondary prevention

- Cervix: the registration of CIN at the cancer registries

Genital tract cancer

- Registration and survival rates by district are reported by stage and site through cancer registries.[104]

9 Targets

Section 7 outlines the shifts in service that are required but due to variations in the current levels of service provision it would not be sensible to set targets apart from those based on current local provision of gynaecological services. Targets could be set for the setting up of a district working party, development of guidelines for the shift of services to primary care, the use of day case surgery and MAS and the development of tertiary level services such as cancer centres. There are however specific targets that can be currently considered in various of the sub-categories of the service.

Subfertility

- Each district should have access to a designated clinical team responsible for the initial investigation of infertility and to specialist IVF or GIFT treatment at a regional or inter-regional level.
- Each district to purchase facilities, or referral of couples for artificial insemination by donor.

Pelvic inflammatory disease and lower genital tract infections

The Health of the Nation targets include several in the area of HIV/AIDS and sexual health that are relevant to PID and lower genital tract infection.[285] The targets are:

To reduce the incidence of gonorrhoea by at least 20% by 1995 (baseline 1990), as an indicator of HIV/AIDS trends. This represents a reduction from 61 new cases per 100 000 population 1990 to no more than 49.

The Faculty of Public Health Medicine have set targets for sexually transmitted diseases.[286]

- A target of 75 cases of chlamydia infection per 100 000 population aged 15–64 by 2000. It would appear from the 1992 returns that this has been achieved already.
- By the year 2000 all middle and secondary schools should, as part of a wider programme of health promotion, provide education on safer sex behaviours and on sexually transmitted diseases and the services available for their treatment.
- Health education must be appropriate to the age and culture of those being targeted and must be conducted in such a way that it does not encourage sexual activity among young adolescents who are not yet sexually active.
- By the year 2000 all health care providers diagnosing sexually transmitted disease should undertake contact tracing as a matter of routine.
- By the year 2000 all physicians and other relevant staff should receive appropriate training in counselling for the prevention of HIV and other sexually transmitted diseases.

Genital tract cancer

The Health of the Nation targets for cervical cancer are:

To reduce the incidence of invasive cervical cancer by at least 20% by the year 2000 (baseline 1986) from 15 per 100 000 population in 1986 to no more than 12 per 100 000. Each district to develop a screening service which has the components outlined in the models of service.

Local targets are essential as populations differ with regard to mobility and ethnic groups and have to be agreed across the sectors contributing to the service locally.

The national target will be achieved by taking the local minimum contribution based on the 20% reduction of their 1986 ICD 180 registrations.

Interim suggested targets for Health of the Nation targets are:

- 90% women aged 20–64 invited for screening
- 80% women aged 20–64 adequately screened at least five-yearly
- all districts to consider the use of the Exeter FHSA system for call/recall programmes.

10 Information

The conditions encompassed in this needs assessment are detailed in Appendix I. These include the ICD 9 codes (Appendix I) which are currently used for reporting primary and secondary care activity and remain similar in ICD 10. There have only been minor changes to the coding for ICD 10 which will only help to clarify certain diseases e.g. carcinoma *in situ* of the cervix and CIN I-III. Diagnostic related groups and health care resource groupings (Appendix I) are appended as they will in the future provide more relevant groupings for commissioning agencies; dividing disease groupings into those with and without interventions and into those requiring minor, intermediate and major levels of intervention.[287,288] The HRGs are groups of finished consultant episodes (FCEs)/cases which are expected to consume similar amounts of resource. These groups are defined on the basis of procedure and diagnoses and each group contains cases with a range of procedures and diagnoses. These are currently coded using ICD 9 and surgical OPCS4R codes. Information on the principal and secondary procedures and the primary and secondary diagnoses, together with information about age, specialty and the method of discharge, is used to assign each record to a particular HRG. The limitation of HRGs is errors in coding and a lack of detailed costing information. The HRGs for gynaecology are divided into procedure HRGs (m1–m13) and medical HRGs for episodes without procedures (m14–m31).[289] The HRG version two *National Statistics for England* contains 10.2 million records covering all NHS inpatient episodes. There are concerns about the quality of the data which are derived from HES. This assessment uses version two which is compiled using the 1993/94 financial year data.[290]

The corresponding surgical OPCS4R codes (three-digit-P-lower female genital tract, Q-upper female genital tract) are similarly enumerated (Appendix I).[291]

The only recent source of data available on the demand for gynaecological consultation is the fourth national survey of morbidity in general practice[31] which is a survey of selected practices in England and Wales. Data are collected by ICD 9 category. Appendix II details the consultation rates per 10 000 person–years at risk by ICD 9 code and the current service availability is considered in more detail in section 5.

There are no data on rates of referral to secondary care for diagnosis and treatment. The only data recorded are the hospital episode statistics (HES) which are published annually. This assessment utilizes the UK HES data for financial year 1993/94.[31] The details of HES for the gynaecology services are considered in section 5.

Unfortunately the only routinely available information in both primary and secondary care is currently by ICD which restricts the analysis in terms of resource groups. Using the routine HES data it is not possible to assess the appropriateness of the interventions as cross-tabulation of ICD and OPCS4R codes is not routinely performed. This is particularly relevant when there are no baseline data on the need for services and hence intervention rates alone are meaningless.

The HRG data are derived from HES. There are inconsistencies between the data sets such that total admissions per 100 000 females remain in doubt. The HRG data are firstly allocated to a procedure code and if admitted and no procedure undertaken allocated a medical code. Appendix III data require further analysis to determine why 16% of women were admitted to hospital without a procedure.

- The number of women admitted with cancer and pregnancy related problems without procedures is the major concern
- In the HRG 1993/94 data supplied by the case-mix office the statistics for HRG by specialty also includes some codes which are suspect: n04: other maternity events, n01: normal delivery, n09: neonatal: low dependency along with f codes which are not gynaecology specific.[290]
- There would appear to be a need to train the relevant clerical and clinical staff to code diagnoses and operations accurately and completely.
- Routine data collection of outpatient attendances by diagnosis should be considered as it is not currently possible to assess the referral patterns of gynaecological problems to secondary care and the proportion of gynaecological outpatients that are subjected to intervention.
- Routine collection of data on 'see and treat' patients should be considered and either incorporated into day case data or produced separately.

Specific concerns regarding the categories of the gynaecology service are outlined as follow.

Pelvic inflammatory disease and lower genital tract infections

- More rapid assimilation by the reporting system of national GUM clinic returns is required. The use of electronic data capture and transfer systems would speed up reporting, and make the collection and analysis of the data easier.
- Surveillance systems should be instituted for monitoring patients with STDs seen by health service providers other than GUM physicians in order that all local cases are captured.
- The current RCGP and HES categories do not allow sensible clinical groupings to be made.

Early pregnancy loss

- Data on medically managed miscarriage should be collected.

Genital tract cancer

- Cancer registration data and SMRs can be obtained from cancer registries and are published by OPCS annually. The accuracy of death certification may be a constraint in using this indicator as coding errors, particularly between the cervix and other parts of the uterus are known to occur.
- A future indicator of the screening service could use cancer registry data as registrations of carcinoma of the cervix become more accurate and timely. Standardized registration ratios could be used as proxies for incidence. If cancer registration data are used constraints such as the completeness and accuracy of ascertainment[292] and the length of time to publication of the data by OPCS need to be considered.

Because of the small number of events in each district or region the 95% confidence intervals of the SMR or standardized registration rates will be wide. Consequently interpretation of these data has to be cautious. The SMR for carcinoma of the cervix varies significantly between regions which may reflect differences in the risk of cervical cancer incidence and/or case fatality. Interpretation of the SMR should be in conjunction with data on risk, such as registration rates. The SMR may also be affected by effectiveness of management of abnormal smears and invasive disease in a district or region.

- The Health of the Nation *Key Area Handbook* on cancer recommends three-yearly registration rates be estimated. For carcinoma *in situ* (ICD 233.1) there is known to be variability between regions and whether this is artefactual is not known.
- Returns and annual analyses of the number of smears, number of abnormal smears are reported in the DH(KC53 and 61) data.

The Health of the Nation *Key Area Handbook* on cancer recommends the following information be prepared annually on the women aged 20–64.

- The proportions of women adequately tested in past systems, ceased from recall, with no computer record, presumed non-responders and waiting times for cytology.
- Currently the cancer registries use a generic stage for all sites. The FIGO gynaecology staging scheme should be adopted for these sites or algorithms developed to convert them accurately.

11 Research

This section outlines broad and specific areas where research is required to enable the need for gynaecology services to be estimated more accurately and the effectivess of interventions assessed in controlled trial settings. The general research themes include the following.

- The incidence and prevalence of the main sub-categories of gynaecology in the UK are unknown and no overall rates of gynaecological disease have been estimated. Such studies would enable needs assessments to be based on more certain grounds.
- With a shift of service provision to primary care being recommended centrally for certain parts of this service, evaluations of this shift and its implications on training, resources and outcome should be undertaken.
- The impact of MAS on service models and resources requires evaluation.

Obstetricians and gynaecologists have been exposed to evidence-based medicine techniques for many years, the forerunner to the Cochrane Collaboration being the National Perinatal Epidemiology Unit at Oxford, which involved clinicians in trials of a wide range of maternity issues.

- This chapter illustrates how little evidence-based medicine data are available for gynaecology and how new techniques are still introduced without formal evaluation.

Areas for research for the various sub-categories of the service are outlined.

Subfertility, PID and lower genital tract infections

- Further detailed epidemiological studies are required to assess the feasibility of preventive strategies to reduce the prevalence of sexually transmitted diseases. This could include defining more precisely the prevalence of PID using relatively cheap, insensitive but specific tests.[293] The evaluation of screening programmes to detect PID should be considered in the UK.
- The development of a vaccine for chlamydia is required.[294]
- The assessment of the prognostic value and cost-effectiveness of different diagnostic techniques is required along with the development of protocols for their use.
- The extent of infertility and fertility problems in the general population requires estimation. Gunnell and Ewing[295] demonstrate how a postal questionnaire can be used to inform purchasing needs for subfertility. However they surveyed women only between the ages of 36–50. There is a need for well designed randomized controlled trials to evaluate the effectiveness of the many medical treatments for different causes of subfertility, particularly for endometriosis.

Endometriosis

- Research into the aetiology and natural history of endometriosis is required. Dose response studies, not only for the new GnRH agonists but also for danazol are necessary.

Menopause

- The influence of ethnicity, diet, physical exercise and smoking on the hormonal status of the menopause require study.
- Substantial RCTs of postmenopausal HRT should be set up, as most of the recommendations to date have been made from observational studies and it is possible that the reported benefits are attributable to lack of similarity between users and non-users. Particular aspects that could be researched include cardiovascular disease and cancer. Assessment of the most effective methods of delivery (e.g. intrauterine, transdermal) of HRT are required.

Urinary incontinence/utero-vaginal prolapse

- Evidence for the effectiveness of interventions for incontinence using multicentre trials is required.
- The aetiology and mechanisms of prolapse require elucidation.
- The effectiveness of HRT in reducing prolapse rates requires assessment.

Menstrual disorders

- Evaluation of different strategies to help women to cope with their perceived heavy periods in order to avoid unnecesary drug or surgical treatment should be undertaken.
- Further assessment of the management of menorrhagia by medical regimens is required using RCTs.
- Long-term follow-up trials of MAS for menstrual disorders should include detailed cost-effectiveness analysis.
- The outcome of repeat endometrial ablation requires investigation.
- Trials of medical treatment versus MAS procedures are required, assessing effectiveness, cost-effectiveness in terms of blood loss, quality of life and patient acceptability.
- Investigation into whether women prefer surgical or medical treatment, or resultant complete amenorrhoea or light bleeding for menstrual disorders should be undertaken.
- Evaluation of 'see and treat' clinics for menstrual disorders should be undertaken.
- An accurate, acceptable and objective method for the routine measurement of menstrual blood loss should be developed.
- Exploration of the different mechanisms and approaches to providing information to woman on treatment options is required.

Premenstrual syndrome

Budeiri *et al.* reviewing the entry criteria and scales for measuring treatment outcomes for PMS, suggest that regulatory authorities could perhaps provide guidance to which scales would be acceptable when drugs for clinical trials for PMS are sumbitted for assessment.[52] Consensus is required given the poor performance of most current treatments of PMS.

Early pregnancy loss

- Trials of medical management versus surgical evacuation are required, including patient acceptability.
- Trials of medical management of miscarriage in primary care should be considered.
- Formal evaluation of early pregnancy assessment units is required.

Genital tract cancer – secondary prevention

Cervix

The current national priorities for health service research in the Health of the Nation *Key Area Handbook*[267] are as follow.

- Evaluation of the effectiveness of the current programme, including issues of cost-effectiveness and efficiency.
- Development of programmes/strategies to establish and monitor standards for screening.
- Evaluation of the effectiveness of different screening intervals including the extra costs of more frequent screening and building on existing estimates, to feed into policy development.
- Identify which groups of women do not come forward for screening. This information would help formulate strategies to improve uptake.
- There is a need for studies to assess the most cost-effective ways of managing abnormal smears.
- A trial to address the issues of the management of women without CIN and possibly CIN I is required.
- Evaluation of the reasons for the regional variations in carcinoma *in situ* registrations.

Other sites

- Multicentre trials of the effectiveness of screening for ovarian and endometrial cancers on survival are required before the development of screening services.

Genital tract cancer

- There will be a need to evaluate the quality of gynaecological oncology services in light of the Expert Advisory Group's suggestions. Measures to assess the co-ordinated service and the type of hospital need to be developed. Health service researchers have failed to determine what aspects of health service delivery influence the variations in survival from cancer, if indeed they do. Research aimed at assessing the quality of care and outcome should be a priority.
- The evaluation of guideline adherence in this subspecialty area of gynaecology and its effect on outcome requires investigation.
- For ovarian cancer multicentre trials of adjuvant therapy with combination therapy are required to answer the questions: which agent, at what dose (particularly with respect to platinum) and in what combination.
- Quality of life measures for gynaecological cancers should be developed which can be used for the routine, as well as research, assessment of outcome.

Appendix I Diagnostic codes

Diagnostic codes, three-digit (ICD 9) from HES data 1993/94

Malignant neoplasm of genitourinary organs:
179	Malignant neoplasm of uterus, part specified
180	Malignant neoplasm of cervix uteri
181	Malignant neoplasm of placenta
182	Malignant neoplasm of body of uterus
183	Malignant neoplasm of ovary and other uterine adnexa
184	Malignant neoplasm of other and unspecified female genital organs

Benign neoplasm:
218	Uterine leiomyoma
219	Other benign neoplasm of uterus
220	Benign neoplasm of ovary
221	Benign neoplasm of other female genital organs

Diseases of other endocrine glands:
256	Ovarian dysfunction

Inflammatory disease of female pelvic organs:
614	Inflammatory disease of ovary, fallopian tube, pelvic cellular tissue and peritoneum
615	Inflammatory diseases of uterus, except cervix
616	Inflammatory disease of cervix, vagina and vulva

Other disorders of female genital tract:
617	Endometriosis
618	Genital prolapse
619	Fistulae involving female genital tract
620	Non-inflammatory disorders of ovary, fallopian tube and broad ligament
621	Disorders of uterus, not elsewhere classified
622	Non-inflammatory disorders of cervix
623	Non-inflammatory disorders of vagina
624	Non-inflammatory disorders of vulva and perineum
625	Pain and other symptoms associated with female genital organs
626	Disorders of menstruation and other abnormal bleeding from female genital tract
627	Menopausal and postmenopausal disorders
628	Infertility, female
629	Other disorders of female genital organs

Pregnancy with abortive outcome:
630	Hydatidiform mole
631	Other abnormal product of conception
632	Missed abortion
633	Ectopic pregnancy
634	Spontaneous abortion
635	Legally induced abortion
636	Illegally induced abortion
637	Unspecified abortion
638	Failed attempted abortion
639	Complications following abortion and ectopic and molar pregnancies

Diagnostic related groups

Diseases and disorders of the female reproductive system (DRG 353–369)
Pregnancy, childbirth and the puerperium (DRGs 370–384)

Major diagnostic category 13 – Medical partitioning

Malignancy age >69 and/or cc	Yes	366
	No	367
Infection		368
Menstrual and other female reproductive system diagnoses		369

Major diagnostic category 13 – Surgical partitioning

Pelvic evisceration, radical hysterectomy and radical vulvectomy		353
Uterine and adnexal		
Ovarian and adnexal malignancy		357
Other malignancy	Yes	354
Age >69 and/or cc	No	355
Non-malignancy	Yes	358
Age >69 and/or cc	No	359
Female reproductive system, reconstructive procedures		356
Vagina, cervix and vulva procedures		360
Laparoscopy and incisional tubal interruption		361
D&C, conization and radio-implant Principle diagnosis malignancy	Yes	363
	No	364
Endoscopic tubal interruption		362
Other female reproductive system OR procedures		365

Major diagnostic category 14

Pregnancy, childbirth and puerperium (relevant codes)		
Postpartum and post-abortion – procedure		377
no procedure		376
Ectopic pregnancy		378
Threatened abortion		379

cc = complication/comorbidity

HRG text labels

HRG	HRG text lable
m01	Minor Procedures Vulva/Labia
m02	Minor Procedures Vagina/Perineum
m03	Minor Procedures Cervix/Uterus
m04	Minor Procedures Uterus/Adnexae
m05	Intermediate Procedures Vulva/Labia
m06	Intermediate Procedures Vagina/Perineum

m07	Intermediate Procedures Vagina/Uterus
m08	Intermediate Procedures Uterus/Adnexae
m09	Major Procedures Vulva/Labia
m10	Major Procedures Uterus/Perineum
m11	Major Procedures Uterus/Adnexae
m12	Complex Major Procedures Vulva/Labia
m13	Complex Major Procedures Uterus
m14	Threatened Abortion
m15	Spontaneous Abortion
m16	Ectopic Pregnancy
m17	Termination of Pregnancy
m18	Contraceptive Care/Sterilization
m19	Infertility
m20	Non-inflammatory Disease of Vulva/Vagina
m21	Inflammatory Disease of Vulva/Vagina/Cervix
m22	Non-inflammatory Disease of Cervix
m23	Ovary/Tube/Pelvic Inflammation
m24	Non-inflammatory Disease of Tube/Ovary
m25	Fibroids/Menstrual Disordes/Endometriosis
m26	Genital Prolapse
m27	Carcinoma of Uterus
m28	Carcinoma of Ovary >69 or w cc
m29	Carcinoma of Ovary <70 w/o cc
m30	Other Gynaecological Malignancy >64 or w cc
m31	Other Gynaecological Malignancy <65 w/o cc
m32	Other Gynaecological Conditions

cc = complication/comorbidity
w = with

Operation codes three-digit OPCS 4R codes

P. LOWER FEMALE GENITAL TRACT

Vulva and female perineum (P01–P13)

p01	Operations on clitoris
p03	Operations on Bartholin gland
p05	Excision of vulva
p06	Extirpation of lesion of vulva
p07	Repair of vulva
p09	Other operations on vulva
p11	Extirpation of lesion of female perineum
p13	Other operations on female perineum

Vagina (P14–P31)

p14	Incision of introitus of vagina
p15	Other operations on introitus of vagina
p17	Excision of vagina
p18	Other obliteration of vagina
p20	Extirpation of lesion of vagina
p21	Plastic operations on vagina
p22	Repair of prolapse of vagina and amputation of cervix uteri

p23	Other repair of prolapse of vagina
p24	Repair of vault of vagina
p25	Other repair of vagina
p26	Introduction of supporting pessary into vagina
p27	Exploration of vagina
p29	Other operations on vagina
p31	Operations on pouch of Douglas

Q, UPPER FEMALE GENITAL TRACT

Uterus (Q01–Q20)

Q01	Excision of cervix uteri
Q02	Destruction of lesion of cervix uteri
Q03	Biopsy of cervix uteri
Q05	Other operations on cervix uteri
Q07	Abdominal excision of uterus
Q08	Vaginal excision of uterus
Q09	Other open operations on uterus
Q10	Curettage of uterus
Q11	Other evacuation of contents of uterus
Q12	Intrauterine contraceptive device
Q13	Introduction of gamete into uterine cavity
Q14	Introduction of abortifacient into uterine cavity
Q15	Introduction of other substance into uterine cavity
Q16	Other vaginal operations on uterus
Q17	Therapeutic endoscopic operations on uterus
Q18	Diagnostic endoscopic examination of uterus
Q20	Other operations on uterus

Fallopian tube (Q22–Q41)

Q22	Bilateral excision of adnexa of uterus
Q23	Unilateral excision of adnexa of uterus
Q24	Other excision of adnexa of uterus
Q25	Partial excision of fallopian tube
Q26	Placement of prosthesis in fallopian tube
Q27	Open bilateral occlusion of fallopian tubes
Q28	Other open occlusion of fallopian tube
Q29	Open reversal of female sterilization
Q30	Other repair of fallopian tube
Q31	Incision of fallopian tube
Q32	Operations on fimbria
Q34	Other open operations on fallopian tube
Q35	Endoscopic bilateral occlusion of fallopian tubes
Q36	Other endoscopic occlusion of fallopian tube
Q37	Endoscopic reversal of female sterilization
Q38	Other therapeutic endoscopic operations on fallopian tube
Q39	Diagnostic endoscopic examination of fallopian tube
Q41	Other operations on fallopian tube

Ovary and broad ligament (Q43–Q56)

Q43	Partial excision of ovary
Q44	Open destruction of lesion of ovary
Q45	Repair of ovary
Q47	Other open operations on ovary
Q48	Oocyte recovery
Q49	Therapeutic endoscopic operations on ovary
Q50	Diagnostic endoscopic examination of ovary
Q52	Operations on broad ligament of uterus
Q54	Operations on other ligament of uterus
Q55	Other examination of female genital tract
Q56	Other operations on female genital tract

Appendix II Morbidity survey in general practice 1991/92 (MSGP4)[31]

Patients consulting and consultation rates per 10 000 female person–years at risk.

Patients consulting rates: rates of patients who consulted at least once during the year at a defined level of diagnostic detail.

Person–years at risk: the sum of the number of days each patient in a particular category was registered with a study practice during the year, divided by the number of days (365) in the year.

Consultation: each diagnosis or reason for contact recorded during a contact; for each contact one or more consultations were recorded.

Condition	ICD	Patients consulting per 10 000 person–years at risk	Consultations per 10 000 person–years at risk
Candidiasis	112	521	690
Trichomoniasis	131	6	7
Malignant neoplasm			
– Uterus, unspecified	179	1	1
– Cervix	120	3	12
– Body uterus	182	2	5
– Ovary + adnexae	183	4	14
Uterine leiomyomata	218	13	16
Other benign neoplasm uterus	219	–	1
Benign neoplasm			
– Ovary	220	1	2
– Other	221	1	1
Pelvic inflammatory disease (PID)	614–616	212	198
Endometriosis	617	11	24
Genital prolapse	618	45	71
Non-inflammatory disorders of ovary, fallopian tube and broad ligament	620	9	14
Disorders of uterus not classified elsewhere	621	5	6
Non-inflammatory disorders cervix	622	22	26
Non-inflammatory disorders vagina	623	64	78

Continued

Continued.

Condition	ICD	Patients consulting per 10 000 person–years at risk	Consultations per 10 000 person–years at risk
Non-inflammatory disorders vulva	624	5	6
Pain associated with female organs	625	278	394
Disorders of menstruation	626	449	676
Menopause/post-menopause	627	328	583
Infertility	628	31	57
Early pregnancy loss	630–639	53	69

Appendix III Hospital episode statistics: financial year 1993/94

The hospital episode statistics cover all specialties and include private patients treated in NHS hospitals. They are based on consultant episodes (a period of care under one consultant within one provider) and the clinical specialty is based on the clinical qualifications of the consultant. The definitions of bed days, episodes and admissions are described in the hospital episode statistics introduction.

Definitions of fields from hospital episode statistics data

Ordinary admissions:
A patient not admitted electively and any patient admitted electively with the expectation that they will remain in hospital for at least one night, including a patient admitted with this intention who leaves hospital for any reason without staying overnight. A patient admitted electively with the intent of not staying overnight but who does not return home as scheduled should be counted as an ordinary admission.

Day case admission:
A patient admitted electively during the course of a day with the intention of receiving care but does not require the use of a hospital bed overnight and who returns home as scheduled. If this original intention is not fulfilled and the patient stays overnight, such a patient should be counted as an ordinary admission.

Bed day episodes:
The period of time in days between start date of the episode and the end date of episode for finished episodes, or the period of time in days between the start date of episode and the end date of the current period for unfinished episodes (i.e. duration of episode). The number of bed days is based on ordinary admissions only

Elective admission:
A patient whose admission date is known in advance, thus allows arrangements to be made beforehand.

Emergency admission:
A patient admitted to hospital at short notice because of clinical need.

Mean waiting time:
This is based on valid cases only and it is calculated for any category as the total waiting times for that category divided by the corresponding number of admission episodes.

Median waiting time:
The waiting time for the middle case when all valid cases in a category are ranked by waiting time.

Number of women per 100 000 female population with gynaecological diagnoses

Diagnostic codes three–digit (ICD 9) from HES data 1993/94.

		Inpatient cases ordinary admission and day cases	Number/ 100 000 females[a]
Malignant neoplasm of genitourinary organs			
179	Malignant neoplasm of uterus, part unspecified	846	4
180	Malignant neoplasm of cervix uteri	8769	344
181	Malignant neoplasm of placenta	376	4
182	Malignant neoplasm of body of uterus	6304	27
183	Malignant neoplasm of ovary and other uterine adnexa	20 010	86
184	Malignant neoplasm of other and unspecified female genital organs	2407	10
Benign neoplasm			
218	Uterine leiomyoma	25 825	111
219	Other benign neoplasm of uterus	591	3
220	Benign neoplasm of ovary	3742	16
221	Benign neoplasm of other female genital organs	625	3
Diseases of other endocrine glands			
256	Ovarian dysfunction	4016	17
Inflammatory disease of female pelvic organs			
614	Inflammatory disease of ovary, fallopian tube, pelvic cellular tissue and peritoneum	20 238	87
615	Inflammatory diseases of uterus, except cervix	1337	6
616	Inflammatory disease of cervix, vagina and vulva	15 063	65
Other disorders of female genital tract			
617	Endometriosis	14 432	62
618	Genital prolapse	31 961	137
619	Fistulae involving female genital tract	1381	6
620	Non-inflammatory disorders of ovary, fallopian tube and broad ligament	17 779	76
621	Disorders of uterus, not elsewhere classified	11 275	48
622	Non-inflammatory disorders of cervix	41 119	176
623	Non-inflammatory disorders of vagina	17 223	74
624	Non-inflammatory disorders of vulva and perineum	6302	27
625	Pain and other symptoms associated with female genital organs	39 448	170
626	Disorders of menstruation and other abnormal bleeding from female genital tract	105 812	455

Continued

Continued.	Inpatient cases ordinary admission and day cases	Number/ 100 000 females[a]
627 Menopausal and postmenopausal disorders	30 757	132
628 Infertility, female	27 099	117
629 Other disorders of female genital organs	2262	10
		1967

Pregnancy with abortive outcome

630 Hydatidiform mole	630–679	1 170 192	5031
631 Other abnormal product of conception			
632 Missed abortion			
633 Ectopic pregnancy			
634 Spontaneous abortion			
635 Legally induced abortion			
636 Illegally induced abortion			
637 Unspecified abortion			
638 Failed attempted abortion			
639 Complications following abortion and ectopic and molar pregnancies			
Total		6998	

[a] OPCS England Population projections: females aged over 15 years

HFS 1993/94 data: admissions, bed days and length of stay by diagnostic shortlist

OA – ordinary admission, DC = day case, OA+DC = inpatients, BD = bed days of ordinary admission, LOS = length of stay

Malignant neoplasm of cervix uteri (diagnostic shortlist 120)

OA		7970
DC		790
OA+DC	=	8769
BD		65 367
mean LOS	=	8.2
median LOS	=	4

Malignant neoplasm of uterus, other and unspecified (diagnostic shortlist 122)

OA		6613
DC		537
OA+DC	=	7150
BD		60 226
mean LOS	=	9.1
median LOS	=	6

Benign neoplasm of uterus (diagnostic shortlist 152)

OA		22 397	
DC		4019	
OA+DC	=	26 416	(98% fibroids)

BD   155 150

mean LOS   =   6.9
median LOS   =   6

Benign neoplasm of ovary (diagnostic shortlist 153)
OA   3712
DC   30
OA+DC   =   3742
BD   30 277

mean LOS   =   8.2
median LOS   =   7

Diseases of female genital organs excluding breast (diagnostic shortlist 37–370)
OA   231 653
DC   151 835
OA+DC   =   383 488
BD   981 353

Subdivisions of diseases of female genital tract

Salpingitis and oophoritis (diagnostic shortlist 371)
OA   2249
DC   356
OA+DC   =   2605
BD   13432

mean LOS   =   6
median LOS   =   6

Inflammatory diseases of pelvic cellular tissues and peritoneum (diagnostic shortlist 371)
OA   14 420
DC   3075
OA+DC   =   17 495
BD   51 723

mean LOS   =   3.6
median LOS   =   2

Inflammatory diseases of uterus, vagina and vulva (diagnostic shortlist 373)
OA   10 945
DC   5455
OA+DC   =   16 400
BD   26 744

mean LOS   =   2.4
median LOS   =   1

Uterovaginal prolapse (diagnostic shortlist 373)
OA   30 842
DC   · 1119
OA+DC   =   31 961
BD   241 826

mean LOS   =   7.8
median LOS   =   6

Menstrual disorders (diagnostic shortlist 375)

OA		45 924
DC		32 220
OA+DC	=	78 144
BD		203 407
mean LOS	=	4.4
median LOS	=	3

Infertility, female (diagnostic shortlist 628)

OA		9738
DC		17 361
OA+DC	=	27 099
BD		17 028
mean LOS	=	1.8
median LOS	=	1

Complications of pregnancy, childbirth and puerperium (diagnostic shortlist 38–41)

OA		1 079 701
DC		90 491
BD		3 284 836
mean LOS	–	1.8
median LOS	=	1

Carcinoma *in situ of cervix* (ICD 233.1)

Total 19 577

Operations by principal operation (three-digit OPCS 4R) OA and DC combined, NHS hospitals, HES, UK 1993/94

P. LOWER FEMALE GENITAL TRACT

Vulva and female perineum (P01–P13)

p01	Operations on clitoris	117
p03	Operations on Bartholin gland	5367
p05	Excision of vulva	5093
p06	Extirpation of lesion of vulva	1485
p07	Repair of vulva	180
p09	Other operations on vulva	6392
p11	Extirpation of lesion of female perineum	660
p13	Other operations on female perineum	2569

Vagina (P14–P31)

p14	Incision of introitus of vagina	304
p15	Other operations on introitus of vagina	810
p17	Excision of vagina	144
p18	Other obliteration of vagina	75
p19	Excision of band of vagina	201
p20	Extirpation of lesion of vagina	2873

p21	Plastic operations on vagina	204
p22	Repair of prolapse of vagina and amputation of cervix uteri	1308
p23	Other repair of prolapse of vagina	19 940
p24	Repair of vault of vagina	505
p25	Other repair of vagina	739
p26	Introduction of supporting pessary into vagina	848
p27	Exploration of vagina	20 538
p29	Other operations on vagina	1758
p31	Operations on pouch of Douglas	296

Q. UPPER FEMALE GENITAL TRACT

Uterus (Q01–Q20)

Q01	Excision of cervix uteri	9416
Q02	Destruction of lesion of cervix uteri	19 622
Q03	Biopsy of cervix uteri	23 031
Q05	Other operations on cervix uteri	1447
Q07	Abdominal excision of uterus	59 376
Q08	Vaginal excision of uterus	14 141
Q09	Other open operations on uterus	1507
Q10	Curettage of uterus	166 146
Q11	Other evacuation of contents of uterus	154 222
Q12	Intrauterine contraceptive device	3404
Q13	Introduction of gamete into uterine cavity	1128
Q14	Introduction of abortifacient into uterine cavity	7223
Q15	Introduction of other substance into uterine cavity	1298
Q16	Other vaginal operations on uterus	430
Q17	Therapeutic endoscopic operations on uterus	9945
Q18	Diagnostic endoscopic examination of uterus	21 853
Q20	Other operations on uterus	1166

Fallopian tube (Q22–Q41)

Q22	Bilateral excision of adnexa of uterus	2650
Q23	Unilateral excision of adnexa of uterus	8281
Q24	Other excision of adnexa of uterus	1867
Q25	Partial excision of fallopian tube	1448
Q26	Placement of prosthesis in fallopian tube	22
Q27	Open bilateral occlusion of fallopian tubes	1856
Q28	Other open occlusion of fallopian tube	136
Q29	Open reversal of female sterilization	1138
Q30	Other repair of fallopian tube	1409
Q31	Incision of fallopian tube	1085
Q32	Operations on fimbria	172
Q34	Other open operations on fallopian tube	485
Q35	Endoscopic bilateral occlusion of fallopian tubes	50 969
Q36	Other endoscopic occlusion of fallopian tube	326
Q37	Endoscopic reversal of female sterilization	433
Q38	Other therapeutic endoscopic operations on fallopian tube	1087
Q39	Diagnostic endoscopic examination of fallopian tube	7169
Q41	Other operations on fallopian tube	12 827

Ovary and broad ligament (Q43–Q56)

Q43	Partial excision of ovary	3372
Q44	Open destruction of lesion of ovary	143
Q45	Repair of ovary	158
Q47	Other open operations on ovary	752
Q48	Oocyte recovery	2039
Q49	Therapeutic endoscopic operations on ovary	3629
Q50	Diagnostic endoscopic examination of ovary	1198
Q52	Operations on broad ligament of uterus	144
Q54	Operations on other ligament of uterus	617
Q55	Other examination of female genital tract	5967
Q56	Other operations on female genital tract	53

Operations by principle operation (OPCS 4R shortlist) ordinary admissions (OA) day cases (DC) and bed days of ordinary admissions (BD), NHS Hospitals, UK, 1993/94

Principal operation shortlist

P	**Lower genital tract**	
OA	42 558	
DC	29 848	
BD	223 571	
PA	**Vulva and female perineum**	
OA	13 651	
DC	8212	
BD	43 835	
PA1	**Operations on Bartholin gland**	
OA	4359	
DC	1008	
BD	5250	
PB	**Vagina**	
OA	28 907	
DC	21 636	
BD	179 736	
PB1	**Repair of prolapse of vagina**	
OA	21 232	
DC	16	
BD	152 978	
Q	**Upper genital tract**	
OA	307 069	
DC	239 718	
BD	973 100	
QA	**Uterus**	
OA	247 541	
DC	187 814	
BD	775 486	

QA1   Operations on cervix uteri
OA   15 659
DC   37 857
BD   26 467

QA2   **Excision of uterus**
OA   73 465
DC   52
BD   527 945

QA3   **Evacuation of contents of uterus**
OA   133 920
DC   126 448
BD   171 790

QB   **Fallopian tube**
OA   48 329
DC   45 031
BD   149 341

QB1   **Excision of adnexa of uterus**
OA   12 782
DC   16
BD   80 617

QB2   **Open occlusion of fallopian tube**
OA   1789
DC   203
BD   5501

QB3   **Endoscopic occlusion of fallopian tube**
OA   19 563
DC   31 732
BD   22 284

QB4   **Other endoscopic operations on fallopian tube**
OA   4466
DC   4223
BD   8463

QC   **Ovary and broad ligament**
OA   11 199
DC   6873
BD   48 273

R   **Female genital tract associated with pregnancy, childbirth and puerperium**
OA   613 740
DC   852
BD   2 126 725

Waiting times: mean and median (days) by main diagnosis (diagnostic shortlist), NHS hospitals, 1993/94

	Waiting time	
	mean	median
Malignant neoplasm of cervix uteri	19.1	13
Malignant neoplasm of uterus and other and unspecified	20.9	14
Benign neoplasm of uterus	95.4	60
Benign neoplasm of ovary	40.4	21
Salpingitis and oophoritis	99.4	60
Inflammatory disease of pelvic cellular tissue and peritoneum	106.4	62
Inflammatory diseases of uterus, vagina and vulva	67.1	40
Utero-vaginal prolapse	146.6	105
Menstrual disorders	90.5	56
Infertility female	101.3	64
Total cases all causes including gynaecology	90.6	41

Waiting times by principal operation (OPCS4 shortlist) UK,1993/94

P. LOWER FEMALE GENITAL TRACT

	Selected codes	
	mean	median
Repair of prolapse of vagina	157.1	117
Excision of uterus	107.1	69
Evacuation of contents of uterus	33.1	11
Total	96.4	54

HRG data 1993/94 section M – female reproductive system

HRG	Label	N cases	% Chap.	% day	% Emerg.	Mean	Std day	Q1	Med	Q3	Trim Pt.	% Trim
m01	Min Pxs Vulva/Labia	1411	0.20	62.7	2.3	1.1	0.8	1	1	2	3	9.5
m02	Min Pxs Vag/Perineum	12 955	1.87	45.8	14.1	1.3	0.8	1	1	2	3	10.0
m03	Min Pxs Cerv/Uterus	42 217	6.10	86.6	1.1	1.0	1.0	0	1	2	5	2.4
m04	Min Pxs Uterus/Adnexae	257 675	37.23	49.3	28.5	1.1	0.8	1	1	1	3	3.6
m05	Inter Pxs Vulva/Labia	14 838	2.14	34.1	33.2	1.3	0.7	1	1	2	3	7.5
m06	Inter Pxs Vag/Perineum	4807	0.69	37.5	8.8	2.3	1.9	1	2	3	8	7.1
m07	Inter Pxs Cerv/Uterus	29 503	4.26	64.9	1.8	1.3	0.9	1	1	2	3	5.9
m08	Inter Pxs Uterus/Adnexae	105 256	15.21	57.3	2.4	1.1	0.8	1	1	2	3	5.8
m09	Maj Pxs Vulva/Labia	1115	0.16	23.6	7.4	12.0	10.5	2	10	18	47	4.5
m10	Maj Pxs Vag/Perineum	22 488	3.25	0.5	1.0	6.6	2.0	5	6	8	12	5.5
m11	Maj Pxs Uterus/Adnexae	86 034	12.43	1.0	12.7	6.1	1.8	5	6	7	10	6.1
m12	Comp Maj Pxs Vulva/Labia	69	0.01	0.0	2.9	22.7	9.8	15	21	32	56	2.9
m13	Comp Maj Pxs Uterus/Adnexae	532	0.08	0.2	4.1	10.2	3.4	8	10	12	20	9.0
m14	Threatened abortion	25 079	3.62	3.8	82.5	1.0	1.1	0	1	2	5	2.5
m15	Spontaneous Abortion	10 899	1.57	2.6	85.6	0.7	0.7	0	1	2	2	7.9
m16	Ectopic Pregnancy	560	0.08	0.2	93.9	1.6	1.9	0	1	2	7	3.9
m17	Termination of Pregnancy	2146	0.31	49.8	11.7	1.0	1.1	0	1	2	5	1.3
m18	Contracept Care/Steril'n	126	0.02	31.7	20.6	2.0	2.2	0	1	4	10	1.2
m19	Infertility	1250	0.18	47.8	15.3	0.5	0.6	0	0	1	2	8.3
m20	Non Infl Dis of Vulva/Vag	8033	1.16	4.5	77.6	1.0	1.1	0	1	1	5	4.3
m21	Infl Dis of Vulva/Vag/Cerv	1490	0.22	7.3	79.8	1.0	1.2	0	1	1	5	9.6
m22	Non Infl Dis of Cerv	1418	0.20	48.3	13.0	0.9	1.1	0	1	1	5	9.8
m23	Ovary/Tube/Pelvic Infl	7018	1.01	0.5	96.1	1.9	1.5	1	2	3	6	4.4
m24	Non Infl Dis of Tube/Ovary	4313	0.62	7.1	81.4	1.7	1.5	1	1	2	6	6.9
m25	Fibs/Menst Disds/End'sis	13 925	2.01	9.8	63.9	1.1	1.2	0	1	2	5	4.2
m26	Genital Prolapse	2778	0.40	15.9	11.1	2.2	2.6	0	1	3	10	7.7
m27	Carcinoma of Uterus	1230	0.18	8.9	40.5	6.7	7.0	2	4	10	29	7.3
m28	Carcinoma of Ovary >69 or w cc	4019	0.58	26.3	35.8	5.1	5.7	1	3	8	23	7.0
m29	Carcinoma of Ovary <70 w/o cc	10 288	1.49	31.7	18.0	1.6	1.4	1	1	2	6	12.2
m30	Oth Gyn Malig >64 or w cc	2201	0.32	5.6	45.2	8.9	8.7	2	6	13	34	6.6
m31	Oth Gyn Malig <65 w/o cc	3389	0.49	18.5	29.3	2.9	2.5	1	2	4	11	12.0
m32	Other Gynae Condns	13 061	1.89	16.6	64.3	1.2	1.2	0	1	2	5	4.8

Appendix IV Outlet of bladder operations in females (M51–M58) (HES, 1990/91), UK

		n	%
M51	Combined abdominal and vaginal operations to support outlet of female bladder	1516	20
M52	Abdominal operations to support outlet of female bladder	4561	61
M53	Vaginal operations to support outlet of female bladder	346	6
M55	Other operations on outlet of female bladder	96	1
M56	Therapeutic operations on outlet of female bladder	265	4
M58	Other operations on outlet of female bladder	700	9
Total		7484	

Appendix V Stratification of laparoscopic procedures by levels of training

(Royal College of Obstetricians and Gynaecologists, 1994)

LEVEL 1 DIAGNOSTIC LAPAROSCOPY

LEVEL 2 MINOR LAPAROSCOPIC PROCEDURES
Laparoscopic sterilization
Needle aspiration of simple cysts
Ovarian biopsy
Minor adhesiolysis (not involving bowel)
Ventro-suspension
Diathermy to endometriosis – Revised AFS Stage I

LEVEL 3 MORE EXTENSIVE PROCEDURES REQUIRING ADDITIONAL TRAINING
Laser/diathermy to polycystic ovaries
Laser/diathermy to endometriosis – Revised AFS Stage II and III
Linear salpingostomy and/or salpingectomy for ectopic pregnancy
Laparoscopic uterosacral nerve ablation
Salpingostomy for infertility
Salpingectomy/salpingo-oophorectomy
Adhesiolysis for moderate and severe adhesions
Adhesiolysis involving bowel laparoscopic ovarian cystectomy
Laparoscopic/laser management of endometrioma
Laparoscopically-assisted vaginal/sub-total hysterectomy (without significant associated pathology)

LEVEL 4 EXTENSIVE ENDOSCOPIC PROCEDURES REQUIRING SUBSPECIALIST OR ADVANCED/TERTIARY LEVEL ENDOSCOPIC SKILLS
Myomectomy
Laparoscopic surgery for revised AFS Stage III and IV endometriosis
Pelvic lymphadenectomy. Pelvic side-wall/ureteric dissection
Presacral neurectomy
Dissection of an obliterated Pouch of Douglas
Laparoscopic incontinence surgical procedures

LEVEL 1 DIAGNOSTIC PROCEDURES
Diagnostic hysteroscopy – plus target biopsy
Removal of simple polyps
Removal of intrauterine contraceptive device (IUD)

LEVEL 2 MINOR OPERATIVE PROCEDURES
Proximal fallopian tube cannulation
Minor Asherman's Syndrome
Removal of pedunculated fibroid or large polyp

LEVEL 3 MORE COMPLEX OPERATIVE PROCEDURES REQUIRING ADDITIONAL TRAINING
Division/resection of uterine septum
Endoscopic surgery for major Asherman's Syndrome
Endometrial resection or ablation
Resection of submucous leiomyoma
Repeat endometrial resection or ablation

Appendix VI Cervical screening Health of the Nation targets

Purchasers

Interventions for NHS purchasers and providers (*Key Area Handbook*).

- Region retains responsibility for monitoring the running of the programme by districts.
- DHAs
  a) health promotion activities
  b) build alliances with other agencies such as the network and HEA
  c) purchasing cervical screening services of high quality
  d) availability of services to eligible population
  e) maximize attendance for screening
  f) set targets for purchasing high quality diagnostic, therapeutic and support services for women with abnormal smears.

Providers

- Health promotion.
- High quality screening, treatment and support services.
- Ensure women with an abnormal smear are followed-up promptly.
- Maintain good liaison with the network.

FHSAs

- Handling the recall system.
- Personal invitation and response to queries.
- Efficient, straightforward methods for checking medical records against the FHSA list.
- Support for practices failing to reach targets, including training for practice nurses.
- Training of practice nurses.

Primary health care team

- Understand and promote the programme.
- Follow-up non-responders.
- Liaise with district co-ordinator.
- Be involved in follow-up and treatment arrangements and model as necessary to provide an efficient and effective service.
- Minimize anxiety in women recalled for further assessment.

(Department of Health, 1993)

Appendix VII Expert Advisory Committee on Cancer. (A policy framework for commissioning cancer services 1994)

The Expert Advisory Committee on Cancer report is a consultative policy framework for commissioning cancer services which will determine the philosophy of purchasing cancer care and where and how much will be purchased. As outlined in this assessment the report focuses on a patient centred approach. Cancer services need to be flexible to respond to emerging technologies and new research findings. The general principles should include the following.

1 Access to uniformly high quality of care in the community or hospital to ensure maximum possible cure rates and best quality of life.
2 Promotion of early recognition of symptoms and availability of screening.
3 Clear information and assistance regarding treatment options and outcomes available.
4 Services to be patient centred.
5 Primary care team is central and continuing element in cancer care and communication between sectors must be of a high quality if the best possible care is to be achieved.
6 Psychosocial aspects of cancer care should be considered at all stages.
7 Cancer registration and careful monitoring of treatment and outcomes is essential.

Recommendation that there must be three levels of care.

1 Primary care as focus of care.
2 Designated cancer units in DGHs to manage commoner cancers (which probably do not include the gynaecological cancers).
3 Designated cancer centres to manage all cancers, including common cancers and less common cancers by referral from cancer units. They will provide specialist diagnostic and therapeutic techniques including radiotherapy.

Element of report for gynaecological services.

1 Need to develop arrangements for the close integration of primary and secondary care, including referral protocols and management protocols.
2 Appropriate training of surgeons (the RCOG subspecialty training scheme for gynaecological oncology).
3 Multi-disciplinary consultation and management requires a minimum of five sessions of the non-surgical oncology type even in the smaller cancer units. The access to specialist nurses with site-specific skills and specialist skills (e.g. lymphoedema management and cytotoxic chemotherapy administration).
4 Chemotherapy if it is to be given in a cancer unit should only be if appropriate facilities and sufficiently experienced multi-disciplinary teams are available. Treatment protocols should be the same as those of the cancer centre. Radiotherapy is usually transferred to the centres.

Contracting

Appropriate contractual arrangements will be reached by purchasing authorities with a cancer centre which will deliver a full range of cancer treatments to encompass treatment programmes for less common and rare cancers and those treatments which are too specialized, technically demanding or capital intensive to be provided in the cancer unit. Chorioncarcinoma is a rare tumour that will be managed in a small number of cancer centres to ensure adequate specialization.

A cancer centre should serve a population of at least 1 000 000 and no less than 750 000.

Specialist centre facilities – paediatric and adolescent cancer services

Assessment and management of rare cancers in multi-disciplinary teams and the accumulation of expertise in these treatments. Specialist surgical services including reconstructive surgery, intensive chemotherapy, full range of radiotherapy, with appropriate number of clinical oncologists to ensure specialist application, medical oncology, sophisticated diagnostic facilities, special expertise in palliative care and rehabilitation.

Contracts should be developed for each site with agreed protocols for referral and diagnosis and co-ordinated delivery of care at all levels.

Appendix VIII Glossary of terms

AID	artificial insemination by donor
CIN	cervical intraepithelial neoplasia
D&C	dilatation and curettage
DRG	diagnostic related groups
DUB	dysfunctional uterine bleeding
ERPC	evacuation of the retained products of conception
GIFT	gamete intra-fallopian transfer
GUM	genitourinary medicine
HES	hospital episode statistics
HIV	human immunodeficiency virus
HRT	hormone replacement therapy
HRG	health care resource grouping
HSG	hysterosalpingogram
ICD	international classification of disease
IUCD	intra-uterine contraceptive device
IVF	*in vitro* fertilization
IVF-ET	*in vitro* fertilization and embryo transfer
LAVH	laparoscopically assisted vaginal hysterectomy
LLETZ	large loop excision of the transformation zone
MAS	minimal access surgery
PID	pelvic inflammatory disease
PMS	premenstrual syndrome
RCOG	Royal College of Obstetricians and Gynaecolgists
TAH	total abdominal hysterectomy
TCRE	transcervical resection of the endometrium

References

1 Ashton JR, Marchbank A, Mawle P *et al.* Family Planning, Abortion and Fertility Services. In *Health Care Assessment Vol. 2* (eds A Stevens, J Raftery). Oxford: Radcliffe Medical Press, 1994, 555–94.

2 Human Fertilisation Embryology Authority. *Annual Report.* London: HFEA, 1992.

3 Taylor-Robinson D. *Chlamydia trachomatis* and sexually transmitted disease. *BMJ* 1994; **308**: 150–1.

4 Ripa T. Epidemiologic control of genital *Chlamydia trachomatis* infections. *Scand J Infect Dis* 1990; **69** (Suppl.): 157–67.

5 Buhang H, Skjeldestag FF, Halvorseule LE *et al.* Should asymptomatic patients be tested for *Chlamydia trachomatis* in general practice? *Br J Gen Prac* 1990; **40**: 142–5.

6 Lugo-Miro VI, Green M, Mazur L. Comparison of different metronidazole regimens for bacterial vaginosis: a meta-analysis. *JAMA* 1992; **268**: 92–5.

7 *Effective Health Care Bulletin 1.* Screening for osteoporosis to prevent fractures. University of Leeds School of Public Health, 1992.

8 Whitehead MI The menopause. (Review). *Practitioner* 1987; **231**: 37–42.

9 Meade TW, Berra A. Hormone replacement therapy and cardiovascular disease. *Br Med Bull* 1992; **48**: 276–308.

10 Hutchinson TA, Polansky SM, Feinstein AR. Postmenopausal oestrogens protect against fractures of hip and distal radius. *Lancet* 1979; **ii**: 705–9.

11 Weiss NS , Ure CL, Ballard JH *et al.* Decreased risk of fractures of the hip and lower forearm with postmenopausal use of estrogen. *N Engl J Med* 1980; **303**: 1195–8.

12 Roche M, Vessey MP. Hormone replacement therapy in the community: risks, benefits and costs. In *HRT and Osteoporosis* (eds JO Drife, JWW Studds). London: Springer-Verlag, 1990.

13 Tapp AJS, Cardozo L, Hills B *et al.* Who benefits from physiotherapy? *Neurol Urodynam* 1988; **7**: 259–61.

14 Jarvis GJ. Surgery for general stress incontinence. *Br J Obstet Gynaecol* 1994; **10**: 371–4.

15 Sculpher MJ, Bryan S, Dwyer N *et al.* An economic evaluation of transcervical endometrial resection versus abdominal hysterectomy for the treatment of menorrhagia. *Br J Obstet Gynaecol* 1993; **100**: 244–52.

16 Raju KS, Auld BJ. A randomised prospective study of laparoscopic vaginal hysterectomy versus abdominal hysterectomy each with bilateral salpingo-oophorectomy. *Br J Obstet Gynaecol* 1994; **101**: 1068–71.

17 Editorial. Pelvic congestion. *Lancet* 1991; **337**: 398–9.

18 O'brien PMS. Helping women with premenstrual syndrome. *BMJ* 1993; **307**: 1471/5.

19 Grimes DA. Frontiers of operative laparoscopy: a review and critique of the evidence. *Am J Obstet Gynecol* 1992; **166**: 1062–71.

20 El Refaey H, Hinshaw K, Smith N. Medical management of missed abortion and anembryonic pregnancy. *BMJ* 1992; **305**: 1399.

21 Henshaw RC, Naji SA, Russell IT. Comparison of medical abortion with surgical vacuum aspiration: women's preferences and acceptability of treatment. *BMJ* 1993; **307**: 714–17.

22 Bonomi P, Blessing JA, Stehman FB *et al.* Randomized trial of three cisplatin dose schedules in squamous-cell carcinoma of the cervix: a Gynecologic Oncology Group Study. *J Clin Oncol* 1985; **3**: 1079–85.

23 Royal College of Obstetricians and Gynaecologists. *Report of the RCOG Working Party on Training in Gynaecological Endoscopic Surgery.* London: RCOG Press, June 1994.

24 Magos AL, Baumann R, Turnbull AC. Managing gynaecological emergencies with laparoscopy. *BMJ* 1989; **299**: 371–4.

25 Department of Health. *Research for Health – a research and development strategy for NHS*. London: Department of Health, 1993.

26 Scottish Needs Assessment Programme. *Improving gynaecological services within existing resources. A programme budgeting and marginal analysis approach*. Scottish Forum for Public Health Medicine, April 1994.

27 NHS Cervical Screening Programme: *First Annual Report*. National Coordinating Network, July 1991.

28 NHS Cervical Screening Programme. *Guidelines on Fail-Safe Actions.* (Pike C, Chamberlain J), June 1992.

29 Salfield NJ, Sharp F. Planning colposcopy and gynaecological laser services. *Community Med* 1989; **11**: 140–7.

30 Department of Health. *A policy framework for commissioning cancer services*. Expert advisory group on cancer. London: Department of Health, 1994.

31 Office of Population Censuses and Surveys. *Morbidity statistics from general practice 1991–1992*. London: HMSO, 1995.

32 Department of Health. *Hospital Episode Statistics. Volumes 1 and 2. England. Financial year 1993–94*. Leeds: Department of Health, 1995.

33 Dowie R. *Patterns of hospital medical staffing. Obstetrics and gynaecology*. London: HMSO, 1991.

34 Audit Commission. *A shortcut to better services: day surgery in England and Wales*. London: HMSO, 1990.

35 Gabbay J, Francis L. How much day surgery? Delphic predictions. *BMJ* 1988; **297**: 1249–52.

36 Department of Health. *New cases seen at NHS genito-urinary medicine clinics in England*. 1992 annual figures. Summary information from form KC60. London: Department of Health, 1993.

37 Sculpher M. *A snip at the price? A review of the economics of minimal access surgery*. Uxbridge: Brunel University Health Economics Research Group, 1993.

38 Royal College of Obstetricians and Gynaecologists Medical Audit Unit. *Medical Audit Unit. Third Bulletin*. Manchester: Royal College of Obstetricians and Gynaecologists, 1991.

39 Department of Health. NHS hospital activity statistics for England 1979–1989/90, summary. *Statistical Bulletin–2/10/90*, 1990.

40 Ferguson JA, Goldacre MJ, Henderson J *et al*. Audit of workload in gynaecology: analysis of time trends from linked statistics. *Br J Obstet Gynaecol* 1991; **98**: 772–7.

41 Dwyer N, Hutton J, Stirrat GM. Randomised controlled trial comparing endometrial resection with abdominal hysterectomy for the surgical treatment of menorrhagia. *Br J Obstet Gynaecol* 1993; **100**: 237–43.

42 *Effective Health Care, Bulletin 3*. The management of subfertility. Leeds: University of Leeds School of Public Health, 1992.

43 Anonymous. Pain of childlessness. *BMJ* 1991; **302**: 134–5.

44 Hager WD, Eschenbach DA, Spence MR *et al*. Criteria for diagnosis and grading of salpingitis. *Obstet Gynecol* 1983; **61**: 113–14.

45 Thomas EJ. Endometriosis. Should not be treated just because it's there. *BMJ* 1993; **306**: 158–9.

46 Studd JWW, Watson NR, Henderson A. Symptoms and metabolic sequelae of the menopause. In *HRT and Osteoporosis* (eds JO Drife, JWW Studd). London: Springer-Verlag, 1990, 23–34.

47 Khaw KT. Epidemiology of the menopause. *Br Med Bull* 1992; **48(No.2)**: 249–61.

48 Fergusson ILC. Genital prolapse. In *Contemporary gynaecology*. London: Butterworth, 1989, 211–18.

49 Hallberg L, Hogdahl A-M, Nilsson L *et al*. Menstrual blood loss – a population study. *Acta Obstet Gynecol Scand* 1966; **45**: 320–51.

50 Reginald PW , Beard RW, Kooner JS *et al*. Intravenous dihydroergotamine to relieve pelvic congestion with pain in young women. *Lancet* 1987; **ii**: 351–3.

51 Beard RW, Highman JW, Pearce S *et al.* Diagnosis of pelvic varicosities in women with chronic pelvic pain. *Lancet* 1984; **ii**: 946–9.

52 Budeiri DJ, Li Wan PoA, Dornan JC. Clinical trials of treatments of premenstrual syndrome: entry criteria and scales for measuring treatment outcomes. *Br J Obstet Gynaecol* 1994; **101**: 689–95.

53 World Health Organization. *International classification of disease.* 9th Revision, Vol.1. London: HMSO, 1977.

54 Regan L. Recurrent miscarriage. *BMJ* 1991; **302**: 543–4.

55 Sagle M, Bishop K, Ridley N *et al.* Recurrent early miscarriage and polycystic ovaries. *BMJ* 1988; **297**: 1027–8.

56 Jordan J. Minor degrees of cervical intra-epithelial neoplasia. *BMJ* 1988; **297** 6.

57 Richardson GS, Scully RE, Nikgu N *et al.* Common epithelial cancer of the ovary. *N Eng J Med* 1985; **312**: 415–23.

58 Campbell S, Bhan V, Royston P *et al.* Transabdominal ultrasound screening for early ovarian cancer. *BMJ* 1989; **299**: 1363–7.

59 Bourne TH, Campbell S, Whitehead MI *et al.* Detection of endometrial cancer in postmenopausal women by transvaginal ultrasonography and colour flow imaging. *BMJ* 1990; **301**: 369.

60 Jacobs I, Prys Davies A *et al.* Prevalence screening for ovarian cancer in postmenopausal women by CA125 measurement and ultrasonography. *BMJ* 1993; **306**: 1030–4.

61 Wilson JMG, Jungner G. *Principles and practice of screening for disease.* Geneva: WHO, 1993.

62 Templeton A, Fraser C, Thompson B. Infertility – epidemiology and referral practice. *Hum Reprod* 1991; **6**: 1391–4.

63 Page H. An economic appraisal of in vitro fertilisation. *J R Soc Med* 1988; **88**: 99–102.

64 Platt R, Rice PA, McCormeck WM. Risk of acquiring gonorrhoea and prevalence of abnormal adnexal findings among women recently exposed to gonorrhoea. *JAMA* 1983; **250**: 3205.

65 Cates W, Rolfs RT, Aral SQ. Sexually transmitted diseases, pelvic inflammatory disease, and infertility: an epidemiologic update. *Epidemiol Rev* 1990; **12**: 199–220.

66 Taylor-Robinson D. *Genital chlamydial infections: clinical aspects, diagnosis, treatment and prevention.* 4th edn. London: Churchill Livingstone, 1991, 219–62.

67 Hopgood J, Mallinson H. Chlamydia testing in community clinics – a focus for accurate sexual health care. *J Family Planning* 1995, **21**: 87–90.

68 Smith JR, Murdoch J, Carrington D. Prevalence of *Chlamydia trachomatis* infection in women having cervical smear tests. *BMJ* 1991; **302**: 1271–83.

69 Fish ANJ, Fairweather DVI, Oriel JD *et al. Chlamydia trachomatis* infection in a gynaecology clinic population identification of high-risk groups and the value of contact tracing. *Eur J Obstet Gynecol Reprod Biol* 1989; **31**: 67–74.

70 Wood PL, Hobson D, Rees E. Genital infections with *Chlamydia trachomatis* in women attending an antenatal clinic. *Br J Obstet Gynaecol* 1984; **91**: 1171–6.

71 Lee NC, Rubin GI, Oey LW *et al.* Type of intra-uterine device and risk of pelvic inflammatory disease. *Obstet Gynecol* 1983; **62**: 1–6.

72 Mead PB. Epidemiolgy of bacterial vaginosis. *Am J Obstet Gynecol* 1993; **169**: 446–9.

73 Hay PE, Taylor-Robinson D, Lamont RF. Diagnosis of bacterial vaginosis in a gynaecology clinic. *Br J Obstet Gynaecol* 1992; **99**: 63–6.

74 Blackwell AL, Thomas PD, Wareham K *et al.* Health gains from screening for infection of the lower genital tract in women attending for termination of pregnancy. *Lancet* 1993; **342**: 206–10.

75 Houston DE, Noller KL, Melton LJ 3rd *et al.* Incidence of pelvic endometriosis in Rochester, Minnesota, 1970–1979. *Am J Epidemiol* 1987; **125**: 959–69.

76 Vessey MP, Villard-Mackintosh L, Painter R. Epidemiology of endometriosis in women attending family planning clinics. *BMJ* 1993; **306**: 182–4.

77 Strathy JH, Molgaard CA, Coulan CB *et al.* Endometriosis and Infertility: a laparoscopic study among fertile and infertile women. *Fertil Steril* 1982; **38**; 667–72.

78 Boyce WJ, Vessey MP. Rising incidence of fracture of the proximal femur. *Lancet* 1985; i: 150–1.

79 Office of Population Censuses and Surveys. *Mortality statistics DH1 (27) 1992*. London: HMSO, 1994.

80 Law MR , Wald NJ , Meade TW. Strategies for prevention of osteoporosis and hip fracture. *BMJ* 1991; **303**: 453–9.

81 Cooper C, Eastell R. Bone gain and loss in premenopausal women. *BMJ* 1993; **306**: 1357–8.

82 Market and Opinion Research Institute. *Survey of prevalence and attitudes to incontinence*. London: MORI, 1991.

83 Thomas TM, Plymat KR, Blannin J *et al.* Prevalence of urinary incontinence. *BMJ* 1980; **281**: 1243–5.

84 Versi E, Cardozo LD. Oestrogens and lower urinary tract function. In *The Menopause* (eds JWW Studd, MI Whitehead). Oxford: Blackwell Scientific Publications, 1988, 76–84.

85 Allen RE, Hosker GL, Smith AR *et al.* Pelvic floor damage and childbirth: a neurophysiological study. *Br J Obstet Gynaecol* 1990; **97**: 770–9.

86 Milton PJD. Utero-vaginal prolapse. In *Progress in Obstetrics and Gynaecology* Vol. 7 (ed. J Studd). Edinburgh: Churchill Livingstone, 1989, 319–30.

87 Rybo G. Menstrual blood loss in relation to parity and menstrual pattern. *Acta Obstet Gynaecol Scand* 1966; **45 (Suppl.)**: 25–45.

88 Smith SK. Menorrhagia In *Progress in Obstetrics and Gynaecology* Vol. 5 (ed. J Studd). Edinburgh: Churchill Livingstone, 1985.

89 Buttram VC, Reiter RC. Uterine leiomyomata: etiology, symptomatology and management. *Fertil Steril* 1981; **36**: 433–45.

90 Vessey M, Villard-Mackintosh L, McPherson K *et al.* The epidemiology of hysterectomy: findings in a large cohort study. *Br J Obstet Gynaecol* 1992; **99**: 402–7.

91 Kuh D, Stirling S. Socioeconomic variation in admissions for diseases of female genital system and breast in a national cohort aged 15–43. *BMJ* 1995; **11**: 840–3.

92 Royal College of Obstetricians and Gynaecologists. Gynaecological laparoscopy. In *Report of the working party of the confidential enquiry into gynaecological laparoscopy* (eds G Chamberlain, D Brown). London: Royal College of Obstetricians and Gynaecologists, 1978.

93 Davies L, Gangar KF, Drummond M *et al.* The economic burden of intractable gynaecological pain. *J Obstet Gynaecol* 1992; **12(Suppl. 2)**: 554–6.

94 Stabile I, Grudzinskas JG. Ectopic Pregnancy: A review of incidence, etiology and diagnostic aspects. *Obstet Gynecol Survey* 1990; **45**: 335–47.

95 Norman SG. An audit of the management of ectopic pregnancy. *Br J Obstet Gynaecol* 1991; **98**: 1267–72.

96 Chow WH, Daling JR, Cates W *et al.* Epidemiology of ectopic pregnancy. *Epidemiol Rev* 1987; **9**: 70–94.

97 Coste J, Job-Spira N, Fernandez H *et al.* Risk factors for ectopic pregnancy: a case control study in France, with special focus on infectious factors. *Am J Epidemiol* 1991; **133**: 839–49.

98 Alberman E. The epidemiology of repeated abortion. In *Early pregnancy loss: mechanisms and treatment* (eds RW Beard, F Sharp). London: Royal College of Obstetricians and Gynaecologists, 1988, 9–17.

99 Warburton D, Fraser FC. Spontaneous abortion risks in man: data from reproductive histories collected in a medical genetic unit. *Hum Genet* 1964; **16**: 1–25.

100 Regan L, Braude PR, Trembath PL. Influence of past reproductive performance on risk of spontaneous abortion. *BMJ* 1989; **299**: 541–5.

101 Chard T. Frequency of implantation and early pregnancy loss in natural cycles. *Balliére's Clin Obstet Gynaecol* 1991; **5**: 179–89.

102 Department of Health. *Summary information from Form KC 61 (England)*, 1993.

103 Office of Population Censuses and Surveys. *Cancer statistics MB1(20) registrations*. London: HMSO, 1993.

104 Office of Population Censuses and Surveys. *Cancer statistics MB1(21) registrations*. London: HMSO, 1994.

105 Villard L, Murphy M. Endometrial cancer trends in England and Wales: a protective effect of oral contraception. *Int J Epidemiol* 1990; **19**: 255–6.

106 FIGO 20th Volume. *Annual results of treatment in gynaecological cancer*. FIGO, 1988.

107 Buchanan H, Vessey M. Epidemiology and trends in hospital discharges for pelvic inflammatory disease in England, 1975 to 1985. *Br J Obstet Gynaecol* 1989; **96**: 1219–23.

108 Buchanan H, Vessey M, Goldacre M *et al.* Morbidity following pelvic inflammatory disease. *Br J Obstet Gynaecol* 1993; **100**: 558–62.

109 McCarthy E. *Inpatient utilisation of short stay hospitals by diagnosis: United States – 1980*. 83rd edn. Hyattsville, Maryland: DHHS, 1982, 83–1735.

110 Barlow DH, Brockie JA, Rees CMP. Study of general practice consultations and menopausal problems. *BMJ* 1991; **302**: 274–6.

111 Wilkes HC, Meade TW. Hormone replacement therapy in general practice: a survey of doctors in the MRC's general practice research framework. *BMJ* 1991; **302**: 1317–20.

112 Draper J, Roland M. Perimenopausal women's views on taking hormone replacement therapy to prevent osteoporosis. *BMJ* 1990; **300**: 786–8.

113 Roberts PJ. The menopause and hormone replacement therapy: views of women in general practice receiving hormone replacement therapy. *Br J Gen Pract* 1991; **41**: 421–4.

114 Coulter A, Bradlow J, Agass M *et al.* Outcomes of referrals to gynaecology outpatient clinics for menstrual problems: an audit of general practice records. *Br J Obstet Gynaecol* 1991; **98**: 789–96.

115 Effective Health Care, Bulletin 9. The management of menorrhagia. Leeds: University of Leeds School of Public Health, 1995.

116 Coulter A, Klassen A, Mackenzie I *et al.* Diagnostic dilatation and curettage: Is it used appropriately? *BMJ* 1993; **306**: 236–9.

117 McPherson K, Strong PM, Epstein A *et al.* Regional variations in the use of common surgical procedures: within and between England and Wales, Canada and the United States of America. *Soc Sci Med* 1981; **15A**: 273–88.

118 Coulter A, McPherson K, Vessey M. Do British women undergo too many or too few hysterectomies? *Soc Sci Med* 1988; **27**: 987–94.

119 Gath D, Osborn M, Bungay G *et al.* Psychiatric disorder and gynaecological symptoms in middle-aged women: a community survey. *BMJ* 1987; **294**: 213–18.

120 Henker FO. Diagnosis and treatment of non organic pelvic pain. *South Med J* 1979; **72**: 1132–4.

121 Gilling-Smith C, Tooz-Hobson P, Potts DJ *et al.* Management of bleeding in early pregnancy in accident and emergency departments. *BMJ* 1994; **309**: 574–5.

122 Henderson J, Godacre MJ, Griffith M *et al.* Day case surgery: geographical variation, trends and readmission rates. *J Epidemiol Comm Hlth* 1989; **43**: 301–5.

123 Morgan M, Beech R. Variations in length of stay and rates of day-case surgery: implications for the efficiency of surgical management. *J Epidemiol Comm Hlth* 1990; **44**: 90–105.

124 Ratcliffe F, Lawson R, Millar J. Day-case laporoscopy revisited: have post-operative morbidity and patients acceptance improved? *Health Trends* 1994; **26**: 47–49.

125 Abbey A, Halman LJ, Andrews FM. Psychosocial, treatment and demographic predictors of stress associated with infertility. *Fertil Steril* 1992; **57**: 122–8.

126 Office of Population Censuses and Surveys. *Congenital Malformation Statistics 1981–85 MB3(2)*. London: HMSO, 1988.

127 Hass GG, Manganiello P. A double blind, placebo-controlled study of the use of methylprednisolone in infertile men with sperm associated immunoglobulins. *Fertil Steril* 1987; **47**: 295–301.

128 Hull MGR, Savage PE, Jacobs HS. Investigation and treatment of amenorrhoea resulting in normal fertility. *BMJ* 1979; **1**: 1257–61.

129 Bury J. *Teenage pregnancy in Britain.* London: Birth Control Trust, 1984.

130 Skjeldestad FE, Tuveng J, Solberg AG *et al.* Induced abortion: *Chlamydia trachomatis* and postabortal complications: a cost benefit analysis. *Acta Obstet Gynecol Scand* 1988; **67**: 525–9.

131 Lee HH, Chernesky MA, Schachter J *et al.* Diagnosis of *Chlamydia trachomatis* genitourinary infection in women by ligase chain reaction assay of urine. *Lancet* 1995; **345**: 213–16.

132 Jones RB. New treatments for *Chlamydia trachomatis. Am J Obstet Gynecol* 1991; **164**: 789–93.

133 Walker CK, Kahn JG, Washington AE *et al.* Pelvic inflammatory diseases: meta-analysis of antimicrobial regimen efficacy. *J Infect Dis* 1993; **168**: 969–78.

134 Department of Health. *The Health of the Nation Key Area Handbook: HIV/AIDS and Sexual Health.* London: Department of Health, 1993.

135 Andersen PG, Christensen S, Detlefsen GU *et al.* Treatment of Bartholin's abscess. Marsupialization versus incision, curettage and suture under antibiotic cover. A randomized study with 6 months' follow-up. *Acta Obstet Gynecol Scand* 1992; **71**: 59–62.

136 Evers JL. The second look laparoscopy for the evaluation of the results of medical treatment of endometriosis should not be performed during ovarian suppression. *Fertil Steril* 1987; **47**: 502–4.

137 Olive DL, Haney AF. Endometriosis-associated infertility: a critical review of therapeutic approaches. *Obstet Gynecol Surv* 1986; **41**: 538–55.

138 Hull ME, Moghissi KS, Magyar DF *et al.* Comparison of different treatment modalities of endometriosis in infertile women. *Fertil Steril* 1987; **47**: 40–4.

139 Rock JA, Truglia JA, Caplan RJ. Zoladex Endometriosis Study Group. Zoladex (goserelin acetate implant) in the treatment of endometriosis: a randomized comparison with danazol. *Obstet Gynecol* 1993; **82**: 198–205.

140 Shaw RW. Zoladex Endometriosis Study Team. An open randomized comparative study of the effect of goserelin depot and danazol in the treatment of endometriosis. *Fertil Steril* 1992; **58**: 265–72.

141 Sutton C, Hill D. Laser laparoscopy in the treatment of endometriosis. A 5-year study. *Br J Obstet Gynaecol* 1990; **97**: 181–5.

142 Schenken RS, Malinak LR. Conservative surgery versus expectant management for the infertile patient with mild endometriosis. *Fertil Steril* 1982; **37**: 183–6.

143 Schmidt CL. Endometriosis: a reappraisal of pathogenesis and treatment. *Fertil Steril* 1985; **44**: 157–73.

144 Bromham DR. Endometriosis in primary care. *Clinical Practice* 1991; **45 (Suppl. 72)**: 54–8.

145 Posthuma WFM, Westendorp RGJ, Vandenbroucke JP. Cardioprotective effect of hormone replacement therapy in postmenopausal women: is the evidence biased? *BMJ* 1994; **308**: 1268–9.

146 Advisory Group on Osteoporosis. Department of Health, 1994.

147 Snow-Harter C, Bouxsein ML, Lewis BT *et al.* Effects of resistance and endurance exercise on bone mineral status of young women: a randomised exercise intervention trial. *J Bone Miner Res* 1992; **7**: 761–9.

148 Prince RL, Smith M, Dick IM *et al.* Prevention of postmenopausal osteoporosis. A comparative study of exercise, calcium supplementation, and hormone-replacement therapy. *N Engl J Med* 1991; **325**: 1189–95.

149 Harlap S. The benefits and risks of hormone replacement therapy. An epidemiologic overview. *Am J Obstet Gynecol* 1992; **166**: 1986–92.

150 Grady D, Rubin SM, Pettiti DB *et al.* Hormone therapy to prevent disease and prolong life in postmenopausal women. *Ann Intern Med* 1992; **117(12)**: 1016–37.

151 Gorsky RD, Koplan JP, Peterson HB *et al*. Relative risks and benefits of long-term estrogen replacement therapy: a decision analysis. *Obstet Gynecol* 1994; **83**: 161–6.

152 Savvas M, Studd JWW, Fogelman I *et al*. Skeletal effects of oral oestrogen compared with subcutaneous oestrogen and testosterone in postmenopausal women. *BMJ* 1988; **297**: 331–3.

153 Weinstein MC, Tosteson AN. Cost-effectiveness of hormone replacement. *Ann NY Acad Sci* 1990; **592**: 162–72, 185–92.

154 Daly E , Roche M , Barlow D *et al*. An analysis of benefits, risks and costs. *Br Med Bull* 1992; **48(2)**: 368–400.

155 Persson I, Adami H, Bergkvist L *et al*. Risk of endometrial cancers after treatment with oestrogens alone or in conjunction with progestogens: results of a prospective study. *BMJ* 1989; **298**: 147–51.

156 Steinberg KK, Thacker SB, Smith SJ et al. A meta-analysis of the effect of estrogen replacement therapy on the risk of breast cancer. *JAMA* 1991; **265**: 1985–90.

157 Versi E, Hyatt J, Anand D. Managing Urinary incontinence in general practice. *The Diplomate* 1994; **1**: 12–17.

158 Jarvis GJ, Hall S, Stamp S *et al*. An assessment of urodynamic examination in incontinent women. *Br J Obstet Gynaecol* 1980; **87**: 893–6.

159 Mantle J, Versi E. Physiotherapy for stress incontinence. A national survey. *BMJ* 1991; **302**: 753–5.

160 Hilton P. Urinary incontinence in women. *BMJ* 1987; **295**: 426–32.

161 Murray K . Medical and surgical management of female voiding difficulty. In *Micturition* (eds JO Drife, P Hilton, SL Stanton). Berlin: Springer-Verlag, 1989; 175–99.

162 Mundy AR, Stephenson TP. 'Clam' ileocystoplasty for the treatment of refractory urge incontinence. *Br J Urol* 1985; **57**: 641–64.

163 Karam MM, Bhatia NN. Management of coexistent stress and urge incontinence. *Obstet Gynecol* 1989; **73**: 4–7.

164 MacKenzie J, Bibby J. Critical assessment of dilatation and curettage of 1029 women. *Lancet* 1978; **ii**: 566–8.

165 Lewis BV. Diagnostic dilatation and curettage in young women. *BMJ* 1993; **306**: 225–6.

166 Rodriguez GC, Gustavo C, Yaqub N *et al*. A comparison of the pipelle device and the vabra aspirator as measured by endometrial denudation in hysterectomy specimens. The pipelle device samples significantly less of the endometrial surface than the vabra aspirator. *Am J Obstet Gynecol* 1993; **168**: 55–9.

167 De Jong P, Doel F, Falconer A. Outpatient diagnostic hysteroscopy. *Br J Obstet Gynaecol* 1990; **97**: 299–303.

168 Cochrane WJ, Thomas MA. Ultrasound diagnosis of gynecologic pelvic masses. *Radiology* 1974; **110**: 649–54.

169 Iles S, Gath D. Psychological problems and uterine bleeding. In *Dysfunctional uterine bleeding and menorrhagia* (ed. JO Drife). London: Balliére Tindall, 1989, 375–89.

170 Drugs for menorrhagia: often disappointing. *Drug Therap Bull* 1990; **28**: 17–18.

171 Cameron IT, Leask R, Kelly RW *et al*. The effects of danazol, mefenamic acid, norethisterone and a progesterone-impregnated coil on endometrial prostaglandin concentrations in women with menorrhagia. *Prostaglandin* 1987; **34**: 99–100.

172 Shaw RW, Fraser HM. Use of superactive luteinising hormone releasing hormone (LHRH) agonist in the treatment of menorrhagia. *Br J Obstet Gynaecol* 1984; **91**: 913–16.

173 Nilsson L, Rybo G. Treatment of menorrhagia. *Am J Obstet Gynecol* 1971; **110**: 713–20.

174 Anderson ABM, Haynes PJ, Guillebaud J *et al*. Reduction of menstrual blood loss by prostaglandin-synthetase inhibitors. *Lancet* 1976; **i**: 774–6.

175 Gillebaud J, Anderson ABM , Turnbull AC. Reduction by mefenamic acid of increased menstrual blood loss associated with intrauterine contraception. *Br J Obstet Gynaecol* 1978; **85**: 53–62.

176 Nilsson L, Rybo G. Treatment of menorrhagia with epsilon aminocaproic acid. A double blind investigation. *Acta Obstet Gynecol Scand* 1965; **44**: 467–83.

177 Ylikorkala O, Niinikka L. Comparison between antifibrinolytic and antiprostaglandin treatment in the reduction of increased menstrual blood loss in women with intrauterine contraceptive devices. *Br J Obstet Gynaecol* 1983; **90**: 78–83.

178 Chimbira TH, Anderson ABM, Naish C *et al.* Reduction pf menstrual blood loss by danazol in unexplained menorrhagia: lack of effect of placebo. *Br J Obstet Gynaecol* 1980; **87**: 1152–8.

179 Magos AL. Management of menorrhagia – hysteroscopic techniques offer a revolution in treatment. *BMJ* 1990; **300**: 1537–8.

180 Coutinho EM, Goncalves MT. Long term treatment of leiomyomas with gestrinone. *Fertil Steril* 1989; **51**: 939–46.

181 West CP. Analogues in the management of uterine fibroids, premenstrual syndrome and breast malignancies. *Balliére's Clin Obstet Gynaecol* 1989; **2**: 689–709.

182 Loffer FD. Hysteroscopic endometrial ablation with the Nd-YAG laser using a non-touch technique. *Obstet Gynecol* 1987; **69**: 679–82.

183 Golan A, Bukovsky I , Pansky M *et al.* Pre-operative gonadotrophin-releasing hormone agonist treatment in surgery for uterine leiomyomata. *Hum Reprod* 1993; **8**: 450–2.

184 Stovall TG, Ling FW, Henry LC *et al.* A randomized trial evaluating leuprolide acetate before hysterectomy as treatment for leiomyomas. *Am J Obstet Gynecol* 1991; **164**: 1420–5.

185 Dicker RC, Greenspan JR, Strauss LT *et al.* Complications of abdominal and vaginal hysterectomy among women of reproductive age in the United States. The collaborative review of sterilization. *Am J Obstet Gynecol* 1982; **144**: 841–8.

186 Wingo PA, Huezo CM, Rubin GL *et al.* The mortality risk associated with hysterectomy. *Am J Obstet Gynecol* 1985; **152**: 803–8.

187 Dennerstein L, Ryan M. The 'post-hysterectomy' syndrome. In *Progress in Obstetrics and Gynaecology Volume 3* (ed. J Studd). Edinburgh: Churchill Livingstone, 1983, 280–91.

188 Clarke A, Rowe P, Black N *et al. Does length of stay affect cost and outcome in hysterectomy?* London: Proceedings Society for Social Medicine, 1993.

189 McKee M, Wilson P. The public health aspects of hysterectomy. *J Royal Soc Med* 1993; **86**: 432–4.

190 Gannon MJ, Holt FM, Fairbank J *et al.* A randomised trial comparing endometrial resection and abdominal hysterectomy for the treatment of menorrhagia. *BMJ* 1991; **303**: 1362–4.

191 Garry R, Erian J, Grochmal SA. A multicentre collaborative study into the treatment of menorrhagia by ND-YAG laser ablation of the endometrium. *Br J Obstet Gynaecol* 1991; **98**: 357–62.

192 Fraser IS, Angsuwathana S, Mahmoud F *et al.* Short and medium term outcomes after rollerball endometrial ablation for menorrhagia. *Med J Aust* 1993; **148**: 454–7.

193 Phipps JH, Lewis BV, Roberts T *et al.* Treatment of functional menorrhagia by radiofrequency-induced thermal endometrial ablation. *Lancet* 1990; **335**: 374–6.

194 Pinion SB, Parkin DE, Abramovitch DR *et al.* Randomised trial of hysterectomy, endometrial laser ablation, and transcervical endometrial resection for dysfunctional uterine bleeding. *BMJ* 1994; **309**: 979–93.

195 Magos AL, Baumann R, Lockwood GM *et al.* Experience with the first 250 endometrial resections for menorrhagia. *Lancet* 1991; **337**: 1074–8.

196 Rankin L, Steinberg LH. Transcervical resection of the endometrium: a review of 400 consecutive patients. *Br J Obstet Gynaecol* 1992; **99**: 911–14.

197 Hunter RW, McCartney AJ. Can laparoscopic assisted hysterectomy safely replace abdominal hysterectomy? *Br J Obstet Gynaecol* 1993; **100**: 932–4.

198 Boike GM, Elfstrand EP, Delpriore G *et al.* Laparoscopically assisted vaginal hysterectomy in a university hospital: report of 82 cases and comparison with abdominal and vaginal hysterectomy. *Am J Obstet Gynecol* 1993; **168**: 1690–7.

199 Summitt RL, Stovase TG, Lipscomb GH *et al.* Randomised comparison of laparoscopy-assisted vaginal hysterectomy with standard vaginal hysteroctemy in an outpatient setting. *Obstet Gynaecol* 1992; **80**: 895–901.

200 Stovall TG, Summitt RL, Bryan DF *et al.* Outpatient vaginal hysterectomy: a pilot study. *Obstet Gynecol* 1992; **80**: 145–9.

201 Clinch J. Length of hospital stay after vaginal hysterectomy. *Br J Obstet Gynaecol* 1994; **101**: 253–4.

202 Farquar CM, Rogers V, Franks S *et al.* A randomised controlled trial of medroxyprogesterone acetate and psychotherapy for the treatment of pelvic congestion. *Br J Obstet Gynaecol* 1989; **96**: 1153–62.

203 Kim DS , Chung SR, Park MI *et al.* Comparative review of diagnostic accuracy in tubal pregnancy. A 14-year survey of 1040 cases. *Obstet Gynecol* 1987; **70**: 547–54.

204 Department of Health. *Report on the Confidential Enquiry into Maternal Deaths in the United Kingdom 1988–1990*. London: HMSO, 1994.

205 Pouly JL, Manhes H, Mage H *et al.* Conservative laparoscopic treatment of 321 ectopic pregnancies. *Fertil Steril* 1986; **46**: 1093–97.

206 De Cherney AH, Diamond MP. Laparoscopic salpingostomy for ectopic pregnancy. *Obstet Gynecol* 1987; **70**: 948–50.

207 Brumsted J, Kessler C, Gibson C *et al.* A comparison of laparoscopy and laparotomy for the treatment of ectopic pregnancy. *Obstet Gynecol* 1988; **71**: 889–92.

208 Goldstein P, Berrier J, Rosen S *et al.* A meta-analysis of randomized control trials of progestational agents in pregnancy. *Br J Obstet Gynaecol* 1989; **96**: 265–74.

209 Daya S. Efficacy of progesterone support for pregnancy in women with recurrent miscarriage: a meta-analysis of controlled trials. *Br J Obstet Gynaecol* 1989; **96**: 275–80.

210 Final Report of the Medical Research Council/Royal College of Obstetricians and Gynaecologists Multicentre randomised trial of cervical cerclage. *Br J Obstet Gynaecol* 1992; **100**: 516–23.

211 McKee M, Priest P, Ginzlet M *et al.* Can out-of-hours operating in gynaecology be reduced? *Arch Emerg Med* 1992; **9**: 290–8.

212 Henshaw RC, Cooper K, El Refaey H *et al.* Medical management of miscarriage: non-surgical uterine evacuation of incomplete and inevitable spontaneous abortion. *BMJ* 1993; **306**: 894–5.

213 UK Multicentre Trial. The efficacy and tolerance of mifepristone and prostaglandin in first trimester termination of pregnancy. *Br J Obstet Gynaecol* 1990; **97**: 480–6.

214 Macrow P, Elstein M. Managing miscarriage medically. *BMJ* 1993; **306**: 876.

215 Bigrigg MA, Read MD. Management of women referred to early pregnancy assessment unit care and cost effectiveness. *BMJ* 1993; **302**: 577–9.

216 Gilling-Smith C, Zelin J, Touquet R *et al.* Management of early pregnancy bleeding in the accident and emergency department. *Arch Emerg Med* 1988; **5**: 133–8.

217 Anderson GH, Boyes DA, Benedet JL *et al.* Organisation and results of the cervical cytology screening programmes in British Columbia, 1955–85. *BMJ* 1988; **296**: 975–8.

218 Laara E. Trends in mortality from cervical cancer in the Nordic countries: association with organised screening programmes. *Lancet* 1987; **1**: 1247–9.

219 Macgregor JE, Campbell MK, Mann EMF *et al.* Screening for cervical intra-epithelial neoplasia in north-east Scotland shows fall in incidence and mortality from invasive cancer with concomitant rise in preinvasive disease. *BMJ* 1994; **305**: 1407–11.

220 Coleman D, Day N, Douglas G *et al.* European guidelines for quality assurance in cervical cancer screening. Europe against cancer programme. *Eur J Cancer* 1993; **29A (Suppl. 4)**.

221 Kitchener HC. United Kingdom Colposcopy Survey. British Society for colposcopy and cervical pathology. *Br J Obstet Gynaecol* 1991; **98**: 1112–6.

222 Johnson N, Sutton J, Thornton JG *et al.* Decision analysis for best management of mildly dyskaryotic smears. *Lancet* 1993; **342**: 91–6.

223 Wolfe CDA, Doherty I, Raju KS *et al.* First steps in the development of an information and counselling service for women with an abnormal smear result. *Eur J Obstet Gynaecol Reprod Biol* 1992; **45**: 201–6.

224 NHS Cervical Screening Programme. *The role of genito-urinary medicine cytology and colposcopy in cervical screening*. National Coordinating Network, 1994.

225 Williams OE, Bodha M, Alawattegama AB. Outcome of cold coagulation for the treatment of cervical intraepithelial neoplasia in a department of genitourinary medicine. *Genitour Med* 1993; **69**: 63–5.

226 *Royal College of Obstetricians and Gynaecologists News*. January 1994, 8.

227 IARC working group on evaluation of cervical cancer screening programmes. Screening for squamous cervical cancer: duration of low risk after negative results of cervical cytology and the implication for screening policies. *BMJ* 1986; **293**: 659–64.

228 La Vecchia C, Franceschi S, Decarli A *et al.* 'Pap' smear and the risk of cervical neoplasia; quantitative estimates from a case-control study. *Lancet* 1984; **ii**: 779–82.

229 Aristizabal N, Cuello C, Correa P *et al.* The impact of vaginal cytology on cervical cancer risk in Cali, Colombia. *Int J Cancer* 1984; **34**: 5–9.

230 Flannelly G, Anderson D, Kitchener HC *et al.* Management of women with mild and moderate cervical dyskaryosis. *BMJ* 1994; **308**: 1399–403.

231 Luesley DM, Cullimore J, Redman CW *et al.* Loop diathermy excision of the cervical transformation zone in patients with abnormal cervical smears. *BMJ* 1990; **300**: 1690–3.

232 Bigrigg A, Haffenden DK, Sheehan AL *et al.* Efficacy and safety of large-loop excision of the transformation zone. *Lancet* 1994; **343**: 32–4.

233 Robertson JH, Woodend BE, Crozier EH *et al.* Risk of cervical cancer associated with mild dyskariosis. *BMJ* 1988; **297**: 18–21.

234 Cooper P, Kirby AJ, Spiegerlhalter DJ *et al.* Management of women with a cervical smear showing a mild degree of dyskariosis: a review of policy. *Cytopathology* 1992; **3**: 331–9.

235 Cuzick J, Terry G, Ho L *et al.* Human papilloma virus type 16 DNA in cervical smears as predictors of high-grade cervical cancer. *Lancet* 1992; **339**: 959–60.

236 Tawa K, Forsythe A, Cove K *et al.* A comparison of the papanicolaou smear and the cervigram: sensitivity, specificity and cost analysis. *Obstet Gynecol* 1988; **71**: 229–35.

237 Chappatte OA, Byrne DL, Raju KS *et al.* Histological differences between colposcopic-directed biopsy and loop excision of the transformation zone(LLETZ): a cause for concern. *Gynecol Oncol* 1991; **43**: 46–50.

238 Montz FJ, Holschneider CH, Thompson LD. Large-loop excision of the transformation zone: effect on the pathologic interpretation of resection margins. *Obstet Gynecol* 1993; **81**: 976–82.

239 Gunasekera PC, Phipps JH, Lewis BV. Large loop excision of the transformation zone (LLETZ) compared with carbon dioxide laser in the treatment of CIN: a superior model of treatment. *Br J Obstet Gynaecol* 1990; **97**: 995–8.

240 Oyesanya OA, Amerasinghe CN, Manning EA. Outpatient excisional management of cervical intraepithelial neoplasia. A prospective, randomised comparison between loop diathermy excision and laser excisional conisation. *Am J Obstet Gynecol* 1993; **168**: 485–88.

241 Woodman CBJ, Byrne P, Kelly KA *et al.* A randomized trial of laser vaporisation in the management of cervical intraepithelial neoplasia associated with human papillomatosis infection. *J Public Health Med* 1993; **15**: 327–31.

242 Pearson SE, Whittaker J, Ireland D et al. Invasive cancer of the cervix after laser treatment. *Br J Obstet Gynaecol* 1989; **96**: 486–8.

243 Bourne TH, Campbell S, Reynolds KM *et al.* Screening for early familial ovarian cancer with transvaginal ultrasonography and colour blood flow imaging. *BMJ* 1993; **306**: 1025 9.

244 Bourne TH, Whitehead MI, Campbell S *et al.* Ultrasound screening for familial ovarian cancer. *Gynaecol Oncol* 1991; **43**: 92–7.

245 Parkes CA, Smith D, Wald NJ *et al.* Feasibility study of a randomised trial of ovarian cancer screening among the general population. *J Med Screen* 1994; **1**: 209–14.

246 Standing Subcommittee on Cancer of the Standing Medical Advisory Committee. *Management of ovarian cancer.* Current Clinical Practices (1991). Report of a Working Group. Chairman: Professor JS Scott. Leeds: Standing Subcommittee on Cancer of the Standing Medical Advisory Committee, 1991, 1–50.

247 Finn CB, Luesley DM, Buxton EJI *et al.* Is Stage I epithelial ovarian cancer overtreated both surgically and systematically? Results of a five-year cancer registry review. *Br J Obstet Gynaecol* 1992, **99**: 54–8

248 Mayer AR, Chambers SK, Graves E *et al.* Cancer staging: does it require a gynecologic oncologist? *Gynecol Oncol* 1992: **47**: 223–7.

249 Eisenkop SM, Spirtos NM, Montag TW *et al.* The impact of subspecialty training on the management of advanced ovarian cancer. *Gynecol Oncol* 1992; **47**: 203–9.

250 Medical Research Council Gynaecological Cancer Working Party, An overview in the treatment of advanced ovarian cancer. *Br J Cancer* 1990; **61**: 495–6.

251 Advanced Ovarian Trialists Group. Chemotherapy in advanced ovarian cancer: an overview of randomised clinical trials. *BMJ* 1991; **303**: 884–93.

252 McGuire WP, Hoskins WJ, Brady MF *et al.* Cyclophosphamide and cisplatin compared with paclitaxel and cisplatin in patients with stage III and stage IV ovarian cancer. *N Engl J Med* 1996; **334**: 1–6.

253 Gillis CR, Hole DJ, Still RM *et al.* Medical audit, cancer registration, and survival in ovarian cancer. *Lancet* 1991; **337**: 611–12.

254 Grant PT, Beischer NA, Planner RS. The treatment of gynaecological malignancy in a general public hospital. *Med J Aust* 1992; **157**: 378–80.

255 Hudson CN, Potsides P, Curling OM. An audit of surgical treatment of ovarian cancer in a metropolitan health region. *J Roy Soc Med* 1991; **84**: 206–9.

256 De Palo G, Mangioni C, Periti P *et al.* Treatment of FIGO (1971) Stage I endometrial carcinoma with intensive surgery, radiotherapy and hormonotherapy according to pathological prognostic groups. Long-term results of a randomised multicentre study. *Eur J Cancer* 1993; **29A**: 1113–40.

257 Morgan PR, Anderson MC, Buckley CH *et al.* The Royal College of Obstetricians and Gynaecologists micro-invasive carcinoma of the cervix study. preliminary results. *Br J Obstet Gynaecol* 1993; **100**: 664–8.

258 Saunders N. Pelvic exenteration: by whom and for whom? *Lancet* 1995; **345**: 5–6.

259 Royal College of Obstetricians and Gynaecologists. Report on the Audit Committee's Working Group on Communication Standards. *Gynaecology: Surgical Procedures*, 1995.

260 Stott NCH. Day case surgery generates no increased workload for community based staff. True or false? *BMJ* 1992; **304**: 825–6.

261 Royston CMS, Lansdown MRJ, Brough WA. Teaching laparoscopic surgery: the need for guidelines. *BMJ* 1994; **308**: 1023–5.

262 Lewis B. Guidelines for endometrial ablation. *Br J Obstet Gynaecol* 1994; **101**: 470–3.

263 Reniers J, Collet M, Leclerc A *et al.* Chlamydial antibodies and tubal infertility. *Int J Epidemiol* 1989; **18**: 261–3.

264 Emslie C, Grimshaw J, Templeton A. Do clinical guidelines improve general practice management and referral of infertile couples? *BMJ* 1993; **306**: 1728–31.

265 Royal College of Obstetricians and Gynaecologists. Fertility Sub-Committee. *Infertility: guidelines for practice.* London: RCOG, 1992.

266 Redmayne S , Klein R. Rationing in practice: the case of in-vitro fertilisation. *BMJ* 1993; **306**: 1521–3.

267 Bull A, Lyons C. Purchasing (and rationing) an *in vitro* fertilisation service. *Br J Obstet Gynaecol* 1994; **101**: 759–61.

268 Department of Health. *The Health of the Nation Key Area Handbook: Cancer.* London: Department of Health, 1993.

269 Garnett T, Mitchell A, Studd J. Patterns of referral to a menopause clinic. *J Royal Soc Med* 1991; **84**: 128–30.

270 Maclennan AH. Running a menopause clinic. *Balliére's Clin Endocrinol Metab* 1993; **7(1)**: 243–53.

271 Intercollegiate working party on cervical cytology screening. Report. London: Royal College of Obstetricians and Gynaecologists, 1987.

272 Elkind A, Eardley A, Thompson R *et al. Operating Cervical Screening: The experience of District Health Authorities.* NHS Cervical Screening Programme. Applied Epidemiology Publications, Oxford, 1990.

273 Ellman R, Chamberlain J. Improving the effectiveness of cervical cancer screening. *J Royal Coll Gen Pract* 1984; **34**: 537–42.

274 Beardow R, Oerton J, Victor C. Evaluation of the cervical cytology screening programme in an inner city health district. *BMJ* 1989; **299**: 98–100.

275 Department of Health. *Summary information from Form KC 53 (England)*, 1993.

276 Department of Health and Social Security. *Health Services: Management: Cervical Cancer Screening.* HC(88)1. London: Department of Health and Social Security, 1988.

277 Majeed FA, Cook DG, Anderson HR *et al.* Using patient and general practice characteristics to explain variations in cervical smear uptake rates. *BMJ* 1994; **308**: 1272–6.

278 Giles JA, Hudson E, Crow J *et al.* Colposcopic assessment of the accuracy of cervical cytology screening.*BMJ* 1988; **296**: 1099–2.

279 National Audit Office. *Cervical and Breast Screening in England.* London: HMSO, 1992.

280 Campion MJ, Singer A, Mitchell HS. Complacency in diagnosis of cervical cancer. *BMJ* 1987; **294**: 1337–9.

281 Wolfe CDA, Tilling K, Bourne HM *et al.* Variations in the screening history and appropriateness of management of cervical cancer in south-east England. *European Journal of Cancer* 1996; **32**: 1198–1204.

282 Garratt AM, Ruta DA, Abdalla M *et al.* The SF 36 health survey questionnaire: an outcome measure suitable for routine use within the NHS? *BMJ* 1993; **306**: 440–4.

283 Ruta DA, Garratt AM, Chodha YC *et al.* Assessment of patients with menorrhagia: how valid is a structured clinical history as a measure of health status? (In press.)

284 Higham JM, Shaw RW. *Measured menstrual blood losses – normal population and 'menorrhagia' patients.* Carnforth: Parthenon,1990, 69–82.

285 Department of Health. *The Health of the Nation: A strategy for health in England.* London: Department of Health, 1992.

286 *UK Levels of Health.* The Faculty of Public Health Medicine of the Royal College of Physicians. First Report, June 1991.

287 World Health Organization. Recommended definitions, terminology and format for statistical tables related to the perinatal period. *Acta Obstet Gynecol Scand* 1977; **56**: 247–53.

288 Health Systems International. *Diagnosis Related Groups.* 3rd Revision. Definitions manual. New Haven, Connecticut: Health Systems International, 1986.

289 Information Management Group. *Health Care Resource Groups.* London: NHS Executive, 1994.

290 National Casemix Office. *HRG Version 2.0 national statistics 1993–94.* Winchester: National Casemix Office, 1995.

291 Office of Population Censuses and Surveys. *Tabular list of the classification of surgical operations and procedures.* 4th Revision. Consolidated version. London: HMSO, 1990.

292 Choyce A, McAvoy B R. Cervical cancer screening and registration – are they working? *J Epidemiol Comm Hlth* 1990; **44**: 52–4.

293 Hay PE, Thomas BJ, Gilchrist C *et al.* The value of urine samples from men with non-gonococcal urethritis for the detection of *Chlamydia trachomatis. Genitourin Med* 1991; **67**: 124–8.

294 Tuffrey M, Alexander F, Conlan W *et al.* Heterotypic protection of mice against chlamydial salpingitis and colonization of the lower genital tract with a human scrovar F isolate of *Chlamydia trachomatis* by prior immunization with recombinant serovar LI major outer-membrane protein. *J Gen Microbiol* 1992; **38**: 1707–15.

295 Gunnell DJ, Ewing P. Infertility prevalence, needs assessment and purchasing. *J Pub Hlth Med* 1994; **16**: 29–35.

Index